DATE DUE

SURGERY FOR PARKINSON'S DISEASE AND MOVEMENT DISORDERS

SURGERY FOR PARKINSON'S DISEASE AND MOVEMENT DISORDERS

Edited by

JOACHIM K. KRAUSS, M.D.

Vice-Chairman
Department of Neurosurgery
University Hospital
Mannheim, Germany

Adjunct Associate Professor
Department of Neurosurgery
Baylor College of Medicine
Houston, Texas

JOSEPH JANKOVIC, M.D.

Professor, Department of Neurology
Baylor College of Medicine
Houston, Texas

ROBERT G. GROSSMAN, M.D.

Professor and Chairman
Department of Neurosurgery
Baylor College of Medicine
Houston, Texas

LIPPINCOTT WILLIAMS & WILKINS
A **Wolters Kluwer** Company

Philadelphia ■ Baltimore ■ New York ■ London
Buenos Aires ■ Hong Kong ■ Sydney ■ Tokyo

Acquisitions Editor: Craig Percy
Developmental Editor: Michelle LaPlante
Production Manager: Toni Ann Scaramuzzo
Production Editor: Michael Mallard
Manufacturing Manager: Colin Warnock
Cover Designer: Mark Lerner
Compositor: TechBooks
Printer: Maple Press

© 2001 by LIPPINCOTT WILLIAMS & WILKINS
530 Walnut Street
Philadelphia, PA 19106 USA
LWW.com

Printed in the USA

Library of Congress Cataloging-in-Publication Data
Surgery for Parkinson's disease and movement disorders / edited by Joachim K. Krauss, Joseph Jankovic, Robert G. Grossman.
p.; cm.
Includes bibliographical references and index.
ISBN 0-7817-2244-6
1. Parkinson's disease—Surgery.   2. Movement disorders—Surgery.   I. Krauss, Joachim K.   II. Jankovic, Joseph.   III. Grossman, Robert G.
[DNLM: 1. Parkinson Disease—surgery. 2. Basal Ganglia—physiopathology.
3. Movement Disorders—surgery. WL 359 S9525 2001]
RC382 .S87   2001
617.4′81—dc21   2001029893

10   9   8   7   6   5   4   3   2   1

To our families, for their support and encouragement

CONTENTS

CONTRIBUTING AUTHORS

Patrick Aebischer, M.D. Professor, Department of Medicine, Lausanne University Medical School; Chief, Division of Surgical Research and Gene Therapy Center, Centre Hospitalier Universitaire Vaudois (CHUV), 1011 Lausanne, Switzerland.

A. Leland Albright, M.D. Professor of Neurosurgery, University of Pittsburgh; Chief of Pediatric Neurosurgery, Children's Hospital of Pittsburgh, Pittsburgh, Pennsylvania 15213.

L. Alvarez, M.D. Centro Internacional de Restauracion Neurologica, Havana, Cuba.

Richard L. Anderson, M.D. Chief, Division of Ophthalmology, Salt Lake Regional Medical Center, Salt Lake City, Utah 84102.

Dalia M. Araujo, Ph.D. Department of Neuroscience, University of California, San Diego, La Jolla, California 92093.

Roy A.E. Bakay, M.D. Professor and Vice-Chairman, Department of Neurosurgery, Rush Presbyterian St. Luke's Medical Center, Chicago, Illinois 60612.

Alim-Louise Benabid, M.D., Ph.D. Professor of Biophysics, Joseph Fourier University Medical School; Head, Department of Neurosurgery, Hôpital Albert Michallon, 38043 Grenoble, France.

Abdelhamid Benazzouz, Ph.D. Hôpital Albert Michallon, 38043 Grenoble, France.

Jean-Charles Bensadoun, Ph.D. Division of Surgical Research and Gene Therapy Center, Centre Hospitalier Universitaire Vaudois (CHUV), 1011 Lausanne, Switzerland.

Veit Braun, M.D. Department of Neurosurgery, University of Ulm, 89312 Günzburg, Germany.

Robert E. Breeze, M.D. Department of Clinical Pharmacology and Toxicology, University of Colorado Health Sciences Center, Denver, Colorado 80262.

Mitchell Brin, M.D. Associate Professor of Neurology, Mount Sinai School of Medicine New York, New York 10029.

P. Cesaro, M.D. Department of Medicine, INSERM U421, Hôpital Henri Mondor 94000 Créteil, France.

Edward D. Clarkson Department of Clinical Pharmacology and Toxicology, University of Colorado Health Sciences Center, Denver, Colorado 80262.

G. Rees Cosgrove, M.D. Associate Professor, Department of Neurosurgery, Harvard Medical School; Massachusetts General Hospital, Boston, Massachusetts 02114.

Fabio Danisi, M.D. Department of Neurology, Mount Sinai School of Medicine, New York, New York 10029.

J. Michael Desaloms, M.D. Staff Neurosurgeon, Presbyterian Hospital of Dallas, Dallas, Texas 75231.

Stephen B. Dunnett, Ph.D. Professorial Research Fellow, School of Biosciences, Cardiff University, Cardiff, CF10 3US, United Kingdom.

Christine Edwards, M.A. Research Coordinator, Center for Neurosciences, North Shore-Long Island Jewish Research Institute, Manhasset, New York 11030.

David Eidelberg, M.D. Professor, Department of Neurology and Neurosurgery, New York University School of Medicine, New York, New York 10016; Head, Center for Neurosciences, North Shore-Long Island Jewish Research Institute, Manhasset, New York 11030.

A. Fève, M.D. Service de Neurochirurgie, Hôpital Henri Mondor 94000 Créteil, France.

J. Stephen Fink, M.D., Ph.D. Professor and Chairman, Department of Neurology, Boston University School of Medicine, Boston, Massachusetts 02118.

Curt R. Freed, M.D. Professor of Medicine and Pharmacology, Department of Clinical Pharmacology and Toxicology, University of Colorado School of Medicine, Denver, Colorado 80262.

Gerhard M. Friehs, M.D. Assistant Professor, Department of Neurosurgery, Brown University; Director, Functional and Stereotactic Neurosurgery, Lifespan-Rhode Island Hospital Providence, Rhode Island 02906.

Isabelle Germano, M.D.   Department of Neurology, Mount Sinai School of Medicine, New York, New York 10029.

Steven S. Gill, F.R.C.P.   Department of Neurology, Frenchay Hospital, Bristol, BS16 ILE, United Kingdom.

Robert G. Grossman, M.D.   Professor and Chairman, Department of Neurosurgery, Baylor College of Medicine, Houston, Texas 77030.

Jorge Guridi, M.D., Ph.D.   Associate Professor, Neurosurgical Department, Navarra University, 31080 Pamplona, Spain.

Peter Heywood, F.R.C.P.   Department of Neurology, Frenchay Hospital, Bristol, BS16 ILE, United Kingdom.

William D. Hutchison, Ph.D.   Assistant Professor, Department of Surgery and Physiology University of Toronto, Toronto Western Hospital, Toronto, Ontario, M5T 2S8, Canada.

Ivan P. Hwang, M.D.   California Eye Clinic, Antioch, California 94509.

Ole Isacson, M.D., Ph.D.   Neuroregeneration Laboratory, Harvard Medical School; McLean Hospital, Boston, Massachusetts 02114.

Joseph Jankovic, M.D.   Professor, Department of Neurology, Baylor College of Medicine; Director, Parkinson's Disease Center and Movement Disorders Clinic, Houston, Texas 77030.

Peter J. Jannetta, M.D.   Walter E. Dandy Professor and Emeritus Chairman, University of Pittsburgh School of Medicine; Department of Neurological Surgery, Presbyterian University Hospital, Pittsburgh, Pennsylvania 15213.

Edward G. Jones, M.D., Ph.D.   Professor, Department of Medicine, University of California, Davis; Director, Center for Neuroscience, Davis, California 95616.

David R. Jordan, M.D.   Professor of Ophthalmology, University of Ottawa Eye Institute, Ottawa, Ontario, K1H 8L6, Canada.

Un Jung Kang, M.D.   Assistant Professor, Department of Neurology, The University of Chicago, Chicago, Illinois 60637.

Y. Keravel, M.D.   Service de Neurochirurgie, Hôpital Henri Mondor, 94000 Créteil, France.

William C. Koller, M.D., Ph.D.   Professor, Department of Neurology, University of Kansas, Kansas City, Kansas 66160.

Adnan Koudsie, M.D.   Hôpital Albert Michallon, 38043 Grenoble, France.

Joachim K. Krauss, M.D.   Vice-Chairman, Department of Neurosurgery, University Hospital, 68167 Mannheim, Germany; Adjunct Associate Professor, Department of Neurosurgery, Baylor College of Medicine, Houston, Texas 77030.

Anthony E. Lang, M.D.   Director, Morton and Gloria Sthulman Movement Disorders Clinic, The Toronto Hospital, Toronto, Ontario, M5T 2S8, Canada.

Paul A. Lapchak, Ph.D.   Research Scientist, Department of Neurosciences, University of California, San Diego, La Jolla, California 92093.

Jean-François Lebas, M.D.   Hôpital Albert Michallon, 38043 Grenoble, France.

C. Leguerinel, M.D.   Service de Neurochirurgie, Hôpital Henri Mondor, 94000 Créteil, France.

Jung-Il Lee, M.D., Ph.D.   Assistant Professor, Department of Neurosurgery, Sungkyunkwan University School of Medicine, Samsung Medical Center, Seoul, 135-710, Korea.

Maureen A. Leehey M.D.   Department of Clinical Pharmacology and Toxicology, University of Colorado Health Sciences Center, Denver, Colorado 80262.

A.J. Lees, M.D.   Reta Lila Weston Institute of Neurological Studies, University College London, London, W1P 6DB, United Kingdom.

Fredrick A. Lenz, M.D., Ph.D.   Professor of Neurosurgery, Johns Hopkins Hospital Baltimore, Maryland 21287.

Martin Lévesque, M.D.   Department of Anatomy and Physiology, Laval University School of Medicine, Beauport, Québec, G1J 2G3, Canada.

Olle Lindvall, M.D., Ph.D.   Professor, Section of Restorative Neurology, Wallenberg Neuroscience Center, University Hospital, 22185 Lund, Sweden.

Andres M. Lozano, M.D., Ph.D.   Division of Neurosurgery, The Toronto Hospital, Western Division, Toronto, Ontario M5T 2S8 Canada.

R. Macias, M.D.   Centro Internacional de Restauracion Neurologica, Havana, Cuba.

Gerhard Marquardt, M.D.   Department of Neurosurgery, University of Frankfurt, 60528 Frankfurt, Germany.

Hans-Michael Meinck, M.D.   Professor, Neurologische Universitätsklinik 69120 Heidelberg, Germany.

Patrick Mertens, M.D., Ph.D.   Associate Professor, Department of Anatomy, Claude Bernard University-Lyon,

Department of Neurosurgery, Hôpital Neurologique P. Wertheimer 69003 Lyon, France.

Jonathan W. Mink, M.D., Ph.D. Associate Professor, Department of Neurology, University of Rochester School of Medicine and Dentistry; Chief, Child Neurology Unit, Strong Memorial Hospital, Rochester, New York 14642.

Fritz Mundinger, M.D. Professor Emeritus, Department of Functional and Stereotactic Neurosurgery, St. Josefs-Krankenhaus, 79114 Freiburg, Germany.

Jean-Paul Nguyen-Buu, M.D. Professor of Neurosurgery, Service de Neurochirurgie Hôpital Henri Mondor, 94000 Creteil, France.

Friedrich A. Nobbe, M.D. Department of Neurology, Klinikum der RWTH, 52057 Aachen, Germany.

Jean-Paul Nguyen, M.D. Professor, Department of Neurosurgery, Hôpital Henri Mondor, 94000 Créteil, France.

José A. Obeso, M.D. Departamento de Neurología y Neurocirugía, Clínica Universitaria, Universidad de Navarra, 31008 Pamplona, Spain.

C. Warren Olanow, M.D. Department of Neurology, Mount Sinai School of Medicine, New York, New York 10029.

William G. Ondo, M.D. Assistant Professor, Department of Neurology, Baylor College of Medicine, Houston, Texas 77030.

Peter Pahapill, M.D. Division of Neurosurgery, The Toronto Hospital, Western Division Toronto, Ontario, M5T 2S8, Canada.

Rajesh Pahwa, M.D. Associate Professor, Department of Neurology, University of Kansas Medical Center; Director, Parkinson's Disease and Movement Disorder Center, Kansas City, Kansas 66160.

André Parent, Ph.D. Professor, Department of Anatomy and Physiology Laval University School of Medicine, Beauport, Québec, G1J 2G3, Canada.

Martin Parent Department of Anatomy and Physiology, Laval University School of Medicine, Beauport, Québec, G1J 2G3, Canada.

Bhupendra C.K. Patel, M.D., F.R.C.S., F.R.C.Ophth. Associate Professor, University of Utah; Moran Eye Center, Salt Lake City, Utah 84132.

Bryan R. Payne, M.D. Department of Neurosurgery, Rush Presbyterian St. Luke's Medical Center, Chicago, Illinois 60612.

Ron W. Pelton, M.D., Ph.D. Salt Lake City, Utah 84132.

Richard D. Penn, M.D. Professor, Department of Neurosurgery, University of Chicago University of Chicago Medical Center, Chicago, Illinois 60637.

Vandhana Pillai, B.S. Program Assistant, Center for Neurosciences, North Shore-Long Island Jewish Research Institute, Manhasset, New York 11030.

Pierre Pollak, M.D. Professor, Department of Neurology, Joseph Fourier University, 38700 La Tronche, France; University Hospital of Grenoble, 38043 Grenoble, France.

B. Pollin Laboratorie de Physiologie de la Manducation, Univeristé Paris VII Denis Diderot, 75251 Paris, France.

Scott L. Rauch, M.D. Associate Professor of Psychiatry, Associate Chief of Psychiatry (for Neuroscience Research), Massachusetts General Hospital, Charlestown, Massachusetts 02129.

Daniel K. Resnick, M.D. Assistant Professor, Department of Neurological Surgery, University of Wisconsin Medical School, Madison, Wisconsin 53792.

Hans-Peter Richter, M.D. Professor and Chairman, Department of Neurosurgery, Ulm University, 89312 Günzburg, Germany.

M.C. Rodriguez-Oroz, M.D. Departamento de Neurología y Neurocirugía, Clínica Universitaria, Universidad de Navarra, 31008 Pamplona, Spain.

Anne Rosser, M.R.C.P, Ph.D. Lister Institute Clinical Research Fellow, Department of Biosciences, Cardiff University, Cardiff, CF1 3US, United Kingdom.

Fumi Sato, Ph.D. Professor, Department of Anatom and Physiology, Laval University School of Medicine, Beauport, Québec, G1J 2G3, Canada.

Richard K. Simpson, Jr., M.D. Associate Professor of Neurosurgery, Baylor College of Medicine, Houston, Texas 77030.

Marc P. Sindou, M.D., D.Sc. Professor and Chairman of Neurosurgery, University of Lyon, Hôpital Neurologique et Neuro-Chirurgical P. Wertheimer, 69003 Lyon, France.

Charles Teo, M.D. Conjoint Lecturer, Department of Neurosurgery, University of New South Wales; Director, Center for Minimally Invasive Neurosurgery, Institute of Neurological Sciences, Prince of Wales Private Hospital, Sydney, NSW 2031, Australia.

Laetitia L. Thompson Department of Clinical Pharmacology and Toxicology, University of Colorado Health Sciences Center, Denver, Colorado 80262.

Volker Tronnier, M.D. Professor, Department of Neurosurgery, University of Heidelberg, 69120 Heidelberg, Germany.

Jerrold L. Vitek, M.D., Ph.D. Associate Professor, Department of Neurology, Emory University School of Medicine, Atlanta, Georgia 30322.

Kevin A. Walter, M.D. Fellow, Department of Neurosurgery, Johns Hopkins Hospital Baltimore, Maryland 21287.

Beverly C. Walters, M.D. Department of Clinical Neurosciences, Brown University School of Medicine, Providence, Rhode Island 02906.

Donald Weisz, M.D. Department of Neurology, Mount Sinai School of Medicine New York, New York 10029.

Knut Wester, M.D., Ph.D. Professor of Neurosurgery, University of Bergen; Chairman, Department of Neurosurgery, Haukeland University Hospital, Bergen, 5021, Norway.

Hans R. Widmer, Ph.D. Director, Research Laboratory, Department of Neurosurgery University Hospital, 3010 Berne, Switzerland.

Michael Zawada Department of Clinical Pharmacology and Toxicology University of Colorado Health Sciences Center, Denver, Colorado 80262.

Vasilios Zerris, M.D. Department of Clinical Neurosciences, Brown University School of Medicine, Providence, Rhode Island 02906.

Anne Zurn, Ph.D., P.D. Head of Research, Division of Surgical Research and Gene Therapy Center, Centre Hospitalier Universitaire Vaudois (CHUV), 1011 Lausanne, Switzerland.

PREFACE

Surgical treatment of Parkinson's disease and other movement disorders, while still in evolution, has become an important therapeutic strategy with dramatic impact on the motor functioning of patients with these chronic and often disabling diseases. Since the early attempts at neurotransplantation in the mid-1980s and the reintroduction of pallidotomy in the United States in the early 1990s, there has been tremendous progress in movement disorders surgery. This progress has been fueled by remarkable advances in neurophysiology, neurobiology, neurology, neurosurgery, neuroimaging and medical technology. As a result of better understanding of the motor physiology and functional anatomy of the basal ganglia and their role in the pathophysiology of Parkinson's disease, new targets such as the subthalamic nucleus have been explored. Deep brain stimulation techniques have furthered and expanded considerably the options of movement disorders surgery. Other targets and new indications are being investigated. It is hard to predict which targets and methods will have the greatest impact within the next few years.

The primary objective of *Surgery for Parkinson's Disease and Movement Disorders* is to provide a critical and scholarly review of the rationales and indications for movement disorders surgery. The volume also reviews the contemporary surgical techniques. Many issues related to the patient selection criteria, the optimal target, surgical methods, and other controversies remain unsolved and, therefore, the reader will note that the authors of some chapters present divergent and even contradictory opinions. Future research will hopefully provide insights into these issues and help to build a consensus.

We very much appreciate the contributions of the international group of authors for their scholarly, timely and up-to-date contributions. We also appreciate the timely manner of the production of this book and we are most grateful to Senior Developmental Editor Michelle LaPlante and Production Editor Michael Mallard from Lippincott Williams & Wilkins.

We hope that this book will be useful for neurologists, neurosurgeons, neurophysiologists, and all health care professionals caring for patients with movement disorders. Furthermore, we hope that the volume will serve as a reference source on the state-of-the-art of contemporary movement disorders surgery.

Joachim K. Krauss
Joseph Jankovic
Robert G. Grossman

AC, Anterior commissure; AD, Anterodorsal nucleus; AM, Anteromedial nucleus; Am, Amygdala; AV, Anteroventral nucleus; BNM, Basal nucleus of Meynert; CeM, Central medial nucleus; CL, Central lateral nucleus; CM, Centre médian nucleus; CN(Cd), Caudate nucleus; F, Fornix; FF, Field of Forel; Gpe, Globus pallidus (external division); Gpi, Globus pallidus (internal division); H, Habenular nuclei; HPT, Habenulopeduncular tract; IC, Internal capsule; IML, Internal medullary lamina; L, Limitans nucleus; LD, Lateral dorsal nucleus; LGd, Dorsal lateral geniculate nucleus; LGv, Ventral lateral geniculate nucleus; LP, Lateral posterior nucleus; L-SG, limitans-suprageniculate nucleus; MD, Mediodorsal nucleus; MG, Medial geniculate complex; ML, Medial lemniscus; MV, Medioventral (reuniens) nucleus; OT, Optic tract; Pa, Paraventricular nuclei; Pc, Paracentral nucleus; Pf, Parafascicular nucleus; Pla, Anterior pulvinar nucleus; Pli, Inferior pulvinar nucleus; Pll, Lateral pulvinar nucleus; Pls, Superior pulvinar nucleus; Po, Posterior nucleus; Pg, Pregeniculate nucleus; PT, Pretectum; Pt, parataenial nucleus; Pu, Putamen; R, Reticular nucleus; Re, Reuniens (medioventral) nucleus; Rh, Rhomboid nucleus; RN, Red nucleus; SB, STN, Subthalamic nucleus; SC, Superior colliculus; SG, Suprageniculate nucleus; SI, Substantia innominata; SN, Substantia nigra; SNc, Pars compacta of substantia nigra; SNr, Pars reticulata of substantia nigra; Sm, Submedial nucleus; Spf, Subparafascicular nucleus; TF, Thalamic fasciculus; VA, Ventral anterior nucleus; Vamc, Magnocellular division of ventral anterior nucleus; VIM, ventrointermediate nucleus; VLa, Anterior ventral lateral nucleus; VLp, Posterior ventral lateral nucleus; VM, Ventral medial nucleus; VMp, Principal ventral medial nucleus; VMb, Basal ventral medial nucleus; VP, Ventral pallidum; VPI, Ventral posterior inferior nucleus; VPM, Ventral posterior medial nucleus; VPL, Ventral posterior lateral nucleus; VPLa, Anterior ventral posterior lateral nucleus; VPLp, Posterior ventral lateral posterior nucleus; VS, Ventral striatum; ZI, Zona incerta.

SURGERY FOR PARKINSON'S DISEASE AND MOVEMENT DISORDERS

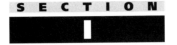

OVERVIEW

Surgery for Parkinson's Disease and Movement Disorders,
edited by J.K. Krauss, J. Jankovic, and R.G. Grossman.
Lippincott Williams & Wilkins, Philadelphia © 2001.

1

CLASSIFICATION AND EPIDEMIOLOGY OF MOVEMENT DISORDERS

JOSEPH JANKOVIC

Movement disorders comprise a group of neurologic symptoms, signs, or diseases manifested by either slowness and poverty of movement, so-called *hypokinesias,* or by excessive, abnormal involuntary movements, so-called *hyperkinesias.* Parkinson's disease (PD) and other parkinsonian disorders are examples of hypokinetic movement disorders, whereas hyperkinetic movement disorders are represented by tremors, dystonia, chorea, tics, myoclonus, and stereotypies. In addition to these primary movement disorders are many miscellaneous disorders that cannot be categorized into any of the major classifications. These miscellaneous movement disorders include gait disorders, ataxias, spasticity, stiff-person syndrome, hemifacial spasm, myokymia, akathisia, restless legs syndrome, periodic movements in sleep, paroxysmal dyskinesias, painful legs and moving toes, automatisms, hyperekplexias and other startle syndromes, apraxias, alien limb, catatonia, and various psychogenic movement disorders. It is beyond the scope of this chapter to review all the movement disorders; only the primary hypokinetic and hyperkinetic disorders are discussed. In addition to phenomenology, classification, and epidemiology, this discussion provides a brief background for the understanding of the mechanisms of these movement disorders by reviewing some relevant aspects of basal ganglia anatomy and function.

FUNCTIONAL ANATOMY OF THE BASAL GANGLIA

The pathophysiology of movement disorders is not fully understood, but a dysfunction in the basal ganglia and their connection has been implicated in most of the primary movement disorders (1). Extraordinary progress has been made in the understanding of the functional neuroanatomy, neurochemistry, and physiology of the basal ganglia, and their

role in motor control, muscle tone, posture, and some cognitive processes is becoming increasingly recognized. These advances have contributed to the development of new pharmacologic and surgical approaches.

Because some knowledge of the functional anatomy of the basal ganglia is critical to understanding the various movement disorders and their treatment, a brief review is appropriate (Fig. 1.1). Basal ganglia, sometimes referred to as the *extrapyramidal system,* include the striatum, globus pallidus (GP), subthalamic nucleus (STN), substantia nigra (SN), and thalamus (2,3). The caudate and putamen are contiguous and comprise the striatum. The cortical input from the prefrontal supplementary motor area, amygdala, and hippocampus is excitatory, mediated by glutamate. Neurons in the SN pars compacta (SNc) provide major dopaminergic input to the striatum and exert both excitatory and inhibitory influences. The interaction between the afferent and efferent pathways is mediated by striatal interneurons, which use acetylcholine as the main neurotransmitter. The SN is a melanin-containing (pigmented) nucleus in the ventral midbrain, and it consists of dopaminergic neurons. Neurons in the SNc provide major dopaminergic input to the striatum. The patchy organization of the striatal neurons divides the striatum into striosomes and matrix, and these subpopulations define the anatomic distribution of DA receptors (4). Five distinct dopamine receptors (D1 to D5) have been cloned and characterized, but the D1 and D2 receptors are best represented in the striatum (5). The D1 receptors are more concentrated in striosomes, whereas the D2 receptors are mostly represented in the matrix of the lateral striatum. The striatal output system is mediated by the inhibitory neurotransmitter γ-aminobutyric acid (GABA). The connection between the STN and the internal (medial) GP (GPi) and between the STN and the lateral (or external) GP (GPe) is excitatory, mediated by glutamate. The two output pathways from the striatum are the indirect pathway, mediated chiefly by the D2 dopamine receptors, and the D1-mediated direct pathway (6). In the indirect pathway, the striatum projects to the neurons in the

J. Jankovic: Department of Neurology, Baylor College of Medicine, Houston, Texas, 77030.

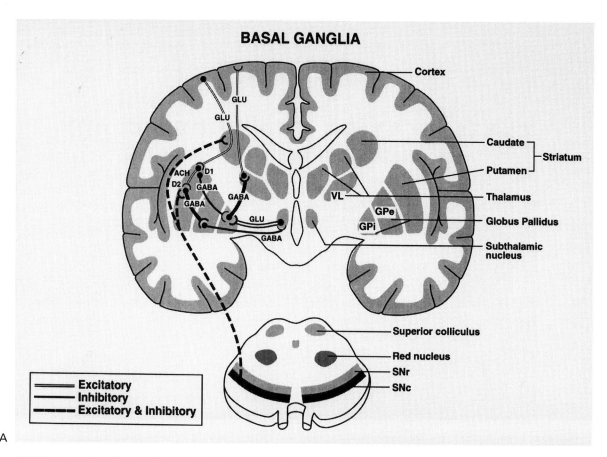

BASAL GANGLIA

Cortex

GLU

GLU

Caudate ⎤ Striatum
Putamen ⎦

ACH D1
D2
GABA
GABA
GABA
GABA
GLU
GABA

VL

GPe
GPi

Thalamus

Globus Pallidus

Subthalamic nucleus

Superior colliculus

Red nucleus

SNr

SNc

	Excitatory
	Inhibitory
	Excitatory & Inhibitory

A

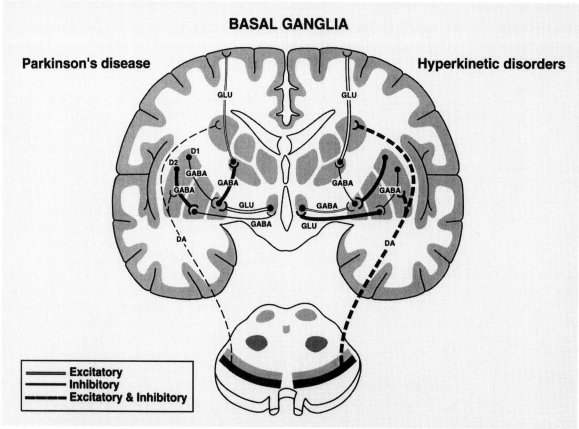

BASAL GANGLIA

Parkinson's disease

Hyperkinetic disorders

GLU

GLU

D1
D2
GABA
GABA
GABA
GLU
GABA
GLU
DA

GABA
GABA
GABA
GABA
DA

	Excitatory
	Inhibitory
	Excitatory & Inhibitory

B

FIGURE 1.1. Schematic diagram of a coronal section of a brain showing some important neuro-transmitter pathways involved in disorders of the basal ganglia (**A**, normal Basal Ganglia) and in Parkinson's disease and hyperkinetic movement disorders (**B**). The thickness of the pathway *lines* indicates activity of the pathway (*thin,* underactive; *thick,* overactive).

GPe using GABA; the GPe, in turn, projects to the STN, which provides excitatory input through glutamate to the GPi and SN pars reticulata (SNr). GPi neurons are GABAergic and synapse in the ventrolateral nucleus of the thalamus. Thalamus provides an excitatory input to the cortex, which, in turn, gives rise to the descending corticospinal pathway.

Electrophysiologic studies show that striatal output neurons are quiescent, with phasic bursts of activity driven by cortical excitatory input, whereas the GPi/SNr neurons are tonically active. In PD, the STN and GPi activity is markedly increased, resulting in suppression of thalamocortical output. The major function of the output nuclei (STN and GPi) is to modify information flow through the corticobasal ganglionic-thalamocortical circuitry and by modulating basal ganglia output to the thalamus to suppress unwanted movements and to facilitate the execution of voluntary movements.

PHENOMENOLOGIC AND ETIOLOGIC CLASSIFICATION

Before a specific cause and treatment can be considered, the movement disorder must be first classified according to its phenomenologic features. This is based on a careful observation of the patient at rest and during nonspecific and specific activities. The clinician must be able first to categorize the movement disorder into one of the three major categories: hypokinetic, hyperkinetic, or miscellaneous. When abnormal involuntary movements are observed (hyperkinesia), it is essential to characterize the movements according to the anatomic distribution, rhythmicity, pattern, influence of a specific activity or a position, suppressibility, effect of sleep and stress, and other factors. Once the phenomenologic features are fully characterized, then various causes and a specific treatment program can be considered.

Many etiologic classifications exist, and these are referred to during reviews of the particular type of movement disorder. The International Classification of Diseases Tenth Revision: Neurological Adaptation, a result of collaboration between the World Health Organization and the Movement Disorder Society (Table 1.1), provides an organized approach to differential diagnosis of movement disorders (7). This classification is in evolution and is periodically revised and updated. Although it is not ideal, it serves to facilitate epidemiologic studies, international communication, education, and clinical research.

The following review emphasizes both phenomenologic and etiologic approaches to classification of movement disorders. Some aspects of the review have been modified from a previous publication (8).

Bradykinesia, the clinical hallmark of hypokinetic (parkinsonian) disorders, is clinically manifested by slowness of limb and body movements, reduced blinking and lack of facial expression, monotonous speech, and slowness in activities of daily living. "Freezing" or "motor blocks" are viewed by some investigators as extreme forms of bradykinesia, but this parkinsonian feature appears to be mediated through a different neurotransmitter system because, in contrast to bradykinesia, it does not improve with dopaminergic therapy. Other features that typically accompany bradykinesia include rigidity, tremor, and gait and balance difficulties. About 75% of patients exhibiting the cardinal signs of parkinsonism have primary (idiopathic) parkinsonism or PD. The others have secondary or heredogenerative forms of parkinsonism (Table 1.2). It is beyond the scope of this chapter to review the clinical, pharmacologic, and imaging features that help to differentiate PD from the atypical forms of parkinsonism (Table 1.3). Features that support a diagnosis of PD include asymmetric onset, presence of resting tremor, and a good (and usually sustained) response to levodopa. In contrast, early falls, oculomotor disturbance, apraxia, and prominent dysautonomia are important clues to an alternative diagnosis (9,10). Of the various parkinsonian signs, bradykinesia correlates best with a reduction in the striatal fluorodopa uptake as measured by positron emission tomography scans and, in turn, with nigral (dopaminergic) damage (11).

Tremor can be defined as a rhythmic, oscillatory movement, and this hyperkinetic movement disorder can be further subdivided according to the position, posture, or motor activity necessary to make it manifest (12). A rest tremor is seen when the body part is in complete repose. This tremor, however, may reappear at the same frequency after a brief latency of several seconds when the limb is held in a sustained posture, the so-called *re-emergent tremor* (13). Maintenance of a posture such as holding the arms in an outstretched, horizontal, position reveals a postural tremor, whereas moving the body part to and from a target brings out kinetic or intention tremor. Occasionally, a tremor is seen only with certain actions or limb positions. *Primary writing tremor* is the most common example of such a task-specific tremor. *Orthostatic tremor,* an example of a position-specific tremor, is an uncommon and frequently unrecognized high-frequency tremor involving the proximal lower limbs and trunk when the patient stands for any period of time. Some patients exhibit tremor only in certain position or when they hold an object of a particular weight. Essential tremor, an autosomal dominant disorder typically manifested as an action-postural-kinetic tremor, is the most common form of tremor encountered in a movement disorders clinic (14). Table 1.4 lists, in addition to the major categories of tremor, various other rhythmic movements that can be sometimes confused with tremor.

Chorea consists of irregular, unpredictable, brief, jerky, continuous movements that move randomly from one part

TABLE 1.1. INTERNATIONAL CLASSIFICATION OF DISEASES TENTH REVISION: NEUROLOGICAL ADAPTATION

Extrapyramidal and Movement Disorders (G20–G29)

G20   *Parkinson's disease*
     Includes: Idiopathic parkinsonism
                  Paralysis agitans
     Excludes: Guamanian type parkinsonism-dementia complex (G23.84)
                  Diffuse Lewy body disease (G31.85)
     G20.-0   Classic type
     G20.-1   Akinetic type
     G20.-2   Tremor type
     G20.-3   Postural instability: gait difficulty (PIGD) type
     G20.-4   Hemiparkinsonism
     Use additional sixth character code, if desired, to indicate whether
        G20.-×0   sporadic
        G20.-×1   familial

G21   *Secondary parkinsonism*
     Excludes: Parkinsonism in diseases classified elsewhere (G22*)

G21.0   Malignant neuroleptic syndrome
     Use additional external cause code, if desired, to identify drug

G21.1   Other drug-induced secondary parkinsonism
     Use additional external cause code, if desired, to identify drug, e.g., dopamine receptor blockers (neuroleptics, Y49.3, .4, .5), antiemetics drugs (Y43.0), dopamine depleters (reserpine tetrabenazine, T46.5), lithium (T43.5), flunarizine (T46.7), cinnarizine (T45.0), diltiazem (T46.1).
     G21.10   Acute drug reaction
     G21.11   Tardive drug reaction

G21.2   Secondary parkinsonism due to other external agents
     Use additional external cause code, if desired, to identify external agent, e.g. manganese poisoning (T57.2), carbon monoxide (T58), cyanide (T57.3), methanol (T51.1), carbon disulfide (T65.4), 1-methyl-4-phenyl-1,2,3,6-tetrahydropyridine (MPTP, T40.94)

G21.3   Postencephalitic parkinsonism
     G21.30   Postencephalitic parkinsonism
                 Encephalitis lethargica
     G21.38   Other postinfectious parkinsonism
              Excludes: Parkinsonism in infectious diseases classified elsewhere (G22.-2*)
                       Slow virus or prion infection of CNS (A81.-)

G21.8   Other secondary parkinsonism
     Excludes: Psychogenic parkinsonism (F44.4+, G22.-3*)
     Use additional code, if desired, to identify the cause, e.g. head injury (S06.-); sequelae of intracranial injury (T90.5)

G21.9   Secondary parkinsonism, unspecified

G22*   *Parkinsonism in diseases classified elsewhere*
     G22.-0*   Parkinsonism in sporadic degenerative diseases classified elsewhere
                [Parkinsonism Plus syndromes]
                Parkinsonism in:
                   Alzheimer's disease (G30.-+)
                   Corticobasal ganglionic degeneration (G23.81+)
                   Dentatorubralpallidoluysian atrophy [DRPLA] (G23.83+)
                   Diffuse Lewy body disease (G31.85+)
                   Guamanian type parkinsonism-dementia complex (G23.84+)
                   Hallervorden-Spatz disease (G23.0+)
                   Olivopontocerebellar degeneration (G11.22+; G11.23+)
                   Pallidopyramidaldentatoluysian degeneration (G23.82+)
                   Progressive supranuclear ophthalmoparesis [Steele-Richardson-Olszewski] (G23.10+)
                   Shy-Drager syndrome (G90.31+)
                   Striatonigral degeneration (G23.2+)
                   Multisystem degeneration with dysautonomia [multiple system atrophy, MSA] (G90.3)
     G22.-1*   Parkinsonism in familial degenerative and metabolic disorders classified elsewhere
                Parkinsonism in:
                   Huntington's disease (G10+)
                   Dopa-responsive dystonia [DRD] (G24.1+)

(continued)

TABLE 1.1. *(continued)*

Extrapyramidal and Movement Disorders (G20–G29)

                    Subacute necrotizing encephalopathy [Leigh's disease] (G31.81+)

                    Wilson's disease [hepatocerebral degeneration] (E83.01+)

G22.-2*   Parkinsonism in infectious diseases classified elsewhere

        Parkinsonism in:

            Acquired immunodeficiency syndrome [AIDS] (B23.8+)

            Creutzfeldt-Jakob disease (A81.0+)

            Gerstmann-Straussler-Scheinker disease (A81.81+)

            Subacute sclerosing panencephalitis (A81.1+)

            Syphilis (A52.1+)

G22.-3*   Parkinsonism in other diseases classified elsewhere

            Brain tumor (C71.-, C79.-, D33.-+)

            Cerebrovascular disease (I60.-I67+)

            Noncommunicating (obstructive) hydrocephalus (G91.1+)

            Normal pressure hydrocephalus (G91.2+)

            Paraneoplastic (C00-D48+)

            Psychogenic (F44.4+)

            Syringomesencephalia (G95.0×3)

G23   *Other degenerative diseases of basal ganglia*

G23.0   Hallervorden-Spatz disease

        G23.00 Pigmentary pallidal degeneration

        G23.08 Other specified pallidal degeneration

G23.1   Progressive supranuclear ophthalmoplegia (opthalmoparesis)

        G23.10 Idiopathic [Steele-Richardson-Olszewski]

        G23.11 Vascular [multiinfarct]

G23.2   Striatonigral degeneration

G23.8   Other specified degenerative diseases of basal ganglia

        Excludes: Multisystem degeneration with dysautonomia [multiple system atrophy, MSA] (G90.3)

        Olivopontocerebellar degeneration (G11.22; G11.23)

        Wilson's disease [hepatolenticular degeneration] (E83.01)

        G23.80 Hemiparkinson-hemiatrophy syndrome

        G23.81 Corticobasal ganglionic degeneration [Corticodentatonigral degeneration with neuronal achromasia]

        G23.82 Pallidopyramidaldentatoluysian degeneration

        G23.83 Dentatorubralpallidolysian atrophy [DRPLA]

        G23.84 Guamanian type parkinsonism

                Parkinsonism-dementia-amyotrophic lateral sclerosis complex of Guam

                Excludes: Western Pacific-type motor neuron disease (G12.24)

        G23.85 Parkinsonism associated with calcification of the basal ganglia

                G23.850 Idiopathic sporadic [Fahr's disease]

                G23.851 With hypoparathyroidism

                G23.852 With pseudohypoparathyroidism

                G23.853 Familial basal ganglia calcifications

G23.9   Degenerative disease of the basal ganglia, unspecified

G24   *Dystonia*

        Excludes: Athetoid cerebral palsy (G80.3)

                   Dystonia (dyskinesia) in diseases classified elsewhere (G26.-0*)

G24.0   Drug-induced dystonia

        Use additional external cause code, if desired, to identify the drug or toxic agent, e.g., manganese (T57.2), carbon disulfide (T65.4), cyanide (T57.3)

        G24.00 Acute drug-induced dystonia

         G24.01 Acute drug-induced dyskinesia

         G24.02 Tardive dystonia

         G24.03 Tardive dyskinesia

         G24.04 Other specified drug-induced dystonia (e.g., drug-induced oculogyric crises)

G24.1   Idiopathic familial dystonia

        G24.10 Autosomal dominant familial dystonia (with DYT1 gene on 9q34)

        G24.11 Nonclassic dystonia

        G24.12 Atypical dystonia

(continued)

TABLE 1.1. *(continued)*

Extrapyramidal and Movement Disorders (G20–G29)

G24.13   Dopa-responsive dystonia (DRD, idiopathic diurnal dystonia, Segawa variant, hereditary progressive dystonia, GTP cyclohydrolase I 14q22.1-q22.2 gene defect)
G24.14   Myoclonic dystonia
G24.15   Rapid-onset dystonia
G24.16   X-linked recessive dystonia-parkinsonism complex [Lubag]
G24.17   Hereditary juvenile parkinsonism-dystonia complex
G24.18   Familial dystonia with other specified inheritance
Use additional sixth character, if desired, to indicate the localization of the dystonia:
G24.1×0   Generalized dystonia, familial
G24.1×1   Hemidystonia, familial
G24.1×2   Axial dystonia, familial
G24.1×3   Cranial dystonia, familial
  G24.1×30   Ocular dystonia, familial
  G24.1×31   Orofacial dystonia, familial
G24.1×4   Laryngeal dystonia, familial
G24.1×5   Cervical dystonia, familial
G24.1×6   Limb dystonia, familial
  G24.1×60   Arm/hand dystonia, familial [writer's/musician/other occupational cramps]
  G24.1×61   Leg/foot dystonia, familial
G24.1×7   Multiple or combined types of idiopathic familial dystonia
G24.1×8   Other types of idiopathic familial dystonia

G24.2   Idiopathic nonfamilial dystonia
G24.20   Generalized dystonia, nonfamilial
G24.21   Hemidystonia, nonfamilial
G24.22   Axial dystonia, nonfamilial
G24.23   Other cranial dystonia, nonfamilial
  Excludes: Blepharospasm (G24.5)
               Idiopathic orofacial dystonia (G24.4)
  G24.230 Ocular dystonia, nonfamilial [idiopathic oculogyric crises]
  Excludes: Drug-induced dystonia (G24.03)
G24.24   Laryngeal dystonia, nonfamilial [isolated spasmodic dysphonia]
G24.25   Limb dystonia, nonfamilial
  G24.250 Arm/hand dystonia, nonfamilial [writer's/musician/other occupational cramps]
  Excludes: Writer's and occupational cramps of psychogenic origin (F44.4)
  G24.251 Leg/foot dystonia, nonfamilial
G24.27   Multiple or combined types of idiopathic nonfamilial dystonia
G24.28   Other types of idiopathic nonfamilial dystonia

G24.3   Spasmodic torticollis [Idiopathic cervical dystonia]
Excludes: Torticollis NOS (M43.6)
          Familial cervical dystonia (G24.1×5)
G24.30   Spasmodic torticollis
G24.31   Spasmodic retrocollis
G24.32   Spasmodic anterocollis
G24.33   Spasmodic laterocollis
G24.38   Other specified cervical dystonia

G24.4   Idiopathic orofacial dystonia
Excludes: Familial orofacial dystonia (G24.1×31)
G24.40   Orofacial dyskinesia
G24.41   Edentulous orofacial dyskinesia
G24.42   Isolated oromandibular dystonia

G24.5   Blepharospasm [idiopathic cranial dystonia, Meige's syndrome]

24.8   Other dystonia
Excludes: Atlantoaxial subluxuation (M43.3, .4)
          Congenital muscular contractions (Q79.8)
          Dystonia in diseases classified elsewhere (G26.-0*)
          Seizure-induced twisting postures (G40.-)
G24.80   Paroxysmal dystonias
  G24.800 Sporadic kinesigenic dystonia
  G24.801 Familial kinesigenic dystonia

(continued)

TABLE 1.1. *(continued)*

Extrapyramidal and Movement Disorders (G20–G29)

G24.802 Sporadic nonkinesigenic dystonia
G24.803 Familial nonkinesigenic dystonia
G24.804 Tonic spasm of multiple sclerosis
G24.805 Paroxysmal nocturnal dystonia
G24.81   Sandifer's syndrome [pseudodystonia with anteroflexion associated with gastrointenstinal reflux in young children]
G24.84   Secondary dystonia NOS
G24.85   Pseudodystonia NOS

G24.9   Dystonia, unspecified

G25   *Other extrapyramidal and movement disorders*

G25.0   Essential tremor
Excludes: Tremor NOS (R25.1)
                      Isolated rest tremor (G25.26)
G25.00   Isolated head tremor
G25.01   Isolated facial tremor
G25.02   Isolated vocal tremor
G25.03   Isolated hand tremor
G25.04   Shuddering attacks of childhood
G25.07   Multiple site tremor
Use additional sixth character, if desired, to indicate whether
   G25.0x0   sporadic
   G25.0x1   familial

G25.1   Drug-induced tremor
Use additional external cause code, if desired, to identify drug

G25.2   Other specified forms of tremor
Excludes: Tremor in diseases classified elsewhere
G25.20   Kinetic [intention] tremor
G25.21   Physiologic tremor
G25.22   Dystonic tremor
G25.23   Orthostatic tremor
G25.24   Task-specific (e.g., handwriting) tremor
G25.25   Midbrain type tremor
G25.26   Isolated rest tremor

G25.3   Myoclonus
Excludes: Ataxia with myoclonus [Ramsay Hunt syndrome] (G11.23)
                      Epilepsia partialis continua (G40.5)
                      Facial myokymia (G51.4)
                      Hemifacial spasm (G51.3)
                      Myoclonic epilepsy (G40.-)
                      Myoclonus in diseases classified elsewhere (G26.-3*)
Use additional external cause code, if desired, to identify drug, if drug-induced
G25.30   Cortical type diffuse myoclonus
G25.31   Focal or multifocal cortical type myoclonus
G25.32   Essential myoclonus [Friedreich's paramyoclonus multiplex]
G25.33   Oculopalatal myoclonus
G25.34   Segmental spinal myoclonus
G25.35   Propriospinal myoclonus
G25.36   Peripheral myoclonus
G25.37   Sleep (hypnic) myoclonus
G25.38   Postanoxic action myoclonus [Lance-Adams]
G25.38   Other specified myoclonic disorders

G25.4   Drug-induced chorea
Use additional external cause code, if desired, to identify drug, e.g., dopamine receptor blockers (neuroleptics, Y49.3, .4, .5), antiemetic drugs (Y43.0), dopaminergic (antiparkinson, Y46.-), psychostimulants (Y49.7), toxins (T51-T65)

G25.5   Other chorea
Chorea NOS
Excludes: Chorea in diseases classified elsewhere (G26.-1*)

(continued)

TABLE 1.1. *(continued)*

Extrapyramidal and Movement Disorders (G20–G29)

		Chorea NOS with heart involvement (I02.0)
		Huntington's disease [Huntington's chorea] (G10)
		Huntington's disease, juvenile onset (less than 20 years) (G10.-1)
		Huntington's disease, late onset (more than 50 years) (G10.-2) rheumatic chorea (I02.-)
		Sydenham's chorea (I02.-)
	G25.50	Chorea gravidarum
2	G25.51	Chorea associated with hormone therapy
	G25.52	Hemichorea
	G25.53	Neuroacanthocytosis [Choreoacanthocytosis]
	G25.54	Benign hereditary chorea
	G25.55	Senile chorea
	G25.56	Kinesigenic choreathetosis

G25.6   Drug-induced tics and other tics of organic origin
       Excludes: Gilles de la Tourette's syndrome (F95.2)
                 Tics NOS (F95.9)
                 Tics in diseases classified elsewhere (G26.-4*)
       G25.60   Drug-induced tics
       Use additional external cause code, if desired, to identify drug
       G25.61   Tics of organic origin not related to drugs
                 Secondary tic NOS

G25.8   Other specified extrapyramidal and movement disorders
       G25.80   Paroxysmal nocturnal limb movement disorder
       G25.81   Painful legs (or arms) moving toes (or fingers) syndrome
       G25.82   Sporadic restless legs syndrome [Ekbom]
       G25.83   Familial restless legs syndrome with or without periodic movements
       G25.84   Stiff-person syndrome [Stiff-man syndrome]
       G25.85   Ballism/hemiballism
                 Use additional code, if desired, when of vascular origin (I63.-)
       G25.86   Opsoclonus-myoclonus syndrome
                 Dancing eyes, dancing feet syndrome
       G25.87   Stereotypies
         Excludes: Edentulous orofacial dyskinesia (G24.41)
                     Epileptic automatisms (G40.-)
                     Gilles de la Tourette syndrome (F95.2)
                     Orofacial dyskinesia (G24.40)
                     Psychogenic stereotypies (F98.4)
                     Restless legs syndrome (G25.82)
                     Stereotyped movement disorder (F98.4)
                     Stereotypies in:
                       Autism (F84.0, .1+, G26.-5*)
                       Diseases classified elsewhere (G26.-5*)
                       Mental retardation (F70-F79+, G26.-5*)
                       Rett's syndrome (F84.2+, G26.-5*)
                       Schizophrenia (F20.-+, G26.-5*)
                       Tardive dyskinesia (G24.02)
       G25.88   Akathisia, not related to drugs
                 Excludes: Akathisia, drug-induced (G21.1)

G25.9   Extrapyramidal and movement disorder, unspecified

G26*   *Extrapyramidal and movement disorders in diseases classified elsewhere*
       G26.-0*   Dystonia in diseases classified elsewhere
                 Hemidystonia in diseases classified elsewhere
                 Dyskinesia in diseases classified elsewhere
                 Dystonia in:
                     Ataxia telangiectasia (G11.30+)
                     Corticobasal ganglionic degeneration (G23.81+)
                     Hallervorden-Spatz disease (G23.0+)
                     Hereditary spastic paraplegia (G11.4+)
                     Huntington's disease (G10+)
                     Joseph's disease (G11.24+)
                     Juvenile neuronal ceroid lipfuscinosis (E75.42+)

(continued)

TABLE 1.1. *(continued)*

Extrapyramidal and Movement Disorders (G20–G29)

    Lesch-Nyhan syndrome (E79.1+)
    Multiple sclerosis (G35+)
    Neuroacanthocytosis (G25.53+)
    Nieman-Pick disease type C (E75.262+)
    Pallidal degeneration (G23.82, G23.83+)
    Parkinson's disease (G20+)
    Progressive supranuclear ophthalmoparesis [Steele-Richardson-Olszewski] (G23.10+)
    Reflex sympathetic dystrophy (G90.83+)
    Rett's syndrome (F84.2+)
    Multisystem degeneration with dysautonomia [multiple system atrophy, MSA] (G90.3)
    Subacute necrotizing encephalopathy [Leigh's disease] (31.81+)
    Wilson's disease [hepatolenticular degeneration] (E83.01+)
G26.-1* Chorea in diseases classified elsewhere
    Hemichorea in diseases classified elsewhere
    Chorea in:
        Hyperthyroidism (E05.-+)
        Neuroacanthocytosis (G25.53+)
        Systemic lupus erythematosus (M32.-+)
    Excludes: Chorea gravidarum (G25.50)
        Chorea NOS with heart involvement (I02.0)
        Huntington's disease (G10)
        Rheumatic chorea (I02.-)
        Sydenham's chorea (I02.-)
G26.-2* Tremor in diseases classified elsewhere
    Tremor in:
        Brain tumor (C71.-, C79.-, D33.-+)
        Cerebrovascular disease (I60-I67+)
        Head injury (S06.-+)
G26.-3* Myoclonus in diseases classified elsewhere
    Myoclonus in:
        Alzheimer's disease (G30.0+)
        Brain tumor (C71.-, C79.-, D33.-+)
        Creutzfeldt-Jakob disease (A81.0+)
        Cerebrovascular disease (I60-I67+)
        Head injury (S06.-+)
        Metabolic encephalopathy (G94.80*)
        Olivopontocerebellar atrophy (G11.22, G11.23+)
        Progressive myoclonic ataxia [Ramsay Hunt syndrome] (G11.13+)
        Toxic encephalopathy (G92+)
G26.-4* Tics in diseases classified elsewhere
G26.-5* Stereotypes in diseases classified elsewhere
    Stereotypes in:
        Autism (F84.0, .1+)
        Mental retardation (F70-F79+)
        Rett's syndrome (F84.2+)
        Schizophrenia (F20.-+)

Modified from Jankovic J. International classification of diseases. Tenth revision: neurological adaptation (ICD-10 NA) extrapyramidal and movement disorders. *Mov Disord* 1995;10:533–540, with permission.

of the body to another (Table 1.5). The movements are brisk and abrupt in some cases, such as in Sydenham's chorea (15), whereas in others, they are slower and more flowing, as in Huntington's disease (16–18). The term *choreoathetosis* has been used in this latter situation in which chorea may be combined with features of dystonia and athetosis. Chorea is typically a manifestation of basal ganglia dysfunction, but in rare cases it is seen in patients with severe proprioceptive dis-

turbance, such as peripheral neuropathy or posterior column dysfunction (19).

Ballism comprises wide-amplitude, flinging movements, usually involving the proximal limbs, most often of only one side of the body *(hemiballism)* (20). Occasionally, bilateral movements occur *(biballism or paraballism)*. Ballism is believed to be at one end of the spectrum of chorea because many patients demonstrate additional distal choreic

TABLE 1.2. CLASSIFICATION OF PARKINSONISM

I. Primary (idiopathic) parkinsonism
  Parkinson's disease
  Juvenile parkinsonism

II. Multisystem degenerations ("parkinsonism plus")
  Progressive supranuclear palsy (PSP)
  Multiple system atrophy (MSA)
    Striatonigral degeneration (SND or MSA-P)
    Olivopontocerebellar atrophy (OPCA or MSA-C)
    Shy-Drager syndrome (SDS)
  Lytico-Bodig or parkinsonism-dementia-ALS complex of
    Guam (PDACG)
  Corticolbasal ganglionic degeneration (CBGD)
  Progressive pallidal atrophy
  Parkinsonism-dementia complex
  Pallidopyramidal disease

III. Heredodegenerative parkinsonism
  Hereditary juvenile dystonia-parkinsonism
  Autosomal dominant Lewy body disease
  Huntington's disease
  Wilson's disease
  Hereditary ceruloplasmin deficiency
  Hallervorden-Spatz disease
  Olivopontocerebellar and spinocerebellar
    degenerations
  Machado-Joseph disease
  Familial amyotrophy-dementia-parkinsonism
  Disinhibition-dementia-parkinsonism-amyotrophy-
    complex
  Gerstmann-Straussler-Scheinker disease
  Familial progressive subcortical gliosis
  Lubag (X-linked dystonia-parkinsonism)
  Familial basal ganglia calcification
  Mitochondrial cytopathies with striatal necrosis
    Ceroid lipofuscinosis
  Familial parkinsonism with peripheral neuropathy
  Parkinsonian-pyramidal syndrome
  Neuroacanthocytosis
  Hereditary hemochromatosis

IV. Secondary (acquired, symptomatic) parkinsonism
  Infectious: postencephalitic, AIDS, subacute scleroding
    pancncephalitis, Creuzfeldt-Jakob disease, prion
    diseases
  Drugs: dopamine receptor blocking drugs (antipsychotic,
    antiemetic drugs), reserpine, tetrabenazine, α-methyldopa,
    lithium, flunarizine, cinnarizine
  Toxins: 1-methyl-4-phenyl-1,2,5,6-tetrahydropyridine,
    carbon monoxide, manganese, mercury, carbon disulfide,
    cyanide, methanol, ethanol
  Vascular: multiinfarct, Binswanger's disease
  Trauma: pugilistic encephalopathy
  Other: parathyroid abnormalities, hypothyroidism,
    hepatocerebral degeneration, brain tumor, paraneoplastic,
    normal pressure hydrocephalus, noncommunicating
    hydrocephalus, syringomesencephalia, hemiatrophy-
    hemiparkinsonism, peripherally induced tremor and
    parkinsonism, and psychogenic

Modified from Jankovic J. Treatment of parkinsonian syndromes. In: Kurlan R, ed. *Treatment of movement disorders.* Philadelphia: JB Lippincott, 1995:95–114, with permission.

movements, and as recovery occurs, hemiballism often transforms into a milder hemichoreic state.

Dystonia can be defined as a disorder dominated by sustained muscle contractions that frequently cause twisting and repetitive movements or abnormal postures (Table 1.6) (21). Dystonic movements may be slow and twisting. Prolonged dystonic spasms result in characteristic posturing of various body parts. In addition, dystonic movements may be rapid, resembling the shocklike jerks of myoclonus (see later), and both dystonia and myoclonus can coexist in families with the *dystonia-myoclonus syndrome.* Dystonia may be also manifested by rhythmic movements, the so-called *dystonic tremor.* Such dystonic tremor can be abolished if the patient is asked to relax and allow the body part to move in the direction of the dystonic pull. The wide range of abnormal movement types that occur in dystonic syndromes is often a source of misdiagnosis. Patients with dystonia may also demonstrate a postural and action tremor of the limbs similar to essential tremor.

The term *action dystonia* refers to dystonic movements and postures that are specific to selected actions or positions. The best example of task-specific dystonia is dystonic writer's cramp and other *occupational spasms.* Many patients use various peculiar tricks to lessen the severity of their abnormal movements. These features have frequently led to a misdiagnosis of dystonia as hysteria. The adult-onset idiopathic focal and segmental dystonias are the most common dystonic disorders seen in neurologic practice. These include cranial dystonia (blepharospasm, oromandibular/lingual dystonia), laryngeal dystonia (spasmodic dysphonia), and cervical dystonia (spasmodic torticollis).

Tics are the most varied of all movement disorders (Table 1.7). Tics are usually abrupt, transient, and at times repetitive and stereotypic, coordinated movements that vary in intensity and occur at irregular intervals (10,22). The movements are most often brief and jerky *(clonic tics);* however, slower, more prolonged movements *(tonic or dystonic tics)* also occur. Patients typically demonstrate a wide array of simple and complex motor or phonic tics as well as associated behavioral symptoms including impulse control problems, hyperactivity and attention deficit disorder, and obsessive-compulsive disorder. Several other features are helpful in distinguishing this movement disorder from other dyskinesias. Patients usually experience an inner urge to make the movement themselves, and this premonitory sensation is temporarily relieved by the execution of the tic. Tics are voluntarily suppressible for variable periods, but this usually occurs at the expense of mounting inner tension and the need to perform the tic. Voluntary suppression, however, is not specific for tics, and several other types of abnormal movements also may be suppressed for short periods of time.

Myoclonus can be defined as a sudden, brief, shocklike involuntary movement that may be caused by both active

TABLE 1.3. PARKINSONISM PLUS SYNDROMES: DIFFERENTIAL DIAGNOSIS

	PD	PSP	SDS	SND	OPCA	CBGD	DLBD	PDACG
Bradykinesia	+	+	+	+	±	+	±	+
Rigidity	+	+	+	+	+	+	±	+
Gait disturbance	+	+	+	+	+	+	±	+
Tremor	+	−	−	−	±	±	−	+
Ataxia	−	−	±	−	+	−	−	±
Dysautonomia	±	±	+	±	±	−	±	±
Dementia	±	+	±	−	−	±	+	+
Dysarthria/dysphagia	±	+	±	+	+	+	±	+
Dystonia	±	±	−	±	−	+	−	−
Eyelid apraxia	−	+	±	±	−	±	−	±
Limb apraxia	−	−	−	−	−	+	±	−
Motor neuron disease	−	−	±	±	−	−	−	+
Myoclonus	±	−	−	±	±	+	±	−
Neuropathy	−	−	±	−	±	−	−	−
Oculomotor deficit	−	+	±	−	+	+	±	±
Sleep impairment	±	±	+	±	±	−	±	−
Asymmetric findings	+	−	−	±	−	+	−	−
Levodopa response	+	±	±	+	±	−	−	−
Levodopa dyskinesia	+	−	−	±	−	−	−	−
Family history	±	−	−	−	−	−	−	−
Putamenal T-2 hypointensity	−	±	+	+	+	−	−	−
Lewy Bodies	+	−	±	±	±	±	+	−

CBGD, cortical-basal ganglionic degeneration; DLBD, diffuse Lewy body disease; OPCA, olivopontocerebellar atrophy (the familial forms of OPCA are included among the genetic forms of spinocerebellar atrophies); PD, Parkinson's disease; PDACG, parkinsonism-dementia-amyotrophic lateral sclerosis complex of Guam; PSP, progressive supranuclear palsy; SDS, Shy-Drager syndrome; SND, striatonigral degeneration.
Modified from Jankovic J. Treatment of parkinsonian syndromes. In: Kurlan R, ed. *Treatment of movement disorders.* Philadelphia: JB Lippincott, 1995:95–114, with permission.

muscle contraction *(positive myoclonus)* and inhibition of ongoing muscle activity *(negative myoclonus)* (Table 1.8) (23,24). *Asterixis* is the most common example of negative myoclonus. The differential diagnosis of myoclonus is broad, and a wide range of clinical patterns of myoclonus is seen. Frequency, amplitude, distribution, rhythmicity, and response to stimuli vary greatly from patient to patient. The frequency varies from an occasional single jerklike movement to constant, repetitive contractions (e.g., epilepsia partialis continua). The amplitude may range from a small contraction that fails to move a joint to a very large jerk that moves the entire body. The distribution ranges from focal involvement of one body part to segmental (involving two or more contiguous regions) to multifocal or even generalized myoclonus. When the jerks occur bilaterally, they may be symmetric or asymmetric. When they occur in more than one region, they may be synchronous in two body parts (within milliseconds) or asynchronous. Myoclonus is usually arrhythmic and irregular, but in some patients it is very regular (rhythmic), and in others, jerky oscillations may last for a few seconds and then fade away (oscillatory). Myoclonic movements may occur spontaneously without a clear precipitant or as a response to a wide variety of stimuli. This stimulus sensitivity may occur in response to sudden noise, light, visual threat, pinprick or touch, or muscle stretch. Attempted movements (or even the intention to move) may initiate the muscle jerks *(action or intention myoclonus).*

Stereotypy is an involuntary, patterned, repetitive, continuous, coordinated, purposeless or ritualistic movement, posture, or utterance (Table 1.9) (25). Stereotypy may be simple, as exemplified by a repetitive tongue protrusion or body rocking movements, or complex, such as self-caressing, crossing and uncrossing of legs, marching in place, and pacing. This movement disorder is typically present in patients with *tardive dyskinesia* (Table 1.10) (7). Other causes of stereotypy include mental retardation, autism, Rett's syndrome, schizophrenia, and other developmental and psychiatric disorders.

Certain types of dyskinesias occur intermittently, rather than in a persistent fashion. This is typical of tics and some forms of myoclonus. Rarely, patients with chorea or dystonia have bouts of sudden-onset, short-lived involuntary movements known as *paroxysmal dyskinesias* (Table 1.11) (26). Action dystonia could be confused with a paroxysmal dyskinesia; however, in the former condition, the abnormal movement consistently occurs in response to the specific action, rather than occurring in a periodic or unpredictable manner.

Abnormal or *excessive startle* occurs in numerous disorders. In some patients, the only problem is an exaggerated response to a startle that habituates poorly after repeated stimuli. Other patients have an abnormal response to the stimuli that normally evoke startle. Hyperekplexia, or *startle disease,* is the best known example of pathologic startle, now

TABLE 1.4. ETIOLOGIC CLASSIFICATION OF TREMORS

I. Rest tremors
   A. Parkinson's disease
   B. Other parkinsonian syndromes
      Multiple system atrophies (striatonigral degeneration, Shy-Drager syndrome, olivopontocerebellar atrophy)
      Progressive supranuclear palsy
      Corticobasal ganglionic degeneration
      Parkinsonism-dementia-amyotrophic lateral sclerosis of Guam
      Diffuse Lewy body disease
      Progressive pallidal atrophy
   C. Heredodegenerative disorders
      Huntington's disease
      Wilson's disease
      Neuroacanthocytosis
      Hallervorden-Spatz disease
      Gerstmann-Strausler-Scheinker disease
      Ceroid lipofuscinosis
   D. Secondary parkinsonism
      Toxic: 1-methyl-4-phenyl-1,2,5,6-tetrahydropyridine, carbon monoxide, manganese, methanol, cyanide, carbon disulfide
      Drug-induced: dopamine receptor blocking drugs (neuroleptics, the "rabbit syndrome"), dopamine-depleting drugs (reserpine, tetrabenazine), lithium, flunarizine, cinnarizine
      Vascular: multiinfarct, Binswanger's, "lower body parkinsonism"
      Trauma: pugilistic encephalopathy, midbrain injury
      Tumor and paraneoplastic
      Infectious: postencephalitic, fungal, AIDS, subacute sclerosing panencephalitis
      Creutzfeldt-Jakob disease
      Metabolic: hypoparathyroidism, chronic hepatic degeneration, mitochondrial cytopathies
      Normal pressure hydrocephalus
   E. Severe essential tremor
   F. Midbrain (rubral) tremor
   G. Tardive tremor
   H. Myorhythmia
   I. Spasmus nutans

II. Action tremors
   A. Postural tremors
      1. Physiologic tremor
      2. Enhanced physiologic tremor
         a. Stress-induced: emotion, exercise, fatigue, anxiety, fever
         b. Endocrine: hypoglycemia, thyrotoxicosis, pheochromocytoma, adrenocorticosteroids
         c. Drugs: β-agonists (theophylline, terbutaline, epinephrine, etc), dopaminergic drugs (levodopa, dopamine agonists), stimulants (amphetamines), psychiatric drugs (lithium, neuroleptics, tricyclics), methylxanthines (coffee, tea), valproic acid, cyclosporine, interferon
         d. Toxins: mercury, lead, arsenic, bismuth, bromine, alcohol withdrawal
      3. Essential tremor
         a. Autosomal dominant
         b. Sporadic
      4. Postural tremor associated with
         a. Dystonia
         b. Parkinsonism
         c. Myoclonus
         d. Hereditary motor-sensory neuropathy (Roussy-Levy)
         e. Kennedy's syndrome (X-linked spinobulbar atrophy)
      5. Parkinson's disease and other parkinsonian syndromes
      6. Tardive tremor
      7. Midbrain (rubral) tremor
      8. Cerebellar hypotonic tremor (titubation)
      9. Neuropathic tremor: motor neuron disease, peripheral neuropathy, peripheral nerve injury, reflex sympathetic dystrophy
   B. Kinetic (intention, dynamic, termination) tremors
      1. Cerebellar disorders (cerebellar outflow): multiple sclerosis, trauma, stroke, Wilson's disease, drugs and toxins
      2. Midbrain lesions
   C. Task- or position-specific tremors
      1. Handwriting
      2. Orthostatic
      3. Other (e.g., occupational) task-specific tremors
   D. Isometric
      1. Muscular contraction during sustained exertion

(continued)

TABLE 1.4. *(continued)*

III. Miscellaneous tremors and other rhythmic movements
  A. Myoclonus: rhythmic segmental myoclonus (e.g., palatal), oscillatory myoclonus, asterixis, minipolymyoclonus
  B. Dystonic tremors
  C. Cortical tremors
  D. Epilepsia partialis continua
  E. Nystagmus
  F. Clonus
  G. Fasciculations
  H. Shivering
  I. Shuddering attacks
  J. Head bobbing (third ventricular cysts)
  K. Aortic insufficiency with head titubation

TABLE 1.5. ETIOLOGIC CLASSIFICATION OF CHOREA

1. Developmental/aging choreas
   a. Physiologic chorea of infancy
   b. Cerebral palsy: anoxic, kernicterus
   c. Minimal cerebral dysfunction
   d. Buccal-oral-lingual dyskinesia and edentulous orodyskinesia in elderly patients
   e. Senile chorea (probably several causes)

2. Hereditary choreas
   a. Huntington's disease
   b. Benign hereditary chorea
   c. Neuroacanthocytosis
   d. Other central nervous system "degenerations": olivoponto cerebellar atrophies (OPCAs), Azorean disease, ataxia telangiectasia, tuberous sclerosis, Hallervorden-Spatz, Dentatorubralpallidoluysian atrophy (DRPLA), familial calcification of basal ganglia, others
   e. Neurometabolic disorders: Wilson's disease, Lesch-Nyhan disease, lysosomal storage disorders, amino acid disorders, Leigh's disease, porphyria

3. Drug induced—neuroleptics (tardive dyskinesia), antiparkinsonian drugs, amphetamines, tricyclics, oral contraceptives, anticonvulsants, anticholinergics, others

4. Toxins—alcohol intoxication and withdrawal, anoxia, carbon monoxide, Mn, Hg, thallium, toluene

5. Metabolic
   a. Hyperthyroidism
   b. Hypoparathyroidism (various types)
   c. Pregnancy (chorea gravidarum)
   d. Hypernatremia and hyponatremia, hypomagnesemia, hypocalcemia
   e. Hypoglycemia and hyperglycemia (latter may cause hemichorea, hemiballism)
   f. Acquired hepatocerebral degeneration
   g. Nutritional, e.g., beriberi, pellagra, vitamin B_{12} deficiency in infants

6. Infectious
   a. Sydenham's chorea
   b. Encephalitis lethargica
   c. Various other infections and postinfectious encephalitides, including Creutzfeldt-Jakob disease

7. Immunologic
   a. Systemic lupus erythematosus (including ANF-negative cases with lupus anticoagulant)
   b. Henöch-Schonlein purpura
   c. Others rarely: sarcoid, multiple sclerosis, Behçet's disease, polyarteritis nodosa, myeloproliferative disorder

8. Vascular (often hemichorea)
   a. Infarction
   b. Hemorrhage
   c. Arteriovenous malformation
   d. Polycythemia rubra vera
   e. Migraine

9. Tumors

10. Trauma, including subdural and epidural hematoma

11. Miscellaneous, including paroxysmal choreoathetosis

TABLE 1.6. ETIOLOGIC CLASSIFICATION OF DYSTONIA

I. Primary Dystonia
  A. Sporadic
  B. Inherited (all autosomal dominant)
      Classic (Oppenheim's) dystonia (common in Ashkenazi Jews, DYT1-9q34)
      Childhood- and adult-onset cranial-cervical-limb dystonia (DYT6-8p21-22)
      Adult-onset cervical and other focal dystonia (DYT7-18p)

II. Secondary Distonia (Dystonia-plus syndromes)
  A. Sporadic
      Parkinson's disease
      Progressive supranuclear palsy
      Multiple system atrophy
      Corticobasal degeneration
  B. Inherited
      1. Autosomal dominant
          Dopa-responsive dystonia (DRD) (DYT5-GTP cyclohydrolase I 14q22.1)
          Dystonia-myoclonus (alcohol responsive, chromosome 18)
      2. Autosomal recessive
          Tyrosine hydroxylase deficiency (chromosome 21)
          Biopterin-deficient diseases
          Aromatic amino acid decarboxylase deficiency (dopamine-agonist responsive dystonia)

III. Heredogenerative diseases
  A. X-linked recessive
      Lubag (X-linked dystonia-parkinsonism, DYT3-Xq13)
      Pelizaeus-Merzbacher disease
      Lesch-Nyhan syndrome
      Deafness, dystonia, retardation, blindness
  B. Autosomal dominant
      Rapid-onset dystonia-parkinsonism (RDP)
      Juvenile parkinsonism-dystonia
      Huntington's disease (IT15-4p16.3)
      Spinocerebellar degenerations (SCA1-SCA8)
      Dentatorubralpallidoluysian atrophy (DRPLA)
      Hereditary spastic paraplegia with dystonia
      Thalamoolivary degeneration with Wernicke's encephalopathy
  C. Autosomal recessive
      Wilson's disease (Cu-ATPase-13q14.3)
      Neurodegeneration with brain iron accumulation type 1 (NBIA 1) (Hallervorden-Spatz disease-20p12.3-p13)
      Hypoprebetalipoproteinemia, acanthocytosis, retinitis pigmentosa, and pallidal degeneration (HARP syndrome)
      Ataxia telangiectasia
      Associated with metabolic disorders
      1. Amino acid disorders
          Glutaric acidemia
          Methylmalonic acidemia
          Homocystinuria
          Hartnup's disease
          Tyrosinosis
      2. Lipid disorders
          Metachromatic leukodystrophy
          Ceroid lipofuscinosis
          Niemann-Pick type C (dystonic lipidosis, "sea blue" histiocytosis)
          Gangliosidoses GM_1-, GM_2-variants
          Hexosaminidase A and B deficiency
      3. Other metabolic disorders
          Tyrosine hydroxylase deficiency (chromosome 21)
          Biopterin deficient diseases
          Triosephosphate isomerase deficiency
          Aromatic amino acid decarboxylase deficiency (dopamine agonist-responsive dystonia)
  D. Unknown inheritance
      Neuroacanthocytosis
      Rett's syndrome
      Intraneuronal inclusion disease
      Infantile bilateral striatal necrosis

(continued)

TABLE 1.6. *(continued)*

      Familial basal ganglia calcifications
      Hereditary spastic paraplegia with dystonia
      Deletion of 18q
  E. Mitochondrial
      Leigh's disease
      Leber's disease
  With a known specific cause
      Perinatal cerebral injury and kernicterus: athetoid cerebral palsy, delayed-onset dystonia
      Infections: Viral encephalitis, encephalitis lethargica, Reye's syndrome; subacute sclerosing panencephalitis; Creutzfeldt-Jakob disease; HIV infection
      Other: tuberculosis, syphilis, acute infectious torticollis
      Drugs: levodopa and dopamine agonists, dopamine receptor-blocking drugs, fenfluramine, anticonvulsants, flecainide, ergots, certain calcium-channel blockers
      Toxins: manganese, carbon monoxide, carbon disulfide, cyanide, methanol, disulfiram, 3-nitroproprionic acid, wasp sting
      Metabolic: hypoparathyroidism
      Paraneoplastic brainstem encephalitis
      Vitamin E deficiency
      Cerebral vascular or ischemic injury
      Multiple sclerosis
      Central pontine myelinolysis
      Brain tumor
      Arteriovenous malformation
      Head trauma and brain surgery (thalamotomy)
      Peripheral trauma (with causalgia)
      Electrical injury

IV. Other hyperkinetic syndromes associated with dystonia
  A. Tic disorders with dystonic tics
  B. Paroxysmal dyskinesias
    1. Paroxysmal kinesigenic dyskinesia
    2. Paroxysmal non-kinesigenic dyskinesia
    3. Paroxysmal exertion-induced dyskinesia
    4. Paroxysmal hypnogenic dyskinesia
  C. Hypnogenic dystonia (probably a seizure disorder)

V. Psychogenic

VI. Pseudodystonia
    Atlantoaxial subluxation
    Syringomyelia
    Arnold-Chiari malformation
    Trochlear nerve palsy
    Vestibular torticollis
    Posterior fossa mass
    Soft tissue neck mass
    Congenital postural torticollis
    Congenital Klippel-Feil syndrome
    Isaac's syndrome
    Sandiffer's syndrome
    Satoyoshi's syndrome
    Stiff-person syndrome
    Ventral hernia

---

known to be associated with a mutation in the gene for a subunit of the glycine receptor on chromosome 5 (27). Various other unusual disorders, first described in the nineteenth century together with Tourette's syndrome, manifest excessive startle, including the jumping Frenchmen of Maine, latah, and myriachit. These latter disorders also demonstrate sudden striking out, echo phenomena, automatic obedience, and several other less common features.

The term *akathisia* refers to a sense of restlessness and the feeling of a need to move (28). This disorder may be accompanied by various "akathisic," stereotypic movements including repetitive rubbing, crossing and uncrossing the arms, stroking the head and face with the hands, repeatedly picking at clothing, abducting and adducting, crossing and uncrossing, swinging the legs or pumping them up and down, shifting weight, rocking, marching in place, or

TABLE 1.7. ETIOLOGIC CLASSIFICATION OF TICS

I. Primary
  A. Sporadic
    1. Transient motor *or* phonic tics (<1 yr)
    2. Chronic motor *or* phonic tics (>1 yr)
    3. Adult-onset (recurrent) tics
    4. Tourette syndrome
    5. Primary dystonia
  B. Inherited
    1. Tourette's syndrome
    2. Huntington's disease
    3. Primary dystonia
    4. Neuroacanthocytosis
    5. Neurodegeneration with brain iron accumulation type 1, NBIA 1 (Hallervorden-Spatz)
    6. Tuberous sclerosis
    7. Wilson's disease
    9. Duchenne's muscular dystrophy

II. Secondary
  A. Infections: encephalitis, Creutzfeldt-Jakob disease, neurosyphilis, Sydenham's chorea
  B. Drugs: amphetamines, methylphenidate, pemoline, levodopa, cocaine, carbamazepine, phenytoin, phenobarbital, lamotrigine, antipsychotics and other dopamine receptor-blocking drugs (tardive tics, tardive tourettism)
  C. Toxins: carbon monoxide, wasp sting encephalopathy
  D. Developmental: static encephalopathy, mental retardation syndromes, chromosomal abnormalities, autistic spectrum disorders (Asperger's syndrome)
  E. Chromosomal disorders: Down's syndrome. Kleinfelter's syndrome, XYY karyotype, fragile X, triple X and 9p mosaicism, partial trisomy 16, 9p monosomy, citrullinemia, Beckwith-Wiedemann syndrome
  F. Other: head trauma, stroke, cardiopulmonary bypass with hypothermia; neurocutaneous syndromes, schizophrenia, neurodegenerative diseases

III. Related manifestations and disorders
    1. Stereotypies/habits/mannerisms
    2. Self-injurious behaviors
    3. Motor restlessness
    4. Akathisia
    5. Compulsions
    6. Excessive startle
    7. Jumping Frenchmen of Maine

Modified from Jankovic J. Differential diagnosis and etiology of tics. Tourette syndrome. *Adv Neurol* 2001;85:15–29, with permission.

pacing while sitting and standing. Patients may even have vocalizations such as moans, grunts, and shouts. Whether true akathisic movements can occur in the absence of the subjective sense of needing to move remains controversial. Akathisia is usually a complication of therapy with dopamine receptor blockers.

Restless legs syndrome is another disorder in which most movements occur secondary to the subjective need to move (29,30). The patient typically complains of a sensory disturbances in the legs (less often in the arms), including pins and needles, creeping or crawling, aching, itching, stabbing, heaviness, tension, burning, or cold. These complaints are usually experienced when patients are lying down or are elevating the legs in the evening. This condition is commonly associated with insomnia and another movement disorder, *periodic movements of sleep* (sometimes inappropriately termed *nocturnal myoclonus*). These periodic, slow, sustained (1- to 2-second) movements range from synchronous to asynchronous extension of the big toes and feet to triple flexion of one or both legs. More rapid myoclonic move-

ments or slower, prolonged dystonic-like movements of the feet and legs also may be present in these patients while they are awake.

Painful legs and moving toes comprise an unusual, but well-defined movement disorder most often involving the lower limbs (31). Rarely, a similar disorder can be seen in the upper limbs. The movements are not usually the main source of disability or concern. Conversely, most of these patients complain of the accompanying deep pulling pain in the lower limb and foot and typically demonstrate continuous, rhythmic, flexing or abducting movements of the toes. In some cases, patients have a history of nerve insult or injury, and the examination may demonstrate evidence of peripheral nerve or root dysfunction.

Hemifacial spasm is one of the best recognized *peripheral movement disorders*. The movement consists of irregular tonic and clonic contractions involving the muscles innervated by the ipsilateral seventh cranial nerve. Eyelid twitching usually is the first symptom, followed at variable intervals by lower facial muscle involvement (32). In rare cases of

TABLE 1.8. ETIOLOGIC CLASSIFICATION OF MYOCLONUS

1. Physiologic myoclonus (normal subjects)
   a. Sleep jerks (hypnic jerks)
   b. Anxiety-induced
   c. Exercise-induced
   d. Hiccough (singultus)
   e. Benign infantile myoclonus with feeding

2. Essential myoclonus (no known cause and no other gross neurologic deficit)
   a. Hereditary
   b. Sporadic

3. Epileptic myoclonus (seizures dominate and no encephalopathy, at least initially)
   a. Fragments of epilepsy
      Isolated epileptic myoclonic jerks
      Epilepsia partialis continua
      Idiopathic stimulus-sensitive myoclonus
      Photosensitive myoclonus
      Myoclonic absences in petit mal
   b. Childhood myoclonic epilepsies
      Infantile spasms
      Myoclonic astatic epilepsy (Lennox-Gastaut)
      Cryptogenic myoclonus epilepsy (Aicardi's)
      Awakening myoclonus epilepsy of Janz
   c. Benign familial myoclonic epilepsy (Rabot's)
   d. Progressive myoclonus epilepsy: Baltic myoclonus (Unverricht-Lundborg)

4. Symptomatic myoclonus (progressive or static encephalopathy dominates)
   a. Storage disease:
      Lafora body disease
      Lipidoses, e.g., GM_2 gangliosidosis, Tay-Sachs, Krabbe's, Ceroid-lipofuscinosis (Batten/Kufs)
      Sialidosis ("cherry-red-spot")
   b. Spinocerebellar degeneration:
      Ramsay Hunt syndrome (several causes)
      Friedreich's ataxia
      Ataxia telangiectasia
   c. Basal ganglia degenerations:
      Wilson's disease
      Torsion dystonia
      Hallervorden-Spatz disease
      Cortico-basal ganglionic degeneration
      Progressive supranuclear palsy
      Huntington's disease
      Parkinson's disease
      Multiple system atrophy
      Dentatorubroluysian atrophy
   d. Mitochondrial encephalopathies
   e. Dementias:
      Creutzfeldt-Jakob disease
      Alzheimer's disease
   f. Viral encephalopathies:
      Subacute sclerosing panencephalitis
      Encephalitis lethargica
      Arbor virus encephalitis
      Herpes simplex encephalitis
      Postinfectious encephalitis
   g. Metabolic:
      Hepatic failure
      Renal failure
      Dialysis syndrome
      Hyponatremia

TABLE 1.8. (continued)

      Hypoglycemia
      Infantile myoclonic encephalopathy (polymyoclonus) (+/- neuroblastoma)
      Nonketotic hyperglycemia
      Multiple carboxylase deficiency
   h. Toxic encephalopathies:
      Bismuth
      Heavy-metal poison
      Methylbromide, dichlorodiphenyltrichloroethane (DDT)
      Drugs including levodopa, tricyclic antidepressants, others
   i. Physical encephalopathies:
      Posthypoxia (Lance-Adams)
      Posttraumatic
      Heat stroke
      Electric shock
      Decompression injury
   j. Focal central nervous system damage:
      Poststroke
      Postthalamotomy
      Tumor
      Trauma
      Olivodentate lesions (palatal myoclonus)
      Spinal cord lesions (segmental/spinal myoclonus)
   k. Rarely root, plexus, or peripheral nerve disorders

Modified from Fahn S, Marsden CD, Van Woert MH. Definition and classification of myoclonus. *Adv Neurol* 1986;43:1–5, with permission.

bilateral involvement, the spasms are asynchronous on the two sides, in contrast to relatively synchronous, although at times asymmetric, contractions seen in patients with *dystonic blepharospasm* (33). In addition to hemifacial spasm, other peripheral movement disorders, such as fasciculations and myokymia, and some movement disorders, particularly dystonia and tremor, can occur after peripheral trauma (34).

TABLE 1.9. ETIOLOGIC CLASSIFICATION OF STEREOTYPIES

Physiologic
   Mannerisms

Pathologic
   Mental retardation
      Autism (Kanner's infantile autism, Asperger's syndrome)
   Rett's syndrome
   Williams' syndrome
   Tardive dyskinesia
   Akathisia
   Neuroacanthocytosis
   Schizophrenia
   Catatonia
   Obsessive-compulsive disorder
   Tourette's syndrome
   Restless legs syndrome
   Epileptic automatism
   Psychogenic

Modified from Jankovic J. Stereotypies. In: Marsden CD, Fahn S, eds. *Movement disorders,* 3rd ed. London: Butterworth-Heinemann, 1994;503–517, with permission.

TABLE 1.10. CLASSIFICATION OF NEUROLEPTIC-INDUCED MOVEMENT DISORDERS

Acute-Transient	Chronic-Persistent
Dystonic reaction	Tardive stereotypy
Parkinsonism	Tardive chorea
Akathisia	Tardive dystonia
Neuroleptic malignant syndrome	Tardive akathisia
	Tardive tics
	Tardive myoclonus
	Tardive tremor
	Persistent parkinsonism
	Tardive sensory syndrome

Modified from Jankovic J. Tardive syndromes and other drug-induced movement disorders. *Clin Neuropharmacol* 1995;18:197–214, with permission.

The nature and extent of the investigation of the patient presenting with a movement disorder vary depending on the clinical circumstances (35). When the historical and clinical features are characteristic of certain idiopathic or genetic conditions (e.g., familial essential tremor, Tourette's syndrome), further investigations may be unnecessary. This approach also applies to certain well-recognized drug-induced movement disorders. The importance of excluding Wilson's disease cannot be overemphasized in view of its treatability and universally fatal outcome if it is left undiagnosed.

EPIDEMIOLOGY

Parkinson's Disease

Epidemiologic studies may provide important clues to potential risk factors associated with PD. Based on a joint analysis of five communities in Europe, the overall prevalence of parkinsonism was estimated to be 2.3% and of PD

TABLE 1.11. CLASSIFICATION OF PAROXYSMAL DYSKINESIAS

1. Paroxysmal kinesigenic dyskinesia (PKD)
2. Paroxysmal nonkinesigenic dyskinesia (PNKD)
3. Paroxysmal exertion-induced dyskinesia (PED)
4. Paroxysmal nocturnal dyskinesia (PND)
5. Paroxysmal psychogenic dyskinesia (PPD)
Each category includes:
   A. Short-lasting ($\leq$5 min)
     1. Idiopathic: familial/sporadic
     2. Secondary
   B. Long-lasting (>5 min)
     1. Idiopathic: familial/sporadic
     2. Secondary

Modified from Demirkiran M, Jankovic J. Paroxysmal dyskinesias: clinical features and classification. *Ann Neurol* 1995;38:571–579, with permission.

1.6% (36). The frequency of the disease increases with age, and it has been estimated that about 3% of people older than age 65 years have PD (37). The overall estimated prevalence of PD in people more than 65 years of age is 34.6% (14.9% for people 65 to 74 years of age, 29.5% for those 75 to 84 years old, and 52.4% for those 85 years old and older) (38). In another epidemiologic study, 108 of 1,056 (10.2%) nondemented persons in upper Manhattan, 65 years of age or older, reported "shaking" (39). Neurologic examination confirmed rest tremor in 8.3% and action tremor in 17.6%, and the prevalence of PD and essential tremor was estimated to be 3.2% and 10.2%, respectively. Bower et al. found 364 incident cases of parkinsonism in Olmsted County, Minnesota between 1976 and 1990: 42% with PD, 20% with drug-induced parkinsonism, and 14% with parkinsonism-dementia (40). The incidence increased with age except in the oldest men, and the diagnosis of parkinsonism was more common in men than in women. Most studies have demonstrated slight male preponderance or no differences in the prevalence by gender (41), but a more recent study from Finland indicated a twofold male preponderance (42). The finding of decreased rates of PD in black populations has led investigators to postulate that melanin may have a neuroprotective function (43). Some investigators have suggested that cutaneous melanin binds potential toxins, as neuronal melanin binds 1-methyl-4-phenyl-1,2,5,6,-tetrahydropyridine (MPTP), before crossing the blood-brain barrier and thereby prevent SN damage (44). A door-to-door population-based survey in Copiah County, Mississippi, a racially balanced community, found a similar prevalence of PD in whites and blacks (45). Other studies have suggested that the disease is less common among Africans and Asians.

Epidemiologic studies have found the disease to be more prevalent in industrial countries and in areas with heavy steel alloy industries and wood pulp mills, and other studies have correlated the occurrence of PD with living in rural areas, vegetable farming, exposure to herbicides and pesticides, and the use of well water (46,47). These findings are supported by many studies, but some studies are flawed by poor design, small sample size, and other methodologic problems; hence a definite relationship between any of these factors and the disease cannot be established. Extensive chemical analyses of well water used in areas of high prevalence of PD in Israel failed to identify any potential neurotoxins (48). Furthermore, only two of 16 pesticide residues were detected in the brains of patients with PD: pp = DDE, a long-lasting residue of dichlorodiphenyltrichloroethane (DDT) and dieldrin, a lipid-soluble, long-lasting mitochondrial poison (49). The first was actually more likely found in Alzheimer's than in PD brain tissue and was also detected in the brains of normal control subjects. Dieldrin was detected in six of 20 brains of patients with PD, and the investigators suggested that further studies of this potential neurotoxin are warranted. We reported on ten patients whose clinical features were consistent with multiple system atrophy and in whom toxins were suspected to play an etiologic role (50). One patient with pathologically confirmed multiple system atrophy was exposed to high concentrations of various toxins including formaldehyde, malathion, and diazinon. The other patients had a history of heavy exposure to various agents, such as *N*-hexane, benzene, methylisobutylketone, and pesticides. Although a cause-and-effect relationship could not be proven, these cases suggest that environmental toxins may play a role in the pathogenesis of some cases of parkinsonism. The methodology of studies showing an inverse correlation between PD and smoking has been questioned, and even if such an inverse relationship does exist, it may be attributed to a "nonsmoking" personality in patients with PD rather than the protective effects of tobacco. Morens et al. analyzed 46 published reports, most of which suggested that frequency of smoking in patients with PD is about half of that in non-PD populations (51). Smoking may be protective in young patients with PD but not in older patients (52). In addition to reviewing the epidemiologic evidence suggesting a possible protective effect of smoking, the authors also provided a critical review of the relevant biologic effects of smoking: (a) nicotine stimulates dopamine release and upregulates postsynaptic nicotine receptors; (b) smoking inhibits monoamine oxidase B (MAO-B) and thus may prevent the generation of toxic metabolites; (c) carbon monoxide, contained in cigarette smoke, also inhibits MAO-B and it may be protective against membrane damage produced by hydrogen peroxide. Gorell et al. concluded that the inverse dose-response relationship between PD and smoking cannot be explained by a bias, and that smoking is "biologically protective" (53).

Epidemiologic studies have thus far failed to uncover clusters of PD that would provide clues to potential environmental factors in the causation of the disease. Studies based on data from death certificates confirmed previous findings that patients with PD may have a lower-than-expected frequency of cancer (54).

Although a cure is not yet in sight, tremendous strides have been made in the treatment of patients with PD, as a result of which the mortality of PD patients has been markedly reduced. Although some studies suggest that the life expectancy of patients with PD is nearly normal (55), others have found two- to fivefold increased risk of mortality (56). In a prospective study of 800 patients who were followed longitudinally from early stages of their disease for an average of 8.2 years, the overall death rate was 2.1% per year, a rate similar to that of an age- and gender-matched United States population without PD (57). PD, along with other neurodegenerative diseases (Alzheimer's disease and motor neuron disease), is expected to surpass cancer as the second most common cause of death by the year 2040 (58).

Essential Tremor

Community-based epidemiologic studies have found the prevalence of essential tremor to range between 0.4 and 3.9% (59), but it may be as high as 5.5% in people more than 40 years old (60) and 14% in people 65 years old or older (37). As indicated above, in one epidemiologic study, 108 of 1,056 nondemented persons in upper Manhattan, 65 year of age or older, reported "shaking" (39). Neurologic examination confirmed rest tremor in 8.3% and action tremor in 17.6%, and the prevalence of PD and essential tremor was estimated to be 3.2% and 10.2%, respectively. Although the amplitude of essential tremor tends to increase with age, the tremor frequency decreases (61).

Dystonia

Based on an epidemiologic study of the population living in Rochester, Minnesota, the incidence of dystonia has been estimated to be two per million persons per year for generalized dystonia and 24 per million per year for focal dystonia (62). The prevalence of dystonia has been estimated to be 3.4 per 100,000 for generalized and 30 per 100,000 for focal dystonia. The prevalence of generalized dystonia among Jews of Eastern European ancestry (Ashkenazi) living in Israel was double that of the United States population (6.8 per 100,000) (63). In the north of England, the prevalence of generalized dystonia is 1.42 per 100,000 and 12.9 per 100,000 for focal dystonia (64).

Tourette's Syndrome

A discovery of a disease-specific marker will be helpful not only in improving our understanding of this complex neurobehavioral disorder, but also in clarifying the epidemiology of Tourette's syndrome. The prevalence rates have varied markedly and have been estimated to be as high as 4.2% when all types of tic disorders are included (65) and one per 83 (1.2%) (66) or as low as 28.7 per 100,000 (0.03%) (67) and one per 10,000 (0.01%) (68). There are many reasons for this wide variation, the most important of which are different ascertainment methods, different study populations, and different clinical criteria. Because about one-third of patients with tics do not even recognize their presence, it is difficult to derive at more accurate prevalence figures for Tourette's syndrome without a well-designed door-to-door survey (69). In one study, 3,034 students in three schools in Los Angeles were monitored over a 2-year period by a school psychologist; the frequency of definite Tourette's syndrome was one per 95 males and one per 759 females (66). In a study my colleagues and I conducted of 1,142 children in the second, fifth, and eighth grades of a general school population, eight (0.7%) had some evidence of Tourette's syndrome (70). In another school-based study, the prevalence of Tourette's syndrome was estimated at 3% (71).

In conclusion, the primary goal of this chapter was to provide an overview of classification and epidemiology of movement disorders. In addition, the functional anatomy of the basal ganglia and the phenomenology of hypokinetic and hyperkinetic movement disorders were reviewed. As the etiology of movement disorders becomes better understood, the classification will change accordingly. For example, the rapidly evolving classification of genetic dystonias now includes genetic forms of dystonia categorized as DYT1 to DYT15. Finally, current knowledge of the epidemiology of the more common movement disorders, PD, essential tremor, dystonia, and Tourette's syndrome, was reviewed.

REFERENCES

1. Jankovic J. Basal ganglia and neurotransmitter disorders. In: McMillan JA, DeAngelis CD, Feigin RD, et al., eds. *Oski's pediatrics: principles and practice,* 3rd ed. Philadelphia: Lippincott Williams & Wilkins, 1999:2005–2016.
2. Alexander GE, Crutcher MD. Functional architecture of basal ganglia circuits: neural substrates of parallel processing. *Trends Neurosci* 1990;13:266–271.
3. Parent A, Parent M, Levesque M. Basal ganglia and Parkinson's disease: an anatomical perspective. *Neurosci News* 1999;2:19–26.
4. Gerfen CR. The neostriatal mosaic: multiple levels of compartmental organization. *Trends Neurosci* 1992;15:133–139.
5. Sibley DR, Monsma FJ. Molecular biology of dopamine receptors. *Trends Pharmacol Sci* 1992;13:61–69.
6. Lang AE, Lozano AM. Parkinson's disease. *N Engl J Med* 1998;339:1044–1053;1130–1143.
7. Jankovic J. International classification of diseases. Tenth revision: neurological adaptation (ICD-10 NA) extrapyramidal and movement disorders. *Mov Disord* 1995;10:533–540.
8. Jankovic J, Lang AE. Classification of movement disorders. In: Germano IM, ed. *Surgical treatment of movement disorders.* Lebanon, NH: American Association of Neurological Surgeons, 1998:3–18.
9. Gelb DJ, Oliver E, Gilman S. Diagnostic criteria for Parkinson's disease. *Arch Neurol* 1999;56:33–39.
10. Jankovic J. Differential diagnosis and etiology of tics. Tourette syndrome. *Adv Neurol* 2001;85:15–29.
11. Vingerhoets FJG, Schulzer M, Calne DB, et al. Which clinical sign of Parkinson's disease best reflects the nigrostriatal lesion? *Ann Neurol* 1997;41:58–64.
12. Deuschl G, Bain P, Brin M, et al. Consensus statement of the Movement Disorder Society on tremor. *Mov Disord* 1998;13:Suppl 3:2–23.
13. Jankovic J, Schwartz, KS, Ondo W. Re-emergent tremor of Parkinson's disease. *J Neurol Neurosurg Psychiatry* 1999;67:646–650.
14. Jankovic J. Essential tremor: clinical characteristics. In: *Current issues in essential tremor.* Somerville, NJ: Embryon, 1999:14–18.
15. Cardoso F, Vargas AP, Oliveira LD, et al. Persistent Sydenham's chorea. *Mov Disord* 1999;14:805–807.
16. Berardelli A, Noth J, Thompson PD, et al. Pathophysiology of chorea and bradykinesia in Huntington's disease. *Mov Disord* 1999;14:398–403.
17. Lacone F, Engel U, Holinski-Feder E, et al. DNA analysis of Huntington's disease: five years of experience in Germany, Austria, and Switzerland. *Neurology* 1999;53:801–806.
18. Reddy PH, Williams M, Tagle DA. Recent advances in understanding the pathogenesis of Huntington's disease. *Trends Neurosci* 1999;22:248–255.
19. Sharp FR, Rando TA, Greenberg SA, et al. Pseudochoreoathetosis: movements associated with loss of proprioception. *Arch Neurol* 1994;51:1103–1109.
20. Vidakovic A, Dragasevic N, Kostic VS. Hemiballism: report of 25 cases. *J Neurol Neurosurg Psychiatry* 1994;57:945–949.
21. Jankovic J, Fahn S. Dystonic disorders. In: Jankovic J, Tolosa E, eds. *Parkinson's disease and movement disorders,* 3rd ed. Baltimore: Williams & Wilkins, 1998:513–551.
22. Jankovic J. Phenomenology and classification of tics: Tourette syndrome. *Neurol Clin* 1997;15:267–275.
23. Mima T, Nagamine T, Nishitani N, et al. Cortical myoclonus: sensorimotor hyperexcitability. *Neurology* 1998;50:933–942.
24. Tassinari CA, Rubboli G, Shibasaki H. Neurophysiology of positive and negative myoclonus. *Electroencephalogr Clin Neurophysiol* 1998;107:181–195.
25. Jankovic J. Stereotypies. In: Marsden CD, Fahn S, eds. *Movement disorders,* 3rd ed. London: Butterworth-Heinemann, 1994:503–517.
26. Demirkiran M, Jankovic J. Paroxysmal dyskinesias: clinical features and classification. *Ann Neurol* 1995;38:571–579.
27. Vergouwe MN, Tijssen MAJ, Peters ACB, et al. Hyperekplexia phenotype due to compound heterozygosity for GLRA1 gene mutations. *Ann Neurol* 1999;46:634–638.
28. Kahn EM, Munetz MR, Davies MA, et al. Akathisia: clinical phenomenology and relationship to tardive dyskinesia. *Compr Psychiatry* 1993;33:233–236.
29. Ondo W, Jankovic J. Restless legs syndrome. In: Appel SH, ed. *Current neurology,* vol 17. Amsterdam: IOS Press, 1998:207–236.
30. Chokroverty S, Jankovic J. Restless legs syndrome: a disease in search of identity. *Neurology* 1999;52:907–910.
31. Dressler D, Thompson PD, Gledhill RF, et al. The syndrome of painful legs and moving toes. *Mov Disord* 1994;9:13–21.
32. Wang A, Jankovic J. Hemifacial spasm: clinical correlates and treatments. *Muscle Nerve* 1998;21:1740–1747.
33. Tan EK, Jankovic J. Bilateral hemifacial spasm: a report of 5 cases and a literature review. *Mov Disord* 1999;14:345–349.
34. Krauss JK, Jankovic J. Posttraumatic movement disorders: head injury and peripheral trauma. 2001 (in press).
35. Anouti A, Koller WC. Diagnostic testing in movement disorders. *Neurol Clin* 1996;14:169–182.
36. De Rijk MC, Tzourio C, Breteler MMB, et al. Prevalence of parkinsonism and Parkinson's disease in Europe: the EUROPARKINSON collaborative study. *J Neurol Neurosurg Psychiatry* 1997;62:10–15.
37. Moghal S, Rajput AH, D'Arcy C, et al. Prevalence of movement disorders in elderly community residents. *Neuropeidemiology* 1994;13:175–178.
38. Bennett DA, Beckett LA, Murray AM, et al. Prevalence of parkinsonian signs and associated mortality in a community population of older people. *N Engl J Med* 1996;334:71–76.
39. Louis ED, Marder K, Cote L, et al. Prevalence of a history of shaking in persons 65 years of age and older: diagnostic and functional correlates. *Mov Disord* 1996;11:63–69.
40. Bower JH, Maraganore D, McDoneel SK, et al. Incidence and distribution of parkinsonism in Olmsted County, Minnesota, 1976–1990. *Neurology* 1999;52:1214–1220.
41. Tanner CM, Goldman SM. Epidemiology of Parkinson's disease. *Neurol Clin* 1996;14:317–336.
42. Kuopio AM, Marttila RJ, Helenius H, et al. Changing epidemiology of Parkinson's disease in southwestern Finland. *Neurology* 1999;52:302–308.
43. Lerner MR, Goldman RS. Skin colour, MPTP and Parkinson's disease. *Lancet* 1987;1:212.

44. D'Amato RJ, Alexander GM, Schwartzman RJ, et al. Evidence for neuromelanin involvement in MPTP-induced neurotoxicity. *Nature* 1987;327:324–327.

45. Schoenberg BS, Anderson DW, Haerer AF. Prevalence of Parkinson's disease in the biracial population of Copiah County, Mississippi. *Neurology* 1985;35:841–845.

46. Ben-Shlomo Y. How far are we in understanding the cause of Parkinson's disease? *J Neurol Neurosurg Psychiatry* 1996;61:4–16.

47. Gorell JM, Johnson CC, Rybicki BA, et al. The risk of Parkinson's disease with exposure to pesticides, farming, well water, and rural living. *Neurology* 1998;50:1346–1350.

48. Goldsmith JR, Herishanu Y, Abarbanel JM, et al. Clustering of Parkinson's disease points to environmental etiology. *Arch Environ Health* 1990;45:88–94.

49. Fleming L, Mann JB, Bean J, et al. Parkinson's disease and brain levels of organochlorine pesticides. *Ann Neurol* 1994;36:100–103.

50. Hanna P, Jankovic J, Kilkpatrick J. Multiple system atrophy: the putative causative role of environmental toxins. *Arch Neurol* 1999;56:90–94.

51. Morens DM, Grandinetti A, Reed D, et al. Cigarette smoking and protection from Parkinson's disease: false association or etiologic clue? *Neurology*? 1995;45:1041–1051.

52. Tzourio C, Rocca WA, Breteler MM, et al. Smoking and Parkinson's disease: an age-dependent risk effect. *Neurology* 1997;49:1267–1272.

53. Gorell JM, Rybicki BA, Johnson CC, et al. Smoking and Parkinson's disease: a dose-response relationship. *Neurology* 1999;52:115–119.

54. Gorell JM, Johnson CC, Rybicki BA. Parkinson's disease and its comorbid disorders: an analysis of Michigan mortality data, 1970 to 1990. *Neurology* 1994;44:1865–1868.

55. Clarke CE. Does levodopa therapy delay death in Parkinson's disease? A review of the evidence. *Mov Disord* 1995;10:250–256.

56. Louis ED, Marder K, Cote L, et al. Mortality from Parkinson disease. *Arch Neurol* 1997;54:260–264.

57. Parkinson Study Group. Mortality in DATATOP: a multicenter trial in early Parkinson's disease. *Ann Neurol* 1998;43:318–325.

58. Lilienfeld DE, Perl DP. Projected neurodegenerative disease mortality in the United States, 1990–1040. *Neuroepidemiology* 1993;12:219–228.

59. Louis ED, Ford B, Pullman S, et al. How normal is "normal"? Mild tremor in a multiethnic cohort of normal subjects. *Arch Neurol* 1998;55:222–227.

60. Rautakorpi I, Takala J, Martilla RJ, et al. Essential tremor in a Finnish population. *Acta Neurol Scand* 1982;66:58–67.

61. Elble RJ, Higgins C, Leffler K, et al. Factors influencing the amplitude and frequency of essential tremor. *Mov Disord* 1994;9:589–596.

62. Nutt JG, Muenter MD, Melton J, et al. Epidemiology of dystonia in Rochester, Minnesota. *Adv Neurol* 1988;50:361–365.

63. Zilber N, Korczyn AD, Kahana E, et al. Inheritance of idiopathic torsion dystonia among Jews. *J Med Genet* 1984;21:13–20.

64. Duffey P, Butler AG, Hawthorne MR, et al. The epidemiology of primary dystonia in the north of England. Dystonia. III. *Adv Neurol* 1998;78:121–125.

65. Costello EJ, Angold A, Burns BJ, et al. The Great Smoky Mountains study of youth: goals, design, methods, and the prevalence of DSM-III-R disorders. *Arch Gen Psychiatry* 1996;53:1129–1136.

66. Comings DE, Himes JA, Comings BG. An epidemiologic study of Tourette's syndrome in a single school district. *J Clin Psychiatry* 1990;51:463–469.

67. Caine ED, McBride MC, Chiverton P, et al. Tourette's syndrome in Monroe County school children. *Neurology* 1988;38:472–475.

68. Singer HS. Neurobiological issues in Tourette syndrome. *Brain Dev* 1994;16:353–364.

69. Kurlan R, Behr J, Medved L, et al. Severity of Tourette's syndrome in one large kindred: implication for determination of disease prevalence rate. *Arch Neurol* 1987;44:268–269.

70. Hanna PA, Janjua FN, Contant CF, et al. Bilineal transmission in Tourette syndrome. *Neurology* 1999;53:813–818.

71. Mason A, Banerjee S, Zeitlin H, et al. The prevalence of Tourette syndrome in a mainstream school population. *Dev Med Child Neurol* 1998;40:292–296.

72. Jankovic J. Treatment of parkinsonian syndromes. In: Kurlan R, ed. *Treatment of movement disorders.* Philadelphia: JB Lippincott, 1995:95–114.

73. Fahn S, Marsden CD, Van Woert MH. Definition and classification of myoclonus. *Adv Neurol* 1986;43:1–5.

74. Jankovic J. Tardive syndromes and other drug-induced movement disorders. *Clin Neuropharmacol* 1995;18:197–214.

Surgery for Parkinson's Disease and Movement Disorders, edited by J.K. Krauss, J. Jankovic, and R.G. Grossman. Lippincott Williams & Wilkins, Philadelphia © 2001.

2

MORPHOLOGY, NOMENCLATURE, AND CONNECTIONS OF THE THALAMUS AND BASAL GANGLIA[1]

EDWARD G. JONES

Several studies of the thalamus and basal ganglia have sought to provide an anatomic substrate for understanding cerebral disturbances leading to involuntary movements and dystonia and for planning neurosurgical interventions aimed at alleviating them. Most of these studies either focus on the thalamus alone or give intimate details of the organization of the basal ganglia that end at the thalamus, largely because of a lack of a corresponding high level of resolution. The present overview, although thalamocentric in its perspective, attempts to set the thalamus more firmly in the context of the circuitry of the basal ganglia than has hitherto been done. The basic premise underlying this account is that a close correspondence exists between the functional divisions of the thalamus and basal ganglia both in humans and in experimental primates, from which most knowledge of anatomic connections and physiologic properties of thalamic cells derives. In the thalamus in particular, transfer of knowledge derived from experimental studies in nonhuman primates to the understanding of human brain organization and function has been hampered by the lack of a common system of nomenclature. The first part of this account therefore deals with nomenclatural issues in the context of the descriptive anatomy of the thalamus of the two species. Later parts deal with the structure and connections of the basal ganglia and how the latter relate to the thalamus. For complete bibliographies dealing with the topics covered, the reader is referred to Parent and Hazrati (1,2), Percheron et al. (3), Macchi and Jones (4), and Jones (5).

NOMENCLATURE AND DIVISIONS OF MONKEY AND HUMAN THALAMI

To understand the pathophysiology of thalamic involvement in movement disorders, to interpret the effects of surgical interventions designed to alleviate them, and to guide stimulating and lesioning devices to their targets under anatomic

and physiologic control, it would obviously be desirable to use a nomenclature that readily permits transfer of information from the experimental primate to man. This has not been easy, for several reasons.

The human thalamus, the largest of the primate thalami, exceeds in size that of the larger apes by at least twice and that of the macaque monkeys by at least five times (5). The larger size is accompanied by greater contrasts in the sizes and packing densities of cells that make up the constituent nuclei of the thalamus, and this leads to greater ease in identifying microscopically the borders between nuclei. Although this feature helps greatly in making correlations or drawing homologies between monkeys, from which experimental anatomic and physiologic data are derived, and the human, it can also present difficulties. In some cases, borders that are clear in the human thalamus are less well defined between corresponding nuclei in the monkey, a factor leading to errors or controversy in assigning homologies. The difficulty in making cross-species correlations is compounded by the finding that variations in cytoarchitecture, myeloarchitecture, or chemoarchitecture that may be minor or even nonexistent in monkeys can be elaborated in the human and thus can invite designation as separate nuclei. The invitation is not one that has been routinely declined by neuroanatomists. The confusion generated by the propensity to divide the human thalamus into more and more nuclei has been further compounded by the use of a nomenclature that is fundamentally different from that customarily used in experimental animals and that has different historical roots. Although some attempts have been made to rationalize usage by introducing a common terminology, these have met with mixed reception and, if accepted at all, have been very slow in entering the vocabularies of most neurosurgeons and neurologists.

Historical Overview

Monkey

The description of the macaque monkey thalamus that probably had most impact historically was that of A. Earl Walker

E.G. Jones: Center for Neuroscience, University of California, Davis, California 95616.

[1] For abbreviations used in this chapter see page xiv.

(6). Walker, in dividing up the ventral nuclear mass of the monkey thalamus into five primary nuclei largely followed an earlier description of Aronson and Papez and, like these predecessors, adopted the nomenclature of what he called the Michigan School of Neuroanatomy. In order, from anterior to posterior, the ventral nuclear group was divided into five nuclei, termed ventralis anterior (VA), ventralis lateralis (VL), ventralis intermedius (VIM), and ventralis posterior (VP), the latter divided into lateral (VPL) and medial (VPM) subnuclei. VIM, intercalated between VL and VP, was originally regarded by Walker as part of VP. Walker's fifth nucleus, his ventralis medialis (MV), lying adjacent to the midline anteriorly, was regarded by him as part of the medial group of nuclei. It is now commonly considered a component of the ventral group and designated by the abbreviation VM.

Later descriptions of the monkey thalamus adopted the parcellation of Walker but often made additional subdivisions of the five basic nuclei of the ventral complex (Table 2.1). In the description of Jerzy Olszewski (7), in which some of the nomenclature owes its origins to the Berlin School of Brain Research, VA was shown to consist of a principal or parvocellular nucleus (VA) and a magnocellular subnucleus (VAmc). VL was identified as a very large nuclear complex that incorporated some of Walker's separate nuclei and further subdivided some of them. VM became a medial subnucleus (VLm) of this large ventral lateral nucleus (VL). The remainder of VL was divided into an anterior or oral subnucleus (pars oralis, VLo), an anteromedial subnucleus (area X), a dorsally placed, caudal subnucleus (pars caudalis, VLc), and an extreme posterodorsal subnucleus (pars postrema, VLps, originally identified by Walker as the pars angularis of the lateral posterior nucleus). Walker's VIM, identifiable by its very large cells, was excluded from the VL complex and was called the oral ventral posterior lateral nucleus (VPLo). Olszewski thus followed Walker in making VIM/VPLo part of the VP nucleus. His reasons for doing so are made clear in his text in which he says (erroneously) that it projected like the rest of VP to the postcentral gyrus, a statement implying that VPLo was part of the somatosensory pathways, although he recognized that its cells had close similarities to those of area X and VLc.

Human

Parcellation of the human thalamus is mainly founded on the description of Hassler (8), which was reproduced by Dewulf (9), Van Buren and Borke (10), and others, as well as appearing in a simpler version in a reclassification by Ohye (11). Hassler's subdivisions, superficially, can appear strikingly different from those of Walker, Olszewski, or others in monkeys (Figs. 2.1 and 2.2). This is the result of two major factors: first, the nomenclature, which derives entirely from the Berlin School, is fundamentally different from that applied to experimental animals, and, second, the nuclei have

many finer subdivisions, giving the impression of a much more complex structure. This nomenclature also suffers from the problem that many of the subdivisions were made in relation to contemporary knowledge of fiber connections that became outdated as the result of studies with modern fiber tracing techniques.

Hassler's subdivision of the human ventral nuclei is as follows: From anterior to posterior there are four primary nuclear divisions, called, in turn, lateropolaris (L.po), ventrooralis (V.o), ventrointermedius (V.im), and ventrocaudalis (V.c). An experienced eye can tell immediately that these are the equivalents of Walker's VA, VL, VIM, and VP of the monkey. Walker's VM is subsumed in Hassler's V.o (see later). However, where Hassler's parcellation becomes complicated is in the subdivisions of each of these major nuclear divisions and in his labeling of transitions between subdivisions as separate nuclei. Later, I attempt to demonstrate that some of Hassler's subdivisions more correctly belong to a different major nucleus.

Description of the Macaque Monkey Ventral Thalamic Nuclei

The anterior pole of the thalamus, immediately posterior to the encircling reticular nucleus, is dominated by the ventral anterior nucleus (VA) (Fig. 2.1). This characteristically consists of medium sized, pale-staining cells that are widely separated from one another, and thus the whole nucleus has a pale, "open" appearance. Medially, VA merges at the midline with the medioventral (reuniens) nucleus (MV), and posteroventrally it merges with the ventral medial (VM) nucleus. The cellular distinctions among these nuclei are not particularly clear, and the exact borders between them are correspondingly difficult to define, a situation leading to disagreement about the locations of the borders. As VA comes to surround the mamillothalamic tract, its cells become large, deeply staining, and more closely packed. This part of VA is customarily referred to therefore as the magnocellular ventral anterior nucleus (VAmc). It is probably more correctly regarded as part of the anterior intralaminar group of nuclei (12). The remainder of VA can be called the principal ventral anterior (VA) nucleus. On moving posteriorly from VA into the VL region, it is evident that the whole ventral lateral complex is especially large in monkeys, a feature that is also characteristic of the human thalamus. Throughout the whole region, nuclear parcellation is very distinct because cell sizes and packing densities differ radically from nucleus to nucleus. In the part of the large VL region lying immediately posterior to VA, cells become smaller and packing density greatly is increased, with clouds and clusters of closely packed, densely-stained neurons that distinguish the ventral lateral anterior nucleus (VLa). For a short distance, this nucleus occupies the full cross-sectional extent of the lateral mass of the thalamus. A little more posteriorly, VLa is displaced laterally by the anteromedial pole of the ventral

TABLE 2.1. COMPARISON OF THE NOMENCLATURES USED BY VARIOUS AUTHORS FOR THE HUMAN AND MACAQUE VENTRAL THALAMIC NUCLEI

Monkeys				Monkeys & Humans	Humans				
Walker (6)	Olszewski (7)	Ilinsky and Kultas-Ilinsky (15)	Percheron et al. (3)	Hirai and Jones (13)	Hassler (8)	Dewulf (9)	Van Buren and Borke (10)	Walker (105)	Ohye (11)
VA	VA	VApc	LRpo LO	**VA**	Dorso-oralis (D.o) internus (D.o.i) externus (D.o.e) Lateropolaris (L.po)	v.a	Lpo	Lpo	Lpo
Vamc	VAmc	VAmc	LRmc	**VAmc**	Latero-polaris magno-cellularis (L.po.mc)	v.o.m.(a)	Lpo(mc)		
VM	VLm	VM	LRvm	**VM**	Ventro-oralis medialis (V.o.m)				
VL	VLo	VAdc	LO	**VLa**	Ventro-oralis anterior (V.o.a)	v.o.a. + d.a.(p)	Voe(a)	Vo	Voe(a)
					Ventro-oralis posterior (V.o.p)	v.o.p.	Voe(p)		Voe(p)
VL	Area X	VL	LIM	**VLp (anteromedial part)**	Ventro-oralis internus (V.o.i)	v.o.m.(p)	Voi	Vo	Voi
VL	VLc	VL	LI	**VLp (dorsal part)**	Dorso-intermedius externus (D.im.e) Dorso-intermedius internus (D.im.i) Dorso-intermedius superior (D.im.s)	d.a.(p)	Do	Vo	
Lppa	VLps	VL	LOd	**VLp (posterodorsal part)**	Dorso-intermedius externus magno-cellularis (D.im.e.mc)				
VIM	VPLo	VL	LI/LIL	**VLp (ventral part)**	Ventro-intermedius internus (V.im.i) Ventro-intermedius externus (V.im.e) Zentro-lateralis intermedius internus (Z.im.i) Zentro-lateralis intermedius externus (Z.im.e)	V.im.	Vimi Vime	VIM	Vim
VPL	VPLc	VPL	LCL	**VPLa** **VPLp**	Zentro-lateralis caudalis internus (Z.c.i) Zentro-lateralis caudalis externus (Z.c.e) Ventro-caudalis anterior externus (V.c.a.e) Ventro-caudalis posterior externus (V.c.p.e)	v.p.l.	Vce	Vce	Vce

LCL, LI, LIL, LIM, LO, LOd, Lppa, LRmc, LRpo, LRvm, VA, ventral anterior nucleus; VAdc, Vamc and VAmc, magnocellular division of ventral anterior nucleus; VApc, ; VL, ventral lateral nucleus; VLa, anterior ventral lateral nucleus; VLc, pars caudalis of ventral lateral nucleus; VLo, pars oralis of ventral lateral nucleus; VLp, posterior ventral lateral nucleus; VLps, pars postrema of ventral lateral nucleus; VM, ventral medial nucleus; VPL, ventral posterior lateral nucleus; VPLa, anterior ventral posterior lateral nucleus; VPLo, oral ventral posterior lateral nucleus; VPLp, posterior ventral lateral posterior nucleus.

From Jones EG. The thalamus of primates. In: Bloom FE, Björklund A, Hökfelt T, eds. *Handbook of chemical neuroanatomy,* vol 14: *The primate nervous system: part II.* Amsterdam: Elsevier, 1998:1–298, with permission.

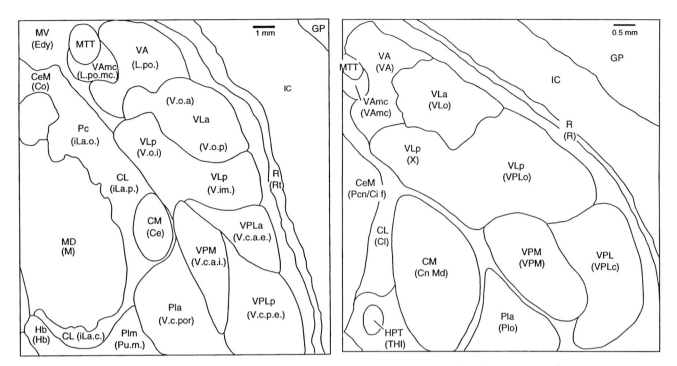

FIGURE 2.1. Camera lucida tracings of horizontal sections of human **(left)** and macaque monkey **(right)** thalami at comparable levels, showing the nuclei of the ventral complex and adjoining regions. Abbreviations indicating the names of the nuclei are the same in each case (13). Abbreviations in parentheses are those of Hassler (8) for the human and of Olszewski (7) for the monkey. (From Jones EG. The thalamus of primates. In: Bloom FE, Björklund A, Hökfelt T, eds. *Handbook of chemical neuroanatomy,* vol 14: *The primate nervous system: part II.* Amsterdam: Elsevier, 1998:1–298, with permission.)

lateral posterior nucleus (VLp), which for a short distance is interposed between VLa and the internal medullary lamina. At the border between VLa and VLp, islands and fingers of densely packed small cells characteristic of VLa interdigitate with extensions of VLp that are clearly recognizable by their larger and more widely dispersed cells. VLp is characterized by these large, deeply staining cells—among the largest in the thalamus—that are widely separated from one another. VLp, followed posteriorly, expands to occupy the full dorsoventral and mediolateral extent of the lateral mass. In sagittal sections, it is sickle-shaped, with a narrow ventral apex and a curved dorsal border expanding anteriorly over VLa and posteriorly over the ventral posterior (VP) nuclei. Cells located in the ventral part of VLp are larger than those in the dorsal part, and this accounts for Olszewski's division of the nucleus into ventral (VPLo) and dorsal (VLc) nuclei. In the human, this practice was also adopted by Hassler (see later). Posterior to VLp is the VP nucleus. It occupies the ventral half of the lateral nuclear mass, narrowing medially to form a tongue lying ventral to the centromedian nucleus (CM) and posteriorly to a pole located dorsal to the medial geniculate complex. Many of its cells are as large as those of VLp, but there are many interspersed smaller cells as well, so the nucleus appears more densely populated than the cell sparse VLp. VP is a complex of two nuclei, the VP lateral

(VPL) and VP medial (VPM) nuclei, separated by a fiber lamina that extends around the circumference of VPM, isolating the nucleus not only from VPL but also from nuclei that lie medial and posterior to it. The cells in VPM are compacted into lobules in frontal sections, although the lobules are really cross sections of elongated rods extending anteroposteriorly through the nucleus. The ventromedial aspect of VPM is separated by a further fiber lamina to form a separate nucleus made up of closely packed smaller cells, traditionally referred to as the parvocellular division of VPM. In recent years, it has come to be called the basal ventral medial nucleus (VMb). Cytologically, VPL consists of a thin anterodorsal shell dominated by large cells and a larger core in which the cell population is more evenly mixed. These divisions may be clearer in some species of monkeys than in others, perhaps warranting their designation as separate subnuclei. They are very much clearer in the human thalamus (13).

The ventral posterior inferior (VIP) nucleus is another subsidiary nucleus intercalated between the ventral aspects of VPM and VPL and the ventral part of the external medullary lamina. It is the region through which most of the fibers of the medial lemniscus enter the thalamus and thus is dominated by neuroglial cells, but it contains numerous small neurons as well.

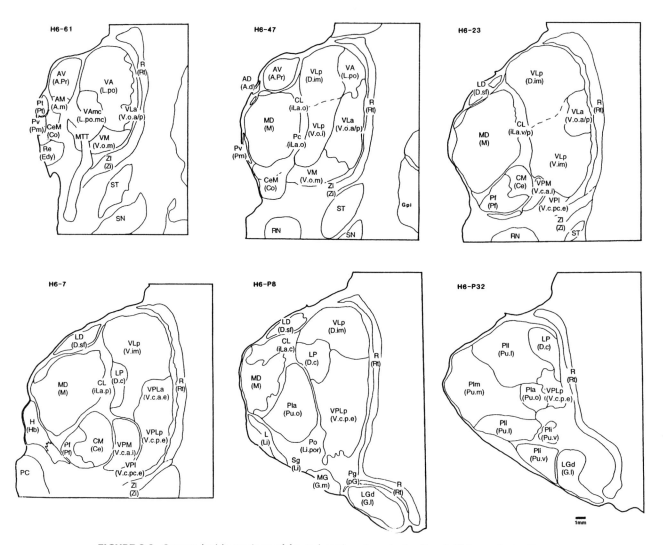

FIGURE 2.2. Camera lucida tracings of frontal sections in anterior **(top left)** to posterior **(lower right)** order, through a human thalamus giving the names of the nuclei (13) and *(in parentheses)* those used by Hassler (8). (From Jones EG. The thalamus of primates. In: Bloom FE, Björklund A, Hökfelt T, eds. *Handbook of chemical neuroanatomy,* vol 14: *The primate nervous system: part II.* Amsterdam: Elsevier, 1998:1–298, with permission.)

Description of the Human Ventral Thalamic Nuclei

The divisions of the lateral nuclear group in the human thalamus closely resemble those of the monkey in relative disposition and cytoarchitecture (Figs. 2.1 and 2.2). Differences are mainly those of size and the distinctness of the borders among nuclei. Clearly defined ventral anterior (VA), ventral medial (VM), ventral lateral anterior (VLa), ventral lateral posterior (VLp), and ventral posterior (VP) nuclei are visible, all with cytologic characteristics similar to those of monkeys. More considerable differences in cell size, in fact, make the borders between the nuclei even more distinct than in the monkey. The interdigitation of small and large celled zones characteristic of the border between VLa and VLp occurs over a greater distance than in monkeys and is very distinct. The division of the VLp nucleus into dorsal and ventral sub-

nuclei, the ventral containing unusually large cells, is also clearly evident. There is a much clearer division of the VPL nucleus into an anterodorsal (VPLa) subnucleus dominated by cells only a little smaller than those of VLp, and a posteroventral (VPLp) subnucleus with a mixed population of large and smaller cells. These two subnuclei represent divisions that are only incipiently visible in monkeys (see earlier). The VMb and VPI nuclei are as distinct as in monkeys.

Chemical Anatomy of the Ventral Nuclei in Monkey and Human Thalami

Histochemical staining for the enzyme acetylcholinesterase is extremely effective in delineating the thalamic nuclei of primates (5,13) (Fig. 2.3). Each nucleus has its own particular histochemical signature, based on the intensity and other

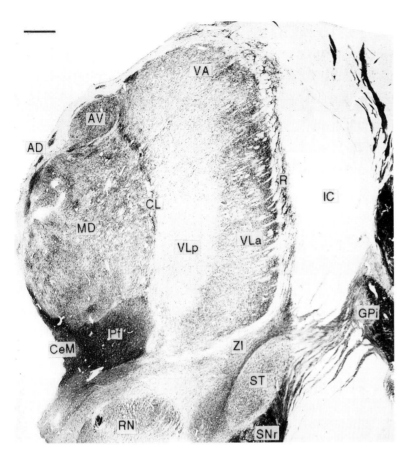

FIGURE 2.3. Photomicrograph of a frontal section through the thalamus of a human stained for acetylcholinesterase and showing the different densities of staining in the three anterior nuclei of the ventral complex (bar = 2 mm).

characteristics of staining. Differences in staining density are often very well defined at nuclear borders, and they can provide a better indication of the location of a border than Nissl or myelin staining alone. In some instances, the staining pattern affirms borders suggested by connection tracing or by physiologic investigation but only indistinctly visible with conventional stains.

Most of the nuclei of the ventral complex can be readily distinguished by different densities of acetylcholinesterase staining in both the human and monkey thalamus. The VA nucleus is characterized by light-to-moderate, clumped staining perforated by bundles of unstained axons. The principal VM nucleus is more homogeneously stained for acetylcholinesterase and extends, tonguelike ventromedial to the VA nucleus, under the internal medullary lamina and toward the mamillothalamic tract. The VAmc surrounding the mamillothalamic tract in this region is the most densely stained.

As VA is traced posteriorly, its clumped acetylcholinesterase staining is replaced by two, radically different zones of staining. A medial zone located adjacent to the internal medullary lamina, extending to the dorsal surface of the thalamus and corresponding to the VLp, is distinguished by very weak acetylcholinesterase staining. A lateral zone corresponding at this level to the VLa is much more heavily stained. As VLp expands posteriorly and replaces VLa, it re-

tains its weak acetylcholinesterase staining. The division of the nucleus into dorsal and ventral subnuclei on the basis of cell size is not distinguishable by histochemical staining.

Further posteriorly, staining becomes denser in the VPM and VPL nuclei. There is no evidence of variations in the density of staining corresponding to the division of the VPL nucleus into VPLa and VPLp subnuclei. The VMb nucleus and the VPI nucleus lying along the external medullary lamina are distinguished by very weak acetylcholinesterase staining.

Nomenclature Concepts of the Human Thalamus

The most commonly used names for the nuclei of the human thalamus derive from the work of Rolf Hassler (8). He divided the ventral nuclear mass into polar (anterior), dorsal, and ventral groups of nuclei. His separation of dorsal and ventral nuclei is one source of confusion in attempting to make correlations of names across species because many of the dorsal nuclei are parts of nuclei recognized in monkeys as ventral nuclei. Hassler further subdivided many of the nuclei he identified into "oral" (anterior), "caudal" (posterior), "internal" (medial), "external" (lateral) and "intermediate" subnuclei, which were sometimes further subdivided. These divisions of divisions commonly led to coupling of the terms *anterior* and *oral, posterior* and *caudal,* or *dorsal* and *superior* in the name of a single nucleus (e.g., *nucleus ventralis caudalis posterior externus*). Where Hassler identified transitions between major nuclear divisions, he called these transitions "zentro" nuclei. The resulting list of lengthy names has little or no relationship with the list of names customarily used in experimental primates It is not only confusing but also tends to impede translation of the results of anatomic and physiologic studies on experimental primates to the understanding and interpretation of interventions in the human thalamus.

Table 2.1 and Figs. 2.1 and 2.2 compare the names applied to the nuclei of the human and monkey thalami. They show that it is possible to rationalize Hassler's nomenclature for the human with that used in other primates and demonstrate that it is relatively easy to apply the more widely used monkey terms to the human thalamic nuclei.

Correlation of Monkey and Human Thalamic Nuclei Given Different Names by Different Investigators

Ventral Anterior Nucleus (VA)

The equivalence of VA across all primate species is controversial because its borders with the more posterior VLa are not clearly defined in Nissl and myelin preparations. However, the chemoarchitecture makes a clear distinction between VA and VLa. Apart from being filled with dispersed, lightly stained, medium-sized cells, VA shows light-to-moderate acetylcholinesterase staining. VLa, by contrast, is characterized by small, densely stained, and closely packed neurons grouped in islands and clouds separated by cell-sparse regions, and it is heavily stained for acetylcholinesterase activity. On these bases, VA corresponds to Hassler's L.po, and VLa corresponds to Hassler's V.o.a and V.o.p together. Later, I consider why Hassler divided VLa (V.o) into anterior and posterior subnuclei.

VAmc of monkeys has an unequivocal and easily recognized architecture, with large, densely staining cells and dense acetylcholinesterase activity. It obviously corresponds to the human nucleus called lateropolaris magnocellularis (L.po.mc) by Hassler.

Ventral Medial Nucleus (VM)

VM (VLm of Olszewski) is recognized by all authors, although its architecture does not differ greatly from that of VA, and not all agree on its exact borders. Parts of it appear to be included in VA of some authors. Its cytoarchitecture and chemoarchitecture are essentially the same as V.o.m of Hassler in humans.

Anterior Ventral Lateral Nucleus (VLa)

VLa of monkeys can be equated on topographic, cytologic, and histochemical grounds with the nucleus ventrooralis anterior (V.o.a) of Hassler. The region identified as V.o.p by Hassler is clearly the region in which islands and fingers of cells proper to VLa (V.o.a) and VLp (V.im) interdigitate. It is not a transitional zone of architecture but truly a region in which the border is "wavy." Hirai and Jones could see no distinction in the region of interdigitation between VLa and VLp, other than that which could be accounted for by the chemoarchitectonic characteristics of the two interdigitating nuclei. Hence V.o.p has no standing as an independent nucleus, and an equivalent name in monkey and human is not needed.

Posterior Ventral Lateral Nucleus (VLp)

VLp is the largest of the ventral nuclei in monkeys and humans (Fig. 2.4). Although containing subnuclear regions of different cell size, these nuclei are linked together by three features: the presence of large cells separated by extensive areas of neuropil (indicative of extensive dendritic ramifications), weak acetylcholinesterase staining, and the finding that all receive the terminations of cerebellothalamic fibers (3,14). All components of VLp can be distinguished from VLa on cytoarchitectonic and chemoarchitectonic grounds.

In monkeys, VLp is represented anteromedially by an extension caught between the internal medullary lamina and the VLa nucleus and called area X by Olszewski. This extension is best appreciated in horizontal sections. In all views, it has the same cytologic appearance and relationship with adjacent nuclei in monkeys and humans. In the latter, it was called nucleus ventrooralis internus (V.o.i) by Hassler. The ventral part of VLp is characterized by extremely large cells, and in the monkey it was called VPLo by Olszewski and VIM by Walker. From cell size alone, it corresponds mainly to Hassler's nucleus ventrointermedius (V.im), which he divided into internal (V.im.i) and external (V.im.e) parts, mainly on the basis of differences in cell size. These may be meaningful in terms of the body topography predicted in VLp (see later).

The dorsal part of VLp in which cells, although still large, are smaller than in the ventral part was called VLc by Olszewski. It is identical in cell structure and position to the nucleus dorsointermedius (D.im) of Hassler in the human, although he divided it into several parts (see later). Where it expands posteriorly over the dorsal surface of the VP nuclei and narrows to a small tail caught dorsolaterally among the external capsule, lateral posterior nucleus, and anterior surface of the medial pulvinar nucleus, it was called VLps by Olszewski and pars angularis of LP by Walker in monkeys. In the human, it can be identified from its location as the nucleus dorsointermedius externus magnocellularis (D.im.e.mc) of Hassler.

The confusing terminology used for the large cerebellar target nucleus (Table 2.1) stems from the finding that each of its cytoarchitectonic components have been given separate names (area X, VLc, VPLo, VLps) in monkeys and because

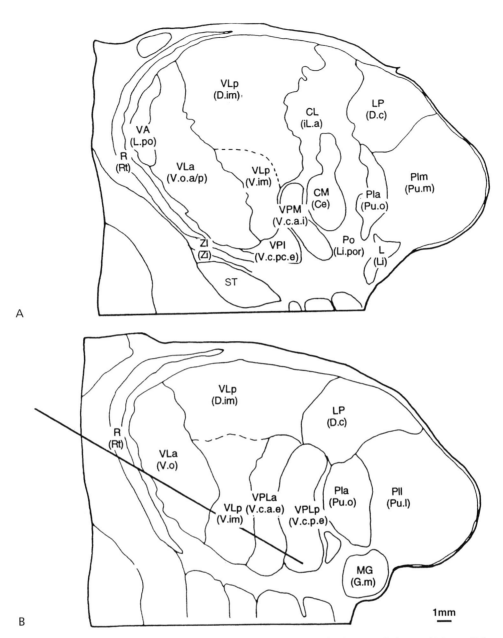

FIGURE 2.4. Camera lucida tracings of parasagittal sections of a human thalamus (**A** is medial to **B**) identifying the nuclei of the ventral complex (13), with the original names of Hassler (8) in parentheses. The *line* on **B** indicates the trajectory of an electrode penetration, as it has been used in stereotactic approaches to the human thalamus and the nuclei that it traverses en route to the somatosensory relay nucleus (VPL). (From Jones EG. The thalamus of primates. In: Bloom FE, Björklund A, Hörkfelt T, eds. *Handbook of chemical neuroanatomy*, vol 14: *The primate nervous system: part II.* Amsterdam: Elsevier, 1998:1–298, with permission.)

the equivalent subnuclei have been relegated to different nuclear groups in both humans and monkeys.

Although Hassler recognized a large number of subnuclei among the ventral nuclei of the human thalamus and gave them lengthy and complex names, it is clear from the foregoing that his basic subdivisions are essentially the same as those made later on cytologic and histochemical grounds by Hirai and Jones. The excessive number of finer nuclear subdivisions made by Hassler can be attributed

to his identification of regions of different cell size or packing density within a nucleus or to transitions among nuclei. Some of these subnuclei are recognizable even in the monkey, for example, the divisions of VLp based on cell size and called D.im and V.im in the human by Hassler, are the same as those called VLc and VPLo in the monkey by Olszewski (7).

Transition zones among nuclei, which Hassler recognized as separate nuclei, can also be seen, for example, in the interdigitation of cells of VLa and VLp, the region that Hassler called V.o.p. Other regions that Hassler identified as regions of cytoarchitectural transition and called "zentro" nuclei include the nucleus zentrolateralis intermedius (Z.im), which is obviously the region of transition between the two differently sized cell populations of VLp mentioned in the preceding paragraph. Many other divisions of the VA (L.po), VLa (V.o.a/p), and VP (V.c) nuclei were made on the same grounds by Hassler. They are listed in Table 2.1. Unless justified by fiber connections, they were eliminated when the major nuclei were renamed by Hirai and Jones.

Ventral Posterior Nucleus (VP)

Immediately posterior to the zone of very large cells that form the ventral part of the VLp nucleus (Olszewski's VPLo and Hassler's V.im) in both monkeys and humans is a region of mixed, very large and smaller cells in which acetylcholinesterase staining is more dense than in VLp. This region is relatively large in humans and was called subnucleus VPLa by Hirai and Jones (13) and the nucleus ventrocaudalis anterior externus (V.c.a.e) by Hassler. A smaller zone with identical cellular characteristics can be recognized in monkeys, in which it forms the proprioceptive shell of the ventral posterior lateral nucleus (see later), but it is insufficiently well defined in monkeys to warrant naming as a separate nucleus. Posterior to VPLa, the cell population becomes more evenly mixed, the large cells outnumbered by small and medium-sized cells, but the moderate density of acetylcholinesterase staining is maintained. These characteristics define the VPLp nucleus of Hirai and Jones, and the cytoarchitecture corresponds to the nucleus ventrocaudalis posterior externus (V.c.p.e) of Hassler. The nucleus called zentrolateralis caudalis (Z.c) by Hassler that extends posteriorly from VPLa (V.c.a.e) over the dorsal surface of the VPL nucleus probably represents the dorsal extension of the proprioceptive shell observed physiologically but not definable anatomically in monkeys. Medial to VPLp is the clearly circumscribed VPM nucleus with tightly packed, medium-sized cells that make it identical to Hassler's nucleus ventrocaudalis anterior internus (V.c.a.i).

More posteriorly, the subsidiary nuclei of the VP complex, VMb, and VPI are the same as Hassler's nucleus ventrocaudalis parvocellularis internus (V.c.pc.i) and nucleus ventrocaudalis parvocellularis externus (V.c.pc.e), respectively.

Divisions of Ventral Thalamic Nuclei Confirmed by Connection Tracing and by Physiologic Properties

Nuclei of Termination of Afferent Fiber Systems

A schematic horizontal section with the major inputs is shown in Fig. 2.5.

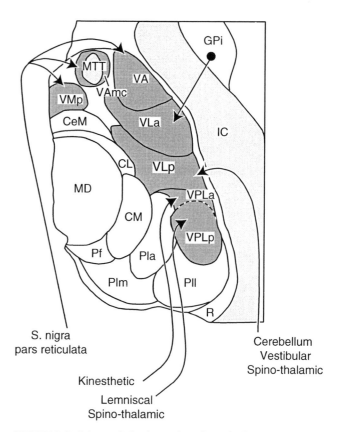

FIGURE 2.5. Schematic horizontal section of a human thalamus with the major inputs to the ventral nuclei indicated by *arrows*. (From Macchi G, Jones EG. Towards an agreement on terminology of nuclear and subnuclear divisions of the motor thalamus. *J Neurosurg* 1997;86:670–685, with permission.)

Terminations of the Projection from the Substantia Nigra

In monkeys, VA, VAmc, and VM are clearly the target of nigral afferents, but investigators disagree about whether all of VA receives nigral fiber terminations or whether some part of it receives fibers from the globus pallidus (3,15,16). This disagreement probably reflects the difficulty authors have in distinguishing the border between VA and VLa.

Terminations of the Projection from the Globus Pallidus

In monkeys, these terminations are largely coextensive with the VLa nucleus, although extensions into VA or VLp have been described (17–21). These appear to be relatively minor and may reflect the difficulty of drawing a border between VA and VLa anteriorly and the interdigitation of islands of cells of VLa and VLp posteriorly. In monkeys, it is now clearly recognized that a topography exists in the pallidothalamic projection (see later) such that ventrolateral parts of the internal segment of the globus pallidus (largely the recipient area for fibers from the putamen, and especially from its large sensorimotor representation) send fibers mainly through the ansa lenticularis to terminate posteriorly in VLa, whereas dorsomedial parts of the internal segment (largely the recipient area for fibers from the caudate nucleus and thus indirectly from the association areas of the cerebral cortex) send fibers mainly through the lenticular fasciculus to terminate more anteriorly in VLa. It would be incorrect, however, to attribute the cytoarchitectonic differentiation of the human equivalent of VLa into anterior (Hassler's V.o.a) and posterior (Hassler's V.o.p) parts as indicative of this division, because V.o.p is a factitious construct.

Region of Projection of the Cerebellum

In the ventral nuclei of monkeys, VLp is the recipient of cerebellar projections (3,14). The three deep cerebellar nuclei project on all components of VLp, the dentate and interpositus contralaterally and the fastigial bilaterally. There is a topography, in that anterior parts of the deep cerebellar nuclei project to the posterolateral parts of VLp (equivalent to VPLo and VLc of Olszewski) and posterior parts project to anteromedial parts of VLp (equivalent to area X of Olszewski) and intervening parts in between. This appears to underlie a representation of body topography, based on the organization of the projections of the different components of VLp to the motor cortex. Thus, a representation of the trunk can be predicted in dorsal regions (VLc and VLps of Olszewski) , a representation of the hand and foot in ventral regions (VPLo of Olszewski), and of the face in anteromedial regions (area X of Olszewski). Evidence indicates a similar somatotopy from stereotactic interventions in this region in the human thalamus (22–24). The larger-celled, ventral and posterior parts of VLp are not only recipients of the deep cerebellar projection, but also they receive spinothalamic and vestibular projections close to the boundary of VPL (5). The inputs from the spinal cord may come specifically from proprioceptive cells in the ventral horn and intermediate zone.

Region of Termination of the Fibers of the Medial Lemniscus

In monkeys, this region is exactly coextensive with the VP nucleus, fibers from the contralateral gracile, and cuneate nuclei ending in somatotopic order in VPL, those from the contralateral principal trigeminal nucleus in the lateral two-thirds of VPM, and those from the ipsilateral principal trigeminal nucleus (which arrive by the dorsal ipsilateral trigeminal pathway) in the medial one-third (17,25–27). The body somatotopy is laid out accordingly and is similar in humans. Cells in the large central core of VPL, corresponding to VPLp in the human, respond specifically to light stimulation of the skin or subcutaneous tissues in a receptor-specific manner (Fig. 2.6). Nociceptive-specific cells can also be found in the core, but these tend to be more concentrated in regions posterior to VPL (28–32).

The anterodorsal large-celled shell of VPL (Hirai and Jones' VPLa and Hassler's V.c.e.a in humans) receives fibers from the dorsal column nuclei and is thus part of the somatosensory thalamus. Single-unit recording reveals that its cells are specifically responsive to stimulation of deep tissues (29), and especially to muscle spindle primary afferents (33),

so it is probably the preferential terminal site for lemniscal fibers arising from the group IA specific relays located at the anterior ends of the gracile and cuneate nuclei. The anterodorsal proprioceptive shell is excluded from the cerebellar relay zone and thus from VLp. It is a part of the lemniscal thalamic relay nucleus and cannot be considered part of VIM.

Divisions of the Ventral Nuclei Based on Physiologic Properties of Their Cells

Although in anesthetized monkeys the anterodorsal shell of VPL is exquisitely sensitive to vibratory stimuli and stimuli that stretch muscles (33–35), VLp, is remarkably silent, its cells showing little spontaneous activity and not responding to peripheral stimuli (25,33). The resolution between borders of the monkey equivalent of V.im (the ventral part of VLp) and the equivalent of VPLa (the proprioceptive shell of VPL) is thus very clear in anesthetized monkeys (24). By contrast, in unanesthetized monkeys, single-unit recordings, made at atlas coordinates corresponding to the ventral part of VLp (Olszewski's VPLo), isolated many cells that responded to passive movements of joints (36–38). In the absence of anesthesia, the neurons of VLp display high spontaneous firing rates, a finding probably reflecting the tonic excitatory input from the cerebellum, and most respond to passive manipulations of joints and muscles, as well as to perturbations imposed on an actively moving limb (37,38). Therefore, resolving the border between VLp and the proprioceptive shell of VPL is very difficult. The inputs from the periphery arrive at relatively short latency, which in the posteroventral, large-celled part of the VLp, may reflect inputs through the spinothalamic tract rather than the cerebellum. In the case of the awake human undergoing recording before stereotactic thalamotomy or placement of chronic stimulating electrodes, in the regions effective for elimination of tremor, many neurons respond to passive movements of joints and microstimulation can elicit sensations referred to deep tissues (39). Although responsivity of the VLp region may be modified in humans undergoing surgical procedures in relation to the neuronal disease that generates tremor or dystonia, resolution of the V.im/VPLa border at operation may not be possible unless more distinguishing features of the movement-related responses in the two (sub)nuclei can be established. This has not yet been examined in detail.

Despite their obvious proprioceptive receptive fields, neurons in VLp generally do not discharge in relation to active movements performed by a monkey. This distinguishes VLp from VLa, because recordings putatively made in VLa in unanesthetized monkeys show that the cells are unlike those in VLp in not usually responding to passive manipulations of muscles and joints, but instead preferentially discharging during active movements (38). Their spontaneous activity is low, a finding probably reflecting the tonic inhibitory input from the globus pallidus. Microstimulation of VLp but not of VLa elicits movements in anesthetized monkeys (40).

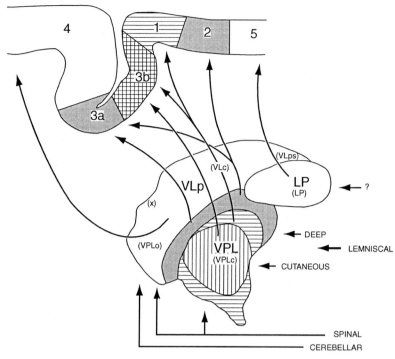

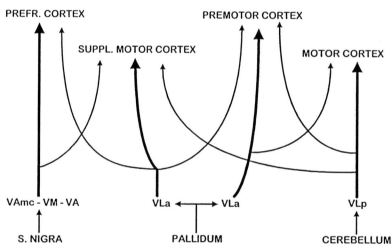

FIGURE 2.6. Cortical projections of the somatosensory **(upper)** and motor **(lower)** relay nuclei of the thalamus. In the **lower figure,** thick lines indicate the predominant and thinner lines subsidiary projections. Abbreviations in parentheses indicate nuclear names of Olszewski (7). **(Upper figure** modified from Jones EG, Friedman DP. Projection pattern of functional components of thalamic ventrobasal complex on monkey somatosensory cortex. *J Neurophysiol* 1982;48:521–544, with permission. **Lower figure** modified from Macchi G, Jones EG. Towards an agreement on terminology of nuclear and subnuclear divisions of the motor thalamus. *J Neurosurg* 1997;86:670–685, with permission.)

More posteriorly in the human thalamus, single-unit recording and microstimulation in regions provisionally identified by atlas coordinates as Hassler's V.c.a.e (VPLa), V.c.p.e (VPLp), and V.c.a.i (VPM) reveal neuronal responses to stimulation of localized peripheral receptive fields, or similarly localized peripheral paresthesias, which follow a somatotopic order according to the part of the nucleus stimulated. The somatotopic body map is thus similar to that in VPM and VPL of monkeys, but it remains uncertain whether this encompasses both VPLa and VPLp (22,23). Early single-unit and multiunit recording studies considered that a single somatosensory map extended without interruption from V.c.a.e and V.c.p.e (VPL) into V.im.e (lateral VLp) and from V.c.a.i (VPM) into V.im.i (medial VLp) (41), but this is unlikely to be correct. Others (22,42) identified an anterior region containing neurons responding to deep stimuli and thought to be V.im (ventral VLp) and an immediately posterior region in which neurons responded to cutaneous stimuli and thought to be within V.c.a.e, V.c.p.e, and V.c.a.i (VPLa, VPLp, and VPM). VPLa (V.c.a.e.) was not therefore identified as a region of deep somatosensory input. In some studies (23,24,30), deep responses were found in a region described as the anterodorsal part of V.c and thus probably equivalent to VPLa and to the anterodorsal shell of VPL of monkeys; cutaneous responses were encountered immediately posterior to this, in a region described as the core of V.c, and therefore probably equivalent to VPLp and to the central cutaneous core of VPL and VPM in monkeys. V.im (ventral VLp) was described as unresponsive to somatosensory stimulation. These results seem to be in line with those obtained by the higher-resolution mapping permitted in monkeys.

In the thalamic regions in which stereotactic lesions or chronic stimulations effectively eliminate tremor in humans (Fig. 2.4), many neurons respond to passive movement of joints, and microstimulation there can elicit sensations referred to deep tissues (11,29,31,32,43). In the eyes of many neurosurgeons, this area is synonymous with Hassler's V.im. The foregoing discussion suggests that it may just as well be VPLa or a combination of VPLa and ventral VLp (V.im). Both of these nuclei could show unusual or heightened neuronal responses in humans with tremor or dystonia on account of neuronal pathology (24,28,44). This could further compound the difficulty of distinguishing between them. The posterior part of the region identified as V.im is regarded by some neurosurgeons as the best target for relieving tremor regardless of its type (11,22,45). VPLa may therefore be the more effective lesion site. This is an issue that should be resolved.

More anteriorly, stereotactic lesions aimed at the V.o.p nucleus of Hassler (the region of interdigitation of VLa and VLp) are reported to be more effective than lesions aimed at V.im in reducing the rigidity, although not the tremor, of Parkinson's disease (46). These lesions primarily interfere with thalamic nuclei receiving pallidal inputs, whereas the more posterior, tremor-effective lesions are likely, as we have seen, to interfere with nuclei receiving proprioceptive or cerebellar inputs.

Divisions of the Thalamus Based on Output Connections

Lack of significant convergence in the terminations of the nigral, pallidal, cerebellar, and lemniscal terminations in the thalamus is now accepted by most workers, although there are holdouts. The nuclei of the ventral complex can thus be considered as relays for parallel motor and sensory channels to the cerebral cortex (Fig. 2.6). The degree of overlap in the projections of the nuclei to the cerebral cortex is still a matter for debate and contains elements of controversy, mainly engendered by a lack of clear-cut experimental results in connection tracing studies, lack of agreement about borders among functional areas of the cortex, and inability to delineate borders among thalamic nuclei. Current

evidence tends to support the view that the principal cortical projections of VA/VMp, VLa, VLp, and VPL/VPM are focused on different cortical areas that may be loosely defined as prefrontal, premotor, motor, and somatosensory, respectively, but the degree of overlap remains to be established definitively.

Cortical Projections of the Nigral and Pallidal Relay Nuclei

The evidence, as it stands, indicates that the nigral territory in the ventral nuclei, VA, VAmc, and VMp, projects diffusely and to an extensive region of the neocortex concentrated in the prefrontal areas, but probably extending into the premotor cortex, including the supplementary motor area, frontal eye field and supplementary eye field, as well as into the anterior cingulate gyrus and even into the posterior parietal cortex. The projections of VLa appear to be more focused and concentrated on the premotor and supplementary motor cortex, but they may extend substantially into the motor cortex, depending on how the border between these two is defined, but not into the prefrontal cortex (4,5).

Cortical Projections of the Cerebellar Relay Nucleus

The projection of the cerebellar territory in the ventral nuclei, VLp, is focused on area 4 with a mediolateral topography that implies a representation of the face in the part of VLp equivalent to Olszewski's area X, of the forelimb and hindlimb successively more laterally in VLp (Olszewski's VPLo), and of the trunk in dorsal VLp (Olszewski's VLc) (14,47), but additional projections have been described to premotor and supplementary motor areas and to posterior parietal areas. Many of the reported differences in the published studies probably depend on the manner in which the borders between cortical fields have been defined by the investigators, coupled with too great a reliance on thalamic atlases and a failure to recognize some of the subtleties in the boundaries between thalamic nuclei, for example, the interdigitation of the cells of VLa and VLp.

A further compounding variable is the presence of two populations of histochemically distinct cell types with different projections to the cerebral cortex distributed through the thalamic nuclei (5). In monkeys, cells expressing the calcium-binding protein, 28-kDa calbindin, are scattered diffusely through all nuclei and project diffusely to superficial layers of the cortex ignoring boundaries between cortical fields. A second population characterized by expression of parvalbumin and found in concentrated numbers only in the principal relay nuclei, including VLa, VLp, and VP, projects in topographic order to middle layers of specific cortical fields. Hence reports of more widespread projections of thalamic nuclei in some studies and not in others are likely to depend on the relative proportions of the two cell types labeled, determined, in turn, by the relative laminar location and extent of injections of tracer in the cortex.

Cortical Projections of the Somatosensory Relay Nuclei

Within the somatosensory relay, the VPL/VPM complex, parallel pathways to the cerebral cortex are also evident in the subdivision of VPL into an anterodorsal, proprioceptive shell and a cutaneous core, a division that is recognized by the parcellation of the human VPL into cytoarchitectonically distinct VPLa and VPLp subnuclei. In monkeys, the neurons of the anterodorsal shell (equivalent to VPLa) respond to inputs, including muscle spindle–specific inputs, from deep tissues and project to areas 3a and 2 of the postcentral gyrus. The neurons of the larger central core (equivalent to VPLp) respond to cutaneous stimuli and project to areas 3b and 1 (26,35). A comparable division of VPM, although likely, has not yet been described.

Intralaminar Nuclei and Motor Pathways through the Thalamus

The intralaminar nuclei are forgotten components of the great loop of connections joining the cerebral cortex through the basal ganglia to the thalamus and back again. They deserve more attention than they have customarily been given. The intralaminar nuclei in both monkeys and humans can be identified histologically by dense histochemical staining for acetylcholinesterase and by the unifying feature of their projection to the striatum (5) (Fig. 2.7). The presence of a striatal projection helps to identify several other nuclei that are not so obviously contained within the internal medullary lamina, for example, the VAmc nucleus, the suprageniculate/limitans nucleus, the paralamellar division of the mediodorsal nucleus, parts of the principal VA nucleus, and the magnocellular medial geniculate nucleus, as parts of the intralaminar or striatally projecting system. Not all intralaminar cells, however, project to the striatum; many project instead to the cerebral cortex, and, as just mentioned, some striatally projecting cells can be found in nuclei outside the classic boundaries of the acetylcholinesterase-stained intralaminar complex.

Apart from γ-aminobutyric acid (GABA)-ergic interneurons, which form approximately 30% of the neuronal population of the intralaminar nuclei in monkeys (48), the intralaminar nuclei consist of largely separate populations of striatally and cortically projecting cells. As in other animals, the striatally projecting group is the largest, and few cells have branched axons to both striatum and cortex (49,50). There is no reason to doubt that it is similar in primates.

The intralaminar nuclei overall can be divided into anterior and posterior groups. In humans, the posterior group, which includes the CM and parafascicular (Pf) nuclei, are traditionally associated with the thalamic projection to the putamen, because vascular lesions of the putamen lead to retrograde cell loss in those nuclei (51,52). The anterior group

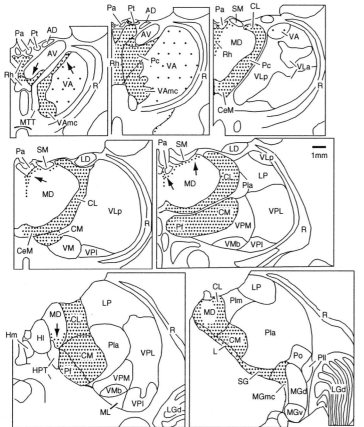

FIGURE 2.7. Camera lucida drawings of frontal sections in anterior **(top left)** to posterior **(bottom right)** order, showing the distribution of the thalamostriatal cells *(dots)* in the intralaminar and adjacent nuclei of the monkey thalamus. *Arrows* indicate extensions of the intralaminar nuclei into adjacent relay nuclei. (From Jones EG. The thalamus of primates. In: Bloom FE, Björklund A, Hökfelt T, eds. *Handbook of chemical neuroanatomy,* vol 14: *The primate nervous system: part II.* Amsterdam: Elsevier, 1998:1–298, with permission.)

of intralaminar nuclei, including the CM, central lateral, paracentral, and midline nuclei, on the basis of retrograde degeneration studies in animals, was traditionally related to the caudate nucleus (53). What we now refer to as the limbic striatum, that is, the nucleus accumbens and adjacent cell groups forming the ventral striatum (see later), from human studies, was thought to be the target of the paracentral nucleus of the anterior intralaminar group (8). Studies in monkeys have revealed much more overlap in the projections of the anterior and posterior groups of intralaminar nuclei within the divisions of the striatum (49,54–57), and this is discussed later.

Inputs to the Intralaminar Nuclei from the Cerebellum, Striatum, and Other Components of the Basal Ganglia

The posterior group of intralaminar nuclei is dominated by inputs from the striatum, whereas the anterior group is dominated by inputs from the cerebellum, with additional inputs from the substantia nigra, other parts of the brainstem such as the superior colliculus, and the spinal cord (Fig. 2.8). The finding that cerebellar, nigral and collicular inputs gain access to the striatum through the intralaminar nuclei, which

therefore form a series of reentrant subcortical loops into the corticostriatopallidothalamic pathways, seems to have escaped the notice of most investigators. The CM nucleus is primarily innervated by the internal segment of the globus pallidus (3,19,20,58–60). The inputs to the parafascicular nucleus have been less well defined but seem to come mainly from brainstem sources, including the vestibular nuclei.

Inputs from the three deep cerebellar nuclei dominate the anterior group of intralaminar nuclei, the dentate and interposed nuclei projecting contralaterally and the fastigial nucleus bilaterally (14). Other inputs come from the spinal cord, the spinal trigeminal nuclei, amygdala, substantia nigra, intermediate layers of the superior colliculus and pretectal nuclei, vestibular and perihypoglossal nuclei, rostral brainstem reticular formation, and periaqueductal gray matter (5). Inputs to the thalamus from the cholinergic, serotoninergic, and noradrenergic brainstem nuclei also tend to be concentrated in the anterior group of intralaminar nuclei.

Cortical Projections of the Intralaminar Nuclei

The cortical projection of the intralaminar nuclei in monkeys and other species is significant although less dense than the projection to the striatum (5). Emphasis has been given to the idea that the cortical projection terminates primarily in layer I of the cortex, but this has not been reliably confirmed in monkeys, and in other species layer VI terminations have been described as well. The cortical projection is not particularly diffuse. Clusters of cells in the intralaminar nuclei project to relatively localized zones of cortex, and relatively few cells branch widely to innervate highly disparate regions. From work done mainly in cats, the anterior group of intralaminar nuclei projects to regions limited to a few functional areas in prefrontal, cingulate, parietotemporal, entorhinal, and prepiriform areas. The paracentral and central lateral nuclei provide most of the projection to lateral areas of the cerebral cortex. In monkeys, this includes most of the superior and inferior parietal lobules (61), consistent with a relationship of the paracentral nucleus with the associational striatum (see later), but it also provides a projection to the cingulate, entorhinal, and periamygdaloid cortex and hippocampus as well (62,63), more in the context of a relationship with the limbic striatum. The central lateral and CM nuclei provide the inputs to the primary somatosensory and motor areas and the anterior parietal cortex, but the projection to the somatosensory areas is weaker than that to the motor areas and much weaker than that to anterior parietal cortex, consistent with a relationship of these nuclei with the sensorimotor striatum. In monkeys, prefrontal and premotor areas may also be targets of the parafascicular nucleus (64). The principal auditory areas and the adjacent insular cortex do not receive a projection from the classic intralaminar nuclei, and in these areas, the suprageniculate/limitans and possibly the magnocellular medial geniculate nuclei provide comparable projections (5).

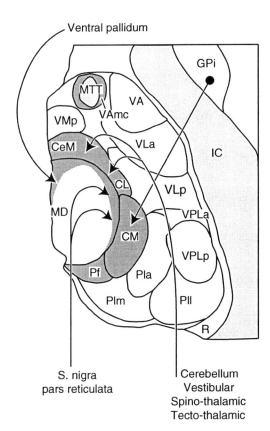

FIGURE 2.8. Schematic horizontal section of a human thalamus showing distribution of inputs *(arrows)* from various sources to the intralaminar nuclei.

PRINCIPAL COMPONENTS OF THE BASAL GANGLIA AND THEIR CIRCUITRY

Brief Overview of the Basal Ganglia

Basal ganglia is a term that throughout the ages has been applied to many different constellations of forebrain nuclei. For the purposes of this account, it will be taken to include the striatum, globus pallidus, substantia nigra, and subthalamic nucleus, a set of forebrain and upper brainstem structures that, along with the thalamus and cerebral cortex, are interlinked in a complex circuitry that underlies the higher cerebral control of movement performance.

The *striatum* is made up of the caudate nucleus and putamen, separated in the human and monkey brain by the an-

terior limb of the internal capsule (Fig. 2.9), but with connecting strands through the capsule, as well as the nucleus accumbens and adjacent regions where the head of the caudate nucleus and putamen merge around and beneath the anterior limb of the internal capsule. This region, called *fundus striati* by Schaltenbrand and Wahren (65), and divided by them, probably under Hassler's influence, into three parts, is now commonly linked with the nucleus accumbens as the *ventral striatum* (66). The fundus striati is now recognized as large and forms much of the deeper part of the olfactory tubercle—probably even reaching the surface of the tubercle in places (Fig. 2.10).

The *globus pallidus* or *pallidum* is separated from the posteromedial part of the putamen and other structures by a fiber

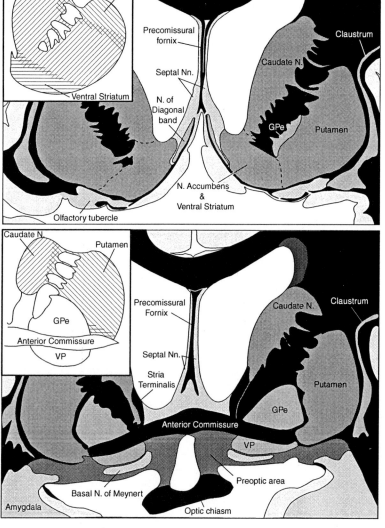

Distribution of cortico-striatal connections in monkeys:

Sensory-motor: Associational: Limbic:

FIGURE 2.9. Camera lucida drawings of frontal sections from a human brain showing the principal components of the basal ganglia at anterior levels of the hemisphere. GPe, external segment of the globus pallidus; VP, ventral pallidum. **Insets** show distributions of corticostriatal fiber terminations on outline drawings of sections from the monkey basal ganglia at comparable levels. The striatum can be divided into three major territories on the basis of the distributions of fibers arising in associational, sensorimotor, and limbic areas of the cerebral cortex.

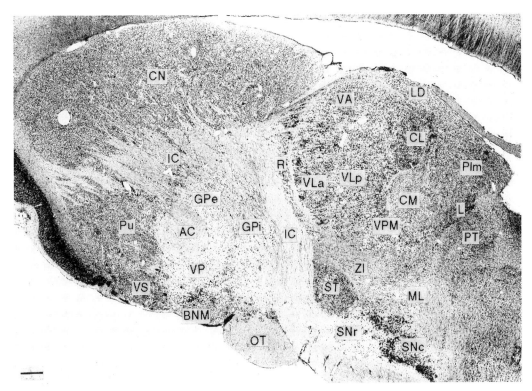

FIGURE 2.10. Photomicrograph from a Nissl-stained parasagittal section through the basal ganglia, thalamus, and upper brainstem of a macaque monkey brain (bar = 1 mm).

lamina and is itself further divided by an additional fiber lamina into the classic external (GPe) and internal (GPi) pallidal segments. These were called *pallidum laterale* and *pallidum mediale,* respectively, by Schaltenbrand and Wahren. In the human, GPi can be partially subdivided by subsidiary laminae into cell groups of uncertain significance but possibly related to different output targets of the GPi (66).

Anteriorly, where the anterior pole of the pallidum sits posterodorsal to the posterior limb of the anterior commissure, the combined GPe and GPi, and especially GPe, send protrusions beneath the anterior commissure and into the ventral striatum. This region, formerly included as part of the substantia innominata by many authors, although recognized by Schaltenbrand and Wahren as part of the GPe, is now customarily referred to as the *ventral pallidum* (66) (Figs. 2.9 and 2.10).

In many nonprimates, the nucleus equivalent to GPi is displaced from the GPe (which is then called the globus pallidus) and becomes embedded in the internal capsule as the entopeduncular nucleus. Here it tends to be continuous with the pars reticulata of the substantia nigra (SNr), and on account of this and the similarity of the (GABA) cell types in both nuclei, some investigators have argued that they are part of a common nucleus. This has also been suggested for primates, including humans, although morphologic continuity of the two nuclei is far more tenuous and is arguably only detectable with unusual stains (66).

The *substantia nigra,* traditionally regarded as part of the upper midbrain, is made up of two divisions, the *pars reticulata* (SNr), primarily composed of GABAergic neurons, and the *pars compacta* (SNc), composed mainly of dopaminergic neurons and more or less continuous with the dopamine cells of the ventral tegmental area (Figs. 2.10 and 2.11). In primates, including humans, the SNr and SNc are essentially layered, the latter lying dorsal to the former, but with fingers and islands of each interdigitating along the border. SNr and SNc are the same terms as those used in the atlas of Schaltenbrand and Bailey (67).

The *subthalamic nucleus* is a large island of small to medium-sized cells clearly identifiable in a medial lacuna of the posterior limb of the internal capsule and insinuated between the zona incerta of the thalamus dorsally and the SNc ventrally (Figs. 2.10 to 2.12). It retains this name or the eponym, *corpus Luysii,* in all brain atlases. The fibrous offshoot of the internal capsule that separates the subthalamic nucleus from the overlying zona incerta is the classically named *lenticular fasciculus* (labeled not quite accurately as Forel's field H2 in the Schaltenbrand and Bailey atlas), into which the subthalamic fasciculus runs, bearing fibers joining the subthalamic nucleus and the GPe. Unlike virtually every other nucleus of the basal forebrain, the subthalamic nucleus is almost completely bereft of GABAergic cells (68).

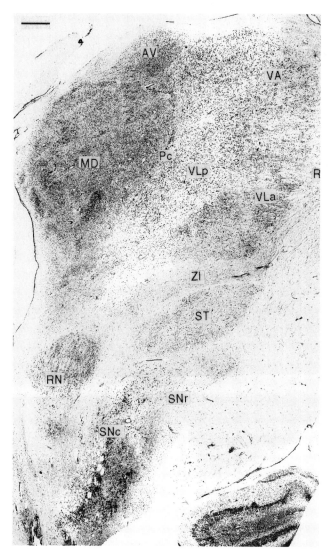

FIGURE 2.11. Photomicrograph of a Nissl-stained frontal section through the human thalamus and upper brainstem (bar = 2 mm).

Parallel Routes Passing through the Basal Ganglia to and from the Thalamus

Pathways Commencing in the Cerebral Cortex

The cerebral cortex imposes an organization on the basal ganglia that is transferred at least in outline to the thalamus. Series of corticostriatopallidothalamocortical loops are engaged, delineated by the origins of corticostriatal fibers in different functional areas of the cerebral cortex and their terminations in different regions of the striatum (Figs. 2.9 and 2.13). This organization is then passed on through each successive synaptic step in the chain of connections leading to the thalamus and back to the cortex. Alexander et al. originally proposed that five such loops could be identified based on the origins of corticostriatal fibers in five different regions of the cortex (69). The names of these loops reflected their cortical origins and putative terminations: motor, oculomotor, dorsolateral prefrontal, lateral orbitofrontal, and anterior

cingulate. More recent research, based on higher-resolution anatomic studies of the basal ganglia in monkeys, has tended toward seeing much more convergence between these seemingly separate parallel pathways. The true situation probably lies somewhere between complete convergence and true parallelism. Nevertheless, three large parallel systems of connections flow from the cerebral cortex through the basal ganglia to the thalamus: sensorimotor, associational, and limbic, the names reflecting the origins of corticostriatal fibers in three large domains of the cerebral cortex.

Corticostriatal fibers arise from all areas of the cerebral cortex, including the neocortex and the medial temporal regions that make up the paleocortex and hippocampal formation (70–78). All areas of the neocortex contribute fibers to the corticostriatal projection, but the greatest contribution is from the sensorimotor areas (73,74,79–82) and the least from the primary visual area (83). In some studies in monkeys, the existence of a corticostriatal projection from the primary visual cortex has been explicitly denied. The projection from the association areas of the frontal, parietal, and temporal lobes, although emanating from a wider area of cortex, is second to that from the sensorimotor areas in terms of its terminal extent in the striatum. The projection from the cingulate and medial temporal areas, in which is included a projection from the amygdala, is third largest in terms of its striatal area of distribution.

The inputs from these three great regions of the cerebral cortex, sensorimotor, associational, and limbic, although overlapping to a considerable extent in the striatum, serve to define three large, functional divisions of the striatum that tend to be preserved in the subsequent links of the chain of connections leading from the striatum through the remainder of the basal ganglia to the thalamus (1).

The sensorimotor zone of the striatum, defined by the extent of terminations of corticostriatal fibers from the sensorimotor regions, is made up of the greater part of the putamen and the dorsolateral rim of the head of the caudate nucleus. The associational zone, as defined by the extent of terminal ramifications of fibers from the frontal, posterior parietal, and temporal cortex, is made up of the greater part of the head, body, and tail of the caudate nucleus and the anterior pole of the putamen. The limbic zone, as defined by the extent of terminations of fibers from cingulate and medial temporal regions, is made up of the nucleus accumbens, fundus striati, and adjacent regions, collectively known as the ventral striatum. Within any of these large zones, inputs from the different contributing areas of the cerebral cortex show a mediolateral and an anteroposterior topography and can interdigitate to a considerable degree, but overlap and convergence are considerable. Inputs from the precentral and postcentral gyri and from the four fields of the somatosensory cortex (areas 3a, 3b, 1, and 2), for example, converge within the sensorimotor zone (73). Within the associational zone, investigators have suggested that inputs from cortical areas that are linked by corticocortical connections in

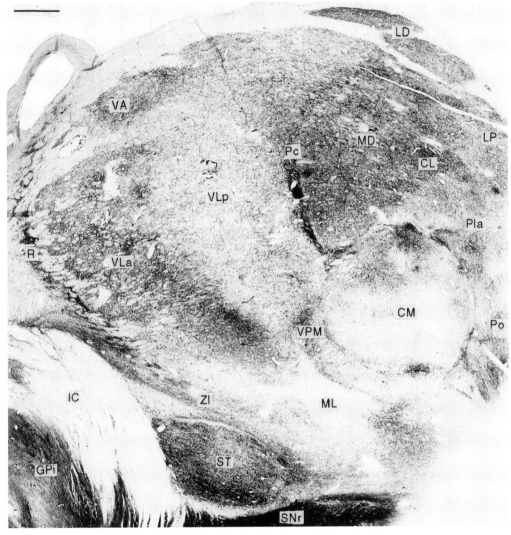

FIGURE 2.12. Photomicrograph from a parasagittal section through the human diencephalon, stained for acetylcholinesterase (bar = 2 mm).

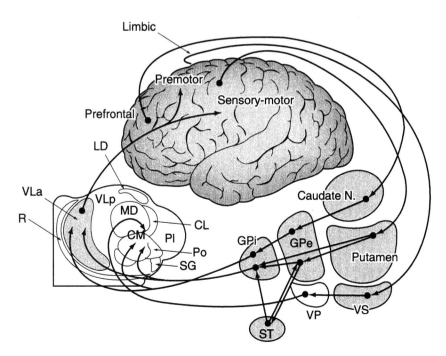

FIGURE 2.13. Parallel limbic, associational, and sensorimotor loops passing through the striatum, globus pallidus, and thalamus and their feedback to prefrontal, premotor, and motor areas of the cortex, based on the topography of the pallidothalamic connections. (Modified from Macchi G, Jones EG. Towards an agreement on terminology of nuclear and subnuclear divisions of the motor thalamus. *J Neurosurg* 1997;86:670–685, with permission.)

the cortex converge, even if the contributing areas are spatially separated, such as in the frontal and parietal lobes (68). This is, however, probably not exclusive.

Retrograde tracing studies indicate that cells in layer V of the neocortex are the principal source of corticostriatal fibers in monkeys (73), but layer III cells also contribute, especially in nonprimates, and especially in the limbic areas. In primates, terminations of corticostriatal fibers from all neocortical areas tend to spread across both the patch and matrix compartments of the striatum. There may be greater segregation in the limbic zone.

Pathways Arising in the Intralaminar Nuclei of the Thalamus

The projections of the anterior and posterior groups of intralaminar nuclei and other striatally projecting cell groups of the thalamus appear to be organized around the divisions of the striatum defined by corticostriatal projections from the sensorimotor, association, and limbic areas of the cerebral cortex. Intralaminar nuclei that are the recipients of corticothalamic fibers arising in a particular cortical area or areas project to the parts of the striatum that receive corticostriatal fibers from the same areas. Hence the striatal projections of the CM nucleus are focused on the sensorimotor striatum (the putamen). The projections of the parafascicular nucleus are focused on the associational striatum (caudate nucleus). The anterior group of intralaminar nuclei are mostly associated with the striatal territory receiving corticostriatal fibers from both the parietotemporal and cingulate cortex, and their projection overlaps from the caudate nucleus into the putamen. The full extent of their terminations has not been mapped in the striatum of primates, but because the projections of the CM and parafascicular nuclei alone fill most of the caudate nucleus and putamen, overlap must be considerable. The limbic or ventral striatum may receive its principal thalamic input from regions ventral to the parafascicular nucleus (49) or from the midline cells of the anterior group of intralaminar nuclei (84). The terminations of the intralaminar axons in the striatum are focused in patches (50,85), which tend to coincide with the matrix of the striatum.

In the matrix compartment, terminals of thalamostriatal fibers converge with those of corticostriatal fibers and of dopaminergic fibers from the SNc on the medium spiny relay cells (86). In monkeys, thalamostriatal synapses, which tend to be concentrated on dendritic shafts, have less intimate associations with the dopaminergic terminals (87) than corticostriatal fibers, which are concentrated on the dendritic spines and end in close proximity to the dopaminergic terminals. Both the thalamic and cortical inputs to the striatum are excitatory. Other subcortical targets of projections from the intralaminar nuclei are reported to be the amygdala (49,88), substantia innominata (49,77), subthalamic nucleus (49), and globus pallidus (49).

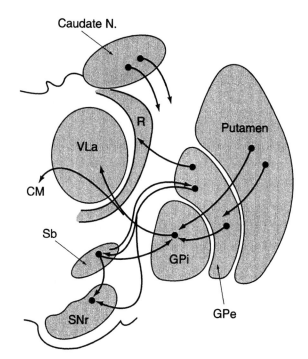

FIGURE 2.14. General scheme of the output connections of the basal ganglia.

Outputs of the Striatum

The principal targets of the striatum are the GPe and GPi and the substantia nigra (predominantly SNr) (Fig. 2.14). In primates, it appears that these three projections arise from different populations of medium spiny striatal cells (89,90). In nonprimates, there may be more collateralization.

The delimitation of three large striatal territories by corticostriatal terminations, coupled with the topographic organization of the striatopallidal and striatonigral projections, ensures that the sensorimotor, associational, and limbic pathways tend to be preserved as parallel streams in the flow of connections through the two divisions of the globus pallidus and the substantia nigra (1). The sensorimotor division of the striatum projects mainly to the posteroventrolateral parts of both the GPe and GPi and to only a restricted part of the SNr. The associational division projects mainly to the anterodorsomedial parts of the GPe and GPi and to the greater part of the SNr. The limbic division projects to the ventral pallidum (divided incompletely into external and internal divisions) and to a restricted part of the SNr.

The smaller sizes of the GPe, GPi, and SNr in comparison with the striatum, their relatively low cell densities, and the far-flung dendrites of their constituent cells, especially in the GPe and GPi, make it likely that much convergence exists between the parallel sensorimotor, associational, and limbic pathways, although studies at the single cell level report some degree of segregation (91).

Outputs of the Two Divisions of the Globus Pallidus and Pars Reticulata of the Substantia Nigra

Globus Pallidus Externus

The principal output target of the GPe is the subthalamic nucleus (58,59,92) (Figs. 2.14 and 2.15), a projection that is directly reciprocated, thus incorporating the subthalamic nucleus to a large extent into a closed loop with the GPe. For the organization of the pallidosubthalamic projection, see later. Other outputs of the GPe, however, are described as passing to the GPi, SNr, and reticular nucleus of the thalamus (91).

Globus Pallidus Internus

The GPi provides the principal basal ganglia input to the relay and intralaminar nuclei of the thalamus. The relay nucleus that forms the principal target of the GPi is the VLa nucleus, as reviewed in an earlier section, furnishing a final relay back mainly to the premotor areas of the frontal lobes, although this is not uncontested. There is a topography in the GPi projection to VLa so that lateral parts of GPi tend to project more anteriorly in VLa and medial parts more posteriorly. This means that the sensorimotor route through the basal ganglia is targeted predominantly posteriorly, and the associational pathway is targeted predominantly anteriorly. In the latter case, some authors see it as extending into VA. The limbic contribution to VLa, if any, has not been defined. Currently, the ventral pallidum is described as projecting to the magnocellular subnucleus of the mediodorsal nucleus of the thalamus (93), although close inspection of published material suggests that the terminations are mainly in paralamellar and midline regions that form parts of the intralaminar system (5). This is an important point considering that the output targets of the magnocellular mediodorsal subnucleus (orbitofrontal cortex) and those of the midline and paralamellar cells (striatum and premotor cortex) are different.

The GPi supplies a heavy projection to the intralaminar nuclei, which, although extensive, is largely confined to the small-celled division of the CM nucleus. This projection, although arising mainly from fibers that are collaterals of those projecting to VLa (94), is diffuse and, unlike the projection to VLa, does not appear to be topographically organized. The GPi also furnishes a projection to the lateral habenular nucleus of the epithalamus and to the pedunculopontine tegmental nucleus of the brainstem.

Substantia Nigra Pars Reticulata

The principal outputs of the SNr are to the thalamus, superior colliculus, and pedunculopontine tegmental nucleus (95–99). Of these, that to the thalamus is greatest and that to the superior colliculus is least. In the thalamus, a continuous zone of terminations of nigral afferents largely defines the lateral components of the anterior group of intralaminar nuclei, namely, the paracentral and central lateral, with continuation into the VAmc (which is probably an intralaminar nucleus, see earlier) and VA, which, like the intralaminar nuclei, contains a population of striatally projecting cells.

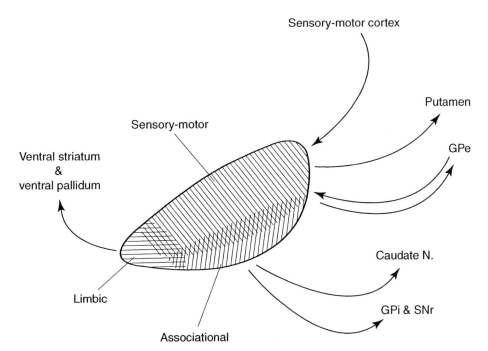

FIGURE 2.15. Sensorimotor, associational, and limbic divisions of the subthalamic nucleus, based on their input and output connections. (Based on Parent A, Hazrati LN. Functional anatomy of the basal ganglia. II. The place of subthalamic nucleus and external pallidum in basal ganglia circuitry. *Brain Res Rev* 1995;20:128–154, with permission.)

Descriptions by some authors place the more posterior parts of the projection within the paralamellar part of the mediodorsal nucleus, which is now regarded as a component of the central lateral nucleus. The important and usually overlooked point is that the SNr targets predominantly thalamic cells, regardless of what an investigator calls them, that project back to the striatum, thus closing a striatopallidothalamostriatal loop subcortically. Other cells in these nuclei project to prefrontal, cingulate, and even parietal cortex, thus forming a nigral relay to these areas.

The projection of the SNr to the superior colliculus ends in the intermediate layers of this structure, and equally neglected is the knowledge that apart from projecting to certain of the pulvinar nuclei of the thalamus, these layers of the colliculus also project extensively to the intralaminar nuclei, more or less overlapping the projection of the SNr, closing another subcortical loop within the basal ganglia circuitry.

Subthalamic Nucleus

As pointed out earlier, the subthalamic nucleus lacks a significant population of GABAergic interneurons (68), so most of its cells are likely to be projection neurons. They are unusual among projection neurons in the forebrain, however, in failing to express the multifunctional protein kinase, α-type II-calcium/calmodulin–dependent protein kinase, an important presynaptic and postsynaptic component of excitatory synapses and expressed almost exclusively in excitatory neurons of the forebrain (68). The subthalamic nucleus is dominated by the sensorimotor cortex, both directly and through the sensorimotor corticostriatopallidosubthalamic pathway (Fig. 2.15).

Cortical efferents terminating in the subthalamic nucleus arise in both the ipsilateral premotor/motor and somatosensory areas, with that from the motor-related areas predominating (92,100,101). There is a topography in the projections, so that fibers from the face representation in the motor cortex terminate dorsolaterally, those from the lower limb representation terminate ventromedially, and those from the upper limb representation terminate in between. Inputs from the supplementary motor area show a reversed topography imposed on this, and inputs from the frontal and supplementary eye fields end more ventrally in the nucleus (102).

The sensorimotor cortical inputs collectively outline a large dorsal region of the subthalamic nucleus and leave a relatively small ventral region unaccounted for. The same large dorsal region is reciprocally connected with the sensorimotor territory of the GPe, both sending fibers to and receiving them back from this region of the GPe. The same dorsal region of the subthalamic nucleus sends other fibers to the putamen, that is, to the sensorimotor division of the striatum (92,103,104).

If the large dorsal part of the subthalamic nucleus can be called the sensorimotor division on grounds just specified, then the smaller ventral part that does not receive inputs from the motor cortex qualifies to be called the associational division because its efferents reach mainly the parts of the GPi and SNr defined as associational on the basis of their connections with the caudate nucleus, as well as the caudate nucleus itself. A small medial tip qualifies to be called a limbic division because of its connections with the ventral pallidum (2,93). Other diffuse inputs to the subthalamic nucleus come from the pedunculopontine tegmental and dorsal raphe nuclei, as well as the SNc.

CONCLUSIONS

Close comparison of the cytoarchitecture and chemoarchitecture of the human and monkey thalamus indicates that it is possible to define equivalent (and undoubtedly truly homologous) nuclei, although past practices mainly based on historical precedent delayed acceptance of a common nomenclature and sometimes engendered controversy. In the basal ganglia and related cell groups such as the substantia nigra and subthalamic nucleus, where the nuclei are circumscribed entities demarcated by fiber laminae, even the untrained eye can discern the obvious similarities between the two species of primate, and no controversy exists. Adopting a common terminology or at least using a thesaurus that permits nomenclatural differences to be resolved out permits the transfer of information from experimental tract tracing and microelectrode investigations in monkeys to the human and thus provides an improved basis for planning neurosurgical interventions, for targeting electrodes, and for using physiologic recordings for exact localization purposes in patients suffering from movement disorders, whether it be in the thalamus or in any other component of the tightly linked circuitry that joins the thalamus and the basal ganglia.

Some issues about this circuitry continue to demand resolution. One of the most disappointing aspects of recent work is the lack of accurate localization of fiber terminations and projecting cells in the thalamus. It is a pity that, despite all the fine-grain organizational anatomy now available for the connections of the basal ganglia in monkeys, often a blank is drawn at the thalamus, to a large extent relating terminal patterns to some ill-defined "VA-VL" complex rather than to nuclei defined in specific cytoarchitectonic terms. High-resolution Nissl or other stained preparations are necessary for delineating thalamic nuclei whose borders can only be identified by visualization of cell populations. Plotting retrogradely labeled cells or anterogradely axonal ramifications on templates derived from an atlas is, regrettably, not good enough, invites controversy, and impedes realization of a satisfactory scheme of the cortical territories on which all the highly organized throughput of the basal ganglia is targeted.

The intralaminar nuclei of the thalamus remain unincorporated into any schemes of basal ganglia circuitry and into any attempt to understand the pathophysiology of movement disorders stemming from pathologic involvement of the basal ganglia or thalamus. Too little attention has been paid to these nuclei as targets of feedback from the substantia nigra, superior colliculus, and diffuse regulatory centers of the lower brainstem and as sources for channeling these feedbacks through subcortical loops back to the striatum and therefore into the corticostriatopallidothalamic loops that so dominate thinking about the pathophysiology of movement disorders.

Finally, the cerebral cortex, although emphasized as the source and organizing principle in the flow of connectivity through the basal ganglia, tends to be mostly neglected in its position as the site to which all the activity flowing through the basal ganglia-thalamic circuitry is ultimately channeled. Part of the reason for this also lies in the lack of resolution and inconsistency of results in studies of thalamocortical connections in the thalamic motor nuclei, a problem that can only be resolved, like the problem of the exact thalamic terminations of the inputs to many of these nuclei, by greater attention to anatomic technique.

ACKNOWLEDGMENTS

This work was supported by grant NS 21377 from the National Institutes of Health, United States Public Health Service.

REFERENCES

1. Parent A, Hazrati LN. Functional anatomy of the basal ganglia. I. The cortico-basal ganglia-thalamo-cortical loop. *Brain Res Rev* 1995;20:91–127.
2. Parent A, Hazrati LN. Functional anatomy of the basal ganglia. II. The place of subthalamic nucleus and external pallidum in basal ganglia circuitry. *Brain Res Rev* 1995;20:128–154.
3. Percheron G, François C, Talbi B, et al. The primate motor thalamus. *Brain Res Rev* 1996;22:93–181.
4. Macchi G, Jones EG. Towards an agreement on terminology of nuclear and subnuclear divisions of the motor thalamus. *J Neurosurg* 1997;86:670–685.
5. Jones EG. The thalamus of primates. In: Bloom FE, Björklund A, Hökfelt T, eds. *Handbook of chemical neuroanatomy*, vol 14: *The primate nervous system: part II.* Amsterdam: Elsevier, 1998:1–298.
6. Walker AE. *The primate thalamus.* Chicago: University of Chicago Press, 1938.
7. Olszewski J. *The thalamus of the Macaca mulatta: an atlas for use with the stereotaxic instrument.* New York: Karger, 1952.
8. Hassler R. Anatomy of the thalamus. In: Schaltenbrand G, Bailey P, eds. *Introduction to stereotaxis with an atlas of the human brain.* Stuttgart: Thieme, 1959:230–290.
9. Dewulf A. *Anatomy of the normal human thalamus: topometry and standardized nomenclature.* Amsterdam: Elsevier, 1971.
10. Van Buren JM, Borke RC. *Variations and connections of the human thalamus.* New York: Springer, 1972.
11. Ohye C. Thalamus. In: Paxinos G, ed. *The human nervous system.* San Diego: Academic, 1990:439–468.
12. Jones EG. Defining the thalamic intralaminar nuclei in primates. In: Gianotti G, Bentivoglio M, Bergonzi P, et al., eds. *Neurologia e scienze di base: scritti in onore di Giorgio Macchi.* Milan: Università Cattolica del Sacro Cuore, 1989:161–194.
13. Hirai T, Jones EG. A new parcellation of the human thalamus on the basis of histochemical staining. *Brain Res Rev* 1989;14:1–34.
14. Asanuma C, Thach WT, Jones EG. Distribution of cerebellar terminations and their relation to other afferent termination in the ventral lateral thalamic region of the monkey. *Brain Res Rev* 1983;5:237–265.
15. Ilinsky IA, Kultas-Ilinsky K. Sagittal cytoarchitectonic maps of the *Macaca mulatta* thalamus with a revised nomenclature of the motor-related nuclei validated by observations on their connectivity. *J Comp Neurol* 1987;262:331–364.
16. Holsapple JW, Preston UB, Strick PL. The origin of thalamic inputs to the "hand" representation in the primary motor cortex. *J Neurosci* 1991;11:2644–2654.
17. Tracey DJ, Asanuma C, Jones EG, et al. Thalamic relay to motor cortex: afferent pathways from brain stem, cerebellum, and spinal cord in monkeys. *J Neurophysiol* 1980;44:532–554.
18. Fenelon G, François C, Percheron G, et al. Topographic distribution of pallidal neurons projecting to the thalamus in macaques. *Brain Res* 1990;520:27–35.
19. Hazrati LN, Parent A. Projection from the external pallidum to the reticular thalamic nucleus in the squirrel monkey. *Brain Res* 1991;550:142–146.
20. Rouiller EM, Liang F, Babalian A, et al. Cerebellothalamocortical and pallidothalamocortical projections to the primary and supplementary motor cortical areas: a multiple tracing study in macaque monkeys. *J Comp Neurol* 1994;345:185–213.
21. Sakai ST, Inase M, Tanji J. Comparison of cerebellothalamic and pallidothalamic projections in the monkey *(Macaca fuscata)*: a double anterograde labeling study. *J Comp Neurol* 1996;368:215–228.
22. Ohye C, Shibazaki T, Hirai T, et al. Further physiological observations on the ventralis intermedius neurons in the human thalamus. *J Neurophysiol* 1989;61:488–500.
23. Lenz FA, Dostrovsky JO, Tasker RR, et al. Single-unit analysis of the human ventral thalamic nuclear group: somatosensory responses. *J Neurophysiol* 1988;59:299–316.
24. Lenz FA, Tasker RR, Kwan HC, et al. Single unit analysis of the human ventral thalamic nuclear group: correlation of thalamic "tremor" cells with the 3–6Hz component of parkinsonian tremor. *J Neurosci* 1988;8:754–764.
25. Jones EG, Friedman DP. Projection pattern of functional components of thalamic ventrobasal complex on monkey somatosensory cortex. *J Neurophysiol* 1982;48:521–544.
26. Jones EG, Friedman DP, Hendry SHC. Thalamic basis of place and modality-specific columns in monkey somatosensory cortex: a correlative anatomical and physiological study. *J Neurophysiol* 1982;48:545–568.
27. Jones EG, Schwark HD, Callahan PJ. Extent of the ipsilateral representation in the ventral posterior medial nucleus of the monkey thalamus. *Exp Brain Res* 1986;63:310–320.
28. Lenz FA, Gracely RH, Rowland LH, et al. A population of cells in the human thalamic principal sensory nucleus respond to painful mechanical stimuli. *Neurosci Lett* 1994;180:46–50.
29. Lenz FA, Kwan HC, Dostrovsky JO, et al. Single unit analysis of the human ventral thalamic nuclear group. *Brain* 1990;113:1795–1821.
30. Lenz FA, Kwan HCV, Martin R, et al. Characteristics of somatotopic organization and spontaneous neuronal activity in the

region of the thalamic principal sensory nucleus in patients with spinal cord transection. *J Neurophysiol* 1994;72:1570–1587.

31. Lenz FA, Dougherty PM. Neurons in the human thalamic somatosensory nucleus (ventralis caudalis) respond to innocuous cool and mechanical stimuli. *J Neurophysiol* 1998;79: 2227–2230.

32. Lenz FA, Seike M, Richardson RT, et al. Thermal and pain sensations evoked by microstimulation in the area of human ventrocaudal nucleus. *J Neurophysiol* 1993;70:200–212.

33. Maendly R, Rüegg DG, Wiesendanger M, et al. Thalamic relay for group I muscle afferents of forelimb nerves in the monkey. *J Neurophysiol* 1981;46:901–917.

34. Mountcastle VB, Poggio GF. The functional properties of ventrobasal thalamic neurons studied in unanesthetized monkeys. *J Neurophysiol* 1963;26:775–806.

35. Friedman DP, Jones EG. Thalamic input to areas 3a and 2 in monkey. *J Neurophysiol* 1981;45:59–85.

36. Anderson ME, Turner RS. Activity of neurons in cerebellar-receiving and pallidal-receiving areas of the thalamus of the behaving monkey. *J Neurophysiol* 1991;66:879–893.

37. Butler EG, Horne MK, Hawkins NJ. The activity of monkey thalamic and motor cortical neurones in a skilled, ballistic movement. *J Physiol (Lond)* 1992;445:25–48.

38. Vitek JL, Ashe J, DeLong MR, et al. Physiological properties and somatotopic organization of the primate motor thalamus. *J Neurophysiol* 1994;71:1498–1513.

39. Ohye C. Rôle des noyaux thalamiques dans l'hypertonie et le tremblement de la maladie de Parkinson. *Rev Neurol* 1986;142:362–367.

40. Miall RC, Price S, Mason R, et al. Microstimulation of movements from cerebellar-receiving, but not pallidal-receiving areas of the macaque thalamus under ketamine anaesthesia. *Exp Brain Res* 1998;123:387–396.

41. Emmers R, Tasker RR. *The human somesthetic thalamus, with maps for physiological target localization during stereotaxic neurosurgery.* New York: Raven, 1970.

42. Ohye C, Narabayashi H. Physiological study of presumed ventralis intermedius neurons in the human thalamus. *J Neurosurg* 1979;50:290–297.

43. Benabid AL, Pollak P, Gao D, et al. Chronic electrical stimulation of the ventralis intermedius nucleus of the thalamus as a treatment of movement disorders. *J Neurosurg* 1996;84:203–214.

44. Vitek JL, Ashe J, DeLong MR. Altered somatosensory response properties of neurons in the "motor" thalamus of MPTP treated parkinsonian monkeys. *Neuroscience* 1990;16:425–438.

45. Yamashiro K, Tasker RR. Stereotactic thalamotomy for dystonic patients. *Stereotact Funct Neurosurg* 1993;60:81–85.

46. Hassler R, Dieckmann G. Stereotaxic treatment for spasmodic torticollis. In: Schaltenbrand G, Walker AE, eds. *Stereotaxy of the human brain: anatomical, physiological and clinical applications,* 2nd ed. Stuttgart: Thieme, 1982:522–531.

47. Stepniewska I, Preuss TM, Kaas JH. Thalamic connections of the primary motor cortex (M1) of owl monkeys. *J Comp Neurol* 1994;349:558–582.

48. Hunt CA, Pang DZ, Jones EG. Distribution and density of GABA cells in intralaminar and adjacent nuclei of monkey thalamus. *Neuroscience* 1991;43:185–196.

49. Sadikot AF, Parent A, François C. Efferent connections of the centromedian and parafascicular thalamic nuclei in the squirrel monkey: a PHA-L study of subcortical projections. *J Comp Neurol* 1992;315:137–159.

50. Sadikot AF, Parent A, Smith Y, et al. Efferent connections of the centromedian and parafascicular thalamic nuclei in the squirrel monkey: a light and electron microscopic study of the thalamostriatal projection in relation to striatal heterogeneity. *J Comp Neurol* 1992;320:228.

51. Le Gros Clark WE, Russell WR. Observations on the efferent connexions of the centre median nucleus. *J Anat* 1939;73:255–262.

52. Vogt C, Vogt O. Thalamusstudien I–III. *J Psychol Neurol (Leipzig)* 1941;50:32–154.

53. Powell TPS, Cowan WM. A study of thalamo-striate relations in the monkey. *Brain* 1956;79:364–389.

54. Fenelon G, François C, Percheron G, et al. Topographic distribution of the neurons of the central complex (centre médian-parafascicular complex) and of other thalamic neurons projecting to the striatum in macaques. *Neuroscience* 1991;45:495–510.

55. Smith Y, Parent A. Differential connections of caudate nucleus and putamen in the squirrel monkey *(Saimiri sciureus)*. *Neuroscience* 1986;18:347–371.

56. Nakano K, Hasegawa Y, Tokushige A, et al. Topographical projections from the thalamus, subthalamic nucleus and pedunculopontine tegmental nucleus to the striatum in the Japanese monkey, *Macaca fuscata. Brain Res* 1990;537:54–68.

57. François C, Percheron G, Parent A, et al. Topography of the projection from the central complex of the thalamus to the sensorimotor striatal territory in monkeys. *J Comp Neurol* 1991;305:17–34.

58. Nauta WJH, Mehler WR. Projections of the lentiform nucleus in the monkey. *Brain Res* 1966;1:3–42.

59. Kim R, Nakano K, Carpenter MB, et al. Projections of the globus pallidus and adjacent structures: an autoradiographic study in the monkey. *J Comp Neurol* 1976;169:263–290.

60. DeVito JL, Anderson ME. An autoradiographic study of efferent connections of the globus pallidus in *Macaca mulatta. Exp. Brain Res* 1982;46:107–117.

61. Pearson RCA, Brodal P, Powell TPS. The projection of the thalamus upon the parietal lobe in the monkey. *Brain Res* 1978;144:143–148.

62. Amaral DG, Cowan WM. Subcortical afferents to the hippocampal formation in the monkey. *J Comp Neurol* 1980;189:573–591.

63. Insausti R, Amaral DG, Cowan WM. The entorhinal cortex of the monkey. II. cortical afferents. *J Comp Neurol* 1987;264:356–395.

64. Huerta MF, Kaas JH. Supplementary eye field as defined by intracortical microstimulation: connections in macaques. *J Comp Neurol* 1990;293:299–330.

65. Schaltenbrand G, Wahren W. Introduction to the plates. In: Schaltenbrand G, Bailey P, eds. *Introduction to stereotaxis with an atlas of the human brain.* Stuttgart: Thieme, 1959.

66. Alheid GF, Heimer L, Switzer III RC. Basal ganglia. In: Paxinos G, ed. *The human nervous system.* San Diego: Academic, 1990:483–582.

67. Schaltenbrand G, Bailey P, eds. *Introduction to stereotaxis with an atlas of the human brain.* Stuttgart: Thieme, 1959.

68. Benson DL, Isackson PJ, Hendry SHC, et al. Differential gene expression for glutamic acid decarboxylase and type II calcium-calmodulin–dependent protein kinase in basal ganglia, thalamus and hypothalamus of the monkey. *J Neurosci* 1991;11:1540–1564.

69. Alexander GE, DeLong MR, Strick PL. Parallel organization of functionally integrated circuits linking basal ganglia and cortex. *Annu Rev Neurosci* 1986;9:357–382.

70. Kemp JM, Powell TPS. The cortico-striate projection in the monkey. *Brain* 1970;93:525–546.

71. Künzle H. Bilateral projections from percentral motor cortex to the putamen and other parts of the basal ganglia: an

autoradiographic study in *Macaca fascicularis*. *Brain Res* 1975;88: 195–210.

72. Goldman PS, Nauta WJH. An intricately patterned prefronto-caudate projection in the rhesus monkey. *J Comp Neurol* 1976; 171:369–386.

73. Jones EG, Coulter JD, Burton H, et al. Cells of origin and terminal distribution of corticostriatal fibers arising in the sensory-motor cortex of monkeys. *J Comp Neurol* 1977;173: 53–80.

74. Künzle H. Projections from the primary somatosensory cortex to basal ganglia and thalamus in the monkey. *Exp Brain Res* 1977;30:481–493.

75. Yeterian EH, Van Hoesen GW. Cortico-striate projections in the rhesus monkey: the organization of certain cortico-caudate connections. *Brain Res* 1978;139:43–63.

76. Selemon LD, Goldman-Rakic PS. Longitudinal topography and interdigitation of corticostriatal projections in the rhesus monkey. *J Neurosci* 1985;5:776–794.

77. Russchen FT, Bakst I, Amaral DG, et al. The amygdalostriatal projections in the monkey: an anterograde tracing study. *Brain Res* 1985;329:241–257.

78. Haber SN, Lund E, Klein C, et al. Topographic organization of the ventral striatal efferent projections in the rhesus monkey: an anterograde tracing study. *J Comp Neurol* 1990;293: 282–298.

79. Künzle H. An autoradiographic analysis of the efferent connections from premotor and adjacent prefrontal regions (areas 6 and 9) in *Macaca fascicularis*. *Brain Behav Evol* 1978;15: 185–234.

80. Flaherty AW, Graybiel AM. Corticostriatal transformations in the primate somatosensory system: projections from physiologically mapped body-part representations. *J Neurophysiol* 1991;66:1249–1263.

81. Flaherty AW, Graybiel AM. Input-output organization of the sensorimotor striatum in the squirrel monkey. *J Neurosci* 1994; 14:599–610.

82. Inase M, Sakai ST, Tanji J. Overlapping corticostriatal projections from the supplementary motor area and the primary motor cortex in the macaque monkey: an anterograde double labeling study. *J Comp Neurol* 1996;373:283–296.

83. Saint-Cyr JA, Ungerleider LG, Desimone R. Organization of visual cortical inputs to the striatum and subsequent outputs of the pallido-nigral complex in the monkey. *J Comp Neurol* 1990; 298:129–156.

84. Giménez-Amaya JM, McFarland NR, Heras SDL, et al. Organization of thalamic projections to the ventral striatum in the primate. *J Comp Neurol* 1995;354:127–149.

85. Kalil K. Patch-like termination of thalamic fibers in the putamen of the rhesus monkey: an autoradiographic study. *Brain Res* 1978;140:333–339.

86. Gerfen CR. The neostriatal mosaic: multiple levels of compartmental organization in the basal ganglia. *Annu Rev Neurosci* 1992;15:1–22.

87. Smith Y, Bennett BD, Bolam JP, et al. Synaptic relationships between dopaminergic afferents and cortical or thalamic input in the sensorimotor territory of the striatum in monkey. *J Comp Neurol* 1994;344:1–19.

88. Mehler WR, Pretorius JK, Phelan KD, et al. Diencephalic afferent connections of the amygdaloid in the squirrel monkey with

observation and comments on the cat and rat. In: Ben-Ari Y, ed. *The amygdaloid complex*. Amsterdam: Elsevier/North Holland, 1981:105–120.

89. Parent A, Bouchard C, Smith Y. The striatopallidal and striatonigral projections: two distinct fiber systems in primates. *Brain Res* 1984;303:385–390.

90. Selemon LD, Goldman-Rakic PS. Topographic intermingling of striatonigral and striatopallidal neurons in the rhesus monkey. *J Comp Neurol* 1990;297:359–376.

91. Hazrati LN, Parent A. The striatopallidal projection displays a high degree of anatomical specificity in the primate. *Brain Res* 1992;592:213–227.

92. Carpenter MB, Carleton SC, Keller JT, et al. Connections of the subthalamic nucleus in the monkey. *Brain Res* 1981;224:1–30.

93. Haber SN, Lynd-Balta E, Mitchell SJ. The organization of the descending ventral pallidal projections in the monkey. *J Comp Neurol* 1993;329:111–128.

94. Parent A, DeBellefeuille L. A pallidointralaminar and pallidonigral projections in primate as studied by retrograde double labeling method. *Brain Res* 1983;278:11–28.

95. Beckstead RM, Frankfurter A. The distribution and some morphological features of substantia nigra neurons that project to the thalamus, superior colliculus and pedunculopontine nucleus in the monkey. *Neuroscience* 1982;7:2377–2388.

96. Beckstead RM. Long collateral branches of substantia nigra pars reticulata axons to thalamus, superior colliculus and reticular formation in monkey and cat: multiple retrograde neuronal labeling with fluorescent dyes. *Neuroscience* 1983;10:767–780.

97. François C, Yelnik J, Percheron G, et al. Topographic distribution of the axonal endings from the sensorimotor and associative striatum in the macaque pallidum and substantia nigra. *Exp Brain Res* 1994;102:305–318.

98. Goldman-Rakic PS, Ilinsky IA, Jouandet ML. Organization of the nigrothalamocortical system in the rhesus monkey. *J Comp Neurol* 1985;236:315–330.

99. Carpenter MB, Nakano K, Kim R. Nigrothalamic projections in the monkey demonstrated by autoradiographic technics. *J Comp Neurol* 1976;165:401–415.

100. Künzle H, Akert K. Efferent connections of cortical area 8 (frontal eye field) in *Macaca fascicularis*: a reinvestigation using autoradiographic techniques. *J Comp Neurol* 1977;173:147–164.

101. Hartmann-von Monakow K, Akert K, Künzle H. Projections of the precentral motor cortex and other cortical areas of the frontal lobe to the subthalamic nucleus in the monkey. *Exp Brain Res* 1978;33:395–403.

102. Nambu A, Takada M, Inase M, et al. Dual somatotopical representations in the primate subthalamic nucleus: evidence for ordered but reversed body-map transformations from the primary motor cortex and the supplementary motor area. *J Neurosci* 1996;16:2671–2683.

103. Nauta HJW, Cole M. Efferent projections of the subthalamic nucleus. *Trans Am Neurol Assoc* 1974;99:170–173.

104. Smith Y, Hazrati LN, Parent A. Efferent projections of the subthalamic nucleus in the squirrel monkey as studied by the PHA-L anterograde method. *J Comp Neurol* 1990;294:306–323.

105. Walker AE. Normal and pathological physiology of the human thalamus. In: Schaltenbrand G, Walker AE, eds. *Stereotaxy of the human brain: anatomical, physiological and clinical applications*, 2nd ed. Stuttgart: Thieme, 1982:181–217.

Surgery for Parkinson's Disease and Movement Disorders,
edited by J.K. Krauss, J. Jankovic, and R.G. Grossman.
Lippincott Williams & Wilkins, Philadelphia © 2001.

3

BASAL GANGLIA ANATOMY AND FUNCTIONAL ORGANIZATION

ANDRÉ PARENT
FUMI SATO
MARTIN PARENT
MARTIN LÉVESQUE

This chapter provides a brief overview of the anatomic and functional organization of the primate basal ganglia. Emphasis is placed on data obtained with single-axon tracing procedures. Each structure that forms the core of the basal ganglia, that is, the striatum, the external segment of the globus pallidus (GPe), the internal segment of the globus pallidus (GPi), and the subthalamic nucleus (STN), has been the subject of single-cell labeling studies in the cynomolgus monkey *(Macaca fascicularis).* The functional significance of the results is discussed in light of the current model of the organization of the basal ganglia. This model is often invoked to explain the effects of stereotactic lesions or high-frequency stimulation of basal ganglia nuclei to alleviate the motor symptoms of Parkinson's disease (PD) and other movement disorders (1–4).

CURRENT MODEL OF THE BASAL GANGLIA

The current model of the organization of the basal ganglia was proposed in the 1980s after key observations were made on animal models of neurodegenerative diseases and patients suffering from hypokinetic or hyperkinetic movement disorders (5–8). It can be summarized as follows: The striatum, the input stage of the basal ganglia, receives multiple afferent projections, the major ones being the glutamatergic excitatory input from the cerebral cortex and the dopaminergic input from the substantia nigra pars compacta (SNc). In contrast, the GPi and the substantia nigra pars reticulata (SNr) represent the major output nuclei of basal ganglia. These structures exert a tonic inhibitory influence mediated

by γ-aminobutyric acid (GABA) on the excitatory premotor neurons located in the ventral tier thalamic nuclei. Between input and output structures, two major projection systems—the so-called direct and indirect pathways—have been identified, arising from separate neuronal populations in the striatum. The direct pathway originates from striatal neurons that contain GABA plus the peptide substance P (SP) or dynorphin (DYN) and project monosynaptically to the GPi/SNr. The indirect pathway arises from striatal neurons that contain GABA and enkephalin (ENK) and whose influence is conveyed to the GPi/SNr polysynaptically through relays in the GPe and the STN. This sequence of connections comprises (a) a GABAergic inhibitory projection from the striatum to GPe; (b) an inhibitory GABAergic projection from the GPe to the STN; and (c) an excitatory glutamatergic projection from the STN to the GPi/SNr (Fig. 3.1A).

At the striatal level, dopamine appears to facilitate transmission along the direct pathway and to inhibit transmission along the indirect pathway, these two opposite effects being mediated apparently by D1 and D2 dopamine receptors, respectively. The imbalance between the activity in the direct and indirect pathways and the resulting alterations in the GPi/SNr are thought to account for the hypokinetic and hyperkinetic features of basal ganglia disorders. Bradykinesia or akinesia observed in PD is postulated to result from increased GABAergic inhibition of thalamic premotor neurons caused by excessiveexcitatory drive from the STN to the GPi/SNr. The loss of striatal dopamine that characterizes PD is thought to cause a disinhibition of GABA/ENK neurons at the origin of the indirect pathway, which leads to a marked hypoactivity of the GPe, followed by a disinhibition of the STN (Fig. 3.1B). At the other end of the spectrum, hyperkinetic movements encountered in Huntington's disease are believed to result from decreased GABAergic inhibition of thalamic premotor neurons caused by a lack of excitatory drive from the STN to the GPi/SNr. In such a case,

---

A. Parent, F. Sato, M. Parent, and M. Lévesque: Laboratoire de Neurobiologie, Centre de recherche Université Laval Robert-Giffard, Beauport, Québec, Canada G1J 2G3.

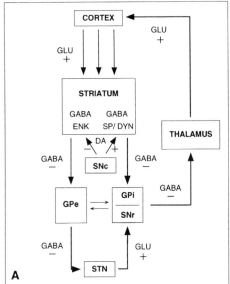

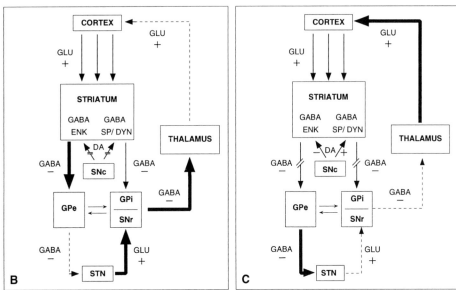

FIGURE 3.1. Functional organization of the basal ganglia in a normal state **(A)** compared with Parkinson's disease **(B)** and Huntington's chorea **(C)**. *Thick and dashed lines* indicate pathways believed to be hyperactive or hypoactive in these pathologic conditions, respectively. DYN, dynorphin; ENK, enkephalin; GABA, γ-aminobutyric acid; GLU, glutamate; GPe, external segment of the globus pallidus; GPi, internal segment of the globus pallidus; SN, substantia nigra; SNc, pars compacta of SN; SNr, pars reticulata of SN; STN, subthalamic nucleus.

degeneration of GABA/ENK striatal neurons that project to the GPe is thought to lead to marked hyperactivity of the GPe, followed by strong inhibition of the STN (Fig. 3.1C). The following section summarizes the results of our own neuroanatomic studies of the primate brain. Some of our results fit perfectly well within the current model, whereas others call for a reevaluation of at least some parts of this scheme of thought.

SINGLE-AXON TRACING EXPERIMENTS

Single axons were traced by using a novel method developed in our laboratory and described in detail elsewhere (9). This procedure involves microiontophoretic injections of the anterograde tracers biocytin or biotin dextran amine (BDA) into small neuronal pools (five to 15 neurons) ("extracellular mode") (Fig. 3.2A,B) or single neurons ("juxtacellular

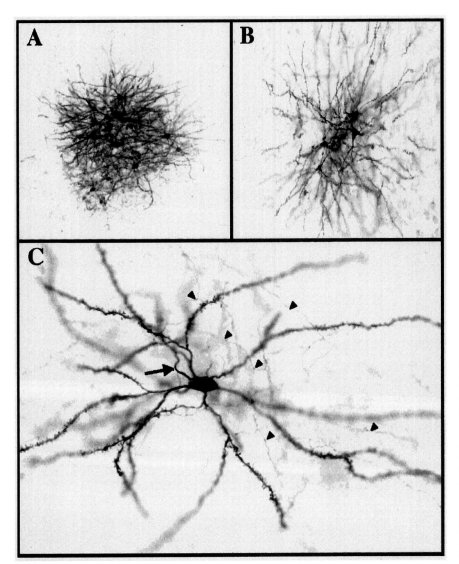

FIGURE 3.2. A and B: Biotin dextran amine (BDA) injection sites in the striatum made by using the extracellular mode of injection. In such a case, the injection size and number of labeled neurons can be modified at will by varying the size of the micropipette tip and the time and amount of current applied to deliver the tracer iontophoretically. The site in **A** contains about ten to 15 labeled neurons, whereas the one in **B** harbors about four to five labeled neurons. **C:** One striatal neuron labeled in a Golgi-like fashion with BDA by using the juxtacellular mode of injection. The *large arrow* points to the initial segment of the axon, whereas the *arrowheads* point to some local collaterals.

mode") (Fig. 3.2C). It allows the electrophysiologic recording of neurons to be injected and yields a detailed view of the entire axonal arborization of the labeled neurons (9,10). These neurons are labeled in a Golgi-like fashion, and their axon can be drawn with a camera lucida from a series of parasagittal sections. A three-dimensional reconstruction of each axon can then be achieved with the help of a computerized image analysis system. The method was applied to the study of the projection neurons in the striatum, GPe, STN, and GPi of cynomolgus monkeys *(Macaca fascicularis).*

Striatum

Striatofugal axons in monkeys are very fine and display numerous, irregularly spaced varicosities along their course. Short, bulblike appendages are also encountered as the striatofugal axons course through the globus pallidus. All putamenofugal fibers penetrate the pallidum by piercing the external medullary lamina, where they give rise to long collaterals arborizing along the inner surface of the lamina. The parent axons continue their course medially to arborize either in the GPe alone or, more commonly, in the GPe and GPi. Axons heading toward the GPi emit numerous collaterals along the outer border of the internal medullary lamina before leaving the GPe. Most axons that arborize profusely in the GPi have a main branch that traverses the peduncular portion of the internal capsule and terminates in the SNr in the form of poorly arborized processes (Fig. 3.3).

Even though most striatofugal axons provided collaterals to the three recipient structures of the striatum in primates, each axon appears to have a preferential target site where it arborizes profusely and forms typical "woolly fibers." Several thin collaterals closely entwine the unstained core of dendrites belonging to pallidal neurons and form these woolly

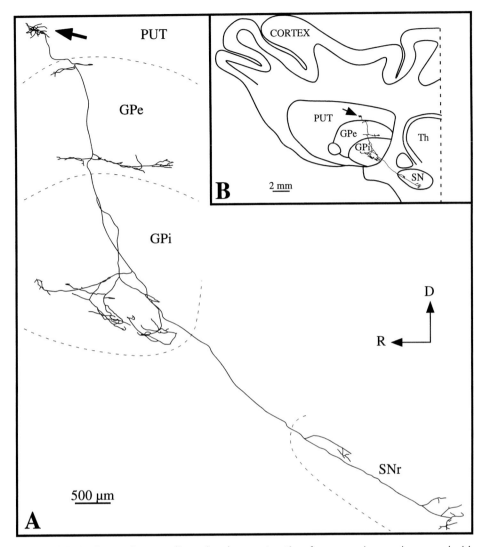

FIGURE 3.3. A: Composite two-dimensional reconstruction from superimposed camera lucida drawings of serial sagittal sections showing the patterns of arborization of a single biocytin-injected striatofugal axon in the external and internal segments of the globus pallidus (GPe and GPi) and the pars reticulata of the substantia nigra (SNr). This particular axon arises from a neuron *(arrow)* located in the middle rostrocaudal third of the putamen (PUT), near the border of the GPe. It arborizes profusely in the GPi and less abundantly in the GPe and SNr. **B:** Overall view of the axon trajectory.

fibers. These thin collaterals are often seen to emerge from a single secondary branch of the main axon.

External Pallidum

Most GPe cells display long, aspiny, and poorly branched dendrites that arborize mostly along the sagittal plane, whereas others show dendrites radiating in all directions. The axons arise from either the cell body or a proximal dendrite. In some cases, axons emit short collaterals that arborize around the cell body. On the basis of their axonal targets, GPe neurons can be subdivided into at least four distinct types: (a) neurons projecting to the GPi, STN, and SNr; (b) neurons projecting to the GPi and STN (Fig. 3.4);

(c) neurons projecting to the STN and SNr; and (d) neurons projecting to the striatum. The degree of arborization varies significantly in the different target structures, and it ranges from a few poorly branched axons in the striatum to numerous, highly branched collaterals in the STN and GPi. In all target structures, however, STN collaterals terminate in the form of large boutons that closely surround the cell bodies and proximal dendrites.

Subthalamic Nucleus

Most STN cells display four to nine long dendrites that cover a large area of the nucleus (Fig. 3.5). The axon arises from the cell body or a proximal dendrite. On the basis of their

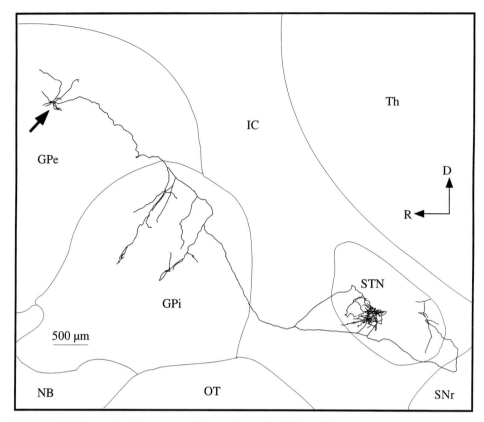

FIGURE 3.4. Camera lucida reconstruction on the sagittal plane of a single biotin dextran amine (BDA)-labeled neuron of the external segment of the globus pallidus (GPe) *(arrow)* projecting to the internal segment of the globus pallidus (GPi) and the subthalamic nucleus (STN). Note the dense but small and highly focussed innervation of the STN. IC, internal capsule; NB, nucleus basalis; OT, optic tract; Th, thalamus.

axonal targets, four distinct types of STN neurons appear to exist: (a) neurons projecting to the SNr, GPi, and GPe (Fig. 3.5); (b) neurons projecting to the SNr and GPe; (c) neurons projecting to the GPi and GPe (the most abundant ones); and (d) neurons projecting to the GPe only. Other STN neurons have a main axon that does not provide collateral to the pallidum. Instead, this axon ascends within the internal capsule as far up as the border of the striatum, where the labeling becomes too faint to allow a faithful tracing of the terminal portion of the axon.

Internal Pallidum

Neurons of the GPi have a large and elongated perikaryon that gives rise to several long, thick, and slightly varicose dendrites. The axon of these neurons emerges either from the perikaryon or a proximal dendrite and branches directly within the GPi. It gives rise first to a long branch that courses caudally to the mesopontine brainstem tegmentum (Fig. 3.6). This branch passes beneath the STN, does not emit collaterals along its way, and terminates principally within the pedunculopontine tegmental nucleus (PPN). Other branches emerge from the main axon of the

pallidal neurons in the GPi. These branches also head toward the brainstem but emit at least one major collateral, which, at the STN level, ascends dorsally within the ventral tier thalamic nuclei (Fig. 3.6). This collateral branches into about ten to 15 thinner collaterals that run throughout large territories of the ventral tier thalamic nuclei. These collaterals, however, develop varicosities only at their terminal tips and only in very specific sectors of the ventral anterior/ventral lateral thalamic nuclei. At these levels, numerous axonal varicosities and terminal boutons closely surround the unstained neurons of the ventral tier thalamic nuclei (Fig. 3.6).

NEURAL NETWORK FUNCTIONAL BASAL GANGLIA ORGANIZATION

The current model of the basal ganglia organization is largely based on the segregation of the striatal output pathways. Early retrograde cell-labeling studies, including ours, have supported such segregation. However, the results of the single-axon tracing studies summarized earlier reveal that striatofugal axons are, in fact, highly collateralized, providing branches to two or even three of the striatal

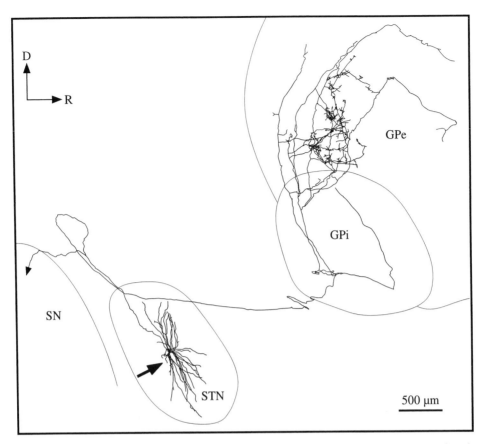

FIGURE 3.5. Camera lucida reconstruction on the sagittal plane of a biotin dextran amine (BDA)-injected subthalamic nucleus (STN) neuron *(arrow)* projecting to the external and internal segments of the globus pallidus (GPe and GPi) and the pars reticulata of the substantia nigra (SNr). Note the profuse arborization in the GPe and the long dendrites covering a large portion of the STN.

recipient structures (GPe, GPi, and SNr). This high degree of collateralization allows striatal neurons to send efferent copies of the information to virtually all striatal targets, a notion that is difficult to reconcile with the current dual model of the basal ganglia.

In the current model, the GPe is considered as a simple relay in the indirect pathway. This view is no longer tenable in view of the data shown earlier, which reveal that the GPe projects to virtually all components of the basal ganglia, including the striatum and the GPi/SNr, through a highly collateralized neuronal system (10,11). Through its direct monosynaptic inhibitory projection to the GPi/SNr, the GPe can markedly alter the functional state of the output structures of the basal ganglia and, as such, must be considered an important integrative structure inserted between the input and output structures of the basal ganglia (12,13). Furthermore, the GPe is likely to be part of a novel disynaptic indirect pathway (striatum-GPe-GPi/SNr), whose activation would reinforce the effect of the postulated trisynaptic indirect pathway (striatum-GPe-STN-GPi/SNr) on basal ganglia output structures.

Although the powerful excitatory influence of the STN on GPi neurons is well established, the common belief that

this effect is a direct function of the level of activity of the GPe appears to be an oversimplification (14–18). As shown earlier, the STN projects to almost all basal ganglia components, including the striatum and the GPe, and it is, in fact, reciprocally linked to the GPe and the striatum. In turn, the STN receives multiple inputs from structures as widely distributed as the cerebral cortex, the SNc, the dorsal raphe nucleus, the PPN, and the centromedian/parafascicular thalamic complex (12,13). Thus, the functional state of STN neurons at any time is likely to be the result of complex neuronal interplay among all these various excitatory and inhibitory influences.

Several important connections have also been left out of the current scheme of the basal ganglia organization. Such is the case for the descending projections of the GPi to the PPN. The data summarized earlier reveal that the principal axonal branches of the GPi projection neurons are those that descend within the brainstem, whereas the GPi innervation of the thalamus is made up of thin collaterals that detach from these thicker descending fibers. The GPi descending fibers arborize principally in the PPN, which projects back to the GPi, STN, and SNc (12,13). The finding that GPi neurons send efferent copies of the information

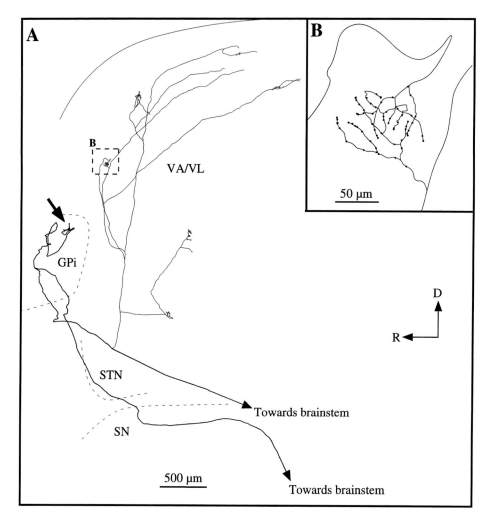

FIGURE 3.6. A: Diagram illustrating in the sagittal plane the course of a single axon of a biotin dextran amine (BDA)-injected neuron of the internal segment of the globus pallidus (GPi) *(arrow)* that branches to the brainstem and thalamus. **B:** High-magnification view of one of the many small terminal fields that characterize pallidothalamic axons *(rectangle* in **A**). VA/VL, ventral anterior/ventral lateral thalamic nuclei.

to premotor neurons located in the thalamus and brainstem could have important functional implications, particularly in respect to dystonia and disturbances of oculomotor movements. The thalamostriatal projections have also been largely ignored, even though these axons arborize densely within the entire striatum (12). Also neglected are the dopaminergic fibers that arborize directly in the STN and the GPi, as well as dopamine that is released within the SNr through the dendrites of SNc neurons (19). This extrastriatal dopamine could directly modulate the activity of the two output structures of the basal ganglia, as well as the STN that drives them, with all three structures expressing D1 dopamine receptors. Extrastriatal dopamine should be taken into account in any model that aims at explaining the pathophysiology of PD.

We believe that the basal ganglia should be viewed as a widely distributed neural network whose individual elements are endowed with a highly patterned set of collaterals whereby each basal ganglia component can interact with

another. The elucidation of this complex microcircuitry is a prerequisite for understanding how cortical information flows through the basal ganglia, particularly in respect to the spatiotemporal sequence of neural events that underlies both normal and abnormal motor behavior.

ACKNOWLEDGMENTS

This research was supported by grant MT-5781 of the Medical Research Council of Canada. Dr. Fumi Sato was on leave of absence from the Department of Anatomy, Faculty of Medicine, Tokyo Medical and Dental University, Tokyo.

REFERENCES

1. Laitinen LV, Bergenheim AT, Hariz MI. Leksell's posteroventral pallidotomy in the treatment of Parkinson's disease. *J Neurosurg* 1992;76:53–61.

2. Limousin P, Pollack P, Benazzouz A, et al. Effect on parkinsonian signs and symptoms of bilateral subthalamic stimulation. *Lancet* 1995;345:91–95.

3. Lozano AM, Lang AE, Galvez-Jimenez N, et al. Effects of GPi pallidotomy on motor function in Parkinson's disease. *Lancet* 1995;346:1383–1387.

4. Baron MS, Vitek JL, Bakay RAE, et al. Treatment of advanced Parkinson's disease by GPi pallidotomy: 1 year pilot-study results. *Ann Neurol* 1996;40:355–3366.

5. Penney JB, Young AB. Speculation on the functional anatomy of basal ganglia disorders. *Annu Rev Neurosci* 1983;6:73–94.

6. Alexander GE, DeLong MR, Strick PL. Parallel organization of functionally segregated circuits linking basal ganglia and cortex. *Annu Rev Neurobiol* 1986;9:357–381.

7. Albin RL, Young AB, Penney JB. The functional anatomy of basal ganglia disorders. *Trends Neurosci* 1989;12:366–375.

8. DeLong MR. Primate model of movement disorders of basal ganglia origin. *Trends Neurosci* 1990;13:281–859.

9. Pinault D. A novel single-cell staining procedure performed *in vivo* under electrophysiological control: morpho-functional features of juxtacellularly labeled thalamic cells and other neurons with biocytin or neurobiotin. *J Neurosci Methods* 1996;65: 113–136.

10. Parent A, Charara A, Pinault D. Single striatofugal axons arborizing in both pallidal segments and in the substantia nigra in primates. *Brain Res* 1995;698:280–284.

11. Kawaguchi Y, Wilson CL, Emson PC. Projection subtypes of rat neostriatal matrix cells revealed by intracellular injection of biocytin. *J Neurosci* 1990;10:3421–3438.

12. Parent A, Hazrati, LN. Functional anatomy of the basal ganglia. I. The cortico-basal ganglia-thalamo-cortical loop. *Brain Res Rev* 1995;20:91–127.

13. Parent A, Hazrati, LN. Functional anatomy of the basal ganglia. II. The place of subthalamic nucleus and external pallidum in basal ganglia circuitry. *Brain Res Rev* 1995;20:128–154.

14. Hassani OK, Mouroux M, Féger J. Increased subthalamic neuronal activity after nigral dopamine lesion independent of disinhibition via the globus pallidus. *Neuroscience* 1996;72: 105–115.

15. Féger J. Updating the functional model of the basal ganglia. *Trends Neurosci* 1997;20:152–153.

16. Levy R, Hazrati LN, Herrero MT, et al. Re-evaluation of the functional anatomy of the basal ganglia in normal and parkinsonian states. *Neuroscience* 1997;76:335–343.

17. Vila M, Levy R, Herrero MT, et al. Consequences of nigrostriatal denervation on the functioning of the basal ganglia in human and nonhuman primates: an *in situ* hybridization study of cytochrome oxidase subunit I. *J Neurosci* 1997;17:765–773.

18. Parent A, Cicchetti F. The current model of the basal ganglia organization under scrutiny. *Mov Disord* 1998;13:199–202.

19. Cossette M, Lévesque M, Parent A. Extrastriatal dopaminergic innervation of the human basal ganglia. *Neurosci Res* 1999;34:51–54.

Surgery for Parkinson's Disease and Movement Disorders,
edited by J.K. Krauss, J. Jankovic, and R.G. Grossman.
Lippincott Williams & Wilkins, Philadelphia © 2001.

4

BASAL GANGLIA MOTOR CONTROL BEFORE AND AFTER SURGERY

JONATHAN W. MINK

The basal ganglia are thought to act in concert with cerebral cortical mechanisms in the control of movement. A significant role of basal ganglia circuits in motor control has been supported historically by several lines of evidence. These include the strong temporal correlation between basal ganglia neuronal discharge patterns and movement, the movement deficits caused experimentally by basal ganglia lesions in nonhuman primates, and the various movement disorders associated with diseases that affect the basal ganglia. More recently, investigators have demonstrated that basal ganglia circuits are involved in aspects of behavior that are not simply motor. Despite the more expanded modern view of the basal ganglia, it is clear that a major function of the basal ganglia is motor (1,2).

What is the motor function of the basal ganglia? Several hypotheses appear to be competing, but they may be complementary. Indeed, there is likely to be participation of the basal ganglia in several different motor functions by virtue of basal ganglia outputs going separately to motor and premotor areas of cerebral cortex (3). In this chapter, the normal motor functions of the basal ganglia are discussed first, followed by a review of motor control in basal ganglia diseases before and after surgical procedures for movement disorders. Finally, the implications of surgery for movement disorders for understanding basal ganglia motor control are discussed.

BASAL GANGLIA NEURONAL ACTIVITY DURING MOVEMENT

DeLong was the first to demonstrate that neuronal activity in the globus pallidus (GP) and striatum correlates with movement, thus providing direct evidence of a motor function of the basal ganglia (4). Since that pioneering work, many investigators have worked to define specifically what

aspects of movement basal ganglia neurons code. The baseline discharge rates, movement-related activity patterns, and the timing of movement-related activity of basal ganglia neurons have provided important clues to understanding basal ganglia motor function.

Striatum

Striatal neurons active in relation to limb movement are located in the putamen (5,6). Movement-related neurons in the putamen are organized somatotopically with the face represented ventromedially, the leg dorsolaterally, and the arm in between in the caudal two-thirds of the putamen (5). Most striatal neurons have low baseline discharge rates of 0.1 to 1 spike per second. When movement direction is dissociated from the pattern of muscle activity, 50% of movement-related putamen neurons fire in relation to direction, and 25% fire in relation to the muscle pattern (7,8). About 40% of movement-related putamen neurons also have somatosensory responses, most of which are related to joint rotation. Correlation of putamen discharge with physical parameters of movement (e.g., velocity, amplitude, force, position, acceleration) has not been demonstrated. Although most putamen cells recorded in movement tasks are "movement-related," 23% to 33% discharge in relation to movement preparation or "set" (9–11). When movement direction is the instructed variable, 50% to 79% of set neurons fire in relation to the intended direction of movement. Putamen neurons with set-related activity are located, on average, anterior to those with movement-related activity in regions that receive input from the prefrontal area, the premotor area, and the supplementary motor area (SMA), rather than from motor cortex (12,13).

Striatal neurons active in relation to eye movements are located in a longitudinal zone in the central part of the caudate nucleus (14). This region receives input from the frontal and supplementary cortical eye fields. Saccade-related neurons have broad movement fields, most of which are located in the contralateral visual field. Just as some putamen neurons discharge in relation to set in limb

J. W. Mink: Department of Neurology, University of Rochester School of Medicine and Dentistry, Rochester, New York 14642.

movement tasks, some caudate neurons have set-related discharge in eye movement tasks (14). The activity of these set-related neurons relates to the direction of the upcoming eye movement.

The timing of neuronal activity in relation to limb or eye movements is important to understanding the function of those neurons in the production of movement. In the putamen, most movement-related activity is late, occurring on average after the onset of muscle activity responsible for producing the movement (7,8). When compared with activity in motor cortex and the SMA, putamen movement-related neurons were found to discharge on average 56 milliseconds after motor cortex and 80 milliseconds after SMA. The timing of set-related activity in putamen is also later than that in motor cortex and the SMA (9,15). For eye movements, the timing of saccade-related caudate discharge precedes saccade onset (14). Saccade-related discharge in the caudate occurs after saccade-related activity in cortical saccade areas (frontal and supplementary eye field) (16,17). The late timing of striatal discharge in relation to movement and in relation to discharge in related cortical areas suggests that the striatum is not primarily involved in the initiation of movement. Instead, it receives information from cortical areas that are responsible for movement generation and may use that information for facilitation or scaling of the cortically initiated movement.

Subthalamic Nucleus

Neurons in the subthalamic nucleus (STN) are tonically active, with average baseline discharge rates of about 20 spikes per second (18). They are organized somatotopically with the lower extremity represented dorsally and the face and eyes represented ventrally (18,19). Most STN neurons increase their discharge rate in relation to eye or limb movement (19,20). For limb movements, most STN movement-related neurons have signals related to movement direction (20,21). Little is known about whether STN neurons discharge in relation to movement parameters or whether they have set-related activity. The timing of STN activity is near the onset of limb movement, but it is late relative to motor cortex and electromyography (EMG) activity (20,21).

Globus Pallidus Pars Interna

The GP pars interna (GPi) is the principal basal ganglia output for limb movement. Neurons in GPi fire tonically at 60 to 80 spikes per second in monkeys maintaining a neutral limb position (22,23). The discharge of many GPi neurons is related to movement direction (24,25). However, for most GPi neurons, discharge is not well correlated with other physical parameters of movement including joint position, force production, movement amplitude, or movement velocity (24,26). Few GPi neurons have activity correlated

with the pattern of muscle activity (23,24). The discharge of GPi neurons is not exclusively related to any one movement mode such as self-paced versus visually guided, ramp versus ballistic, or self-initiated versus externally cued (22,27). Approximately 70% of arm movement–related GPi neurons increase activity and 30% decrease activity from this tonic baseline during movement (23,24,26,28). Because the output from GPi is inhibitory, the large proportion of activity increases during movement translates to broad inhibition of thalamic and brainstem targets with more focal facilitation during movement.

Like striatum, some GPi neurons have set-related activity (29,30). In a reaching task (29), 24% of GP neurons were best related to set and 46% were best related to movement, and many neurons had more than one type of response. In that study, GPi neurons were not considered separately from GP pars externa (GPe) neurons. Most GP neurons responded to electrical stimulation of more than one area of cortex, but most set-related neurons responded to prefrontal and premotor cortex stimulation, and most movement-related neurons responded to premotor and motor cortex stimulation.

The timing of movement-related GPi activity is late compared with the activation of agonist muscles. The average onset of GPi activity is after the onset of EMG but before the onset of movement (23,24,26,28). The tendency is for GPi movement-related increases to occur earlier than decreases (21,28), and this probably reflects the faster speed of the excitatory pathway from cortex to GP through the STN compared with the slower inhibitory pathway from cortex to GP through the striatum (2). The late timing of GPi movement-related activity suggests that the output of the basal ganglia is unlikely to initiate movement.

Some GPi neurons have discharge related to specific components in a sequence of movements. In a task with a sequence of two movements, most GP (GPe and GPi together) neurons had a burst of activity after the onset of the first movement and a second burst after the onset of the second movement (31). However, 33% of GP neurons had an additional burst *preceding* the second movement. In monkeys trained to push buttons in a remembered sequence, about 10% of task-related GP neurons (GPi and GPe were not distinguished) discharged in relation to the specific sequence that was to be performed (32). In a similar task, 8% of SMA neurons had similar sequence-selective discharge (33), but the relative timing of the two areas has not been compared.

Substantia Nigra Pars Reticulata

Substantia nigra pars reticulata (SNr) neurons related to saccadic eye movements are tonically active (34). Unlike GPi neurons during limb movements, virtually all saccade-related SNr neurons decrease activity during the eye movement (35). One-third of SNr cells have activity related to saccades to a visual target. Another one-third of SNr cells have activity related to saccades to a remembered target location (35). SNr neurons that are related to saccades project to the superior colliculus, where they inhibit their targets (36). During saccades, SNr activity change occurs after that in the superior colliculus, a structure that is known to be involved in the initiation of saccades. Thus, for eye movements as well as limb movements, the basal ganglia output acts after other structures initiate movement.

Globus Pallidus Pars Externa

Two types of neurons have been described in GPe based on their baseline activity patterns (4). Most fire at a high frequency (70 spikes per second) that is interrupted with long pauses. Fewer of these neurons fire at a low frequency (10 spikes per second on average) and have frequent spontaneous bursts of activity. Although the baseline discharge patterns in GPe differ from those in GPi, the activity during movement is remarkably similar in the two structures. GPe neurons change activity in relation to limb movement, and for most, these changes are an increase in activity (23,24,28). As in GPi, the coding of movement amplitude, velocity, muscle length, and force is weak in GPe (24,26). Individual GPe neurons may have a preferential relation to one movement mode or movement in a particular context, but overall there is no exclusive activity of GPe in relation to one mode or context. (22,26). The timing of movement-related activity in GPe is late compared with the onset of EMG findings (21,24).

The similarity between GPe and GPi movement-related activity probably reflects the similarity of their inputs. However, their outputs are different: GPe sends inhibitory projections to STN and GPi. It is surprising that most neurons in both GPe and GPi increase because GPe inhibits GPi both directly and indirectly through STN. The similarity of movement-related discharge patterns suggests that GPe activity modulates or focuses GPi activity, rather than being a primary determinant of GPi activity. The specific anatomic relationship among individual GPe and GPi neurons with similar discharge characteristics is not known.

Substantia Nigra Pars Compacta

The striking movement deficits of parkinsonism follow destruction of the SN pars compacta (SNc), yet the discharge of neurons in this structure does not correlate with limb or eye movements (37). SNc neurons fire about 2 Hz at baseline and change activity in relation to sensory stimuli with behavioral significance. The activity of SNc neurons changes in relation to stimuli that predict the attainment of reward (38). Schultz and colleagues showed that the addition of earlier cues that predict the availability of reward leads to earlier discharge of SNc neurons as the significance of those cues is learned (39). During the learning of a new task, 25% of SNc neurons fired shortly after reward delivery, but after the task

was learned, only 9% fired after reward. Conversely, SNc neurons did not respond to trigger stimuli before their significance was learned, but during learning and after the task was learned, nearly 50% responded to instructional cues and trigger stimuli. These data suggest that activity of SNc neurons correlates with the earliest stimulus that reliably predicts the availability of reward. Through the action of dopamine on striatal neurons, SNc neurons can modify the response of striatal neurons to cortical input such that patterns of striatal activity that correlate with task performance resulting in reward are strengthened (2).

Summary

In summary, neuronal activity in most basal ganglia nuclei correlates with movement, with the notable exception of SNc. Movement-related neurons in striatum, STN, GP, and SNr are arranged somatotopically. Neurons in the striatum are quiet at rest and increase during movement. Neurons in the STN are tonically active and increase during movement. Based on the known anatomy (see Chapters 2 and 3), this means that GPi neurons receive a widespread, tonically active excitatory input with phasic increases from STN and a focused, intermittent phasic inhibitory input from striatum. Neurons in GPi and SNr are tonically active; 70% of GPi neurons increase and 30% decrease activity during limb movement. SNr neurons that are related to saccadic eye movements decrease activity during the movement. Basal ganglia neurons do not consistently code parameters of movement, nor do they code muscle activity patterns, but they do code movement direction. Most neurons in SNc discharge in relation to reward and behaviorally relevant stimuli, but not in relation to movement. The timing of activity change in the basal ganglia is late (Table 4.1). Basal ganglia neurons with movement-related discharge before the onset of movement, but after motor cortex and agonist muscles are active. Neurons with set-related discharge are active after neurons with set-related discharge in motor and supplementary motor cortex. These findings suggest that set-related and movement-related activity does not originate in the basal ganglia and thus makes it unlikely that the basal ganglia are primarily involved in the initiation of movement.

TABLE 4.1. TIMING OF BASAL GANGLIA MOVEMENT-RELATED ACTIVITY

Structure	Time before Movement	Time before Muscle Activity
Supplementary motor area	150 msec	
Premotor cortex	130–150 ms	
Cerebellar dentate nucleus	70 ms	29–39 ms
Motor cortex	45–80 ms	14–23 ms
Putamen	20 ms	50 ms after
Subthalamic nucleus	0–50 ms	
Globus pallidus pars interna	30 ms	60 ms after

MOVEMENT DEFICITS ASSOCIATED WITH EXPERIMENTAL FOCAL BASAL GANGLIA LESIONS

Experimental focal lesions in the basal ganglia result in deficits of voluntary movements, involuntary movements, or both. Some older studies concluded that various basal ganglia lesions caused little or no disruption of movement (1), but studies done since the 1970s have reported consistent deficits. These studies are reviewed briefly. A comprehensive review of movement deficits occurring after specific basal ganglia lesions is beyond the scope of this chapter. For a more detailed discussion of movement deficits after basal ganglia lesions, see Mink (2).

Striatum

Lesions in the striatum produce variable results that depend in part on the location of the lesion, in part on the lesion method, and in part on what is measured. Lesions in the putamen are more likely to produce movement deficits than are lesions of the caudate nucleus. Large bilateral electrolytic lesions of the putamen of monkeys result in a parkinsonian syndrome with paucity of movement, severe slowness of movement bilaterally, and postural abnormalities with a loss of righting responses (40). The postural abnormalities include marked flexion of the trunk and extremities, forced grasping, and overactive tonic neck reflexes. Injection of the γ-aminobutyric acid (GABA$_a$) agonist muscimol into the physiologically identified "arm" area of putamen in monkeys causes decreased movement amplitude with cocontraction of agonist and antagonist muscles in visually guided arm movements (41). The cocontraction is present both during maintained posture and during movement. Despite the cocontraction, there appeared to be a period of normal suppression of antagonist EMG during the initial agonist burst, a finding suggesting that the cocontraction was not primarily the result of a loss of reciprocal inhibition. Despite the movement deficit, reaction time is normal. Inactivation of putamen with muscimol has also been shown to impair partially the learning or retention of sequential movements (42).

Subthalamic Nucleus

Monkeys with electrolytic or pharmacologic lesions of STN have involuntary movements of the contralateral arm and leg that are similar to those seen in human patients with STN damage (43,44). Commonly, the chorea or hemiballism resulting from STN lesions involves the lower extremities more than the upper extremities and can persist for days to months. Monkeys with hemiballism are said to be able to make normal voluntary movements (44), but these have not been measured. Hemiballism or hemichorea can also be produced by injecting bicuculline into STN (45). This is para-

doxic because bicuculline is a GABA antagonist and would be expected to cause disinhibition (activation) of STN. However, the behavioral effects are similar to those of STN lesions. Studies with 2-deoxyglucose (2-DG) have shown decreased uptake, presumably reflecting decreased synaptic input, in both segments of GP after bicuculline injection into STN (46), a finding suggesting that the bicuculline causes decreased activity in STN, possibly by inducing depolarization block.

After STN lesion or bicuculline injection into STN, decreased activity occurs in GPe and GPi. This has been shown both with 2-DG autoradiography and with single-unit recording. As noted earlier, Mitchell and colleagues showed that injection of bicuculline into STN unilaterally produces hemiballism or hemichorea that is associated with decreased 2-DG uptake in GPe and GPi (46). There is also decreased uptake in the thalamic targets of GPi. These results were interpreted as showing decreased excitatory input from STN to GPi leading to decreased GPi inhibition of thalamus. However, it is not known whether the changes in 2-DG uptake reflect the cause or the effect of the dyskinesia after STN inactivation; the 2-DG changes may reflect the underlying pathophysiology of chorea or they may be secondary to the increased movements of the animal. After excitotoxic lesions of the STN were induced in monkeys, the activity of both GPe and GPi neurons was decreased during active holding of elbow position as compared with normal subjects (47). The recordings in STN-lesioned monkeys were done after the involuntary movements subsided, so these data do not prove that hemiballism itself is associated with decreased activity in GPi. In fact, these data suggest that hemiballism is not the result of tonic reduction of GPi activity alone, because the tonic reduction remained after the movements ceased. Indeed, hemiballism can be abolished by GPi lesions that eliminate GPi output (48,49). It seems more likely that hemiballism results from an abnormal pattern (e.g., bursting) of GPi activity, rather than a tonically decreased GPi output.

Globus Pallidus Pars Interna

Large bilateral lesions of GP cause slow movement with abnormal postures and increased tone (50). Similar abnormalities have been seen after carbon monoxide or carbon disulfide poisoning, which results in neuronal death in GPi and SNr (51). In these older studies, the large bilateral lesions often involved structures in addition to GP. However, more recent studies with unilateral lesions restricted to GP have shown clear motor deficits. Unilateral combined lesions of GPe and GPi result in slowness of movement but normal reaction time (52–54). Most studies also showed cocontraction of agonist and antagonist muscles with a flexor bias.

Lesions restricted to GPi result in slowness of movement of the contralateral limbs with abnormal cocontraction and flexed posture, but normal reaction time (53,55,56). GPi

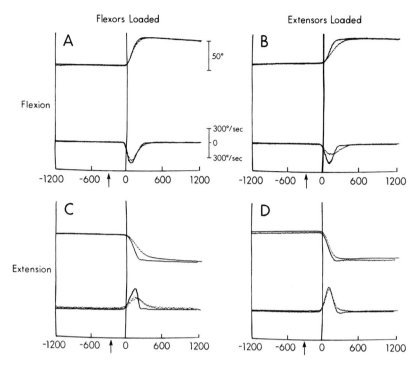

FIGURE 4.1. Slowing of wrist movement after a lesion of the globus pallidus pars interna (GPi). **A** and **D** show movements made by turning on the loaded muscle to make the movement (flexion with flexors loaded and extension with extensors loaded). **B** and **C** show movements made by turning off the loaded muscle to make the movement (flexion with extensors loaded and extension with flexors loaded). The **upper trace** in each graph shows wrist position; the **lower trace** shows wrist velocity. The *solid traces* show control trials; the *dotted traces* show trials 24 days after a kainic acid lesion of the GPi. (From Mink JW, Thach WT. Basal ganglia motor control. III. Pallidal ablation: normal reaction time, muscle cocontraction, and slow movement. *J Neurophysiol* 1991;65: 330–351, with permission.)

lesions cause greater impairment when a movement is made by turning off the active antagonist muscle than when it is made by turning on the agonist (Fig. 4.1) (53). The co-contraction, the inability to turn off the active antagonist, and normal reaction time suggest that the GPi acts not to initiate movement, but to prevent unwanted muscle activity from interfering with voluntary movement initiated by other structures (2,53,57).

Investigators have suggested that reduced activity in GPi is the underlying mechanism of chorea and hemiballism that is seen after ablation of the excitatory input from STN (45,58,59). However, chorea or hemiballism has not been reported after experimental ablation or inactivation of GPi. Although chorea and hemiballism may result from diminished excitation of GPi by STN, elimination of GPi activity does not produce these movements. As noted earlier, ablation of GPi eliminates choreic dyskinesia after STN lesions in monkeys and people and may eliminate choreic dopa-induced dyskinesia in Parkinson's disease (PD). One way to explain these findings is to postulate that partial reduction of GPi activity causes target neurons in the thalamus and brainstem to become unstable and to fire in bursts, ultimately leading to the bursts of muscle activity that underlie chorea. Elimination of GPi activity results in a more stable state of the thalamic and brainstem target neurons.

Substantia Nigra Pars Reticulata

Inactivation of SNr causes eye movement deficits. Injection of muscimol into the lateral SNr causes involuntary saccades and an inability to maintain visual fixation (60). After SNr inactivation, voluntary saccades to the contralateral visual field are increased in amplitude, and saccades to the ipsilateral field are decreased. When the monkeys make spontaneous eye movements after SNr inactivation, the eyes tend to assume an abnormal position in the contralateral field. Thus, just as GPi inactivation results in an inability to inhibit unwanted limb and trunk muscle activity, SNr inactivation results in an inability to inhibit unwanted eye movements (60).

Globus Pallidus Pars Externa

Few reports of lesions restricted to GPe have been published. Injection of muscimol into GPe at one site in one monkey resulted in abnormally flexed posture of the arm with agonist-antagonist cocontraction (41). These results are similar to the results of combined GPe and GPi lesions (52,54) and also lesions of GPi alone (53,55,56). Injection of the bicuculline into GPe produces chorea that is similar to that seen with STN lesions (61,62). Investigators have thought that the mechanism of the chorea after bicuculline injection in GPe is disinhibition of GPe, which leads to inhibition of STN. Thus, when chorea is produced by injecting bicuculline into GPe, 2-DG activity is increased in STN and is decreased in GPi (62). As expected, most GPe neurons increase activity after injection of bicuculline, but unexpectedly, most GPi neurons also increase activity after the bicuculline injection (61). In addition, many GPe and GPi neurons develop abnormal bursts and pauses in association with the dyskinesia. These results suggest that chorea results from abnormal patterns of activity in GPi and not from globally decreased GPi output.

Substantia Nigra Pars Compacta

Experimental lesions of SNc in monkeys cause parkinsonism that is an excellent model of human PD. Currently, the most commonly used method for lesioning SNc dopamine neurons is the neurotoxin 1-methyl-4-phenyl-1,2,5,6-tetrahydropyridine (MPTP). MPTP produces parkinsonism in several species of monkeys (63–66). The parkinsonism in MPTP-affected monkeys has been associated with nearly complete degeneration of dopamine neurons in the SNc and adjacent ventral tegmental area with variable degeneration in the locus caeruleus (64). Primates given MPTP unilaterally develop transient dystonia before the onset of chronic parkinsonism (67). However, to date, there have been no quantitative studies of movement physiology in this animal model of dystonia.

Monkeys with MPTP-associated parkinsonism have both slow movement and prolonged reaction times (68). The slowing of movement may be accompanied by cocontraction of agonist and antagonist muscles (63). The increased reaction time is associated with increased latency from the cue to move to the onset of EMG activity showing that the deficit was not just one of muscle contraction rate. The reaction times tend to recover over time, but the slowness of movement does not improve (68). When monkeys with MPTP-associated parkinsonism were given levodopa, the reaction times, movement speed, and rigidity improved (66,68).

The MPTP model of PD has been useful for determining changes in the physiology of downstream structures that are associated with the parkinsonism. These results are reviewed extensively elsewhere (45,58,59). MPTP-affected monkeys have increased 2-DG activity in GPe, the pedunculopontine area, and ventral anterior/ventral lateral thalamus with slightly increased activity in GPi and markedly reduced activity in STN (69). Because 2-DG uptake is thought to correlate with the activity of nerve terminals, uptake in a structure presumably reflects the activity of the afferents to that structure. Accordingly, the pattern of 2-DG uptake in the MPTP-affected monkey was interpreted as reflecting increased striatal inhibition of GPe with resulting disinhibition of STN and excessive activation of GPi (45). This scheme is supported by findings of increased levels of met-enkephalin immunoreactivity in the striatum and increased met-enkephalin mRNA levels in GPe of MPTP-affected monkeys (70) and in 6-hydroxydopamine treated rats (71). Investigators have suggested that increased striatal inhibition of GPe and decreased striatal inhibition of GPi are mediated by the differential effect of dopamine on these two pathways.

Electrophysiologic evidence has tended to support the idea that parkinsonism is associated with decreased activity in GPe and increased activity in STN, GPi, and SNr (72–75). However, some monkeys with parkinsonism after MPTP administration have no significant change in the average discharge rate of GPi neurons (73). GPe and GPi neurons also have abnormally increased responses to somatosensory stimuli, passive limb movement, and electrical stimulation of the striatum (73,76). A test of the hypothesis that parkinsonism is associated with decreased activity of GPe and increased activity of GPi and STN comes with focal lesions of the presumed overactive structures. Ablation or inactivation of STN in MPTP-affected monkeys reverses the symptoms of MPTP-associated parkinsonism (77, 78). Similarly, blockade of the excitatory input from STN to GPi with kynurenate reverses parkinsonism in the MPTP-affected monkey (79). Symptomatic improvement after STN inactivation is not accompanied by normalization of baseline discharge in GPi (78). This finding suggests that increased tonic discharge in GPi is not of primary importance in the pathophysiology of parkinsonism.

Abnormally increased GPi activity should lead to excessive inhibition of thalamic targets and reduced activity in motor cortical areas. In parkinsonian monkeys, motor cortex neurons have reduced activity in relation to movement, and the timing of the movement-related changes is more variable, but there is not a consistent delay in the onset of motor cortex activity (80–82). These results are consistent with excessive inhibition from GPi to thalamus, which would be reflected in decreased excitability of motor cortex. However, dopamine input to motor cortex also occurs (83), and the abnormal motor cortex discharge may result from the loss of that input in addition to the abnormal GPi discharge.

Overall, the evidence generally supports the model that abnormally increased GPi discharge contributes to the pathophysiology of parkinsonism (58,59). However, the findings that average baseline discharge of GPi neurons in some parkinsonian monkeys is normal and that reversal of parkinsonism by STN is not accompanied by normalization of GPi activity suggest that the model is incomplete. Furthermore, little is known of the change in movement-related STN or GP activity in parkinsonism. It also appears that abnormal temporal patterns of neuronal discharge may be more important than abnormal tonic discharge rate (49,73,76).

Summary

In summary, damage to any basal ganglia structure may cause slowness of voluntary movement, involuntary movements, involuntary postures, or a combination of these. Damage to the striatum causes voluntary movement to be slow and may produce involuntary movements or postures, depending on the mechanism of damage. Damage to the STN causes large-amplitude involuntary limb movements. Damage to the GP causes slowness of movement, abnormal postures, and difficulty in relaxing muscles, but it does not delay movement initiation. Damage to SNr causes abnormal eye movements, but it does not delay the initiation of eye movements. Damage to SNc causes parkinsonism with tremor at rest, slowness of movement, rigidity, and postural instability.

SPECIFIC MOTOR DEFICITS ASSOCIATED WITH HUMAN MOVEMENT DISORDERS

Most studies investigating the effect of surgical therapies for movement disorders have used clinical rating scales to evaluate the outcome. Whereas the commonly used rating scales have been validated and proven reliable, they do not provide quantitative measures of voluntary movement. Mechanisms of voluntary movement and posture control have been studied extensively in PD, but less so in dystonia and chorea. These mechanisms have now been studied after surgical treatment by a few groups. In this section, the motor physiology of PD, dystonia, and chorea will be reviewed. In the following section, the effect of surgical treatments on motor physiology will be discussed.

Parkinson's Disease

The main symptoms of PD include (a) tremor at rest, (b) slowness of movement (bradykinesia), (c) paucity of movement (akinesia), (d) muscular rigidity, and (e) postural instability. Although these cardinal signs are present to some degree in most patients with advanced PD, considerable variability exists among individual patients. Some patients may have severe bradykinesia with minimal rigidity, others may have the opposite, and still others may have both equally. Although it is well established that PD results from degeneration of SNc neurons that provide dopamine innervation to the striatum, the different manifestations of PD may reflect differential involvement of separate basal ganglia circuits (84–86). There also may be involvement of neural systems (noradrenergic locus coeruleus neurons, cholinergic pedunculopontine neurons, dopaminergic mesocortical and mesolimbic neurons) in addition to the nigrostriatal dopamine system. Thus, some of the motor abnormalities in PD may not reflect nigrostriatal dopamine depletion alone. Most physiologic studies have focused on individual manifestations of PD; few have investigated the degree to which common or separate mechanisms may cause these manifestations.

Parkinsonian Tremor

The pathophysiology of *tremor* in PD is poorly understood. It is generally agreed that parkinsonian tremor largely results from central tremor generators, possibly located in the thalamus (87, 88). Evidence indicates that peripheral afferent activity can modulate and even entrain tremor in PD (88). However, parkinsonian tremor persists after deafferentation (89). Thus, although there may be some modulation of PD tremor by muscle afferent activity, central mechanisms are responsible for its production. One hypothesis states that parkinsonian tremor is caused by hyperpolarization of thalamic neurons that results in rebound bursting when the resting potential of these neurons returns to baseline (87).

Increased inhibitory output from GP to thalamus in PD could set up such a mechanism. Alternatively, abnormal high-frequency periodic GPi activity could be transformed in the thalamus to the lower-frequency periodicity of parkinsonian tremor (73). The most effective site for thalamic stimulation or thalamotomy in the treatment of parkinsonian tremor is the thalamic target of cerebellar, rather than pallidal, efferents. This finding suggests that corticothalamic or cerebellothalamic circuits may participate in the pathophysiology of parkinsonian tremor.

Bradykinesia

It is well known that *slowness of movement* is a hallmark of PD. However, voluntary movements are slow in almost any disease that affects part of the motor system. What distinguishes the different conditions is the quality of the impairment. In PD, patients have slowness and reduced amplitude of individual movements that typically worsen in repetitive movements as the movements progress. The classic example of this is the micrographia of PD in which handwriting can be near normal at the beginning of a line, but the size of letters and the velocity of strokes decrease as the writing continues.

The slowness of movement in PD has been associated with reduced magnitude of agonist muscle activity during movement (90). The reduced agonist amplitude often results in a succession of multiple, small-amplitude submovements instead of a larger-amplitude single movement. In addition to decreased agonist activation, patients often have excessive cocontraction of the antagonist during movement (91) and muscular cocontraction at rest (92). This abnormal cocontraction can combine with the abnormally reduced contraction of the agonist to cause slowing of movement. People with PD are often more impaired when relaxing muscles to reduce force than when activating muscles to generate force (Fig. 4.2) (93–95). Thus, the ability to "turn off" muscles may be more impaired than the ability to "turn on" muscles.

Although PD causes a slowing of movement generally, movement may be more severely impaired when visual cues are absent. People with PD are slower when making self-initiated movements than when making stimulus-triggered movements (96–98). They are also more severely impaired when they are deprived of visual feedback of ongoing movement (99), particularly if they cannot see the moving body part (100). This increased dependence on visual information is often seen clinically as "freezing" when a visual border is approached, improved walking when the patient is given lines to step on, or improved handwriting on lined paper. Why does PD cause more difficulty making movements in the absence of visual feedback? One possible explanation is that the basal ganglia are preferentially involved in the control of self-initiated movements or movements without visual feedback. This concept seems unlikely because movements performed

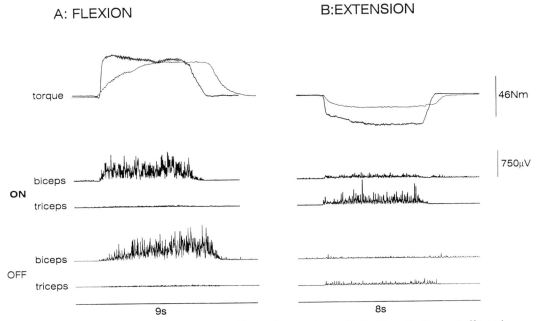

A: FLEXION   B:EXTENSION

FIGURE 4.2. Voluntary isometric elbow flexion in a patient with Parkinson's disease "off" and "on" L-dopa. Torque, biceps, and triceps electromyograms are shown. **A:** Active flexion with active return to baseline force. **B:** Active flexion with passive return to baseline force. Note the delayed relaxation time in the "off" condition. (From Corcos DM, Chen CM, Quinn NP, et al. Strength in Parkinson's disease: relationship to rate of force generation and clinical status. *Ann Neurol* 1996;39:79–88, with permission.)

with visual feedback are also impaired in PD and in animals with basal ganglia lesions. It is also possible that people with PD have an increased dependence on all modalities of feedback to try to compensate for their deficit. When they are deprived of one modality of information, the remaining modalities are insufficient to allow them to compensate.

Several studies have shown that patients with PD have more difficulty performing sequences of movements than individual movements (101,102). When patients with PD disease performed a task involving a grasp and elbow flexion separately, simultaneously, or sequentially, they were slower than healthy individuals in all conditions. However, they were slower on simultaneous and sequential movements than they were on the individual components (101,102). When these patients performed the movements sequentially, there was a greater latency to begin the second movement than in healthy persons. However, other studies have been unable to demonstrate specific deficits in tasks involving movement sequences (103,104). Another study showed that patients with PD were equally slow when they drew the sides of a pentagon sequentially as when they repeatedly drew one side five times, a finding indicating progressive slowing of movement with repetition, but not a specific sequencing deficit (105). The different results among these studies may have been caused by task differences. It is also not known whether sequential movement of a single body part is affected differently from sequential movements across body parts. Even though sequential movements and self-paced movements are most severely impaired in PD, even single stimulus-triggered

movements are slow (90,106). This finding suggests that the fundamental deficit in PD may not be one of sequencing, but that tasks requiring sequential or repetitive movements may exacerbate the deficit.

Akinesia

The *paucity of movement* and "freezing" in PD have been attributed to a defect of movement initiation. Many, but not all, people with PD do have prolonged reaction times in stimulus-triggered movements, a finding indicating that initiation of movement is delayed in some cases (106). However, it is not clear that the delayed initiation results from basal ganglia dysfunction. Instead, the delayed initiation may result from the loss of dopamine input to prefrontal, premotor, or motor cortex (83,107,108). Animals with focal lesions of the dopamine input to prefrontal cortex have prolonged reaction times (109), but animals with lesions of the basal ganglia output (GPi or SNr) usually do not (see earlier). It is also possible that the prolonged reaction time in PD does not result from dysfunction of movement initiatory systems. Muscle activity may begin at the normal time in relation to movement, but the magnitude of the initial muscle activity may not be sufficient to overcome inertial and viscoelastic forces rapidly (106), and the mechanically detected onset of movement is delayed. Alternatively, an inability to inhibit unwanted posture-holding mechanisms may delay the onset of movement because of competition of antagonistic motor mechanisms. In either case, the initiatory commands may be normal, but other factors cause the onset of movement to be delayed.

Rigidity

The *rigidity* of PD has been attributed in part to hyperactivity of the transcortical stretch reflex. When a muscle is stretched during active maintained limb position, two or three identifiable reflex components are seen with EMG (110). The first is a short-latency response that corresponds to the spinal monosynaptic stretch reflex. The second and third reflect a longer-latency polysynaptic reflex that involves motor cortex and possibly other supraspinal mechanisms (111,112). Normally, the transcortical stretch reflex is active to resist displacement from an actively held posture and is inhibited when patients are instructed not to resist the displacement (110). In PD, transcortical stretch reflexes are increased, and there is an inability to suppress them completely in response to instruction (92,110,113). The monosynaptic stretch reflex is normal in PD.

Postural Instability

People with PD have an inability to inhibit long-latency reflexes other than the transcortical stretch reflex. Although it is often stated that PD is accompanied by a loss of postural reflexes, it appears that an inability to *inhibit* long-latency postural reflexes contributes to the postural instability of PD. When healthy persons are subjected to perturbations while they are standing, they have stereotyped patterns of muscle activity in the legs and trunk that maintain upright stance. If these persons then sit down and are subjected to the same perturbation, this activity no longer occurs. By contrast, patients with PD have an inappropriate cocontraction of leg and back muscles in response to perturbation from upright stance (Fig. 4.3). When the same persons are subjected to a perturbation in a sitting position, they continue to have the same pattern of muscle activity (114). Thus, they are not able to inhibit appropriately the postural reflexes that were active during stance. These data, together with the proposed mechanism of rigidity and the finding that many "primitive reflexes" are abnormally active in PD (115), suggest a possible inability to suppress unwanted reflex activity generally.

Gait

The *gait abnormalities* in PD are of several types. These include small steps, diminished armswing, propulsion or retropulsion, freezing, *en bloc* turns, and excessive flexion of the trunk and limbs. The gait abnormalities probably result from the same combination of factors that impair movement of individual limbs (bradykinesia, rigidity, akinesia), in addition to postural instability and difficulty inhibiting postural reflexes, and possibly mechanisms unique to gait. Few quantitative studies of parkinsonian gait have been performed. Kinematic studies have shown that walking velocity is slow and that a short stride length contributes more than decreased cadence (steps per minute) to that slowing

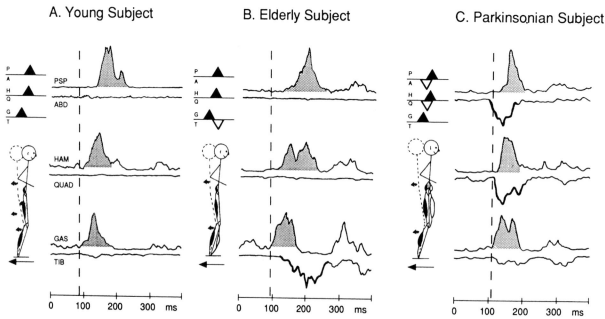

A. Young Subject   **B. Elderly Subject**   **C. Parkinsonian Subject**

FIGURE 4.3. Pattern of muscle activation in response to backward surface translation in young persons **(A)**, normal elderly persons **(B)**, and patients with Parkinson's disease (PD) **(C)**. Note the coactivation of muscles in the patient with PD. ABD, abdominals; GAS, gastrocnemius; HAM, hamstrings, PSP, paraspinous; QUAD, quadriceps; TIB, anterior tibialis. (From Horak FB, Nutt JG, Nashner LM. Postural inflexibility in parkinsonian subjects. *J Neurol Sci* 1992;111:46–58, with permission.)

(116,117). Patients with PD increase their walking speed by increasing cadence rather than stride length (116,117). Preliminary data also show that the increased speed of walking after levodopa treatment is largely the result of increased stride length (118).

Dystonia

Dystonia is a movement disorder characterized by sustained involuntary muscle contraction that results in abnormal postures, often with a twisting character (torsion dystonia). Dystonia can involve individual body parts (focal, segmental, or hemidystonia) or the entire body (generalized dystonia). There have been many fewer studies of motor physiology in dystonia than in PD. Most studies of movement physiology in dystonia have been in people with idiopathic focal or segmental dystonia, but some studies have been conducted in patients with idiopathic generalized dystonia. There is no generally accepted animal model of dystonia, but abnormalities resembling dystonia have been reported after lesions of GPi (53), putamen (40,41), and SNc (67) in monkeys. An interesting animal model of focal dystonia was developed by Byl et al. by "overtraining" monkeys to perform a complex sensory-motor task (119). After thousands of repetitions, the monkeys developed hand cramps with dystonic posturing. The development of dystonic posturing was accompanied by expanded representation of the dystonia digits in somatosensory cortex. A study of human dystonia provided evidence for a similar type of expanded cortical representation of dystonic body parts (120).

Studies of dystonia have revealed abnormal cocontraction of agonist and antagonist muscles at rest that is often exacerbated by movement (121). At rest, the abnormal contractions can be sustained or intermittent. The intermittent contractions usually last 1 to 2 seconds, although some are as short as 100 milliseconds. During voluntary movement, excessive voluntary contractions are seen in muscles that would not normally be active in the task. In addition to the excessive activity of nearby muscles, agonist muscle activity is prolonged (122), and movement-related cortical potentials are reduced just before movement (123). The combination of slight reduction in agonist activity and excessive activity in antagonist muscles causes movement to be slow. As with PD, movement sequences are relatively more severely impaired than are the individual components (124).

In dystonia, the monosynaptic and long-latency stretch reflexes are normal at rapid rates of stretch, but with slower stretches, the long-latency reflex is prolonged compared with the normal state (125). Stretch of one muscle group often results in overflow activation of other muscle groups (121), and investigators have suggested that people with dystonia have impaired reciprocal inhibition on a supraspinal basis (126–128). People with dystonia often have paradoxic activation of a passively shortened muscle (the so-called shortening reaction) (121). Thus, various mechanisms may contribute to

the abnormal muscle activity seen in dystonia. What these mechanisms may have in common is an inability to inhibit unwanted reflex activity in response to stretch. This view is supported by evidence that focal dystonia can be decreased by blocking δ-motor neuron drive to spindles with lidocaine (129).

The data summarized earlier suggest that dystonia results from abnormal basal ganglia function, which, in turn, causes altered regulation of cortical, spinal, and probably brainstem mechanisms. The results are abnormal muscular cocontraction and overflow of activity to muscle adjacent to the prime movers for any given task. Reviews of dystonia (67,130) and of normal basal ganglia function (2) have suggested that abnormality is one of selective activation of desired movements and inhibition of competing motor mechanisms.

Chorea and Ballism

Chorea is characterized by involuntary movements consisting of frequent, brief, sudden, random, twitchlike movements that involve any body part and sometimes resemble fragments of normal voluntary movement. *Ballism* is characterized by larger-amplitude flinging movements of the limbs, most commonly on one side of the body (hemiballism). Although chorea and ballism have been regarding separately in many texts, good evidence indicates that they form a spectrum of dyskinesias with similar underlying anatomic and pathophysiologic mechanisms (45,58,59). Hemiballism most commonly accompanies damage to the STN. Chorea accompanies many different disorders, but the physiology of chorea has been studied mostly in Huntington's disease (HD). In early adult-onset HD, chorea is the predominate abnormality, but as the disease progresses, rigidity, dystonia, and parkinsonism can also occur. Like PD, HD is associated with degeneration of neurons outside the basal ganglia, so it cannot be concluded with certainty that all features of HD result from basal ganglia dysfunction.

In HD, the EMG bursts underlying the choreic movements are sudden, brief, and unpredictable, like the involuntary movements themselves. The EMG bursts vary from less than 50 to 300 milliseconds in duration. The magnitude, duration, and muscle location of bursts vary from moment to moment unpredictably (131). There have been relatively few studies, but investigators have shown that voluntary movements are slow and reaction times are prolonged in HD (132–134). Voluntary movements are accompanied by prolonged agonist and antagonist EMG activity (131). As in PD and dystonia, patients with HD may be more severely impaired when they perform movement sequences than when they perform the individual components (124,134).

In contrast to PD, the long-latency stretch reflex is reduced or absent in HD (135–137). The segmental stretch reflex is normal, but somatosensory-evoked potentials are markedly reduced (136), a finding suggesting that the abnormality lies in supraspinal component of the afferent limb of the long-latency transcortical reflex. Patients with advanced or juvenile-onset HD develop rigidity similar to that in PD (138). However, the studies of long-latency reflexes have all been in people with early HD and not in those with prominent rigidity. Furthermore, people with chorea caused by diseases other than HD have normal long-latency stretch reflexes (135), a finding suggesting that there may be no specific relationship between chorea and long-loop reflexes.

The pathologic hallmark of HD is a marked loss of neurons in the striatum. Medium spiny neurons are most severely affected, and within that population it is the enkephalin-containing neurons that project to GPe that are lost first (139) The substance P–containing medium spiny striatal neurons that project to GPi and SNr are relatively preserved until later in the disease, when rigidity typically appears. This specific pattern of striatal cell loss may explain why experimental lesions of the striatum in monkeys rarely result in chorea, because they would involve both groups of cells. An association of chorea with the loss of GPe-projecting neurons and of rigidity with the loss of both GPe- and GPi-projecting striatal neurons has been a major factor in models of basal ganglia pathophysiology (45,58,59). In these models, loss of striatal inhibition of GPe neurons results in excessive inhibition of STN from GPe and, ultimately, underactivity of GPi and SNr.

Investigators have long recognized that damage to STN by ischemic stroke or hemorrhage results in a bizarre involuntary movement that is characterized by large-amplitude, flinging (ballistic) movements of the contralateral extremities. The movement abnormality is usually present immediately after the lesion and improves over time. The voluntary movements of people with hemiballism have not been studied in detail. Voluntary limb movements are performed with superimposed involuntary movements, but it is not known whether the underlying voluntary movements are impaired. It is also unknown whether there is greater impairment of some types of movement over others. Likewise, whether long-loop reflexes are normal in hemiballism is unknown.

Summary

In summary, basal ganglia movement disorders are associated with difficulty in producing normal voluntary movement and in preventing unwanted movement. Even in PD, which is generally viewed as a disorder with decreased motor output, patients have difficulty in suppressing unwanted excessive motor output. One scheme of basal ganglia function that includes both facilitation of wanted movement and inhibition of unwanted or competing movements is shown in Fig. 4.4 (2). According to this scheme, cerebral cortical mechanisms that are responsible for the generation of movement send corollary signals to striatum and STN. Acting in GPi and SNr, the signal from striatum acts to reduce the inhibitory basal ganglia output and thus to facilitate the desired motor pattern. The signal from STN acts to maintain or

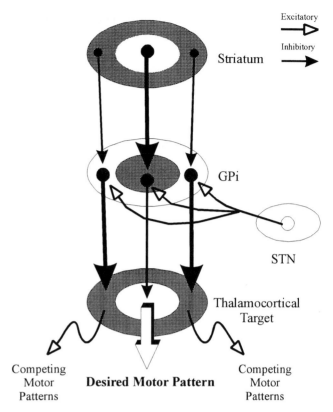

FIGURE 4.4. Focused selection and inhibition of competing motor patterns. During voluntary movement, excitatory subthalamopallidal neurons increase the activity of the pallidal neurons in the territory surrounding a functional center. Inhibitory striatopallidal neurons inhibit the functional center, resulting in a focused output pattern. The pallidal activity changes are conveyed to the targets in the thalamus and pedunculopontine area *(not shown)*, causing disinhibition of neurons involved in the desired motor program and inhibition of surrounding neurons involved in competing motor programs. *Open arrows* indicate excitatory projections; *filled arrows* indicate inhibitory projections. The relative magnitude of activity is represented by line thickness.

increase the inhibitory basal ganglia output of surrounding areas in GPi or SNr and to inhibit potentially competing motor patterns. Dysfunction of either component can contribute to difficulty with movement. Abnormal phasic discharge in either striatal output or the STN output could contribute to phasic involuntary movement such as chorea or dystonia.

MOTOR PHYSIOLOGY AFTER SURGICAL TREATMENT OF MOVEMENT DISORDERS

Subsequent chapters of this book address the individual surgical procedures for treatment of movement disorders and relevant clinical outcome studies. This section focuses on motor physiology and quantitative studies of movement after surgical treatment. Most published studies on surgical treatments have used well-established clinical rating scales, but few have used direct quantification of movement deficits before and after surgical treatment. No quantitative studies of voluntary movement have been performed to date in patients with dystonia, chorea, or hemiballism. Studies have investigated different aspects of movement after pallidotomy, but there are no reports yet of the effect of STN or pallidal stimulation on specific movement tasks. Hence, the emphasis in this section is on PD and *pallidotomy*.

Parkinsonian Tremor

Most studies of pallidotomy for PD report significant and lasting reduction of tremor (140–144). These studies used the Unified Parkinson Disease Rating Scale, which includes a clinical assessment of tremor amplitude and constancy (145). Thus, it is apparent that tremor amplitude is reduced after pallidotomy, but it is not known whether the frequency or response of tremor to peripheral perturbation changes with pallidotomy.

Bradykinesia

Most reports of pallidotomy in PD have shown that bradykinesia improves significantly contralateral to the lesion (140–144). The improvement in bradykinesia has been demonstrated with the Unified Parkinson Disease Rating Scale, which uses repetitive movements of fingers, hands, and feet or with counts of finger tapping in a set time period. More recently, several investigators quantified performance of several different movement tasks and showed that the improvement of bradykinesia after pallidotomy may be specific to certain tasks. Movement time is decreased in the arm contralateral to pallidotomy on simple and choice reaction time tasks, isometric and isotonic ballistic movements (146), and repetitive movements movement between two adjacent targets (147). Similarly, movement time improves in sequential arm movements contralateral to pallidotomy (146,148), with one study showing a bilateral improvement in the latency between the two components of the sequence (148).

Reaching speed was shown to improve after pallidotomy, but there was abnormal patterning of the movement during a reach to grasp objects of differing sizes (149). Performance on the Purdue peg-board task improved in one study (147), but not in another (146). Despite improvements in other tasks, two studies showed no improvement in rhythm, amplitude, or speed of repetitive finger movements (146,148). These studies suggest that the improvement of movement after pallidotomy may be limited to certain types of movement. However, it is also possible that lesion size, lesion location, or both may be important determinants of which types of movement improve.

The quantitative movement studies described earlier evaluated patients after withholding levodopa overnight. At present, no reports exist of the interaction of levodopa and pallidotomy on these tasks. However, one report showed no improvement in "on" levodopa performance of an elbow flexion task after pallidotomy (150). Clinical rating scales have likewise shown little additive effect of levodopa and pallidotomy (143,150). Because clinical signs and symptoms that do not improve with levodopa tend not to improve with pallidotomy (143), these findings suggest that levodopa and pallidotomy affect common mechanisms. However, levodopa remains effective after pallidotomy, so the mechanisms of the two therapies must not be identical.

Akinesia

The effect of pallidotomy on reaction time has been variable. In one study, surgery had no effect on movement initiation in unwarned simple and choice reaction time tasks, but a precued choice reaction time task was slightly improved (146). The slope of the late component of movement-related cortical potentials was increased when the patients performed joystick movements with the hand contralateral to the pallidotomy. Improved reaction time in a paced joystick movements task was accompanied by increased activation of the SMA and dorsal prefrontal cortex (151). Another study showed significant improvement in simple and choice reaction times for the arm contralateral to the pallidotomy (147). No study to date has reported the time to EMG onset as opposed to the time from EMG onset to movement onset. This will be important in assessing changes in central timing after pallidotomy. The freezing phenomenon does not improve significantly after pallidotomy (143), a finding that is relevant to the degree that freezing reflects a deficit of movement initiation. However, freezing is a complex phenomenon that may also involve faulty inhibition of posture-holding mechanisms (2).

Rigidity

Rigidity has been shown to improve after pallidotomy (140–144). Although parkinsonian rigidity is defined clinically, it has been shown to be correlated with increased activity of the long-latency stretch reflex as described earlier. One study evaluated the long-latency stretch reflex after pallidotomy and found a decrease in the amplitude with no change in the spinal stretch reflex (146).

Postural Stability and Gait

The effect of pallidotomy on postural stability and gait has been variable across studies (140–144). Few quantitative studies of postural stability and gait have been conducted, and these have involved small numbers of subjects. Balance was found to be improved after pallidotomy, based on measures of sway in patients standing on a foam surface (152). In a study of multiple tasks involving activities of daily living, it was found that tasks involving standing and walking were more greatly improved than tasks involving limb movement (153). My colleagues and I have shown that stride length and walking speed improve significantly after pallidotomy and that there may be an additive effect of pallidotomy and levodopa (118).

IMPLICATIONS OF BASAL GANGLIA SURGERY FOR BASAL GANGLIA MOTOR CONTROL

The beneficial effects of surgical ablation of GPi or chronic stimulation of STN or GPi are well established and are consistent with the popular models of PD pathophysiology that emphasize increased tonic activity of STN and GPi (58,59). However, some results of surgical treatment are contrary to what would be predicted by the models, and the results of surgical treatment for movement disorders are different from the effects of similar lesions in neurologically normal animals. Understanding the basis for these differences is important for fully understanding normal and abnormal basal ganglia function.

Pallidotomy is especially effective for eliminating dopa-induced dyskinesia (140–144), yet this is opposite to what would be predicted by the models. The models predict that decreased GPi output would be associated with increased and not decreased dyskinesia. However, the reduced dyskinesia is consistent with older data in monkeys showing that dyskinesia resulting from STN lesions is eliminated by GPi lesions (43,154) and a more recent report of hemiballism improving after pallidotomy (155). It also appears that the temporal pattern of GPi discharge may be more important in the pathophysiology of dyskinesia than is the tonic discharge rate. Thus, although the effect of pallidotomy on dopa-induced dyskinesia is contrary to the models, it is consistent with other existing data.

It is more difficult to reconcile the effects of pallidotomy and STN stimulation in PD with the effects of lesions in neurologically normal subjects. As described earlier, GPi lesions in normal monkeys causes slowness of movement (bradykinesia) and flexor rigidity, but pallidotomy improves these symptoms in PD. This apparent paradox was noted by Denny-Brown in the 1960s and has been emphasized again more recently. Furthermore, strokes involving GP can produce parkinsonism (156), and syndromes with pallidal degeneration result in many features of parkinsonism (157,158). Differences of lesion location or cause may explain some of the differences, but they are unlikely to be the primary factors. Investigators have shown that different locations of pallidotomy lesions or stimulator placement may produce different effects on rigidity and bradykinesia, but none has been shown to worsen the cardinal signs (84–86). As noted earlier, some movement tasks do not improve after pallidotomy, but those that do improve are similar to the tasks that are impaired after GPi lesions in monkeys. STN stimulation in patients with parkinsonism and STN

stimulation or ablation in monkeys improves all aspects of parkinsonism, but it does not cause significant dyskinesia (77,78,159–161). However, STN lesions in previously normal monkeys or people produces dramatic dyskinesia (43). These results suggest a significant reorganization of basal ganglia circuits in PD.

Several lines of evidence support the idea that basal ganglia circuits undergo substantial reorganization in PD. First, it appears that dopamine depletion alone is not sufficient to cause parkinsonism. Baboons with unilateral MPTP-induced lesions of SNc develop transient dystonia at a time when there is nearly complete striatal dopamine denervation (67). The subsequent development of parkinsonism appears to be associated with changes in dopamine receptors without further changes in striatal dopamine content. This finding suggests that factors in addition to dopamine denervation are important in the pathophysiology of PD and that these factors may occur in response to chronic rather than acute dopamine depletion. The importance of factors in addition to striatal dopamine depletion is also suggested by the spontaneous recovery of some primates after MPTP administration despite persistent depletion of more than 90% of striatal dopamine content (66). Second, long-term treatment of PD with levodopa is associated with the development of dopa-induced dyskinesia. Although this is likely to result from an interaction between disease duration and long-term treatment, it appears to reflect a significant functional change in the response of basal ganglia circuits to levodopa (162). This may be related to changes in dopamine receptor regulation in the setting of chronic treatment with levodopa (163,164). Third, behavioral and physiologic studies have shown that there are different responses to dopamine (165) or μ-opoid (166) receptor agonists in the dopamine-depleted animals compared with normal animals.

In summary, the effects of neurosurgical treatment of basal ganglia movement disorders are not completely explained by current physiologic and pathologic models of the basal ganglia. It is clear that these treatments are effective, sometimes dramatically so. It is less clear why these treatments work. One explanation is that an abnormal signal pattern causes greater deficits than the absence of that signal (49). This explanation is consistent with results of surgery, but it does not explain why there are greater deficits from lesions in neurologically normal subjects than from the same lesions in the setting of basal ganglia disease. It is likely that chronic basal ganglia diseases are accompanied by fundamental and significant physiologic changes so the effects of lesions in different conditions may vary and may also be different, even opposite, from the effects of lesions in neurologically normal subjects. It is tempting to discard models of basal ganglia function that do not explain all the phenomena, but it may be appropriate to have different models for normal and pathologic conditions until there is better understanding of the physiologic changes that accompany the different disorders.

It has become clear that simple changes in tonic neuronal firing rates are not sufficient to explain the clinical syndromes or response to surgical treatment. Better knowledge of phasic neuronal discharge patterns is required, both of temporal discharge patterns at rest and of movement-related discharge patterns. Little is known of how movement-related discharge patterns change in basal ganglia diseases, yet this is critical information if we are fully to understand basal ganglia function and the neural mechanisms of surgical therapy for movement disorders. Further study in animal models and during intraoperative neuronal recording in human diseases will enhance our understanding of these complex neural systems and disorders.

ACKNOWLEDGMENT

This work was supported by National Institutes of Health grant K08 NS01808, the McDonnell Center for Higher Brain Function, and the American Parkinson Disease Association.

REFERENCES

1. DeLong MR, Georgopoulos AP. Motor functions of the basal ganglia. In: Brooks VB, ed. *Handbook of physiology: the nervous system.* Bethesda, MD: American Physiological Society, 1981: 1017–1062.
2. Mink JW. The basal ganglia: focused selection and inhibition of competing motor programs. *Prog Neurobiol* 1996;50:381–425.
3. Hoover JE, Strick PL. Multiple output channels in the basal ganglia. *Science* 1993;259:819–821.
4. DeLong MR. Activity of pallidal neurons during movement. *J Neurophysiol* 1971;34:414–427.
5. Crutcher MD, DeLong MR. Single cell studies of the primate putamen. I. Functional organization. *Exp Brain Res* 1984;53:233–243.
6. Alexander GE, DeLong MR. Microstimulation of the primate striatum. II. Somatotopic organization of striatal microexcitable zones and their relation to neuronal response properties. *J Neurophysiol* 1985;53:1417–1430.
7. Crutcher MD, DeLong MR. Single cell studies of the primate putamen. II. Relations to direction of movements and patterns of muscular activity. *Exp Brain Res* 1984;53:244–258.
8. Crutcher MD, Alexander GE. Movement-related neuronal activity selectively coding either direction or muscle pattern in three motor areas of the monkey. *J Neurophysiol* 1990;64:151–163.
9. Alexander GE, Crutcher MD. Preparation for movement: neural representations of intended direction in three motor areas of the monkey. *J Neurophysiol* 1990;64:133–150.
10. Jaeger D, Gilman S, Aldridge JW. Primate basal ganglia activity in a precued reaching task: preparation for movement. *Exp Brain Res* 1993;95:51–64.
11. Schultz W, Romo R. Role of primate basal ganglia and frontal cortex in the internal generation of movements. I. Preparatory activity in the anterior striatum. *Exp Brain Res* 1992;91:363–384.
12. Flaherty AW, Graybiel AM. Two input systems for body representations in the primate striatal matrix: experimental evidence in the squirrel monkey. *J Neurosci* 1993;13:1120–1137.
13. Goldman PS, Nauta WJH. An intricately patterned prefronto-caudate projection in the rhesus monkey. *J Comp Neurol* 1977;171:369–386.
14. Hikosaka O, Sakamoto M, Usui S. Functional properties of monkey caudate neurons. I. Activities related to saccadic eye movements. *J Neurophysiol* 1989;61:780–798.
15. Romo R, Schultz W. Role of the primate basal ganglia and frontal cortex in the internal generation of movements. III. Neuronal activity in the supplementary motor area. *Exp Brain Res* 1992;91:396–407.
16. Bruce CJ, Goldberg ME. Primate frontal eye fields. I. Single neurons discharging before saccades. *J Neurophysiol* 1985;53:603–635.
17. Schlag J, Schlag-Rey M. Evidence for a supplementary eye field. *J Neurophysiol* 1987;57:179–200.
18. DeLong MR, Crutcher MD. Georgopoulos AP. Primate globus pallidus and subthalamic nucleus: functional organization. *J Neurophysiol* 1985;53:530–543.
19. Matsumura M, Kojima J, Gardiner TW, et al. Visual and oculomotor functions of the monkey subthalamic nucleus. *J Neurophysiol* 1992;67:1615–1632.
20. Wichmann T, Bergman H, DeLong MR. The primate subthalamic nucleus. I. Functional properties in intact animals. *J Neurophysiol* 1994;72:494–506.
21. Georgopoulos AP, DeLong MR, Crutcher MD. Relation between parameters of step-tracking movements and single cell discharge in the globus pallidus and subthalamic nucleus of the behaving monkey. *J Neurosci* 1983;3:1586–1598.
22. Mink JW, Thach WT. Basal ganglia motor control. I. Nonexclusive relation of pallidal discharge to five movement modes. *J Neurophysiol* 1991;65:273–300.
23. Mitchell SJ, Richardson RT, Baker FH, et al. The primate globus pallidus: neuronal activity related to direction of movement. *Exp Brain Res* 1987;68:491–505.
24. Mink JW, Thach WT. Basal ganglia motor control. II. Late pallidal timing relative to movement onset and inconsistent pallidal coding of movement parameters. *J Neurophysiol* 1991;65:301–329.
25. Turner RS, Anderson ME. Pallidal discharge related to the kinematics of reaching movements in two dimensions. *J Neurophysiol* 1997;77:1051–1074.
26. Brotchie P, Iansek R, Horne MK. Motor function of the monkey globus pallidus. 1. Neuronal discharge and parameters of movement. *Brain* 1991;114:1667–1683.
27. Hamada I, DeLong MR, Mano NI. Activity of identified wrist-related pallidal neurons during step and ramp wrist movements in the monkey. *J Neurophysiol* 1990;64:1892–1906.
28. Anderson ME, Horak FB. Influence of the globus pallidus on arm movements in monkeys. III. Timing of movement-related information. *J Neurophysiol* 1985;54:433–448.
29. Nambu A, Yoshida S, Jinnai K. Discharge of pallidal neurons with input from various cortical areas during movement in the monkey. *Brain Res* 1990;519:183–191.
30. Neafsey EJ, Hull CD, Buchwald NA. Preparation for movement in the cat. II. Unit activity in the basal ganglia and thalamus. *Electroencephalogr Clin Neurophysiol* 1978;44:714–723.
31. Brotchie P, Iansek R, Horne MK. Motor function of the monkey globus pallidus. II. Cognitive aspects of movement and phasic neuronal activity. *Brain* 1991;114:1685–1702.
32. Mushiake H, Strick PL. Pallidal neuron activity during sequential arm movements. *J Neurophysiol* 1995;74:2754–2758.
33. Mushiake H, Inase M, Tanji J. Selective encoding of motor sequence in the supplementary motor area of the monkey cerebral cortex. *Exp Brain Res* 1990;82:208–210.
34. Hikosaka O, Wurtz RH. Visual and oculomotor functions of

monkey substantia nigra pars reticulata. I. Relation of visual and auditory responses to saccades. *J Neurophysiol* 1983;49:1230–1253.

35. Hikosaka O, Wurtz RH. Visual and oculomotor functions of monkey substantia nigra pars reticulata. III. Memory-contingent visual and saccade responses. *J Neurophysiol* 1983;49:1268–1284.

36. Hikosaka O, Wurtz RH. Visual and oculomotor functions of monkey substantia nigra pars reticulata. IV. Relation of substantia nigra to superior colliculus. *J Neurophysiol* 1983;49:1285–1301.

37. DeLong MR, Crutcher MD, Georgopoulos AP. Relations between movement and single cell discharge in the substantia nigra of the behaving monkey. *J Neurosci* 1983;3:1599–1606.

38. Romo R, Schultz W. Dopamine neurons of the monkey midbrain: contingencies of responses to active touch during self-initiated arm movements. *J Neurophysiol* 1990;63:592–606.

39. Schultz W, Romo R, Ljungberg T, et al. Reward-related signals carried by dopamine neurons. In: Houk JC, Davis JL, Beiser DG, eds. *Models of information processing in the basal ganglia.* Cambridge: MIT Press, 1995:233–249.

40. Denny-Brown D, Yanagisawa N. The role of the basal ganglia in the initiation of movement. In: Yahr MD, ed. *The basal ganglia.* New York: Raven Press, 1976:115–149.

41. Kato M, Kimura M. Effects of reversible blockade of basal ganglia on a voluntary arm movement. *J Neurophysiol* 1992;68:1516–1534.

42. Miyachi S, Hikosaka O, Miyashita K, et al. Differential roles of monkey striatum in learning of sequential hand movement. *Exp Brain Res* 1997;115:1–5.

43. Carpenter MB, Carpenter CS. Analysis of somatotopic relations of the corpus Luysi in man and monkey. *J Comp Neurol* 1951;95:349–370.

44. Hamada I, DeLong MR. Excitotoxic acid lesions of the primate subthalamic nucleus result in transient dyskinesias of the contralateral limbs. *J Neurophysiol* 1992;68:1850–1858.

45. Crossman AR. Primate models of dyskinesia: the experimental approach to the study of basal ganglia–related involuntary movement disorders. *Neuroscience* 1987;21:1–40.

46. Mitchell IJ, Sambrook MA, Crossman AR. Subcortical changes in the regional uptake of [3H]-2-deoxyglucose in the brain of the monkey during experimental choreiform dyskinesia elicited by injection of a gamma-aminobutyric acid antagonist into the subthalamic nucleus. *Brain* 1985;108:405–422.

47. Hamada I, DeLong MR. Excitotoxic acid lesions of the primate subthalamic nucleus result in reduced pallidal neuronal activity during active holding. *J Neurophysiol* 1992;68:1859–1866.

48. Carpenter MB, Whittier JR, Mettler FA. Analysis of choreoid hyperkinesia in the rhesus monkey: surgical and pharmacological analysis of hyperkinesia resulting from lesions in the subthalamic nucleus of Luys. *J Comp Neurol* 1950;92:293–331.

49. Vitek J, Chockkan V, Zhang JY, et al. Neuronal activity in the basal ganglia in patients with generalized dystonia and hemiballismus. *Ann Neurol* 1999;46:22–35.

50. Denny-Brown D. *The basal ganglia and their relation to disorders of movement.* London: Oxford University Press, 1962.

51. Richter R. Degeneration of the basal ganglia in monkeys from chronic carbon disulphide poisoning. *J Neuropathol Exp Neurol* 1945;4:324–353.

52. Hore J, Vilis T. Arm movement performance during reversible basal ganglia lesions in the monkey. *Exp Brain Res* 1980;39:217–228.

53. Mink JW, Thach WT. Basal ganglia motor control. III. Pallidal ablation: normal reaction time, muscle cocontraction, and slow movement. *J Neurophysiol* 1991;65:330–351.

54. Horak FB, Anderson ME. Influence of globus pallidus on arm movements in monkeys. I. Effects of kainic acid-induced lesions. *J Neurophysiol* 1984;52:290–304.

55. DeLong MR, Coyle JT. Globus pallidus lesions in the monkey produced by kainic acid: histologic and behavioral effects. *Appl Neurophysiol* 1979;42:95–97.

56. Inase M, Buford JA, Anderson ME. Changes in the control of arm position, movement, and thalamic discharge during local inactivation in the globus pallidus of the monkey. *J Neurophysiol* 1996;75:1087–1104.

57. Mink JW, Thach WT. Basal ganglia intrinsic circuits and their role in behavior. *Curr Opin Neurobiol* 1993;3:950–957.

58. Albin RL, Young AB, Penney JB. The functional anatomy of basal ganglia disorders. *Trends Neurosci* 1989;12:366–375.

59. DeLong MR. Primate models of movement disorders of basal ganglia origin. *Trends Neurosci* 1990;13:281–285.

60. Hikosaka O, Wurtz RH. Modification of saccadic eye movements by GABA-related substances. II. Effects of muscimol in monkey substantia nigra pars reticulata. *J Neurophysiol* 1985;53:292–308.

61. Matsumura M, Tremblay L, Richard H, et al. Activity of pallidal neurons in the monkey during dyskinesia induced by injection of bicuculline in the external pallidum. *Neuroscience* 1995;65:59–70.

62. Mitchell IJ, Jackson A, Sambrook MA, et al. The role of the subthalamic nucleus in experimental chorea: evidence from 2-deoxyglucose metabolic mapping and horseradish peroxidase tracing studies. *Brain* 1989;112:1533–1548.

63. Benazzouz A, Gross C, Dupont J, et al. MPTP induced hemi-parkinsonism in monkeys: behavioral, mechanographic, electromyographic and immunohistochemical studies. *Exp Brain Res* 1992;90:116–120.

64. Crossman AR, Clarke CE, Boyce S, et al. MPTP-induced parkinsonism in the monkey: neurochemical pathology, complications of treatment and pathophysiological mechanisms. *Can J Neurol Sci* 1987;14:428–435.

65. Jenner P, Rupniak NMJ, Rose S, et al. 1-Methyl-4-phenyl-1,2,3,6-tetrahydropyridine–induced parkinsonism in the common marmoset. *Neurosci Lett* 1984;50:85–90.

66. Schneider JS, Unguez G, Yuwiler A, et al. Deficits in operant behaviour in monkeys treated with N-methyl-4-phenyl-1,2,3,6-tetrahydropyridine (MPTP). *Brain* 1988;111:1265–1285.

67. Perlmutter JS, Tempel LW, Black KJ, et al. MPTP induces dystonia and parkinsonism: clues to the pathophysiology of dystonia. *Neurology* 1997;49:1432–1438.

68. Schultz W, Studer A, Romo R, et al. Deficits in reaction times and movement times as correlates of hypokinesia in monkeys with MPTP-induced striatal dopamine depletion. *J Neurophysiol* 1989;61:651–668.

69. Mitchell IJ, Clarke CE, Boyce S, et al. Neural mechanisms underlying parkinsonian symptoms based upon regional uptake of 2-deoxyglucose in monkeys exposed to 1-methyl-4-phenyl-1,2,3,6-tetrahydropyridine. *Neuroscience* 1989;32:213–226.

70. Augood SJ, Emson PC, Mitchell IJ, et al. Cellular localization of Enk. gene expression in MPTP-treated cynomolgus monkeys. *Mol Brain Res* 1989;6:85–92.

71. Gerfen CR, Engber TM, Mahan LC, et al. D1 and D2 dopamine receptor-regulated gene expression of striatonigral and striatopallidal neurons. *Science* 1990;250:1429–1432.

72. Wichmann T, Bergman H, Starr PA, et al. Comparison of MPTP-induced changes in spontaneous neuronal discharge the internal pallidal segment and in the substantia nigra pars in primates. *Exp Brain Res* 1999;125:397–409.

73. Bergman H, Wichmann T, Karmon B, et al. The primate subthalamic nucleus. II. Neuronal activity in the MPTP model of parkinsonism. *J Neurophysiol* 1994;72:507–520.

74. Miller WC, DeLong MR. Parkinsonian symptomatology: an anatomical and physiological analysis. *Ann NY Acad Sci* 1988;515: 287–302.

75. Filion M, Tremblay L. Abnormal spontaneous activity of globus pallidus neurons in monkeys with MPTP-induced parkinsonism. *Brain Res* 1991;547:142–151.

76. Tremblay L, Filion M, Bedard PJ. Responses of pallidal neurons to striatal stimulation in monkeys with MPTP-induce parkinsonism. *Brain Res* 1989;498:17–33.

77. Bergman H, Wichmann T, DeLong MR. Reversal of experimental parkinsonism by lesions of the subthalamic nucleus. *Science* 1990;249:1436–1438.

78. Wichmann T, Bergman H, DeLong MR. The primate subthalamic nucleus. III. Changes in motor behavior and neuronal activity in the internal pallidum induced by subthalamic inactivation in the MPTP model of parkinsonism. *J Neurophysiol* 1994;72:521–530.

79. Brotchie JM, Mitchell IJ, Sambrook MA, et al. Alleviation of parkinsonism by antagonism of excitatory amino acid transmission in the medial segment of the globus pallidus in rat and primate. *Mov Disord* 1991;6:133–138.

80. Doudet DJ, Gross C, Arluison M, et al. Modifications of precentral cortex discharge and EMG activity in monkeys with MPTP-induced lesions of DA nigral neurons. *Exp Brain Res* 1990;80:177–188.

81. Gross C, Feger J, Seal J, et al. Neuronal activity in area 4 and movement parameters recorded in trained monkeys after unilateral lesion of the substantia nigra. *Exp Brain Res* 1983;7[Suppl]:181–193.

82. Watts RL, Mandir AS. The role of motor cortex in the pathophysiology of voluntary movement deficits associated with parkinsonism. *Neurol Clin* 1992;10:451–469.

83. Gaspar P, Stepniewski I, Kaas JH. Topography and collateralization of the dopaminergic projections to motor and lateral prefrontal cortex in owl monkeys. *J Comp Neurol* 1992;325:1–21.

84. Bejjani B, Damier P, Arnulf I, et al. Pallidal stimulation for Parkinson's disease: two targets? *Neurology* 1997;49:1564–1569.

85. Krack P, Pollak P, Limousin P, et al. Opposite motor effects of pallidal stimulation in Parkinson's disease. *Ann Neurol* 1998;43: 180–192.

86. Gross RE, Lombardi WJ, Lang AE, et al. Relationship of lesion location to clinical outcome following microelectrode-guided pallidotomy for Parkinson's disease. *Brain* 1999;122:405–416.

87. Pare D, Curro'Dossi R, Steriade M. Neuronal basis of the parkinsonian resting tremor: a hypothesis and its implications for treatment. *Neuroscience* 1990;35:217–226.

88. Rack PMH, Ross HF. The role of refes in the resting tremor of Parkinson's disease. *Brain* 1986;109:115–141.

89. Foerster O. Resection of the posterior roots of spinal cord. *Lancet* 1911;2:76–79.

90. Hallett M, Khoshbin S. A physiological mechanism of bradykinesia. *Brain* 1980;103:301–314.

91. Hayashi A, Kagamihara Y, Nakajima Y, et al. Disorder in reciprocal innervation upon initiation of voluntary movement in patients with Parkinson's disease. *Exp Brain Res* 1988;70:437–440.

92. Berardelli A, Sabra AF, Hallett M. Physiological mechanisms of rigidity in Parkinson's disease. *J Neurol Neurosurg Psychiatry* 1983;46:45–53.

93. Corcos DM, Chen CM, Quinn NP, et al. Strength in Parkinson's disease: relationship to rate of force generation and clinical status. *Ann Neurol* 1996;39:79–88.

94. Kunesch E, Schnitzler A, Tyercha C, et al. Altered force release control in Parkinson's disease. *Behav Brain Res* 1995;67:43–49.

95. Wing AM. A comparison of the rate of pinch grip force increases and decreases in parkinsonian bradykinesia. *Neuropsychologia* 1988;26:479–482.

96. Freeman JS, Cody FWJ, Schady W. The influence of external timing cues upon the rhythm of voluntary movements in Parkinson's disease. *J Neurol Neurosurg Psychiatry* 1993;56:1078–1084.

97. Martin JP. *The basal ganglia and posture.* Philadelphia: JB Lippincott, 1967.

98. Robertson C, Flowers KA. Motor set in Parkinson's disease. *J Neurol Neurosurg Psychiatry* 1990;53:583–592.

99. Flowers KA. Visual "closed-loop" and "open-loop" characteristics of voluntary movement in patients with parkinsonism and intention tremor. *Brain* 1976;99:269–310.

100. Klockgether T, Dichgans J. Visual control of arm movement in Parkinson's disease. *Mov Disord* 1994;9:48–56.

101. Benecke R, Rothwell JC, Dick JPR, et al. Performance of simultaneous movements in patients with Parkinson's disease. *Brain* 1986;109:739–757.

102. Benecke R, Rothwell JC, Dick JPR, et al. Simple and complex movements off and on treatment in patients with Parkinson's disease. *J Neurol Neurosurg Psychiatry* 1987;50:296–303.

103. Canavan AGM, Passingham RE, Marsden CD, et al. Sequencing ability in parkinsonians, patients with frontal lobe lesions and patients who have undergone unilateral temporal lobectomies. *Neuropsychologia* 1989;27:787–798.

104. Rafal RD, Inhoff AW, Friedmen JH, et al. Programming and execution of sequential movements in Parkinson's disease. *J Neurol Neurosurg Psychiatry* 1987;50:1267–1273.

105. Agostino R, Berardelli A, Formica A, et al. Analysis of repetitive and nonrepetitive sequential arm movements in patients with Parkinson's disease. *Mov Disord* 1994;9:311–314.

106. Evarts EV, Teravainen H, Calne DB. Reaction time in Parkinson's disease. *Brain* 1981;104:167–186.

107. Gaspar P, Duyckaerts C, Alvarez C, et al. Alterations of dopaminergic and noradrenergic innervations in motor cortex in Parkinson's disease. *Ann Neurol* 1991;30:365–374.

108. Sawaguchi T, Goldman-Rakic PS. The role of D1-dopamine receptor in working memory: local injections of dopamine antagonists into the prefrontal cortex of rhesus monkeys performing and oculomotor delayed response task. *J Neurophysiol* 1994;71:515–528.

109. Hauber W, Bubser M, Schmidt WJ. 6-Hydroxydopamine lesion of the rat prefrontal cortex impairs motor initiation but not motor execution. *Exp Brain Res* 1994;99:524–528.

110. Tatton WG, Lee RG. Evidence for abnormal long-loop reflexes in rigid parkinsonian patients. *Brain Res* 1975;100:671–676.

111. Evarts EV, Tanji J. Reflex and intended responses in motor cortex pyramidal tract neurons of monkey. *J Neurophysiol* 1976;39:1069–1080.

112. Matthews PBC. The human stretch reflex and the motor cortex. *Trends Neurosci* 1991;14:87–91.

113. Rothwell JC, Obeso JA, Traub MM, et al. The behavior of the long-latency stretch reflex in patients with Parkinson's disease. *J Neurol Neurosurg Psychiatry* 1983;46:35–44.

114. Horak FB, Nutt JG, Nashner LM. Postural inflexibility in parkinsonian subjects. *J Neurol Sci* 1992;111:46–58.

115. Vreeling FW, Verhey FRJ, Houx PJ, et al. Primitive reflexes in Parkinson's disease. *J Neurol Neurosurg Psychiatry* 1993;56:1323–1326.

116. Morris ME, Iansek R, Matyas TA, et al. The pathogenesis of gait hypokinesia in Parkinson's disease. *Brain* 1994;117:1169–1181.

117. Morris M, Iansek R, Matyas T, et al. Abnormalities in the stride length-cadence relationship in parkinsonian gait. *Mov Disord* 1998;13:61–69.

118. Bastian AJ, Mink JW, Kelly V, et al. Additive effects of l-dopa and pallidotomy on the kinematics of walking but not reaching. *Soc Neurosci Abstr* 1998;24:409.

119. Byl NN, Merzenich MM, Jenkins WM. A primate genesis model of focal dystonia and repetitive strain injury. I. Learning-induced dedifferentiation of the representation of the hand in the primary somatosensory cortex in adult monkeys. *Neurology* 1996;47:508–520.

120. Bara-Jimenez W, Catalan MJ, Hallett M, et al. Abnormal somatosensory homunculus in dystonia of the hand. *Ann Neurol* 1998;44:828–831.

121. Marsden CD, Rothwell JC. The physiology of idiopathic dystonia. *Can J Neurol Sci* 1987;14:521–527.

122. van der Kamp W, Berardelli A, Rothwell JC, et al. Rapid elbow movements in patients with torsion dystonia. *J Neurol Neurosurg Psychiatry* 1989;52:1043–1049.

123. Deuschl G, Toro C, Matsumoto J, et al. Movement-related cortical potentials in writer's cramp. *Ann Neurol* 1995;38:862–868.

124. Agostino R, Berardelli A, Formica A, et al. Sequential arm movements in patients with Parkinson's disease, Huntington's disease and dystonia. *Brain* 1992;115:1481–1495.

125. Tatton WG, Redingham W, Verrier MC, et al. Characteristic alterations in responses to imposed wrist displacements in parkinsonian rigidity and dystonia musculorum deformans. *Can J Neurol Sci* 1984;11:281–287.

126. Nakashima K, Rothwell JC, Day BL, et al. Reciprocal inhibition between forearm muscles in patients with writer's cramp and other occupational cramps, symptomatic hemidystonia and hemiparesis due to stroke. *Brain* 1989;112:681–697.

127. Panizza M, Lelli S, Nilsson J, et al. H-reflex recovery curve and reciprocal inhibition of H-reflex in different kinds of dystonia. *Neurology* 1990;40:824–828.

128. Chen R, Wassermann EM, Canos M, et al. Impaired inhibition in writer's cramp during voluntary muscle activation. *Neurology* 1997;49:1054–1059.

129. Kaji R, Rothwell JC, Katayama M, et al. Tonic vibration reflex and muscle afferent block in writer's cramp. *Ann Neurol* 1995;38:155–162.

130. Berardelli A, Rothwell JC, Hallett M, et al. The pathophysiology of primary dystonia. *Brain* 1998;121:1195–1212.

131. Marsden CD, Obeso JA, Rothwell JC. Clinical neurophysiology of muscle jerks: myoclonus, chorea, and tics. *Adv Neurol* 1983;39:865–881.

132. Bradshaw JL, Phillips JG, Dennis C, et al. Initiation and execution of movement sequences in those suffering from and at-risk of developing Huntington's disease. *J Clin Exp Neuropsychol* 1992;14:179–192.

133. Brown RG, Jahanshahi M, Marsden CD. The execution of bimanual movements in patients with Parkinson's, Huntington's and cerebellar disease. *J Neurol Neurosurg Psychiatry* 1993;56:295-297.

134. Thompson PD, Berardelli A, Rothwell JC, et al. The coexistence of bradykinesia and chorea in Huntington's disease and its implications for theories of basal ganglia control of movement. *Brain* 1988;111:223–244.

135. Deuschl G, Lucking CH, Schenck E. Hand muscle reflexes following electrical stimulation in choreatic movement disorders. *J Neurol Neurosurg Psychiatry* 1989;52:755–762.

136. Noth J, Friedemann H, Podoll K, et al. Absence of long-latency reflexes to imposed finger displacements in patients with Huntington's disease. *Neurosci Lett* 1983;35:97–100.

137. Noth J, Podoll K, Friedemann HH. Long-loop reflexes in small hand muscles studied in normal subjects and in patients with Huntington's disease. *Brain* 1985;108:65–80.

138. Homberg V, Huttunen J. Muscle tone in Huntington's disease. *J Neurol Sci* 1994;121:147–154.

139. Reiner A, Albin RL, Anderson KD, et al. Differential loss of striatal projection neurons in Huntington disease. *Proc Natl Acad Sci USA* 1988;85:5733–5737.

140. Baron MS, Vitek JL, Bakay RAE, et al. Treatment of advanced Parkinson's disease by posterior GPi pallidotomy: 1-year results of a pilot study. *Ann Neurol* 1996;40:355–366.

141. Dogali M, Fazzini E, Kolodny E, et al. Stereotactic ventral pallidotomy for Parkinson's disease. *Neurology* 1995;45:753–761.

142. Samii A, Turnbull IM, Kishore A, et al. Reassessment of unilateral pallidotomy in Parkinson's disease: a 2-year follow-up study. *Brain* 1999;122:417–425.

143. Lang AE, Lozano AM, Montgomery E, et al. Posteroventral medial pallidotomy in advanced Parkinson's disease. *N Engl J Med* 1997;337:1036–1042.

144. Laitinen LV, Bergenheim AT, Hariz MI. Leksell's posteroventral pallidotomy in the treatment of Parkinson's disease. *J Neurosurg* 1992;76:53–61.

145. Lang A, Fahn S. Assessment of Parkinson's disease. In: Munsat T, ed. *Quantification of neurologic deficit.* Boston: Butterworth, 1989:285–309.

146. Limousin P, Brown RG, Jahanshahi M, et al. The effects of posteroventral pallidotomy on the preparation and execution of voluntary hand and arm movements in Parkinson's disease. *Brain* 1999;122:315–327.

147. Jankovic J, Ben-Arie L, Schwartz K, et al. Movement and reaction times and fine coordination tasks following pallidotomy. *Mov Disord* 1999;14:57–62.

148. Kimber TE, Tsai CS, Semmler J, et al. Voluntary movement after pallidotomy in severe Parkinson's disease. *Brain* 1999;122:895–906.

149. Bennett KM, O'Sullivan JD, Peppard RF, et al. The effect of unilateral posteroventral pallidotomy on the kinematics of the reach to grasp movement. *J Neurol Neurosurg Psychiatry* 1998;65:479–487.

150. Pfann KD, Penn RD, Shannon KM, et al. Pallidotomy and bradykinesia: implications for basal ganglia function. *Neurology* 1998;51:796–803.

151. Samuel M, Ceballos-Baumann AO, Turjanski N, et al. Pallidotomy in Parkinson's disease increases supplementary motor area and prefrontal activation during performance volitional movements an H2(15)O PET study. *Brain* 1997;120:1301–1313.

152. Masterman D, DeSalles A, Baloh RW, et al. Motor, cognitive, and behavioral performance following unilateral ventroposterior pallidotomy for Parkinson disease. *Arch Neurol* 1998;55:1201–1208.

153. Meyer CH. Unilateral pallidotomy for Parkinson's disease promptly improves a wide range of voluntary activities—especially gait and movements. *Acta Neurochir Suppl (Wien)* 1997;68:37–41.

154. Carpenter MB, Whittier JB. Study of methods for producing experimental lesions of the central nervous system with special reference to the stereotaxic technique. *J Comp Neurol* 1952;97:73–131.

155. Suarez JI, Metman LV, Reich SG, et al. Pallidotomy for hemiballismus: efficacy and characteristics of neuronal activity. *Ann Neurol* 1997;42:807–811.

156. Bhatia KP, Marsden CD. The behavioural and motor consequences of focal lesions of the basal ganglia in man. *Brain* 1994;117:859–876.

157. Aizawa H, Kwak S, Shimizu T, et al. A case of adult onset pure pallidal degeneration. I. Clinical manifestations and neuropathological observations. *J Neurol Sci* 1991;102:76–82.

158. Katayama S, Watanabe C, Khoriyama T, et al. Slowly progressive L-DOPA nonresponsive pure akinesia due to nigropallidal degeneration: a clinicopathological case study. *J Neurol Sci* 1998;161:169–172.

159. Benazzouz A, Gross C, Feger J, et al. Reversal of rigidity and improvement in motor performance by subthalamic high-frequency stimulation in MPTP-treated monkeys. *Eur J Neurosci* 1993;5:382–389.

160. Kumar R, Lozano A, Kim Y, et al. Double-blind evaluation of subthalamic nucleus deep brain stimulation in advanced Parkinson's disease. *Neurology* 1998;51:850–855.

161. Krack P, Pollak P, Limousin P, et al. Subthalamic nucleus or internal pallidal stimulation in young onset Parkinson's disease. *Brain* 1998;121:451–457.

162. Hershey T, Black K, Stambuk M, et al. Altered thalamic response to levodopa in Parkinson's patients with dopa-induced dyskinesias. *Proc Natl Acad Sci USA* 1998;95:12016–12021.

163. Dumartin B, Caille I, Gonon F, et al. Internalization of D1 dopamine receptor in striatal neurons *in vivo* as evidence of activation by dopamine agonists. *J Neurosci* 1998;18:1650–1661.

164. Muriel MP, Bernard V, Levey A, et al. Levodopa induces a cytoplasmic localization of D1 dopamine receptors in striatal neurons in Parkinson's disease. *Ann Neurol* 1999;46:103–111.

165. Kreiss DS, Mastropietro CW, Rawji SS, et al. The response of subthalamic nucleus neurons to dopamine receptor stimulation. *J Neurosci* 1997;17:6807–6819.

166. Churchill L, Klitenick MA, Kalivas PW. Dopamine depletion reorganizes projections from the nucleus accumbens ventral pallidum that mediate opioid-induced motor activity. *J Neurosci* 1998;18:8074–8085.

Surgery for Parkinson's Disease and Movement Disorders,
edited by J.K. Krauss, J. Jankovic, and R.G. Grossman.
Lippincott Williams & Wilkins, Philadelphia © 2001.

5

PRINCIPLES AND TECHNIQUES OF MOVEMENT DISORDERS SURGERY

JOACHIM K. KRAUSS
ROBERT G. GROSSMAN

The renaissance of movement disorders surgery has resulted both in the introduction of new techniques and in the refinement of operative methods that have been known for decades. Although surgical options include various techniques targeting the central nervous system, peripheral nerves, and affected muscles, for treatment of specific movement disorders, the mainstay of movement disorders surgery is functional stereotactic neurosurgery. The basic principles of this discipline were established in the early twentieth century (1). Functional stereotactic neurosurgery was introduced into clinical practice in the late 1940s (2), and many innovative concepts were developed in the 1950s (3). The tremendous progress made in surgical techniques since the early 1980shas been paralleled and stimulated by the development of new methods in neuroimaging and neurophysiology, leading to much better accuracy in definition of the target.

Here we briefly summarize the principles and techniques of contemporary functional stereotactic neurosurgery for treatment of movement disorders. For detailed description of other techniques, the reader is referred to the corresponding chapters. There are many different ways to perform movement disorders surgery. Depending on the complexity of the movement disorder, the techniques used for anatomic and physiologic definition of the target, and the experience of the surgeon, operative time may vary considerably. It may range between 1 and 2 hours for thalamotomy in a patient with tremor, and it may take more than 10 hours for implantation of bilateral subthalamic nucleus (STN) electrodes in a patient with akinetic-rigid Parkinson's disease (PD). The widespread use of chronic deep brain stimulation (DBS) has furthered the spectrum of movement disorders surgery and has been instrumental in exploring new indications. The basic principles of functional

stereotactic neurosurgery apply to both lesioning techniques and DBS.

PRINCIPLES OF STEREOTACTIC SURGERY

The principles of stereotactic surgery include the acquisition of data from various imaging modalities and their transfer to a Cartesian coordinate system. In functional stereotactic surgery, these coordinates are generally referenced to an apparatus, the stereotactic frame, which is rigidly fixed to the patient's head. *Stereotaxis* has been derived from the Greek, meaning "three-dimensional arrangement." At the 1973 meeting of the World Society for Stereotactic and Functional Neurosurgery in Tokyo, members agreed to use the term *stereotactic* surgery instead of the formerly used *stereotaxic* surgery, to refer also to the Latin word *tactus,* to touch (4). So far, the accuracy of frameless stereotactic systems has not been sufficient to envision their application in functional neurosurgery for the treatment of movement disorders.

Stereotactic Coordinate Space

Stereotactic surgery is based on a *Cartesian coordinate system* that implies that any point in space can be determined by three coordinates *(x, y,* and *z),* which are defined with regard to three intersecting orthogonal planes (Fig. 5.1). These three planes, the abscissa, ordina, and applicata, intersect at one point, which is commonly defined as zero (5,6). This three-dimensional coordinate space was first discussed by the French philosopher and mathematician René Descartes in the seventeenth century. By convention, the *x* coordinate defines the distance to the midsagittal plane (right to left), the *y* coordinate defines the distance to a reference point along the rostrocaudal axis (anterior to posterior), and the *z* coordinate defines the distance to a reference point in the coronal plane (superior to inferior) (Fig. 5.2). An alternative method to describe the location of a point in space is by using a *polar coordinate system* (7,8), specifying its distance

J.K. Krauss: Department of Neurosurgery, University Hospital, Klinikum Mannheim, 68167 Mannheim, Germany.
R.G. Grossman: Department of Neurosurgery, Baylor College of Medicine, Houston, Texas 77030.

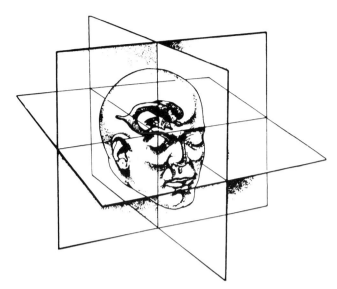

FIGURE 5.1. Cartesian coordinate system with three orthogonal intersecting planes as used to define the coordinates of a target in stereotactic neurosurgery. (From *Todd-Wells Manual of stereotaxic procedures.* Randolph: Codman and Shurtleff, 1967, with permission.)

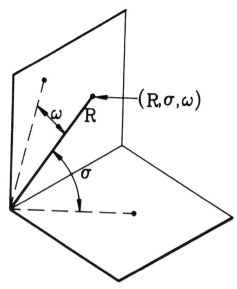

FIGURE 5.3. Definition of a point in space by using a polar coordinate system. A straight line is drawn from the zero point to the target point. The distance between these two points is defined as *R*. The inclination of the line from the horizontal plane is σ, and the angle from the vertical plane is ω. (From Kelly PJ. *Tumor stereotaxis.* Philadelphia: WB Saunders, 1991, with permission.)

and direction from a reference point that involves the calculation of a line and its two angles to the horizontal and vertical plane (Fig. 5.3).

Ventricular Landmarks and Anatomic Target Definition

Because stereotactic positive-contrast ventriculographywas the method of choice in functionalstereotactic neurosurgery long before the advent of computed tomography (CT) and of magnetic resonance imaging (MRI),it has been generally accepted to refer the coordinates of a target in the basal gan-

glia or in the thalamus to anatomic landmarks in the third ventricle (Fig. 5.4). Initially, the calcification of the pineal gland and the foramen of Monro (FM) as defined by pneumencephalography were used for internal reference points (9). Later, the posterior commissure (PC) was introduced to replace the pineal gland. Subsequently, target coordinates have been referred either to the FM-PC line or to the connecting line between the anterior commissure (AC) and the PC (6,10). To compare the differences in the *y* and *z* coordinates, a correction factor for the angle between the FM-PC line and the AC-PC line has to be considered (11) (Fig. 5.5).

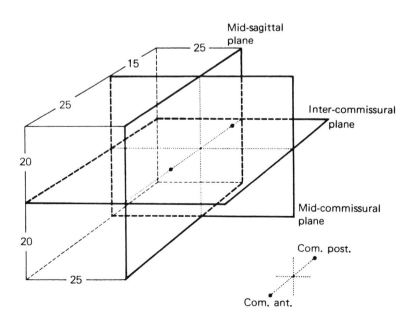

FIGURE 5.2. Diagram of Schaltenbrand and Wahren showing the relation of the three reference planes to the anterior and posterior commissures. In this diagram, the stereotactic coordinates *x, y,* and *z* are defined with regard to the midsagittal plane, the intercommissural plane, and the midcommissural plane. The figure also shows the central block of the brain (in millimeters), which was used to prepare the plates in the Schaltenbrand-Wahren stereotactic atlas. (From Schaltenbrand G, Wahren P. *Atlas for stereotaxy of the human brain.* Stuttgart: Thieme, 1977, with permission.)

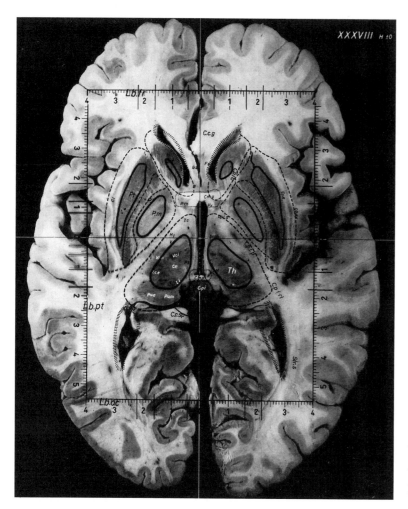

FIGURE 5.4. Macroscopic axial section of a "standard brain" through the anterior and posterior commissures of the third ventricle that demonstrates the spatial relationship between the thalamus and the basal ganglia and the intercommissural line. (From Schaltenbrand G, Bailey P. *Introduction to stereotaxis with an atlas of the human brain.* Stuttgart: Thieme, 1959, with permission.)

Furthermore, the definition of the AC-PC line varies among different investigators. The intercommissural line has been used most widely, and several investigators demonstrated that there is relatively little anatomic variation in the morphology of various basal ganglia nuclei and their relative distance to the intercommissural line among individual patients. Nevertheless, spatial variability requires intraoperative physiologic confirmation of the target (12). Factors that need to be considered with the indirect method of anatomic target definition are the length of the AC-PC line and the height and width of the third ventricle. In patients with very short or very long AC-PC lines, the target coordinates should be adjusted by a proportional correction procedure (13). The method of Guiot uses a geometric technique to adjust for variations in the length of the intercommissural line and the thalamic height (Fig. 5.6) (14,15). This method has been used primarily with ventriculography. It is also applicable, however, to other imaging modalities.

STEREOTACTIC TECHNOLOGY

Various stereotactic frame systems, instruments, and software packages are used in contemporary functional stereo-

tactic neurosurgery. The stereotactic frame not only serves as a reference base for the calculation of the stereotactic coordinates, but it also provides intraoperative fixation of the skull. Immobility of the head is pivotal for stereotactic imaging and the avoiding of artifacts. The mechanical accuracy of current frames is in the range of less than 1 mm.

Stereotactic Head Frames

Stereotactic frames have been classified according to their design and working principles into four different systems: (a) rectilinear systems; (b) arc systems; (c) bur-hole mounted systems; and (d) a system with interlocking arcs (16). Nowadays, targeting in functional stereotactic surgery is performed mainly with translational types of stereotactic devices and arc-centered frames. With the arc-centered type, the target point is constantly at the center of the arc regardless of changing of the location of the entry point at the skull and the angles of the trajectory (17). One should note the differences in the trajectories when multiple parallel pathways are obtained for microelectrode recording with these two different types. The Riechert-Mundinger frame II and the Talairach frame, for example, are based on the translational principle, whereas

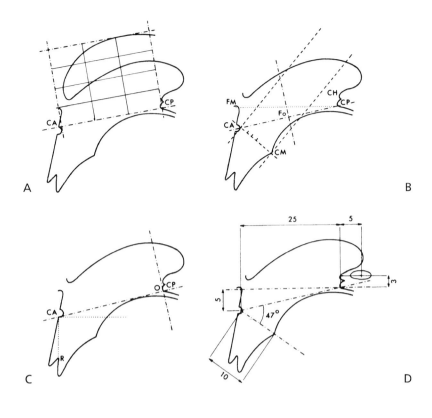

Surgery for Parkinson's Disease and Movement Disorders, edited by J.K. Krauss, J. Jankovic, and R.G. Grossman. Lippincott Williams & Wilkins, Philadelphia © 2001.

FIGURE 5.5. Differences in reference points in the third ventricle in functional stereotactic surgery as used by Talairach **(A),** Guiot, Riechert and Hassler, Schaltenbrand, and Bailey **(B),** and Remond and Delmas and Pertuiset **(C). D:** Measures and angles to compare the different systems. (From Van Manen J. *Stereotactic methods and their application in disorders of the motor system.* Assen: van Gorcum, 1967, with permission.)

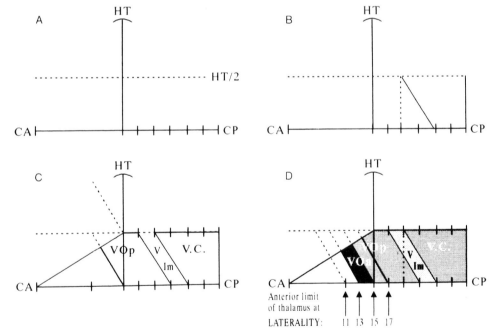

FIGURE 5.6. Guiot's geometric method for target determination that adjusts for variations in the length of the intercommissural line and the thalamic height. In this example, the calculation of a target in the thalamic ventralis intermedius (VIM) based on ventriculography is shown. **A:** The anterior and posterior commissures (CA and CP) are determined on a lateral ventriculogram. After the intercommissural line (IC) has been drawn, a perpendicular line is drawn at its midpoint extending to the floor of the lateral ventricle. This is the thalamic height (HT). Another line is drawn at the midpoint of the thalamic height (HT/2) parallel to and of equal length than the IC. **B:** Both the IC and the HT/2 lines are divided into twelfths. Then, a line is drawn from 2/12 IC to 4/12 HT/2 (with the CP being defined as 0/12). **C:** A second line is drawn from 3/12 IC to 5/12 HT/2. The ventralis oralis posterior (VOP), the VIM, and the VC (ventrocaudalis) are defined by these schematic outlines. The structures of the anterior thalamus are delineated by drawing a line between CA and the midpoint of HT/2. **D:** Whereas the y and z coordinates are defined by the lateral ventriculogram, additional information from the anteroposterior ventriculogram is necessary to derive the x coordinate. In this drawing, the anterior limit of the ventrolateral thalamus is shown at different lateralities. (From Burchiel KJ. Thalamotomy for movement disorders. *Neurosurg Clin North Am* 1995;6:55–71, with permission.)

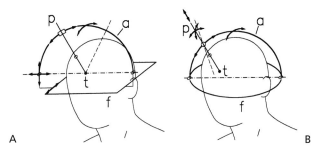

FIGURE 5.7. The translational and the center-of-arc principles to reach a calculated target in functional stereotactic surgery. **A** and **B:** a, arc; f, frame; p, probe; t, target. **A:** With the arc-centered type, the target is always at the center of the arc regardless of the choice of the entry point and of the trajectory, which can be modified as needed intraoperatively. **B:** With the translational principle, the direction of the trajectory is determined by the position of the electrode carrier along the arc, and the depth of the probe has to be calculated in addition. The trajectory is not as variable as compared with the arc-centered type. (From Struppler A. The history of stereotactic and functional neurosurgery techniques. In: Gildenberg PL, Tasker RR, eds. *Textbook of stereotactic and functional neurosurgery.* New York: McGraw-Hill, 1998:1233–1243, with permission).

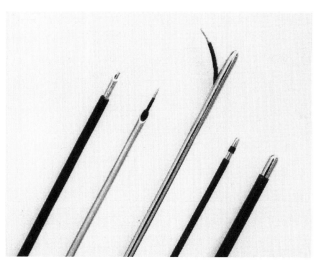

FIGURE 5.8. Samples of radiofrequency electrodes for temperature-controlled lesioning in functional neurosurgery. From **left** to **right:** electrodes used for rhizotomy and cordotomy, a chord electrode, and bipolar and monopolar straight electrodes for basal ganglia surgery. (Courtesy of Stryker-Leibinger, Frisburg, Germany.)

the Leksell frame and the Riechert-Mundinger system with the Zamorano-Dujovny 3/8-arc present arc-centered types (Fig. 5.7). In our experience, arc-centered systems provide better flexibility and more versatility in functional stereotactic neurosurgery. With these types of frames, intraoperative movement along all three axes of the stereotactic coordinate space is possible without the need for repeated target calculation. In general, it is advantageous to use shorter instruments (guiding cannulas and electrodes) because the risk of deviation at the target site is lower than with longer instruments. The length of such probes used in stereotactic surgery often equals 19 cm, which is the distance from the arc to the target. The Leksell G frame is useful because it has a relatively small profile as compared with other stereotactic frames. Most contemporary available stereotactic frames are both CT and MRI compatible.

Stereotactic Instruments and Software

The same electrodes are used commonly for *macrostimulation* at the anatomically defined target and lesioning. These electrodes are coupled to electrical devices that usually serve multiple purposes such as impedance monitoring, on-line documentation of temperature, stimulation, and high-frequency coagulation. With contemporary commercially available systems, it is possible to set different pulse durations and trains for stimulation. The frequency and the voltage used for stimulation at the target may either be changed gradually or stepwise incrementally. Most systems allow temperature-controlled radiofrequency coagulation.

High-frequency electrodes most commonly have a diameter of 1 to 2 mm and a 1- to 4-mm uninsulated tip (Figs. 5.8 and 5.9). Such electrodes are available both for monopolar and bipolar lesioning (Fig. 5.10). The chord electrode is

a specially designed electrode with a sheath and a central core that can be protruded perpendicular to the axis of the electrode in a semicircular fashion (Figs. 5.8 and 5.9). This type of electrode allows exploration of the area adjacent to the electrode without the need for repeated puncture (18). These electrodes are also available both in monopolar and bipolar mode. With temperature-controlled radiofrequency lesioning, the desired coagulation temperature is preselected at the console of the lesion generator. High-frequency energy passes through the electrode until the preselected temperature is reached and is then kept constant throughout the time of coagulation. This is achieved by a thermosensor built into the electrode tip, which measures the temperature in the adjacent tissue, and transmits it back to the lesion generator (Fig. 5.11).

For stereotactic imaging localization, attachments with fiducials of different materials depending on the imaging modality are mounted onto the head ring (Fig. 5.12). The calculations may be performed directly on the console of the imaging devices or with workstations as described later. A digitizing tablet is helpful when the reference points are determined on lateral and anteroposterior ventriculograms. Console software or software packages for target calculation are commercially available. However, many surgeons use additional software or prefer their own software for this purpose.

STEREOTACTIC ATLASES

The general acceptance in functional stereotactic surgery of referring the coordinates of a target to anatomic landmarks of the third ventricle has resulted in the generation

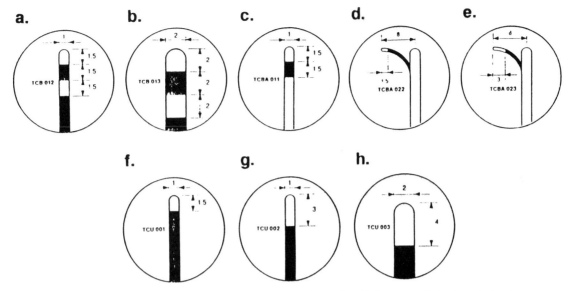

FIGURE 5.9. Dimensions in millimeters of commonly used radiofrequency lesioning electrodes (**A–C**: bipolar electrodes; **D** and **E**: chord electrodes; **F–H**: monopolar electrodes). (Courtesy of Stryker-Leibinger, Frisburg, Germany.)

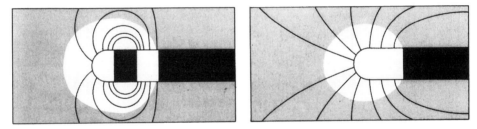

FIGURE 5.10. Principles of bipolar (**left**) and monopolar (**right**) high-frequency coagulation. Note the differences in the distribution of the current. (Courtesy of Stryker-Leibinger, Frisburg, Germany.)

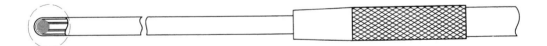

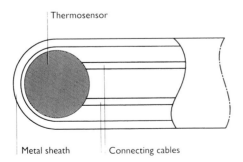

FIGURE 5.11. Thermocontrolled coagulation is achieved by a thermosensor that is built into the electrode tip measuring the temperature in the surrounding tissue and transmitting it back to the lesion generator. (Courtesy of Stryker-Leibinger, Frisburg, Germany.)

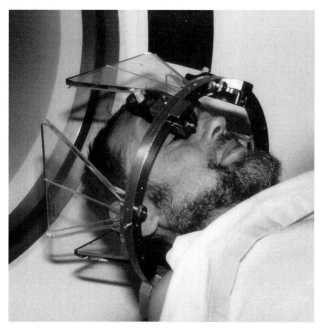

FIGURE 5.12. Four transparent plates with fiducials are mounted onto the stereotactic ring for stereotactic computed tomography imaging localization.

of several stereotactic atlases (19). The first *stereotactic brain atlas* was published by Spiegel and Wycis in 1952 (20). Human stereotactic brain atlases present mean values for the three-dimensional location of a target and show exemplary anatomic specimens. The most widely used stereotactic atlases are the atlases of Talairach and colleagues (1957) (21), Schaltenbrand and Bailey (1959) (10), and its newer version, the Schaltenbrand-Wahren atlas (1977) (6). The Schaltenbrand-Bailey atlas was the major reference for AC-PC based three-dimensional coordinates for decades. The Schaltenbrand-Wahren atlas was planned as a second, revised, and enlarged edition of the Schaltenbrand-Bailey atlas. In response to renewed interest in functional stereotactic neurosurgery, the Schaltenbrand-Wahren atlas was reprinted in the late 1990s. It contains series of myelin-stained brain sections 1 to 4 mm thick in each of three orthogonal planes. Each photographic section is presented with a transparent overlay providing the contours and anatomic nomenclature of the thalamic and basal ganglia and their circuitry (Fig. 5.13). In addition, a grid on the overlay allows the determination of the stereotactic coordinates for a given structure. The newest stereotactic atlas is by Talairach and Tournoux, published in 1988 (22); this atlas uses a novel approach, dividing the brain into orthogonal parallelograms (Fig. 5.14). As indicated by Lozano et al., a potential source of error in target determination may derive from the stereotactic atlas that is used for reference (23). Pallidal coordinates, for example, differ between the Schaltenbrand-Bailey atlas and the Schaltenbrand-Wahren atlas. The lateral coordinates differ by 1 to 2 mm, and the vertical coordinates differ by 2 to 3 mm. According to Lozano et al., the coordinates in the Schaltenbrand-Wahren edition match more closely

with physiologic mapping, and this finding accords with our experience.

Electronic versions of the Schaltenbrand-Wahren atlas and the Talairach atlas are also available on CD ROM. These digitized stereotactic atlases can be used both with stereotactic CT or MRI. The atlas maps are superimposed on the patient's scans, and the maps can be stretched or reduced in relation to the length of the patient's AC-PC line.

TARGETS IN CONTEMPORARY MOVEMENT DISORDERS SURGERY

Since the 1950s, various thalamic and basal ganglia nuclei have been targeted for treatment of movement disorders. In the early years of functional stereotactic surgery, *target selection* was often made empirically, and models to understand the rationales choosing a specific target were poorly developed (24). Nowadays, the range of targets that are commonly used is much more limited than before. In summary, contemporary targets for treatment of parkinsonian symptoms include the thalamic ventralis intermedius (VIM), which corresponds to the ventral part of the posterior ventral lateral nucleus (VLp) according to the classification of Hirai and Jones (see Chapter 2), the posteroventral lateral globus pallidus internus (GPi), and the STN. Tremors other than those caused by PD are treated almost exclusively by targeting the thalamic VIM and the thalamic ventralis oralis posterior (VOP) nucleus. As outlined by Jones, the concept of delineating the VOP as a proper nucleus is probably not justified because this thalamic area presents a region of interdigitation between two other nuclei, the VLa and VLp in Jones' terminology. For choreic and dystonic movement disorders, pallidal or thalamic targets are used. Subthalamic structures such as the fields of Forel or the zona incerta are still being used by some neurosurgeons to include thalamic input in placing lesions in thalamotomy to treat various movement disorders (Fig. 5.15). The STN proper, so far, has not been considered a target for movement disorders other than PD. It is surprising to see that some nuclei that were described as effective targets for treatment of movement disorders in the past are now almost completely neglected. In particular, medial thalamic structures such as the centrum medianum/nucleus parafascicularis complex are relevant in this context (25,26). Likewise, targeting cerebellar nuclei for treatment of spasticity and dystonia has been almost completely abandoned (27).

Thalamic subnuclei show a clear somatotopic organization. Basically, the concept of Hassler's thalamic homunculi is still valid today (Fig. 5.16). The leg is presented more lateral in the thalamic VIM than the arm. The x coordinate in a patient with tremor undergoing thalamic DBS or thalamotomy thus will differ depending on whether the patient has also prominent tremor of the leg. The choice of the coordinates for a specific target furthermore depends on the preference and experience of the neurosurgeon. When

Laitinen asked 16 neurosurgeons in 1985 about their preferred target coordinates for treatment of parkinsonism, a considerable variety was evident (28). The somatotopy of the GPi is much less clear than that of the thalamic VIM. With microelectrode techniques, investigators have shown that one cell often responds to multiple joints (29). According to the observations by Hoover and Strick, an individual patient may have several somatotopic maps with different cortical projections (30). Guridi and colleagues found that most of the neurons in patients with PD responsive to passive manipulation or active movements of the limbs were in the lateral portion of the GPi (31). The upper limb and the axial body were presented more frequently in the more lateral portion and in its ventral one-third. Lower limb responses were recorded more frequently in the dorsal one-third, in contrast. There was no clear somatotopy in the vertical axis for the distribution of tremor-related cells.

The AC-PC based anatomic coordinates now used by most neurosurgeons are shown in Table 5.1. The choice of the corresponding coordinates in a given patient considers various aspects including individual morphology, the specific movement disorder to be treated, and the method used, that is, radiofrequency lesioning versus DBS. However, once again, such coordinates should be considered only preliminary, and further intraoperative confirmation or modification by neurophysiologic investigations is absolutely mandatory in our opinion.

PREOPERATIVE NEUROLOGIC AND RADIOLOGIC ASSESSMENT

Most patients with movement disorders have a long history of medical treatment before they are considered candidates

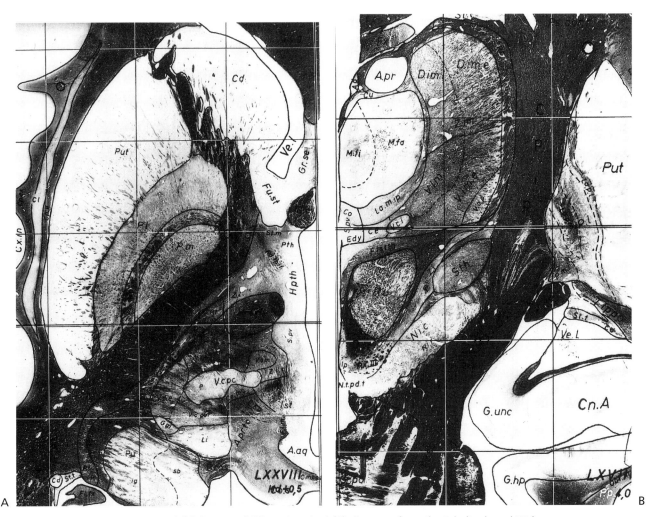

FIGURE 5.13. Axial **(A)**, coronal **(B)**, and sagittal **(C)** diagrams from the Schaltenbrand-Wahren atlas. This example demonstrates the stereotactic morphology of the ventralis intermedius in the three orthogonal planes based on the intercommissural line. The axial diagram is 0.5 mm above the intercommissural plane, the coronal diagram is 4 mm behind the midcommissural plane, and the sagittal diagram is 13 mm lateral to the midsagittal plane. (From Schaltenbrand G, Wahren P. *Atlas for stereotaxy of the human brain.* Stuttgart: Thieme, 1977, with permission.)

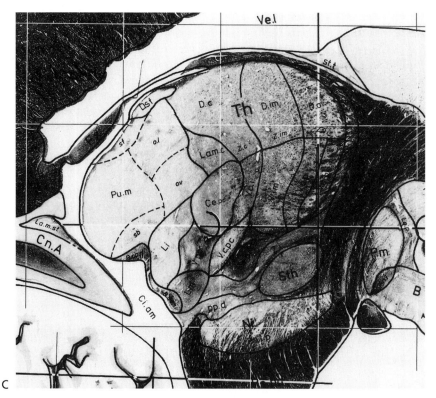

C

FIGURE 5.13. Continued.

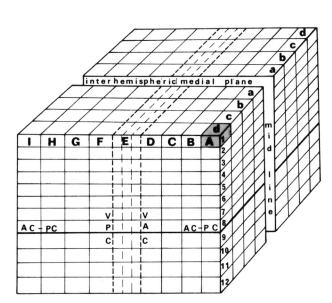

FIGURE 5.14. With the method of Talairach and Tournoux, the brain is divided into orthogonal parallelograms based on the intercommissural line. The volumes of these parallelograms are defined by a capital letter, a lowercase letter, and a number, each (e.g., A-d-1, which is shown as a *shaded area*). (From Talairach J, Tournoux P. *Co-planar stereotaxic atlas of the human brain: 3-dimensional proportional system: an approach to cerebral imaging.* Stuttgart: Thieme, 1988, with permission.)

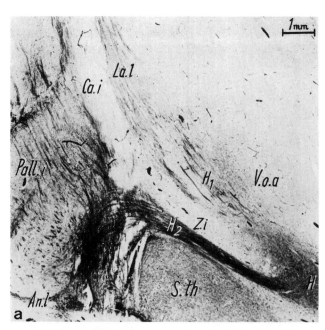

FIGURE 5.15. Morphology of the subthalamic area demonstrated by a coronal section through the anterior thalamus of an 8-month old fetus. An.l, ansa lenticularis; Ca.i, internal capsule; H, H1 and H2, Forel's fieds; La.l, lamella lateralis thalami; Pall.i, globus pallidus internus; S.th, subthalamic nucleus; V.o.a, ventralis oralis anterior; Z.i, zona incerta. (From Hassler R, Mundinger F, Riechert T. *Stereotaxis in Parkinson syndrome.* Berlin: Springer, 1979, with permission.)

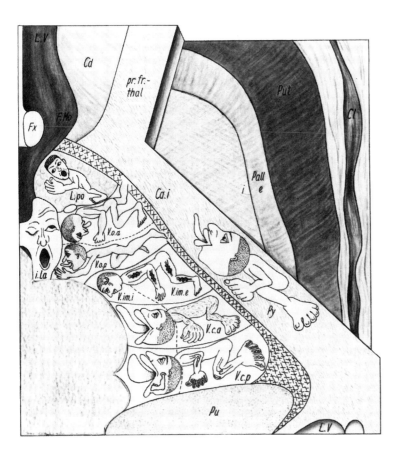

FIGURE 5.16. Somatotopic representation of the ventrolateral and ventrocaudal thalamus. The homunculi demonstrate the somatotopy of different thalamic subnuclei according to Hassler's nomenclature: Ca.i, internal capsule; Cd, caudate; Cl, claustrum; F.Mo, foramen of Monro; Fx, fornix; L.po, lateropolaris; L.V, lateral ventricle; Pall e and i, external and internal segment of globus pallidus; Pu, pulvinar; Put, putamen; Py, pyramidal tract; V.c.a and V.c.p, ventralis caudalis (anterior and posterior); V.im.i and V.im.e, ventralis intermedius (internus and externus); V.o.a, ventrooralis anterior; V.o.p, ventrooralis posterior. (Modified from Hassler R, Mundinger F, Riechert T. *Stereotaxis in Parkinson syndrome.* Berlin: Springer, 1979, with permission.)

for surgery. As discussed elsewhere in this volume, the selection of the target structure and the choice of the operative method, that is, ablative lesioning versus DBS, depend on the specific symptoms of the individual patient. It is highly recommended that clinicians see patients with PD preoperatively both "off" and "on" levodopa medication. In our opinion, procedures such as neurotransplantation for treatment of PD or Huntington's disease should be performed only in the framework of stringent clinical protocols, whereas other techniques such as thalamic DBS or thalamotomy for tremor have become routine in clinical practice. Nevertheless, numerous questions in movement disorders surgery remain unanswered and require further study. Therefore, it is desirable to collect prospective data and standardized documentation whenever possible. It is feasible to obtain independent assessment of outcome by movement disorders specialists. Formal neurologic assessments should be performed within days preoperatively. Ideally, two formal examinations should be obtained. Because of restrictions in staffing and financing, however, this is rarely possible.

Standardized assessment of movement disorders surgery became available only after the introduction of adequate rating scales that addressed treatment-related changes specifically. Useful scales, which provide a global view on the severity of PD and the limitations in daily living activities, that have been available since the 1960s include the Hoehn and Yahr staging system, the Webster scale, and the Schwab and England activities of daily living scale (32–34). A major impetus for the refinement of instruments to evaluate surgical outcome was the growing interest in transplantation programs for PD in the late 1980s. The Core Assessment Program for Intracerebral Transplantation (CAPIT) was published first in 1992 and has been used widely since then (35). A newer protocol was developed and published to allow comparison of different surgical interventions, the Core Assessment Program for Surgical Interventional Therapies in PD (CAPSIT-PD) (36). The CAPSIT-PD includes cognitive screening tests, evaluation of self-reporting

TABLE 5.1. STEREOTACTIC TARGET COORDINATES BASED ON THE INTERCOMMISSURAL LINE USED IN CONTEMPORARY SURGICAL TREATMENT OF MOVEMENT DISORDERS[a]

	x	y	z
Ventralis intermedius thalami	12–15	–3––7	+2––1
Globus pallidus pars interna	19–22	+2–+3	–4––6
Subthalamic nucleus	12–13	–4	–4––6

[a]The ranges given differ both with regard to differences in individual morphology and preferences of different surgeons. These anatomic coordinates are considered only preliminary, and physiologic target definition is essential.

by a patient diary, and assessment of quality of life (37). Furthermore, the protocol includes ratings of dyskinesias and dystonias, timed tests, and the Unified Parkinson's Disease Rating Scale (UPDRS). The UPDRS has become the most important rating scale to evaluate the impact of treatment of PD. The UPDRS assesses four domains including the following: mentation, behavior, and mood; activities of daily living; motor examination; and complications of therapy. The section on motor examination is administered both in the "off" state (usually, the "practically defined off" after a 12-hour washout of antiparkinsonian drugs in the morning) and in the "on" state (usually, the "best on" as assessed after the patient has taken the individual standard levodopa dose). Videotaping of the motor examination both "off" and "on" levodopa allows blinded evaluation and comparison of preoperative and follow-up examinations. Various rating scales to assess postoperative outcome are available for movement disorders other than PD.

We require *preoperative multiplanar MRI* of the brain in all patients who are considered candidates for functional stereotactic surgery. This approach allows exclusion of patients with symptomatic movement disorders who can be treated otherwise and permits assessment of the degree of cortical atrophy, ventriculomegaly, and ischemic encephalopathy. Severe cerebral atrophy may be a contraindication for surgery. We have shown, however, that patients with PD who have mild to moderate degrees of cerebral atrophy are not predisposed to a less favorable outcome after unilateral pallidotomy (38). Patients with cervical or truncal dystonia should also have plain radiographs in anteroposterior and lateral projections, to detect and document degenerative spine disease.

PREOPERATIVE PREPARATION OF THE PATIENT

With regard to the cost of the hospital stay and the current practice of reimbursement of health insurance carriers, patients are often admitted 1 day preoperatively or on the same day the surgical procedure is performed. Medication should have been stable for at least 1 month preoperatively. In patients who have difficulty in sleeping, a short-acting benzodiazepine not interfering with the movement disorder may be administered in the evening the day before the surgical procedure. Routine preoperative laboratory investigations include tests to detect clotting or bleeding disturbances. Any medication that may interfere with coagulation such as aspirin should be stopped 10 days preoperatively. Because cooperation of the patient is needed during the surgical procedure to guide placement of the lesion or of the electrode, it is important that patients are informed and understand each step of the operative procedure.

Functional stereotactic neurosurgery for treatment of movement disorders is performed using local anesthesia with few exceptions. General anesthesia may be necessary in patients with severe dystonia or ballism and in children (39, 40). In particular, under such circumstances, intraoperative microelectrode recording is clearly advantageous. Communication with the patient and neurologic assessment are essential during neurophysiologic confirmation of the target. Furthermore, the therapeutic effect can be assessed immediately, such as in patients with tremor, and the risk of side effects can be minimized. We do not give "premedication" or sedating or centrally acting analgesic drugs before or during any phase of the procedure. Laitinen has administered a combination of pethidine (meperidine) and atropine 15 minutes before the stereotactic device is mounted in pallidal surgery for PD (41). Some surgeons sedate patients for fixation of the stereotactic head frame by intravenous administration of propofol or short half-life benzodiazepines. Propofol may not ideally be suited for this purpose, because it may elicit abnormal movements, and it can interfere with parkinsonian symptoms (42). Investigators have also shown that propofol may suppress the firing of human pallidal neurons (43). We have tested the influence of the short-acting opioid remifentanil on single-unit recording and have not found significant changes with analgesic nonsedating dosages (Krauss and Koller, unpublished data).

Usually, any drugs used for treatment of the movement disorders are withheld preoperatively. In almost all centers, patients with PD are operated on in their "off" state. This allows the surgeon more easily to monitor the efficacy of stimulation or lesioning on parkinsonian target symptoms such as bradykinesia, rigidity, and tremor, which may guide the decision whether an electrode should be repositioned or a lesion should be enlarged or additional lesions be made. Furthermore, dyskinesias occurring while the patient is taking levodopa may interfere with fixation of the stereotactic head frame and stereotactic imaging, and they can cause artifacts during microelectrode recording. We usually give the last dose of antiparkinsonian medication at 6 p.m. on the day before the operation. Patients who suffer from very severe "off" periods may have single injections of subcutaneous apomorphine during the night if needed.

Corticosteroids are administered routinely in the perioperative period in many centers to reduce edema along the trajectory of the electrode and around the lesion in cases of radiofrequency lesioning. No hard data, however, are available to demonstrate the efficacy of this prophylaxis. We usually give a single bolus of 20 mg dexamethasone or 100 mg prednisolone directly before the skin incision is made. Other surgeons start with corticosteroids the night before the operation and taper the dosage over several days postoperatively (44).

The perioperative use of prophylactic anticonvulsants is controversial. The risk of postoperative seizures is probably reduced with CT and MRI localization of the target as compared with positive-contrast ventriculography. Occasionally, preoperative "loading" with relatively high doses

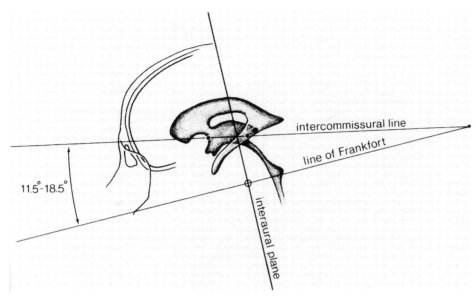

FIGURE 5.17. Relation between the intercommissural line and the "Frankfurter horizontale" (orbitomeatal line). The intercommissural line is angled at 11.5 to 18.5 degrees above the orbitomeatal line. (From Van Manen J. *Stereotactic methods and their application in disorders of the motor system.* Assen: van Gorcum, 1967, with permission.)

may contribute to postoperative lethargy and confusion. In particular, in elderly patients, these drugs may be poorly tolerated. Intravenous antibiotic prophylaxis is given before the procedure and may be maintained for 24 hours. We use third-generation cephalosporins such as cefuroxime or cefotiam.

We place an intravenous line, and in addition an arterial line to obtain accurate measurement of arterial blood pressure. Careful intraoperative and perioperative monitoring of the blood pressure is helpful for immediately recognizing and counteracting blood pressure rises or hypotension. Arterial hypertension may occur any time during the procedure, in particular when sedatives have not been given. Presumably, the risk of intracerebral hemorrhage is reduced when hypertension is corrected promptly. Occasionally, arterial hypotension may be seen during the procedure. Before we routinely placed arterial lines, we had to abort the operation in a patient because of the occurrence of vasovagal syncope during macrostimulation. Monitored care by an anesthesiologist experienced in functional stereotactic surgery has proved to be very valuable in our practice.

Fixation of the Stereotactic Head Frame

The head frame can be fixed to the patient's head in the operating room, in the ward, or in the radiology suite. The stereotactic frame is fixed rigidly to the skull, usually with four screws. The points of attachment are scrubbed and anesthetized with local anesthetic. We use a mixture of a long-acting and short-acting local anesthetic such as 2% lidocaine and 0.25% bupivacaine. The frame is attached to the patient's head to avoid any rotation or tilt of the head relative to the frame axes. The base line (y axis) should be as nearly parallel to the intercommissural line as possible. To achieve this alignment, the stereotactic frame is usually tilted slightly above the orbitomeatal line (Fig. 5.17). When one uses the Leksell G frame, the earbars are helpful for this purpose. For lesioning procedures, it is sufficient to shave the patient's hair only at the site of the incision, which is prepared with an antiseptic and is infiltrated with local anesthetic. The head is shaved more thoroughly in patients undergoing DBS both for subcutaneous tunneling of the lead and for minimizing the risk of infection.

STEREOTACTIC IMAGING AND ANATOMIC TARGET DEFINITION

There are divergent opinions on which stereotactic imaging method is most suitable for target determination in functional stereotactic surgery. For decades, *stereotactic ventriculography* was used to identify the AC and the PC. To avoid parallax effects, ventriculography was ideally performed with fixed x-ray tubes with long projection lines (teleradiology). These systems are rarely available now. The use of standard radiographs makes tedious calibrations necessary. Although ventriculography allows precise identification of the commissures, direct visualization and confirmation of the target are not possible. Ventriculography has largely been replaced by *stereotactic CT or MRI.* Investigators have demonstrated that CT- and MRI-guided localization of the commissures is accurate and is even superior to ventriculography (45,46).

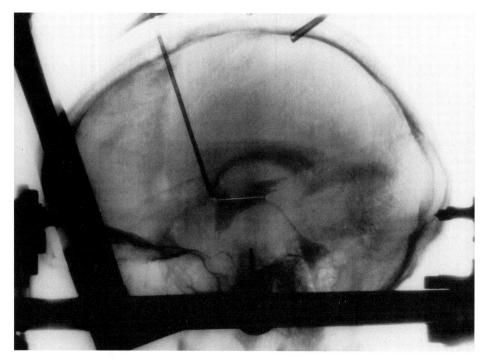

FIGURE 5.18. Stereotactic ventriculography. Lateral ventriculogram with the cannula in the frontal horn of the lateral ventricle close to the foramen of Monro. In this case, the line between the foramen of Monro and the posterior commissure has been marked *(white line)*.

Stereotactic Ventriculography

Positive-contrast ventriculography is still used by many surgeons for target calculation. Some obtain intraoperative ventriculography as an adjunct to CT- or MRI-based stereotactic determination of the targetcoordinates. Stereotactic ventriculography is currently performed with nonionic contrast media (Fig. 5.18). The contrast medium is injected into the lateral ventricle, for example, 10 mL iohexol (240 mg I/mL). To perform ventriculography, an additional tract to the anterior horn of the lateral ventricle is needed. In contemporary operating suites, ventriculograms in lateral and anteroposterior projections are obtained using C-arms. Image magnification has to be corrected with standard arithmetic algorithms. In rare cases, ventriculography may result in acute encephalopathy (47).

Stereotactic Computed Tomography

CT is considered the most geometrically accurate imaging modality for stereotactic localization. Over the years, it has replaced ventriculography as standard imaging technique in functional stereotactic neurosurgery. Several studies have shown the very high spatial accuracy of CT-guided stereotactic surgery (48,49). CT imaging has the relative disadvantage as compared with MRI in being inferior in the display of anatomic detail. For several years, we have used stereotactic CT as the primary method to identify the commissures. With regard to accuracy in the z axis and the resolution of

the reformations in the coronal and sagittal planes, it is advantageous to obtain contiguous 1-mm axial scans through the third ventricle and the basal ganglia (Fig. 5.19A). Depending on the software used for target calculation, it is best to coincide the z and the y axes of the scanner with the frame by using the laser light in the gantry. The imaging data can be transferred to a workstation where the axial scans are displayed simultaneously with the coordinated reformatted sagittal and coronal images (50). The simultaneous and multiplanar display allows visualization and accurate confirmation of the localization of the commissures in three planes. The most posterior margin of the AC and the most anterior margin of the PC are determined (Fig. 5.19B). When the commissures are present on more than one axial scan, the images displaying the largest diameter of the AC and the PC are selected, respectively.

Stereotactic Magnetic Resonance Imaging

Stereotactic MRI offers the advantage of demonstrating the morphology of the basal ganglia and of their circuitry much better than any other method. Therefore, in addition to defining the target by its spatial relation to the AC-PC line, MRI can also be used to obtain the target coordinates directly from visualization of the target structure (51). In the past, however, the use of stereotactic MRI localization in functional neurosurgery was limited because of various factors resulting in nonlinear image distortion (52). Magnetic

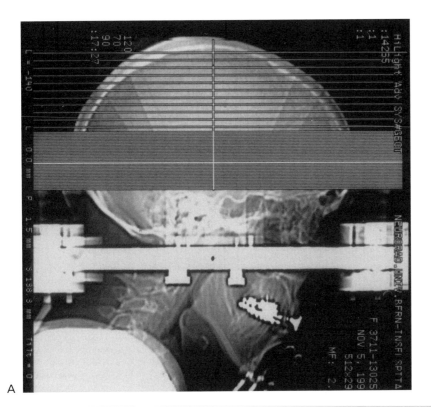

A

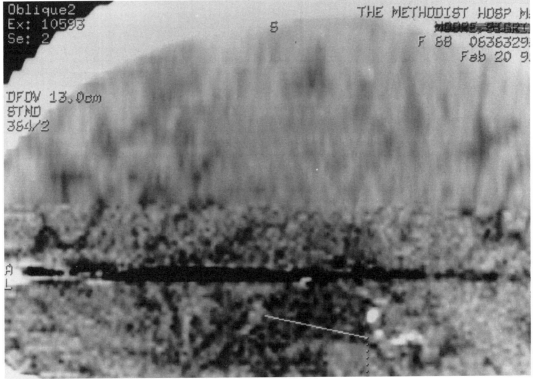

B

FIGURE 5.19. Stereotactic computed tomography for determination of the coordinates of the anterior and posterior commissures. **A:** Scout with prescribed 1-mm axial scans. **B:** Reformatted sagittal image through the anterior and posterior commissures. The tilt of the intercommissural line needs to be considered for target calculation.

distortions result from both gradient field nonlinearities and resonance offsets, including field inhomogeneities and chemical shift (53,54). To overcome these limitations, distortion correction methods have been developed. There are several techniques to reduce MRI distortion. Phantom measurements have been used routinely to detect spatial distortions for a given system and to improve its performance (55). Advances in correcting gradient and magnetic field inhomogeneities have yielded a geometric accuracy of about 1 mm, which is comparable to that of CT scanning. Frame-related factors are also of great importance for image distortion. In general, it appears to be advantageous for the fiducial system of the head frame to be close to the patient's head. The Leksell frame has been found to be relatively free of geometric distortion as compared with other frames (56). Resolution and accuracy can be further improved by obtaining narrow slice thicknesses and volume acquisitions. Three-dimensional data sets with magnetization prepared rapid gradient echoes have been shown to be of particular advantage (57). With three-dimensional MRI reconstructions, it is also possible to obtain multiplanar views of the AC-PC line. It is desirable to increase the matrix size to 512×512 pixels. Studies comparing the spatial accuracy of MRI-based localization systems and CT stereotaxy have shown that both machine-related and object-related MRI distortions can be minimized to acceptable levels by using distortion-resistant stereotactic instruments, contemporary scanning machinery, and improved scanning algorithms. Under such optimized conditions, the average difference between CT and MRI stereotactic coordinates of external fiducials, intracerebral target points, and anatomic landmarks is in the order of 1 pixel size. In one study, statistically significant but relatively small differences were found between MRI- and CT-derived target coordinates for patients undergoing thalamotomy or pallidotomy. The MRI-based calculations of the target coordinates differed from the CT-based calculations by a mean of 0.41 mm on the x axis, 0.06 mm on the y axis, and 0.34 mm on the z axis (58). With regard to the differences in reference point selection, the authors concluded that stereotactic MRI is an acceptable method that can be used alone to determine the anatomic target in functional stereotactic surgery. Another study also found agreement between ventriculography-derived coordinates and three-dimensional MRI-based calculation of thalamic and pallidal targets (59).

Some magnetic distortion with MRI appears to be inevitable, and continued vigilance is necessary with MRI stereotactic localization. It is recommended that one check the measurement of the fiducial system on the MRI console on a daily basis.

Coregistration and Image Fusion

Cross registration of stereotactic MRI and CT imaging has been used to take advantage of both the better spatial accuracy of CT technology and the higher anatomic resolution

of MRI scanning (60,61). The disadvantage of such image fusion algorithms that can be performed with commercially available software is the higher investment of time for acquisition of the images for operative planning. Available software allows coregistration of nonstereotactic MRI images with stereotactic CT scans.

Algorithms for Target Determination and Alignment Correction

Misalignment correction for the target calculation must be applied when the AC-PC line is not in perfect alignment with the three orthogonal axes of the stereotactic frame. Misalignment of the intercommissural line may best be envisioned by analogy to the motions of a sailboat, that is, pitch, yaw, and roll. *Pitch* refers to the elevation or depression of the bow of the boat (tilt of the intercommissural line in the anteroposterior axis), *yaw* describes turning of the bow to the right or the left (rotation of the intercommissural line), and *roll* indicates heeling of the boat (tilting of the head relative to the frame that results in changes in the positions of structures lateral to the intercommissural line, with reference to the frame base). Tilting of the AC-PC line relative to the y axis, which means that the AC and the PC are shown on different axial images, is encountered most frequently. Roll is infrequently a problem, in our experience. Various methods have been used to correct for misalignment (62,63). We have developed a computerized misalignment correction algorithm that has been implemented on a personal computer with a spreadsheet program (64). Basically, this algorithm corrects for deviations of the axis of the AC-PC line in relation to the stereotactic frame by rotating the target vector by different angles (Fig. 5.20). The frame coordinates of the preliminary target are then retranslated to CT coordinates, and its position is checked on multiplanar images with the interactive software (Fig. 5.21). If the target appears to be too close to adjacent structures such as the internal capsule or the choroid fissure, it is moved further away by 1 or 2 mm. The target coordinates are calculated independently by the neurosurgeon directly from the imaging data set and by the neuroradiologist using the programmed algorithm.

OPERATIVE PROCEDURE AND PHYSIOLOGIC TARGET DEFINITION

Despite the high resolution of contemporary neuroimaging techniques, physiologic confirmation and exploration of the target before placement of a lesion or implantation of a DBS electrode are essential to improve the accuracy of the procedure and to reduce side effects. Individual spatial variability may have a significant impact on physiologic target definition (12,65). Techniques that have been widely used for physiologic target determination in functional stereotactic

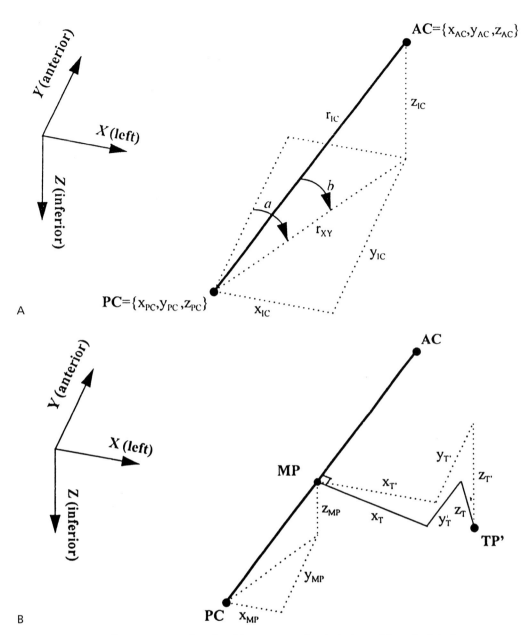

FIGURE 5.20. Alignment correction algorithm to correct for deviations of the axis of the intercommissural line (IC) in relation to the stereotactic frame. **A:** In this example, the anterior commissure (AC) lies above and to the left of the posterior commissure (PC), and it causes the IC line to deviate from the image *y* axis by the angle *a* in the *x-y* plane and by the angle *b* in the perpendicular plane. **B:** The diagram shows the displacements from the midpoint of the IC line parallel to the stereotactic atlas axes and calculated offsets from the midpoint to the target point in the CT image taking into account the deviation from the image *y* axis. The calculated offsets parallel the CT image axes. (From Krauss JK, King DE, Grossman RG. Alignment correction algorithm for transformation of stereotactic anterior commissure/posterior commissure-based coordinates into frame coordinates in image-guided functional neurosurgery. *Neurosurgery* 1998;42:806–812, with permission.)

neurosurgery include impedance monitoring, microelectrode recording, semimicroelectrode recording, microstimulation, and macrostimulation. Opinions differ about which neurophysiologic methods should be considered the "gold standard" in movement disorders surgery. Microelectrode recording and stimulation are methods used complementary to macrostimulation.

Surgical Technique

Once the coordinates of the tentative target have been calculated, the patient is brought to the operating room. With Laitinen's stereoadapter, the frame can be refixed, and the procedure may also be done another day (Fig. 5.22). In the operating room, the patient is positioned comfortably

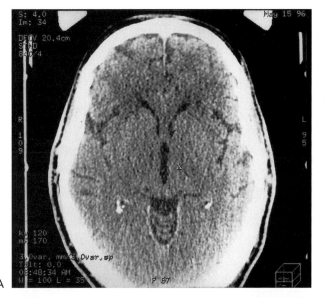

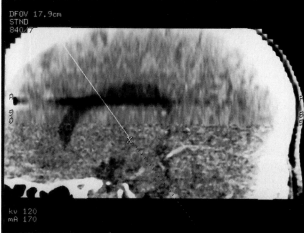

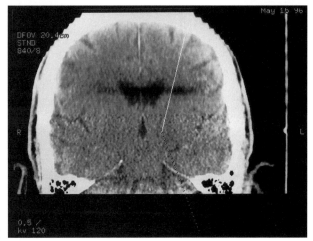

FIGURE 5.21. Confirmation of the target coordinates for the thalamic ventralis intermedius nucleus in a patient with tremor. The preliminary target and the electrode trajectory are shown simultaneously on coordinated axial **(A)** and reformatted tilted coronal **(B)** and sagittal **(C)** views. These views also allow correction of the target coordinates if necessary. (Modified from Krauss JK, Grossman RG. Surgery for hyperkinetic movement disorders. In: Jankovic J, Tolosa E, eds. *Parkinson's disease and movement disorders,* 3rd ed. Baltimore: Williams & Wilkins, 1998:1017–1047, with permission.)

in a semisitting position. The stereotactic frame is fixed to the table with a Mayfield adapter. This position avoids intraoperative cerebrospinal fluid leakage and reduces the possibility of "brain shift" (Fig. 5.23). Targets are reached usually through a frontal approach. The location of the bur hole depends mainly on the structure to be approached. We place the bur hole 2 cm lateral to the midline and 7 to 8 cm above the orbital rim, that is, usually just behind the hairline, for a pallidal procedure, and 3 cm lateral and 2 cm anterior to the coronal suture with a thalamic target. Some surgeons have used a much lower approach for pallidal procedures (66). The longitudinal incision is prepared with an antiseptic and is infiltrated with local anesthetic. The cranial opening may also be made with a twist drill (67). Typically, 3-mm twist drills are used. In our opinion, operating through a bur hole has several advantages. It allows better visualization and subsequent preservation of cortical vessels. Furthermore, multiple pathways for microelectrode recording can be made without the need for drilling a new opening. The dura is

coagulated and incised in a cruciate fashion. Any coagulation of even small bridging veins should be avoided because this may result in venous infarctions. A guiding cannula that allows passing of microelectrodes, macroelectrodes, and DBS electrodes is inserted into the brain at the crown of a gyrus after coagulation and incision of the arachnoid.

Impedance Recording

Impedance recording has been used to identify subcortical target nuclei since the early days of functional stereotactic surgery (68,69). Impedance reliably distinguishes gray matter from white matter and from cerebrospinal fluid spaces. In its present form, however, it is of only limited clinical usefulness in thalamic and basal ganglia surgery. Impedance is a complex phenomenon reflecting not only the resistance of tissue to current flow but also the properties of the system with which it is determined. Electrical impedance (Z) in tissue is defined as total opposition to a constant alternating

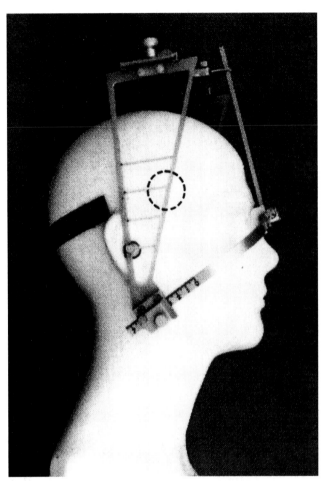

FIGURE 5.22. Laitinen's stereoadapter mounted onto a dummy. This relocatable device may be used for biopsies or functional stereotactic neurosurgery.

current. According to *Ohm's law* (Z = E/I), it is measured as the ratio of the voltage E (measured in volts) to the intensity of the current (I) that is generated in the tissue (measured in amperes). The impedance also depends on the capacitance, the frequency of the current, and the resistance of the tissue. Most standard radiofrequency lesion generators allow measuring electrical impedance. The electrical impedance of the brain structures that are traversed can be measured while the macroelectrode is forwarded to the target. The signal changes can be displayed acoustically with speakers. The change of the impedance on entering the basal ganglia yields a characteristic change in the sound. Typically, the impedance raises from about 300 to about 600 ohm with a 1.1 × 3-mm electrode. There are some variations of the impedance when the probe is advanced, for example, from the putamen to the GPi while traversing the medullar laminae between the external segment of the GP (GPe) and the GPi as well as within the internal pallidum (i.e., between the more lateral and the more medial portion of the GPi). The impedance abruptly drops when the choroidal fissure is entered. Laitinen et al. used impedance recording in conjunction with macrostimulation to guide the ventral extension of

a pallidotomy lesion (41,70). No further lesioning was performed when the impedance dropped to less than 400 ohm. According to some studies, impedance measurements with bipolar electrodes at frequencies between 8,000 and 10,000 Hz could be an interesting adjunct for physiologic target definition (71).

Microelectrode Recording

Microelectrode recording is a very efficient and elegant technique, and it offers a unique opportunity for the electrophysiologic study of the basal ganglia (72–76). The issue whether microelectrode recording is necessary to enhance the precision and the safety of targeting thalamic and basal ganglia nuclei in movement disorders surgery is still a matter of debate (31,77–80). Although some investigators are convinced that single-unit recording is a prerequisite for optimal targeting, others argue that the results using macrostimulation alone are comparable, and thus microelectrode recording is dispensable. Arguments against the use of microelectrode recording that are brought forward frequently include increased operating time and dependence on a neurophysiologist during the operation. These objections, however, are not necessarily valid. Although microelectrode recording in the context of scientific neurophysiologic studies may be time consuming, its use in clinical routine adds little to operative time. Techniques and the interpretation of the signals are easily learned by specialists in functional neurosurgery. Microelectrode recording is not accompanied by a higher risk of intracerebral hemorrhage, as has been argued by some of its opponents. One study using microelectrode recording to define the final target in 50 patients with PD who were undergoing pallidotomy demonstrated that the target determined by mapping was 2.3 mm more lateral and 3 mm more posterior than the target that had been defined by MRI (31). In this study, the actual lesion overlapped the initial target in only 45% of patients. The authors concluded that defining the target by anatomic imaging alone was not sufficient to determine reliably the position of the lesion to be made. Nevertheless, similar clinical outcomes after pallidotomy were reported without the use of microelectrode recording (41,70,81,82). A comparison of the relative advantages and disadvantages of microelectrode recording versus macrostimulation is shown in Table 5.2.

We find it very helpful to integrate microelectrode recording in procedures targeting the GPi and the STN. In particular, although macrostimulation in the GPi allows one to determine thresholds to assess the proximity of the neighboring internal capsule and optic tract, there is no way to determine exactly where within the pallidum, whether in the GPi or in the GPe, the electrode is located. Conversely, we do not perform single-unit mapping in thalamic procedures for tremor. Here, the goal to be achieved—the suppression of tremor—is more straightforward, and it is immediately assessable during the surgical procedure. The rationales and

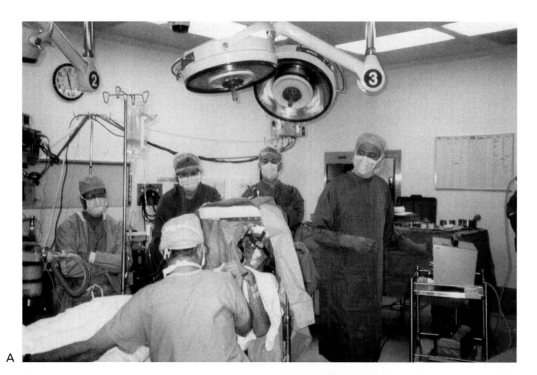

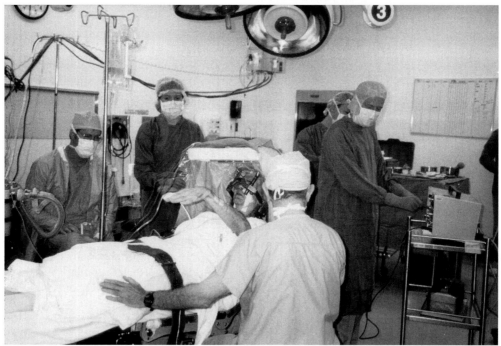

FIGURE 5.23. Positioning of a patient for a functional stereotactic procedure. The stereotactic frame is fixed to a Mayfield adapter, and the patient is in a comfortable semisitting position throughout the procedure. **A:** Testing of rigidity during pallidal macrostimulation. **B:** The patient holds up the left arm while a contralateral radiofrequency lesion is placed.

techniques of recording of single-unit discharges and of microstimulation are detailed by Hutchison in Chapter 6. We discuss only few general aspects in this section. High-impedance microelectrodes can be advanced either mechanically by a micrometer screw, manually by a hydraulic microdrive or electronically by switch buttons. We prefer

the hydraulic microdrive, which allows very fine movements of the electrode tip. The trajectory should allow sufficient recording of the area above and below the target structure and should seek identification of the adjacent optic tract in pallidal surgery. The signals are displayed on speakers and on an oscilloscope and are analyzed on line. The relative position

TABLE 5.2. PHYSIOLOGIC TARGET DEFINITION IN SURGICAL TREATMENT OF MOVEMENT DISORDERS: MICROELECTRODE RECORDING COMPARED WITH MACROSTIMULATION

	Macrostimulation	Single-Unit Recording
Safety	High	High
Time for exploration	Minutes	30 minutes to hours
Patient cooperation	Necessary	Not necessary
Resolution of spatial morphology of the explored area	Medium	Excellent
Identification of subnuclei	Medium	Excellent
Mapping of somatotopy	Good	Excellent
Identification of adjacent structures	Good	Not possible
Cost of equipment	Moderate	High
Setup of equipment in the operating room	Unproblematic	Time consuming
Sophistication of backup equipment required	Low	High
Durability of electrode	High	Low
Difficulties in solving technical problems	Medium	Complex

Modified from Tasker RR, Kiss ZHT. The role of the thalamus in functional neurosurgery. *Neurosurg Clin North Am* 1995;6:73–104, with permission.

of the units with regard to the tentative target is mapped on graph paper, and we take into account the firing pattern and frequency. We investigate only a few cells for their response to movement-related activity. In the early studies after the reintroduction of pallidotomy, many investigators used multiple microelectrode passes (72,79). Sometimes up to 6.8 trajectories were investigated on average. Over the past few years, however, most groups have reduced the number of pathways to explore the target structure. Currently, we usually obtain only one or two pathways in routine pallidal procedures in patients with PD. When the first trajectory yields satisfactory localization with identification of striatal cells, GPe pausers and bursters, laminar border cells, and abundant high-frequency discharge GPi cells, with adequate and proportionate spatial distribution, no additional tracts are made. Nevertheless, in single patients, more trajectories are necessary to identify the target precisely.

Microstimulation

Microstimulation by high-impedance electrodes *in situ* is a useful supplementary method to microelectrode recording (23,83). As in *macrostimulation,* intrinsic responses (i.e., modification of electrical activity at the target site) and extrinsic responses to spread of the current to neighboring structures can be achieved. In pallidal surgery, microstimulation is performed at 3 to 4 mm below the ventral pallidal border, with the room light dimmed to identify the optic tract. Visual sensations such as seeing stars or "Christmas lights" in different colors are reported by most, but not all, patients. At this location, we also perform photic stimulation by switching a flash light on and off in front of the patient's eyes. Frequently, this maneuver results in slight changes of the basic firing rate of the optic tract. Microstimulation of the corticospinal tract can evoke tetanic contractions of the contralateral extremities. In our experience, the use of microstimulation is restricted by its inherent technical limitations. Stimulation with increasingly higher voltage to evoke extrinsic responses often results in marked

reduction of the electrode impedance, and this may hamper its subsequent performance for microelectrode recording. It is necessary then to wait several minutes until the impedance of the electrode has recovered or it needs to be replaced.

Semi-microelectrode Recording

Semimicroelectrodes have tip diameters of 25 μm or more. These electrodes do not allow recording of single units, but they record background mass electrical activity, which has been called "neural noise" (84,85). The technique is simpler than microelectrode recording and requires less specialized technical equipment. In experienced hands, it allows differentiation of the putamen, the GPe, the GPi, the internal capsule, and the optic tract (Fig. 5.24). It may also be used to detect movement-related discharges in the thalamus and

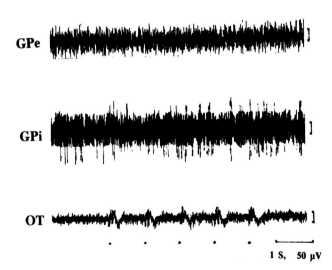

FIGURE 5.24. Semi-microelectrode recording in the globus pallidus externus (GPe) and internus (GPi). Below, the signals obtained from the optic tract (OT) are shown (From Ohye C. Neural noise recording in functional neurosurgery. In Gildenberg PL, Tasker RR, eds. *Textbook of stereotactic and functional neurosurgery.* New York: McGraw-Hill, 1998:941–947, with permission.)

the GPi. The spatial resolution, however, is less accurate as compared with high-impedance microelectrode recording.

Macrostimulation

Macrostimulation with monopolar or bipolar electrodes is the most frequently used method for target confirmation. Stimulus parameters vary from surgeon to surgeon, according to individual preference and experience. Often, rectangular monophasic pulses are used with a pulse width of 100 microseconds.

On insertion of the macroelectrode, a *setzeffekt* consisting of temporary improvement of the movement disorder of the contralateral extremity may occur. This effect is most pronounced in thalamic surgery for tremor and may result in complete and prolonged disappearance of contralateral tremor. In this setting, it has also been designated the *microthalamotomy effect*. The *setzeffekt* is much less consistent and weaker in the pallidum, where it may result in mild amelioration of contralateral bradykinesia. Some slight improvement may occasionally also be seen in dystonic movement disorders. We consider the *setzeffekt* a useful sign for good electrode location.

Macrostimulation is used to assess the threshold for the amelioration of the movement disorder and for spread of current to adjacent structures (24,86,87). The threshold is variable and depends on several factors such as the type of electrode, the waveform, the pulse width, and other parameters. Thus, it is not possible to compare thresholds directly, as reported by different surgeons. In the ventrolateral thalamus, low-frequency stimulation has no intrinsic effect or may even drive the tremor, whereas stimulation with frequencies higher than 80 Hz are effective in suppressing it. Macrostimulation is used to identify the internal capsule by evoking muscle twitches or tetanic contractions, the sensory relay thalamus (ventroposterolateralis and ventroposteromedialis) by producing paresthesias, and the optic tract by eliciting the perception of flashes or of phosphenes in the contralateral visual field. We perform macrostimulation first at a frequency of 5 Hz and then at 100 Hz. The voltage is increased incrementally from 0 v until a response is elicited. The occurrence of intrinsic and extrinsic responses is monitored by continuously watching and talking to the patient and is being protocolled (Fig. 5.23A). If no response of the tremor below a threshold of 2 v is obtained in thalamic surgery, we relocate the electrode until a satisfactory effect is noted. The appearance of capsular responses at a low voltage indicates that the electrode should be placed more medially, whereas early provocation of paresthesias suggests that a more anterior location should be sought. In pallidal surgery, the occurrence of phosphenes below a certain threshold indicates close proximity to the optic tract. Then, the electrode may be withdrawn in 0.5-mm increments, and the stimulation may be repeated in case a lesion is planned. In the

pallidum and the STN, both improvement of contralateral parkinsonian symptoms and the appearance of dyskinetic movements may be evoked at higher frequencies. An intense feeling of fear can be elicited in the patient by stimulation at 100 Hz at a threshold of 3 to 4 v in the GPi (88). This effect, which was always obtained when the voltage was increased to the threshold with the electrode properly placed at the final target site, appears to be an intrinsic pallidal response that is possibly related to the stimulation of pallidal neurons or circuitries related to emotion.

Intraoperative Evoked Potentials

In his pivotal report on posteroventral pallidotomy in 1992, Laitinen et al. reported postoperative homonymous visual field defects in 14% of patients (70). In subsequent studies, this incidence was markedly reduced. *Visual-evoked potentials* have been found a helpful adjunct to macrostimulation (89,90). Monocular stimulation with flash stimuli has been used alternating epochs between ipsilateral and contralateral eyes (89).

LESIONING TECHNIQUES

Various methods were used earlier for *lesioning* in functional stereotactic surgery (3,91–93). Electrolytic lesioning was the first technique to be applied (91). With electrical lesions, however, it was difficult to avoid charring of tissue around the electrode, and the final size of the lesion was unpredictable. Other methods that were used and that are mainly of historical interest include chemical lesioning, cryogenic lesion making, insufflation of balloons, induction heating of small implanted metal rods, ultrasound-induced lesions, and the implantation of radioactive isotopes (3,92,93). Currently, *thermocontrolled radiofrequency lesioning* is the technique that is used almost exclusively.

Radiofrequency Lesioning

The lesion is made, in general, with the electrode that has been used for macrostimulation. Some surgeons place *test lesions* before the final lesion is made (94). Test lesions usually are produced by heating up the electrode to 45° to 60°C for 10 to 60 seconds. Rarely, higher temperatures limited for only few seconds are applied, for example, 84°C for 10 seconds. Test lesions, however, may also result in irreversible tissue damage (95).

There are numerous variations how the lesions in thalamotomy or pallidotomy are created among different surgeons (96). In pallidotomy we place the lesion within 1 mm of the ventral border of the lateral GPi according to the microelectrode mapping. We perform pallidotomy with a monopolar 1.1 × 3-mm electrode. Usually, we place two

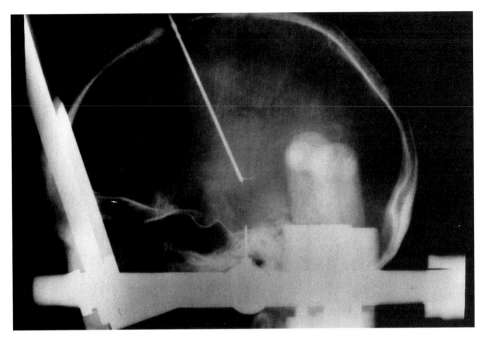

FIGURE 5.25. Intraoperative lateral radiograph demonstrating the use of the chord electrode.

lesions spaced 1.5 to 2 mm apart along the same trajectory by subsequently withdrawing the electrode. The lesions are created with the temperature controlled at 75°C for 60 seconds. During lesioning, strength and mobility of the contralateral arm, speech, and visual fields are monitored (Fig. 5.23B). This approach allows early detection of possible adverse effects and, if such effects occur, discontinuation of the radiofrequency lesioning. Some groups place serial lesions not in a ventral to dorsal direction but instead forward the electrode after the first lesion has been made (81). Other investigators make lesions along different parallel tracts, with the aim of reducing the activity of the physiologically defined sensorimotor region (78). Instead of using a fixed temperature for lesioning, the electrode may also be heated stepwise starting at 70° to 80°C and finally to 90°C for 60 seconds (23). The time of lesioning also varies with the thresholds at which capsular or optic responses are evoked by macrostimulation (85). For additional lesions, smaller electrodes with a diameter of 1.1 × 1 are useful. Some patients develop transient involuntary movements during pallidotomy or immediately thereafter. These movements usually are confined to the extremities contralateral to the side of the lesion. Most frequently, these movements appear choreic or choreoathetotic, but dystonic or hemiballistic hyperkinesias may also occur. Their appearance has been considered to predict a more favorable clinical outcome in patients with PD (97).

For thalamotomy, we use a monopolar 2 × 4-mm electrode to create a single lesion with the tip located just at the thalamic base. Again, the electrode is heated up to 70°C for 60 seconds, during which time the patient is monitored

for speech and motor symptoms. Even when the tremor is completely arrested after the electrode has been inserted, an appropriate lesion should be made to achieve long-term control. The subthalamic area including the zona incerta and the fields of Forel may be reached with the help of the chord electrode, which allows one to make additional smaller lesions (Fig. 5.25).

Radiofrequency lesioning is thought to be superior to all other methods used in the past to create therapeutic lesions in functional stereotactic surgery because it allows better definition of the lesion by varying parameters such as the diameter of the electrode, the exposed length of the electrode tip, and modulation of the time and temperature of the lesion making. The predictability of radiofrequency lesions has been shown in experimental lesioning studies in egg white (Fig. 5.26) (24, 98, 99). Furthermore, a computer model using finite element analysis has been introduced to study the spatial configuration of lesions created by varying different parameters (Fig. 5.27) (100). However, although the lesion may be predicted accurately by such models, there is some variation in the size of the final lesion in clinical functional stereotactic surgery. In an MRI study of 36 patients who underwent pallidotomy for treatment of PD, we found a lack of correlation in the volumes of pallidal lesions in the immediate postoperative phase and at 6-month follow-up (101).

MRI examinations of radiofrequency lesions performed within days after the surgical procedure typically show a three-zoned lesion (101,102) (Fig. 5.28). The lesion has an ellipsoid shape, with the longer diameter along the axis of the electrode tract. The inner zone of the lesion is hyperintense

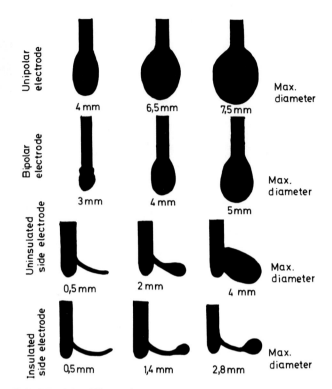

FIGURE 5.26. Different forms and sizes of radiofrequency lesions in egg white according to electrode type and diameter at a fixed temperature of 73°C. (From Hassler R, Mundinger F, Riechert T. *Stereotaxis in Parkinson syndrome.* Berlin: Springer, 1979, with permission.)

on T2-weighted images, the middle zone is hypointense, and the outer zone is hyperintense. The MRI appearance of these three zones is related to specific forms of hemoglobin and to the cellular and interstitial water content. Inversion recovery sequences are helpful to delineate the precise anatomic location of the lesion (Fig. 5.29). The middle zone of the

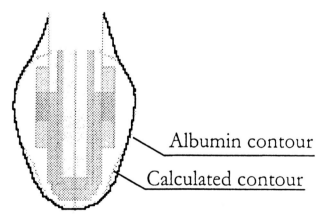

Albumin contour

Calculated contour

FIGURE 5.27. The power distribution of a radiofrequency lesion (60°C isotherm) predicted by a finite element model as compared with the contour of a nongelatinous albumin lesion. (From Eriksson O, Wren J, Loyd D, et al. A comparison between *in vitro* studies of protein lesions generated by brain electrodes and FEM simulations. *Med Biol Eng Comput* 1999;37:737–741, with permission.)

lesion is thought to correspond to the area of the hemorrhagic coagulation necrosis, and the outer zone is thought to present perilesional edema. There is additional edema beyond this zone that is not concentric and is less hyperintense than the outer zone of the lesion, which may spread along the longitudinal direction of axons (Fig. 5.29). In pallidotomy, such edema may spread along the internal capsule or the fibers of the optic tract (Fig. 5.30). In general, the lesions shrink over time, and investigators have assumed that healing and repair of the lesion occur over few months (Fig. 5.31). The late-phase lesion is hyperintense on T2-weighted MRI images and most likely indicates permanent tissue necrosis or gliosis (Figs. 5.31 and 5.32). An exponential rate for the shrinkage has been postulated, but most likely the kinetics of the shrinkage differs in different patients. The stage of the evolution of a radiofrequency lesion is critical when correlations between lesion volume and clinical improvement are made (101,103). Lesions should be of sufficient size to control movement disorders in the long term (104). The ideal size of the lesion, however, depends on several issues. We have seen some patients with good outcome after pallidal or thalamic surgery in whom the lesion could not be detected by MRI follow-up months or years after the operation.

Chemical Target Control and Perspectives

Chemical lesioning was performed earlier by alcohol or procaine oil injections at the target (105,106). Because both the lesion configuration and the clinical effects were difficult to control, this technique was subsequently abandoned. However, interest in chemical target control techniques has been renewed. Convection-enhanced delivery of quinolinic acid to the GPi specifically for lesioning of neurons expressing the *N*-methyl-D-aspartate receptor in MPTP (1-methyl-4-phenyl-1,2,3,6-tetrahydropyridine) parkinsonian monkeys yielded significant improvement of parkinsonian symptoms. Histologic examination showed selective damage to GPi neurons with complete sparing of white matter tracts (107–109). Temporary tremor arrest has been demonstrated after thalamic microinjections of muscimol in patients with essential tremor (110). Transient depression of neuronal activity at the target can be achieved by microinjection of local anesthetics such as lidocaine (111).

The use of short-pulsed lasers to achieve nonthermal ablation of neural tissue with laser pulses in the picosecond to femtosecond range may be an alternative lesioning method in the future (112).

Postoperative Care

Dural closure is not necessary because the bur hole is located close to the vertex. We place a small piece of gelatin such as

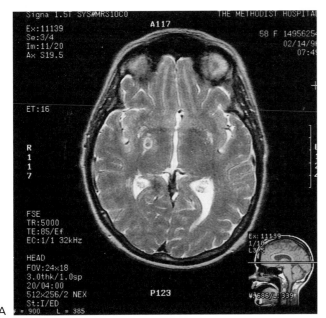

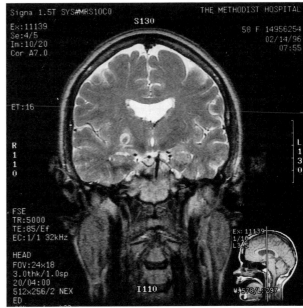

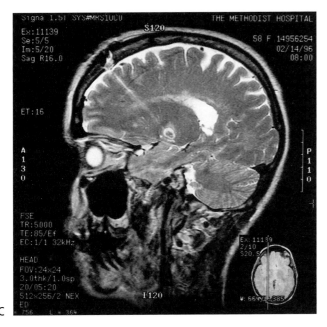

FIGURE 5.28. Magnetic resonance T2-weighted sequences of a 58-year-old patient 2 days after a right-sided pallidotomy. The axial **(A)**, coronal **(B)**, and sagittal **(C)** images show the elliptoid shape of the lesion and its three-zoned composition. (From Krauss JK, Desaloms MJ, Lai EC, et al. Microelectrode-guided posteroventral pallidotomy for treatment of Parkinson's disease: postoperative magnetic resonance imaging analysis. *J Neurosurg* 1997;87:358–367, with permission.)

Gelfoam in the dural opening. The bur hole can be covered by a plastic bur hole cover or a miniplate to achieve satisfactory cosmesis. The skin is closed with a two-layer suture. Patients are observed in an intermediate care unit overnight. Although this regimen probably is not necessary with regard to the risk of postoperative bleeding, intense monitoring and care are very supportive for patients, in particular parkinsonian patients who were "off" levodopa for several hours. In patients with PD, we usually do not administer levodopa directly postoperatively. Commonly, we start with levodopa on the first postoperative day with about one-half of the preoperative dosage. The usual preoperative dosage is given the following day, and adjustments are made subsequently. We

obtain postoperative MRI or CT scans routinely on the first or second postoperative day to confirm appropriate lesion placement or to check the position of the DBS electrode. Patients usually are discharged between 2 and 4 days postoperatively.

CHRONIC DEEP BRAIN STIMULATION

Chronic DBS has been used for decadesin the treatment of intractable pain (113). The techniques have evolved basically from cardiac pacemaker technology. As early as the 1970s, the place of DBS in the therapeutic management

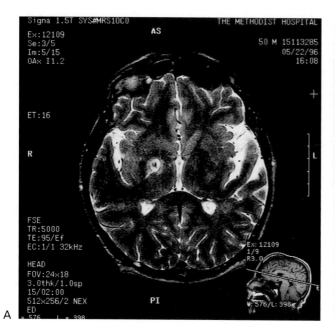
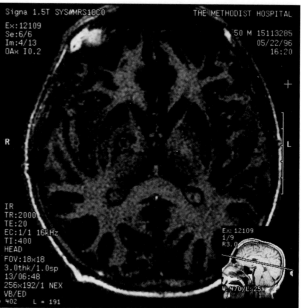

FIGURE 5.29. Axial T2-weighted **(A)** and inversion recovery **(B)** Magnetic resonance images in a 50-year-old man 3 days after a right-sided pallidotomy. The inversion recovery sequences show clearly that the lesion is confined to the globus pallidus internus. Additional perilesional edema spreads into the adjacent internal capsule. (From Krauss JK, Desaloms MJ, Lai EC, et al. Microelectrode-guided posteroventral pallidotomy for treatment of Parkinson's disease: postoperative magnetic resonance imaging analysis. *J Neurosurg* 1997;87:358–367, with permission.)

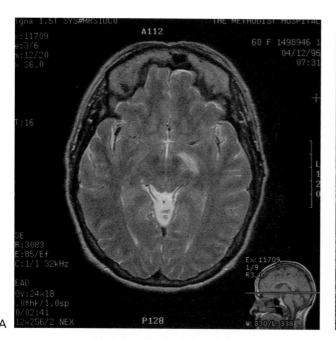
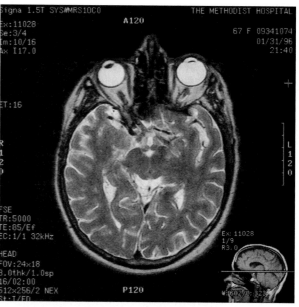

FIGURE 5.30. Axial T2-weighted magnetic resonance images obtained 2 days postoperatively. In both patients, asymptomatic edema of the optic tract is detected, and it is more marked in **(A)** than in **(B)**. (From Krauss JK, Desaloms MJ, Lai EC, et al. Microelectrode-guided posteroventral pallidotomy for treatment of Parkinson's disease: postoperative magnetic resonance imaging analysis. *J Neurosurg* 1997;87:358–367, with permission.)

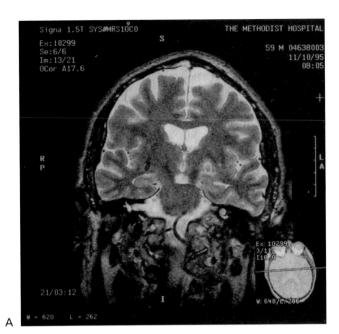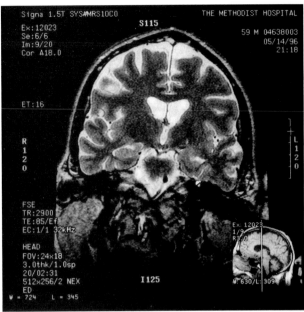

A   B

FIGURE 5.31. Coronal T2-weighted magnetic resonance images of a 59-year-old man after left-sided posteroventral pallidotomy 2 days postoperatively **(A)** and at 6-month follow-up **(B).** There is considerable shrinkage of the lesion, which is composed of three characteristic zones in the early phase and presents as a small hypertense lesion in the late phase. Nevertheless, the beneficial clinical effect was sustained.

of movement disorders was investigated (114–116). However, it was not until Benabid and colleagues in Grenoble and Siegfried in Zürich demonstrated the efficacy of thalamic DBS in larger series of patients that it became widely accepted as a therapeutic option for the treatment of movement disorders (117–120). Although the thalamic VIM is

the major target for tremor, the GPi and the STN are targeted for treatment of other parkinsonian symptoms and dystonia.

Here, we will not discuss the advantages and relative disadvantages of DBS as compared to lesioning (120–122). Recently, Schuurman and colleagues conducted a prospective

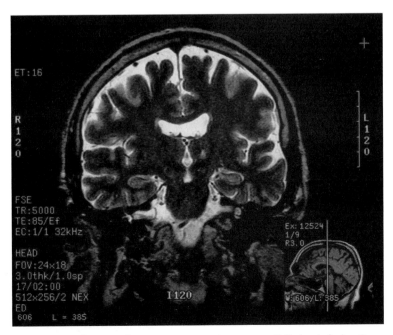

FIGURE 5.32. A coronal magnetic resonance scan shows a small thalamic lesion 3 years after a successful thalamotomy for the treatment of tremor.

randomized study showing that thalamic stimulation and thalamotomy are equally effective for the suppression of tremor, but thalamic stimulation had fewer adverse effects and resulted in a greater improvement in function (123). Chronic DBS has been pivotal in developing simultaneous bilateral basal ganglia surgery further (124–126). One of the major qualities of DBS is that it is principally reversible. The use of DBS technology is also more forgiving than radiofrequency lesioning when the target has not been identified with absolute precision. In that regard, DBS is easier to perform, and slight deviations from reaching the ideal target can be compensated for by combining different electrode contacts. Among the major drawbacks of DBS are higher expenses, mainly related to the cost of the hardware. Furthermore, with the present technology, the pulse generator needs to be replaced after 2 to 7 years of use.

Technology

Contemporary DBS systems consist of four elements: the electrode which is guided stereotactically to the selected target, an extension wire, an implantable pulse generator (IPG), and external programming devices. At this time, the hardware for DBS that is used most widely in clinical routine is manufactured and distributed by Medtronic, Minneapolis. Two different types of electrodes are currently available for DBS for treatment of movement disorders (Fig. 5.33). The electrodes are 1.2 mm in diameter. The unipolar electrode

is either 23 or 30 cm long, and the quadripolar electrodes are 28 or 40 cm long. The flexible electrode is shielded by a plastic sheath on the outside and is stabilized by a removable stylet within the electrode. In most cases, quadripolar electrodes are used (Figs. 5.34 and 5.35). The "standard" quadripolar electrode (model 3387) has four contacts, each 1.5-mm long, at a 1.5-mm distance from each other. There is a dead space of 1.5 mm at the tip of the lead. The most distal contact has been designated as contact 0, and the most proximal is termed contact 3. Principally, quadripolar electrodes allow two different modalities of stimulation. With monopolar cathodal stimulation, the IPG serves as the anode. Any of the electrode contacts or a combination of adjacent contacts may be selected for chronic DBS. Bipolar stimulation uses one of the electrode contacts as the anode and another one as the cathode. Again, a combination of electrode contacts may be chosen. With bipolar stimulation, the polarity of the contacts may be switched. A variant of the standard quadripolar electrode, the reduced space electrode (model 3389), with the contacts closer together, has been developed for chronic STN DBS (127,128). The monopolar electrode (model 3388) has a single contact at the tip of the wire and is free of the 1.5-mm dead space. This electrode has been used by some surgeons for GPi stimulation in patients with PD (129). The extension wires connect the DBS electrode to the IPG and are available in different lengths to allow implantation of the IPG in a subcutaneous pocket below the patient's clavicle or in the subcutaneous tissue of the abdominal wall.

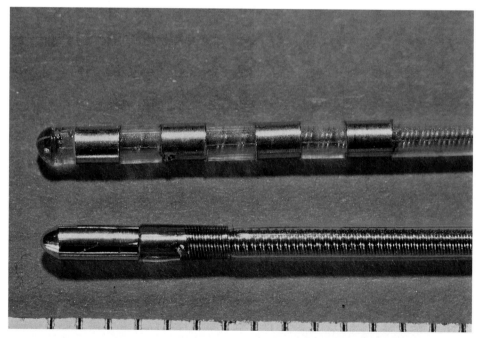

FIGURE 5.33. Two different types of electrodes for chronic deep brain stimulation. The quadripolar electrode has four contacts, each 1.5 mm long at a 1.5 mm distance from each other, and a dead space at the tip of the lead. The unipolar electrode has a single larger contact at the tip of the lead. **Below:** Scale in millimeters.

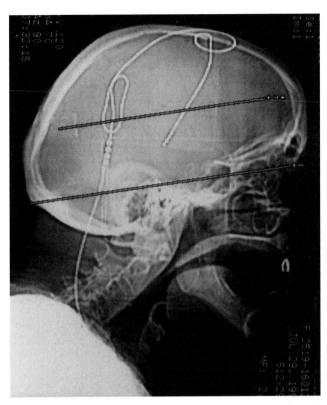

FIGURE 5.34. Lateral radiograph showing an implanted quadripolar deep brain stimulation electrode in the thalamic ventralis intermedius (VIM) for treatment of unilateral tremor.

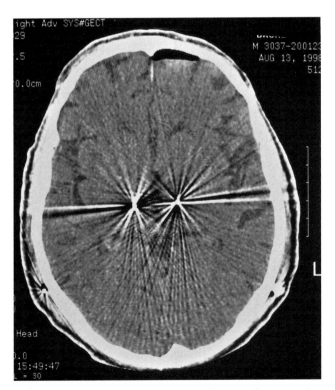

FIGURE 5.35. Axial computed tomography scans demonstrating bilateral deep brain stimulation of the ventralis intermedius (VIM) in a patient with tremor.

The first IPG that was used regularly in movement disorders surgery was the Itrel I. The Itrel I has an oval shape (10 mm thick, 21 cc, and 36 g) and is smaller than the other IPG models. There are several limitations when using the Itrel I with regard to programming of stimulation parameters. One has few choices of amplitude of the voltage, of frequency of the stimulation, and of pulse width. Stimulation frequencies higher than 130 pulses per second cannot be programmed with early models, and fine tuning of the parameters is not possible. Therefore, we generally replace the Itrel I with an Itrel II when the batteries have run down. The Itrel II has been used in most clinical trials so far (10 mm thick, 23 cc, and 49 g). It is slightly larger than the Itrel I, but it allows for much more variability in selecting stimulation parameters (Fig. 5.36). The amplitude that can be programmed ranges from 0 to 10.5 v, the frequency from 2 to 185 Hz (depending on the software used for programming), and the pulse width from 60 to 450 microseconds. The Itrel II has been further developed, and is now available as the *Soletra*. The IPGs may be operated either in electrical mode or in a magnet mode. Other features that are available include programming of different patterns of stimulation delivery continuously or cycling between on and off with given time frames, a lower amplitude at the onset of stimulation, and other functions to tailor the parameters to the needs of the individual patient. These features are seldom used in movement disorders surgery but are much more commonly used in the treatment of chronic pain. More recently, the Kinetra has entered the market. The Kinetra allows stimulation of two DBS electrodes, and thus can be implanted unilaterally in patients with bilateral procedures instead of two Itrel IIs. It is bulkier, however, and it tends to be more visible in the subclavicular region in very thin persons. The Kinetra and the Itrel III have several new programming features that are interesting for future investigations.

The IPG is usually programmed once it has been implanted and the patient is fully awake postoperatively. This is achieved noninvasively with a console programmer operating by telemetry (model 7432) (Fig. 5.37). A programming head connected to the console by a cable is placed directly over the subcutaneous IPG. Optimal parameters are determined by varying the electrode contacts, the stimulation mode (monopolar versus bipolar), pulse width, frequency, and amplitude.

There are several possibilities for patients to control the performance of their IPGs (Fig. 5.37). For many patients, we think that it is advantageous to have continuous stimulation. This is particularly true for patients with dystonia and patients with PD who are severely akinetic at night or who wake up because of intermittent bursts of resting tremor. In other patients with essential tremor or PD-related tremor, however, it is useful to switch the stimulation off overnight to increase battery life. The IPGs are turned off by a handheld magnet and are turned on the same way. The Access Therapy Controller (model 7436) is available for use with

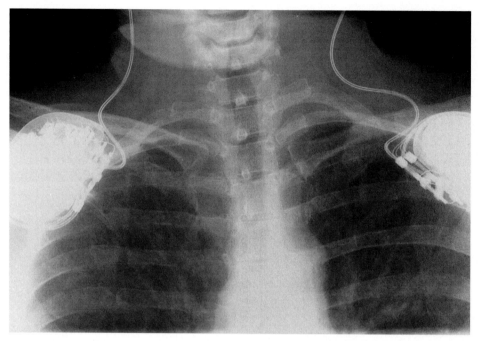

FIGURE 5.36. Bilateral implantations of pulse generators (Itrel II) in a subcutaneous pocket below the clavicle.

the Kinetra stimulation system. It can be used to turn the stimulator on or off, and it allows the patient to modify stimulation amplitude, pulse width, and rate within given limits preprogrammed by the physician.

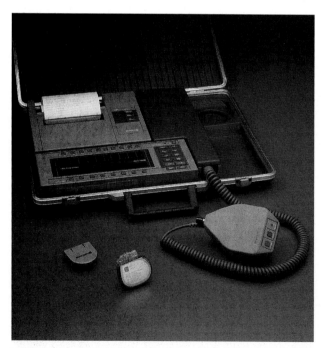

FIGURE 5.37. Devices to program and control the performance of an implanted pulse generator (console programmer with programming head and magnet). (Courtesy of Medtronic, Minneapolis.)

Operative Technical Aspects

The principles of anatomic and physiologic definition of the target in chronic DBS are essentially identical to those used for radiofrequency lesioning. There are some differences in technique for implantation of the DBS hardware among specialists in functional neurosurgery (130–137). The IPG may be implanted in the same operative session after the patient has undergone induction of general anesthesia, or the electrode may be externalized to perform test stimulations. Opinions differ with regard to the usefulness and the necessity of interoperative test stimulation.

We generally perform the two successive steps of the procedure in the same operative session. The first step involves fixation of the stereotactic frame, stereotactic imaging, and placement of the DBS electrode by using local anesthesia. As with radiofrequency lesioning, we consider physiologic target definition with microelectrode recording very useful for targeting the GPi. Because of its small size, this technique is also extremely valuable for identification of the STN. Subsequently, macrostimulation is usually performed with the same electrodes that are used for radiofrequency lesioning. An alternative is to perform macrostimulation directly with the DBS electrodes (137). For this purpose, the electrodes are directly advanced through the guiding cannula by locating the tip of the quadripolar lead (dead space) 1.5 mm below the target with all four contacts free or, if a unipolar electrode is used, directly at the target (Fig. 5.38). Improvement of tremor during thalamic procedures on insertion of the lead (the microthalamotomy effect or *setzeffekt*) is considered a sign indicating good positioning of the electrode the tremor is not adequately controlled below a threshold of 1 to 2 v or when persistent extrinsic responses are observed below a threshold of 2 to 4 v (depending on the screening device used), different combinations of electrode contacts or monopolar trials through the different electrode contacts are tested. If these trials do not yield adequate relief or still elicit persistent extrinsic responses, then the electrode is repositioned, guided by the effects that have been observed during stimulation with regard to all three dimensions.

Appropriate positioning of the electrode is much more difficult to confirm in patients with dystonic movement disorders and in the GPi and the STN. Some surgeons find it helpful to demonstrate adequate anatomic positioning of the electrode by intraoperative radiography or ventriculography (130). When a satisfactory position has been achieved, the stylet of the lead and the guiding cannula are carefully removed. During this process, the electrode is stabilized with a lead holder and rubber-shod forceps. The electrode then is secured to a plastic ring that has been placed in the bur hole (Fig. 5.39). Permanent fixation is achieved by placing a bur hole cap into the ring. Because this maneuver may result in a slight downward dislocation of the electrode, several alternatives have been developed for electrode fixation. These techniques include the use of a hollow double screw that can be fixed to the bur hole, the Straumann screw (Waldenburg, Switzerland), fixation with titanium miniplates, and the use of methylmethacrylate (139,140). Finally, the lead is coiled under the galea. If the electrode is externalized, a special extension wire is used that can be cut later at the site where it exits the scalp, to guarantee sterility. External test stimulations are usually performed over several days.

The patient undergoes induction of general anesthesia while the stereotactic head frame is removed. The IPG is implanted in a subcutaneous infraclavicular pouch after it is connected to the DBS electrode with the subcutaneous extension wire. It is advisable to fix the IPG to the muscle fascia with a nonabsorbable suture because subcutaneous switching of the IPG around its axis may impede programming later or may render it impossible. The extension wire

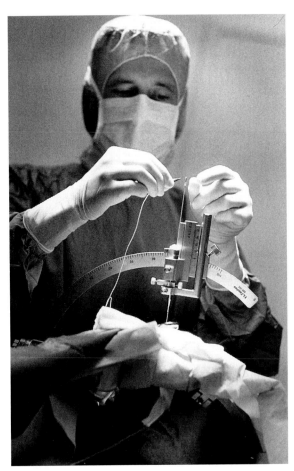

FIGURE 5.38. Intraoperative test stimulation through a unipolar deep brain stimulation electrode. (Courtesy of Michael Schneeberger, Bern.)

in the *x* and *y* axes. Thresholds for both intrinsic and extrinsic evoked responses are determined directly through the implanted electrode with a screening device (model 3625). Intraoperative screening may also be performed with a modified IPG (MIPG) consisting of an Itrel II, which allows finer determination of the thresholds by using the console programmer (138). Intraoperative test stimulation through DBS electrodes is performed with stimulation parameters similar to those of radiofrequency lesioning electrodes. The major advantages of stimulating directly through the DBS leads are that the effects can be assessed more directly with the system that will be used later on, and there is no risk of differences in the physiologic definition of the target and the final location of the electrode (137). In thalamic procedures, stimulation is performed in all patients even when the tremor has been completely abolished by insertion of the lead. The thresholds for arrest of the tremor of the arm and leg are determined at 130 Hz. The voltage then is increased until paresthesias of the contralateral face, hand, or fingers are elicited, or until tetanic contractions of the hand or corner of the mouth are noted. When

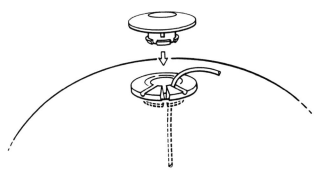

FIGURE 5.39. The electrode is fixed in a slot of the bur hole ring by gently pressing a cap into the ring. (Courtesy of Medtronic, Minneapolis.)

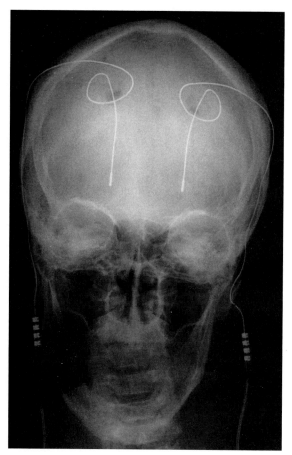

FIGURE 5.40. Fracture of the left deep brain stimulation lead above the connector in a patient with dystonia.

is tunneled subcutaneously with a tunneling device similar to that used in shunt surgery. The extension wire is coiled behind the IPG. The connector should be placed between the intracranial electrode and the extension wire on the patient's skull because placing it in the neck can result in an increased likelihood of fracture of the DBS electrode close to the connector. This is particularly the case in patients with dystonic head movements (Fig. 5.40). In our experience, operative time for both steps from fixation of the head frame until extubation, including stereotactic image acquisition and target calculation, insertion of the lead and neurophysiologic determination of the target, and implantation of the IPG, totals about 2.5 to 4 hours for unilateral thalamic surgery for control of tremor. Operative times can be considerably longer with other movement disorders and bilateral procedures targeting the GPi or the STN. The IPGs can be programmed immediately postoperatively. When a prolonged microthalamotomy-like effect is present, the IPG is programmed on reappearance of the tremor.

When the MIPG has been used intraoperatively, the recorded parameters can be used as a basis for programming. Although programming is straightforward in patients with unilateral tremor, it may be time consuming in patients with

dystonia or PD. Several postoperative visits can be necessary to achieve the optimal parameter setting in patients with GPi or STN stimulation. It is essential to see patients with PD both off and on levodopa, to optimize the effects of stimulation with GPi or STN electrodes. The effect of thalamic DBS on tremor is observed within a second or so after programming of the IPG, whereas the effect of GPi and STN stimulation may need longer to be assessed appropriately. In dystonia, some early response is usually noted, but optimal clinical improvement is typically delayed, and it may take months to be fully appreciated. Switching the stimulators on can elicit brief flashes in the contralateral visual field in GPi stimulation and paresthesias in thalamic stimulation that are clinically irrelevant.

Specific Issues

Operative side effects of positioning of the electrode are similar to those for positioning of lesion-making electrodes (141,142). Stimulation-specific side effects include paresthesias, gait ataxia, and dysarthria (143). Rarely, patients develop focal dystonia with thalamic stimulation. The advantage of DBS is that these unwanted effects can be reduced be decreasing the intensity of stimulation. Chronically implanted foreign bodies may subserve the delayed occurrence of infections, which, however, are very rare in DBS for treatment of movement disorders in our experience. Tolerance to the stimulation can develop over time, but it is usually compensated for by adjustment of stimulation parameters, in particular by increasing amplitude. When the stimulators are switched off, rebound phenomena may occur. These may consist of increased tremor amplitudes with thalamic stimulation (130) and "super offs" with cessation of STN stimulation (144). A neuroprotective effect of chronic STN stimulation has been hypothesized (145).

The mechanisms of DBS are not entirely clear (146–148). Because chronic DBS has a clinical effect similar to that of a lesion, investigators have assumed that DBS causes a functional ablation of neurons by blocking their activity. In addition, other mechanisms could be involved, such as orthodromic activation of efferent fibers or antidromic driving of inhibitory fibers (147). In movement disorders such as dystonia in which a delayed response is seen, reorganization of central neural circuitries may also be relevant. There is little experience with the long-term effect of chronic DBS on adjacent neural elements. Postmortem studies in patients with thalamic stimulation for PD-related tremor revealed only small areas of gliosis and spongiosis around the tract (149,150).

Lead fracture may occur primarily at two sites: at the DBS electrode close to the connection of the extension wire, as outlined earlier, and on the extension wire just close to the site where it is plugged into the IPG (Fig. 5.41). Overall, however, this complication is rare, observed in about 3% of

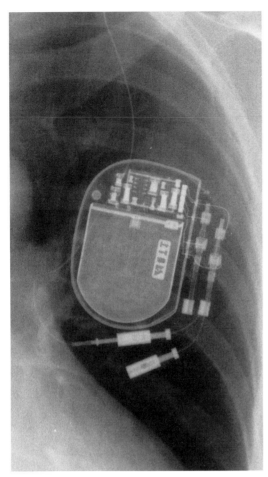

FIGURE 5.41. Cable fracture of the extension wire close to the implanted pulse generator.

luck. Theft-detecting devices can also switch stimulators off or on. They have been described as a safety hazard in patients with spinal stimulation electrodes. MRI appears to pose no particular risk in patients with externalized DBS electrodes. The issue whether patients with implanted DBS systems can undergo MRI investigations is under discussion (151,152). Further investigations are necessary.

The time after which the batteries need to be replaced depends on various factors. Battery life is mainly shortened by high amplitudes, but stimulation frequency and pulse width are also relevant (Fig. 5.42). Rechargeable IPGs would be desirable. Most likely, we will see major improvements in existing systems with progress in technology over the next few years.

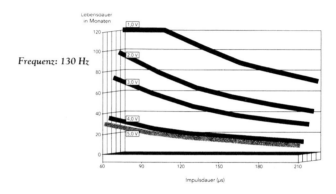

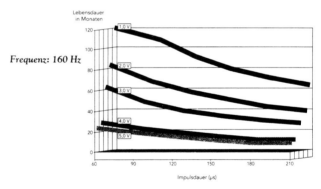

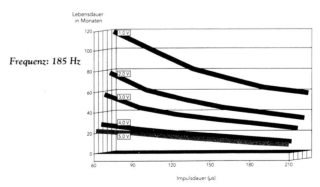

FIGURE 5.42. Battery life in months of an Itrel II pulse generator at different frequencies in chronic deep brain stimulation depending on the amplitude and the pulse widths used (16 hours daily). (Courtesy of Medtronic, Minneapolis.)

our patients at a mean follow-up of more than 2 years. In the first case, the complete DBS electrode has to be explanted and repositioned under stereotactic guidance. Unfortunately, there is no way to repair the DBS electrode at the site of the fracture. The site of the fracture is usually well visualized on lateral and anteroposterior radiographs.

Patients with cardiac pacemakers have been considered not to be candidates for chronic DBS. With special precautions, however, the operation of both systems in a patient is possible. When the DBS system is implanted in such patients, continuous electrocardiographic monitoring by a cardiologist is necessary intraoperatively and during the initial programming. Both the cardiac pacemaker and the DBS have to be programmed in bipolar stimulation mode, for the patient's safety.

The IPGs can be switched off by static electromagnetic fields or by magnets. Sometimes, IPGs may also switch from electrical stimulation mode to magnet stimulation mode. This may occur, for example, with door-locking magnets built into refrigerators. We had one patient whose IPG was switched on before programming by a large horseshoe that he had fixed at the rail of his bed to bring him good

REFERENCES

1. Horsley V, Clarke RH. The structure and function of the cerebellum examined by a new method. *Brain* 1908;31:45–124.
2. Spiegel EA, Wycis HT. Thalamotomy and pallidotomy for treatment of choreic movements. *Acta Neurochir* 1952;2:417–422.
3. Krauss JK, Grossman RG. Historical review of pallidal surgery for treatment of parkinsonism and other movement disorders. In: Krauss JK, Grossman RG, Jankovic J, eds. *Pallidal surgery for the treatment of Parkinson's disease and movement disorders.* Philadelphia: Lippincott–Raven, 1998:1–23.
4. Bullard DE, Nashold BS. Evolution of principles of stereotactic neurosurgery. *Neurosurg Clin North Am* 1995;6:27–41.
5. *Todd-Wells manual of stereotaxic procedures.* Randolph: Codman and Shurtleff, 1967.
6. Schaltenbrand G, Wahren P. *Atlas for stereotaxy of the human brain.* Stuttgart: Thieme, 1977.
7. Birg W, Mundinger F. Computer calculations of target parameters for a stereotactic apparatus. *Acta Neurochir* 1973;29:123–129.
8. Kelly PJ. *Tumor stereotaxis.* Philadelphia: WB Saunders, 1991.
9. Talairach J, Hecaen H, David M, et al J. Recherches sur la coagulation thérapeutique des structures souscorticales chez l'homme. *Rev Neurol* 1949,81:4–24.
10. Schaltenbrand G, Bailey P. *Introduction to stereotaxis with an atlas of the human brain.* Stuttgart: Thieme, 1959.
11. Van Manen J. *Stereotactic methods and their application in disorders of the motor system.* Assen: van Gorcum, 1967.
12. Kelly PJ, Derome P, Guiot G. Thalamic spatial variability and the surgical results of lesions placed with neurophysiologic control. *Surg Neurol* 1978;9:307–315.
13. Grossman RG, Hamilton WJ. Surgery for movement disorders. In: Jankovic J, Tolosa E, eds. *Parkinson's disease and movement disorders,* 2nd ed. Baltimore: Williams & Wilkins, 1993:531–548.
14. Taren J, Guiot G, Derome P, et al. Hazards of stereotaxic thalamectomy: added safety factor in corroborating x-ray target localization with neurophysiological methods. *J Neurosurg* 1968;29:173–182.
15. Burchiel KJ. Thalamotomy for movement disorders. *Neurosurg Clin North Am* 1995;6:55–71.
16. Gildenberg PL, Tasker RR, eds. *Textbook of stereotactic and functional neurosurgery.* New York: McGraw-Hill, 1998.
17. Struppler A. The history of stereotactic and functional neurosurgery techniques. In: Gildenberg PL, Tasker RR, eds. *Textbook of stereotactic and functional neurosurgery.* New York: McGraw-Hill, 1998:1233–1243.
18. Mundinger F. Stereotaxic interventions on the zona incerta area for treatment of extrapyramidal motor disturbances and their results. *ConfinNeurol* 1965;26:222–230.
19. Coffey RF. Stereotactic atlases in printed formats. In: Gildenberg PL, Tasker RR, eds. *Textbook of stereotactic and functional neurosurgery.* New York: McGraw-Hill, 1998:237–248.
20. Spiegel EA, Wycis HT. *Stereoencephalotomy: thalamotomy and related procedures. Part I: methods and stereotaxic atlas of the human brain.* New York: Grune & Stratton, 1952.
21. Talairach J, David M, Tournoux P, et al. *Atlas d'anatomie stéréotaxique.* Paris: Masson, 1957.
22. Talairach J, Tournoux P. *Co-planar stereotaxic atlas of the human brain: 3-dimensional proportional system: an approach to cerebral imaging.* Stuttgart: Thieme, 1988.
23. Lozano A, Hutchison W, Kiss Z, et al. Methods for microelectrode-guided posteroventral pallidotomy. *J Neurosurg* 1996;84:194–202.
24. Hassler R, Mundinger F, Riechert T. *Stereotaxis in Parkinson syndrome.* Berlin: Springer, 1979.
25. Jeanmonod D, Magnin M, Morel A. Low-threshold calcium spike bursts in the human thalamus: common physiopathology for sensory, motor and limbic positive symptoms. *Brain* 1996;119:363–375.
26. Markham CH, Rand RW. Stereotactic surgery in Parkinson's disease. *Arch Neurol* 1963;8:621–631.
27. Siegfried J. Stereotaxic cerebellar surgery. *Confin Neurol* 1971;33:350–360.
28. Laitinen LV. Brain targets in surgery for Parkinson's disease. *J Neurosurg* 1985;62:349–351.
29. Taha JM, Favre J, Baumann TK, et al. Characteristics and somatotopic organization of kinesthetic cells in the globus pallidus of patients with Parkinson's disease. *J Neurosurg* 1996;85:1005–1112.
30. Hoover JE, Strick PL. Multiple output channels in the basal ganglia. *Science* 1993;259:819–821.
31. Guridi J, Gorospe A, Ramos E, et al. Stereotactic targeting of the globus pallidus internus in Parkinson's disease: imaging versus electrophysiological mapping. *Neurosurgery* 1999;45:278–287.
32. Hoehn MM, Yahr MD. Parkinsonism, onset, progression, and mortality. *Neurology* 1967;17:427–442.
33. Webster DD. Critical analysis of the disability in Parkinson's disease. *Mod Treat* 1968;5:257–282.
34. Schwab RS, England AC. Projection technique for evaluating surgery in Parkinson's disease. In: Gillingham FJ, Donaldson MC, eds. *Third symposium on Parkinson's disease.* Edinburgh: Livingstone, 1969.
35. Langston JW, Widner H, Goetz CG, et al. Core assessment program for intracerebral transplantations (CAPIT). *Mov Disord* 1992;7:2–13.
36. Defer GL, Widner H, Marie RM, et al. Core assessment program for surgical interventional therapies in Parkinson's disease (CAPSIT-PD). *Mov Disord* 1999;14:572–584.
37. Jenkinson C, Fitzpatrick R, Peto V. Health-related quality-of-life measurement in patients with Parkinson's disease. *Pharmacoeconomics* 1999;15:157–165.
38. Desaloms JM, Krauss JK, Lai EC, et al. Posteroventral medial pallidotomy for treatment of Parkinson's disease: preoperative magnetic resonance imaging features and clinical outcome. *J Neurosurg* 1998;89:194–199.
39. Krauss JK, Mohadjer M, Nobbe F, et al. Bilateral ballism in children. *Childs Nerv Syst* 1991;7:342–346.
40. Ondo WG, Desaloms JM, Jankovic J, et al. Pallidotomy for generalized dystonia. *Mov Disord* 1998;13:693–698.
41. Laitinen LV. Pallidotomy for Parkinson's disease. *Neurosurg Clin North Am* 1995:6:105–112.
42. Krauss JK, Akeyson EW, Giam P, et al. Propofol-induced dyskinesias in Parkinson's disease. *Anesth Analg* 1996;83:420–422.
43. Heit G, Murphy G, Jaffe R, et al. Effects of propofol on human globus pallidus neurons. *Stereotact Funct Neurosurg* 1996–1997;67:74.
44. Bie RMA de, Schuurman PR, de Haan PS, et al. Unilateral pallidotomy in advanced Parkinson's disease: a retrospective study of 26 patients. *Mov Disord* 1999;14:951–957.
45. Alterman RL, Kall BA, Cohen H, et al. Stereotactic ventrolateral thalamotomy: is ventriculography necessary? *Neurosurgery* 1995;37:717–722.
46. Hariz MI, Bergenheim AT. A comparative study on ventriculographic and computerized tomography-guided determinations of brain targets in functional stereotaxis. *J Neurosurg* 1990;73:565–571.
47. Schuurman PR, Speelman JD, Ongerboer de Visser BW, et al. Acute encephalopathy after iohexol ventriculography in functional ster—eotaxy. *Acta Neurochir* 1998;140:98–99.
48. McKean JD, Allen PB, Filipow LJ, et al. CT guided functional stereotaxic surgery. *Acta Neurochir* 1987;87:8–13.
49. Kondziolka D, Dempsey PK, Lunsford LD, et al. A comparison between magnetic resonance imaging and computed

tomography for stereotactic coordinate determination. *Neurosurgery* 1992;30:402–407.

50. Krauss JK, Grossman RG. Surgery for hyperkinetic movement disorders. In: Jankovic J, Tolosa E, eds. *Parkinson's disease and movement disorders,* 3rd ed. Baltimore: Williams & Wilkins, 1998:1017–1047.

51. Starr PA, Vitek JL, DeLong M, et al. Magnetic resonance imaging-based stereotactic localization of the globus pallidus and subthalamic nucleus. *Neurosurgery* 1999;44:303–314.

52. Walton L, Hampshire A, Forster DMC, et al. A phantom study to assess the accuracy of stereotactic localization, using Tl-weighted magnetic resonance imaging with the Leksell stereotactic system. *Neurosurgery* 1996;38:170–178.

53. Smith RC, Lange RC, McCarthy SM. Chemical shift artifact: dependance on shape and orientation of the lipid-water interface. *Radiology* 1991;181:225–229.

54. Sumanaweera TS, Adler JR Jr, Napel S, et al. Characterization of spatial distortion in magnetic resonance imaging and its implications for stereotactic surgery. *Neurosurgery* 1994;35:157–166.

55. Orth RC, Sinha P, Madsen EL, et al. Development of a unique phantom to assess the geometric accuracy of magnetic resonance imaging for stereotactic localization. *Neurosurgery* 1999;45:1423–1431.

56. Burchiel KJ, Nguyen TT, Coombs BD, et al. MRI distortion and stereotactic neurosurgery using the Cosman-Roberts-Wells and Leksell frames. *Stereotact Funct Neurosurg* 1993;60:210–214.

57. DiPierro CG, Francel PC, Jackson TR, et al. Optimizing accuracy in magnetic resonance image-guided stereotaxis: a technique with validation based on the anterior commissure-posterior commissure line. *J Neurosurg* 1999;90:94–100.

58. Holtzheimer PE 3rd, Roberts DW, Darcey TM. Magnetic resonance imaging versus computed tomography for target localization in functional stereotactic neurosurgery. *Neurosurgery* 1999;45:290–297.

59. Schuurman PR, de Bie RMA, Majoie CBL, et al. A prospective comparison between three-dimensional magnetic resonance imaging and ventriculography for target-coordinate determination in frame-based functional stereotactic neurosurgery. *J Neurosurg* 1999;91:911–914.

60. Alexander E III, Kooy HM, van Herk M, et al. Magnetic resonance image-directed stereotactic neurosurgery: use of image fusion with computerized tomography to enhance spatial accuracy. *J Neurosurg* 1995;83:271–276.

61. Cohen DS, Lustgarten JH, Miller E, et al. Effects of coregistration of MR to CT images on MR stereotactic accuracy. *J Neurosurg* 1995;82:772–779.

62. Patil AA, Gelber P. Accuracy of thalamotomy target determination using axial images only. *Stereotact Funct Neurosurg* 1991;56:104–108.

63. Spiegelmann R, Friedman WA. Rapid determination of thalamic CT-stereotactic coordinated: a method. *Acta Neurochir* 1991;110:77–81.

64. Krauss JK, King DE, Grossman RG. Alignment correction algorithm for transformation of stereotactic anterior commissure/posterior commissure–based coordinates into frame coordinates in image-guided functional neurosurgery. *Neurosurgery* 1998;42:806–812.

65. Sugita K, Takaoka Y, Mutsuga N, et al. Correlation between anatomically calculated target point and physiologically determined point in stereotaxic surgery. *Confin Neurol* 1972;34:84–93.

66. Dogali M, Fazzini E, Kolodny E, et al. Stereotactic ventral pallidotomy for Parkinson's disease. *Neurology* 1995;45:753–761.

67. Taha JM, Favre J, Baumann TK, et al. Tremor control after pallidotomy in patients with Parkinson's disease: correlation with microrecording findings. *J Neurosurg* 1997;86:642–647.

68. Bullard DE, Nashold BS Jr. Impedance recording in functional neurosurgery. In: Gildenberg PL, Tasker RR, eds. *Textbook of stereotactic and functional neurosurgery.* New York: McGraw-Hill, 1998:949–953.

69. Laitinen LV, Johansson GG. Locating human cerebral structures by the impedance method. *Confin Neurol* 1967;29:197–201.

70. Laitinen LV, Bergenheim AT, Hariz MI. Leksell's posteroventral pallidotomy in the treatment of Parkinson's disease. *J Neurosurg* 1992;76:53–61.

71. Axer H, Stegelmeyer J, Graf von Keyserlingk D. Comparison of tissue impedance measurements with nerve fiber architecture in human telencephalon: value in identification of intact subcortical structures. *J Neurosurg* 1999;90:902–909.

72. Hutchison WD, Lozano AM, Davis KD, et al. Differential neuronal activity in segments of globus pallidus in Parkinson's disease patients. *Neuroreport* 1994;5:1533–1537.

73. Vitek JL, Bakay RAE, DeLong MR. Microelectrode-guided pallidotomy for medically intractable Parkinson's disease. In: Obeso JA, DeLong MR, Ohye C, et al., eds. The basal ganglia and new surgical approaches for Parkinson's disease. *Adv Neurol* 1997;74:183–198.

74. Gross RE, Lombardi WJ, Hutchison WD, et al. Variability in lesion location after microelectrode-guided pallidotomy for Parkinson's disease: anatomical, physiological, and technical factors that determine lesion distribution. *J Neurosurg* 1999;90:468–477.

75. Sterio D, Beric A, Dogali M, et al. Neurophysiological properties of pallidal neurons in Parkinson's disease. *Ann Neurol* 1994;35:586–591.

76. Hutchison WD, Allan RJ, Opitz H, et al. Neurophysiological identification of the subthalamic nucleus in surgery for Parkinson's disease. *Ann Neurol* 1998;44:622–628.

77. Alterman RL, Sterio D, Beric A, et al. Microelectrode recording during posteroventral pallidotomy: impact on target selection and complications. *Neurosurgery* 1999;44:315–323.

78. Bakay RAE. Comment on: Sutton JP, Couldwell W, Lew MF, et al. Ventroposterior medial pallidotomy in patients with advanced Parkinson's disease. *Neurosurgery* 1995;36:1116–1117.

79. Baron MS, Vitek JL, Bakay RAE, et al. Treatment of advanced Parkinson's disease by posterior GPi pallidotomy: 1-year results of a pilot study. *Ann Neurol* 1996;40:355–366.

80. Tasker RR, Kiss ZHT. The role of the thalamus in functional neurosurgery. *Neurosurg Clin North Am*er 1995;6:73–104.

81. Johansson F, Malm J, Nordh E, et al. Usefulness of pallidotomy in advanced Parkinson's disease. *J Neurol Neurosurg Psychiatry* 1997;62:125–132.

82. Kishore A, Turnbull IM, Snow JB, et al. Efficacy, stability and predictors of outcome of pallidotomy for Parkinson's disease: six-month follow-up with additional 1-year observations. *Brain* 1997;120:729–737.

83. Yamashiro K, Mukawa J. Correlation of microstimulation, single-unit recording, and averaged evoked potentials. In: Gildenberg PL, Tasker RR, eds. *Textbook of stereotactic and functional neurosurgery.* New York: McGraw-Hill, 1998:925–933.

84. Ohye C. Neural noise recording in functional neurosurgery. In: Gildenberg PL, Tasker RR, eds. *Textbook of stereotactic and functional neurosurgery.* New York: McGraw-Hill, 1998:941–947.

85. Iacono RP, Shima F, Lonser RR, et al. The results, indications, and physiology of posteroventral pallidotomy for patients with Parkinson's disease. *Neurosurgery* 1995;36:1118–1127.

86. Schaltenbrand G, Spuler H, Prucker G, et al. Electroanatomical observations on the ventral caudal parts of the thalamus according to the facts of stereotactic stimulation in man. *Z Neurol* 1974,206:287–308.

87. Tasker RR, Organ LW, Hawrylyshyn PA. *The thalamus and midbrain of man: a physiological atlas using electrical stimulation.* Springfield, IL: Charles C Thomas, 1982.

88. Riechert T. *Stereotactic brain operations.* Bern: Huber, 1980.

89. Bonaroti EA, Rose RD, Kondziolka D, et al. Flash visual evoked potential monitoring of optic tract function during macroelectrode-based pallidotomy. In: Lunsford LD, ed. Controversies in movement disorder surgery. *Neurosurg Focus* 1997;3:2.

90. Yokoyama T, Sugiyama K, Nishizawa S, et al. Visual evoked potentials during posteroventral pallidotomy for Parkinson's disease. *Neurosurgery* 1999;44:815–824.

91. Carpenter MB, Whittier JR. Study of methods for producing experimental lesions of the central nervous system with special reference to stereotaxic technique. *J Comp Neurol* 1952;97:73–131.

92. Iskandar BJ, Nashold BS Jr. History of functional neurosurgery. *Neurosurg Clin North Am* 1995;6:1–25.

93. Walker AE. Stereotaxic surgery for tremor. In: Schaltenbrand G, Walker AE, eds. *Stereotaxy of the human brain.* Stuttgart: Thieme, 1982:515–521.

94. Favre J, Taha JM, Nguyen TT, et al. Pallidotomy: a survey of current practice in North America. *Neurosurgery* 1996;39:883–890.

95. Lunsford LD. Comment on Favre J, Taha JM, NguyenTT, et al. Pallidotomy: a survey of current practice in North America. *Neurosurgery* 1996;39:890–892.

96. Cosman ER. Radiofrequency lesions. In: Gildenberg PL, Tasker RR, eds. *Textbook of stereotactic and functional neurosurgery.* New York: McGraw-Hill, 1998:973–985.

97. Merello M, Cammarota A, Betti 0, et al. Involuntary movements during thermolesion predict a better outcome after microelectrode guided posteroventral pallidotomy. *J Neurol Neurosurg Psychiatry* 1997;63:210–213.

98. Dieckmann G, Gabriel E, Hassler R. Size, form and structural peculiarities of experimental brain lesions obtained by thermocontrolled radiofrequency. *Confin Neurol* 1965;26:134–142.

99. Eriksson O, Wardell K, Bylund NE, et al. *In vitro* evaluation of brain lesioning electrodes (Leksell) using a computer-assisted video system. *Neurol Res* 1999;21:89–95.

100. Eriksson O, Wren J, Loyd D, et al. A comparison between *in vitro* studies of protein lesions generated by brain electrodes and FEM simulations. *Med Biol Eng Comput* 1999;37:737–741.

101. Krauss JK, Desaloms JM, Lai EC, et al. Microelectrode-guided posteroventral pallidotomy for treatment of Parkinson's disease: postoperative magnetic resonance imaging analysis. *J Neurosurg* 1997;87:358–367.

102. Tomlinson FH, Jack CR Jr, Kelly PJ. Sequential magnetic resonance imaging following stereotactic radiofrequency ventralis lateralis thalamotomy. *J Neurosurg* 1991;74:579–584.

103. Lehman RM, Mezrich R, Sage J, et al. Peri- and postoperative magnetic resonance imaging localization of pallidotomy. *Stereotact Funct Neurosurg* 1994;62:61–70.

104. Hirai T, Miyazaki M, Nakajima H, et al. The correlation between tremor characteristics and the predicted volume of effective lesions in stereotaxic nucleus ventralis intermedius thalamotomy. *Brain* 1983;106:1001–1018.

105. Cooper IS. *Parkinsonism: its medical and surgical therapy.* Springfield, IL: Charles C Thomas, 1961.

106. Narabayashi H, Okuma T, Shikiba S. Procaine oil blocking of the globus pallidus. *Arch Neurol Psychiatry* 1956;75:36–48.

107. Gogate N, Corthesy ME, Lonser RR, et al. Convection-enhanced superselective excitotoxic pallidal lesioning for Parkinson's disease. *Neurosurgery* 1997;41:739.

108. Lieberman DM, Corthesy ME, Cummins A, et al. Reversal of experimental parkinsonism by using selective chemical ablation of the medial globus pallidus. *J Neurosurg* 1999;90:928–934.

109. Lonser RR, Corthesy ME, Morrison PF, et al. Convection-enhanced selective excitotoxic ablation of the neurons of the globus pallidus internus for treatment of parkinsonism in nonhuman primates. *J Neurosurg* 1999;91:294–302.

110. Pahapill PA, Levy R, Dostrovsky JO, et al. Tremor arrest with thalamic microinjections of muscimol in patients with essential tremor. *Ann Neurol* 1999;46:249–252.

111. Dostrovsky JO, Sher GD, Davis KD, et al. Tasker RR. Microinjection of lidocaine into human thalamus: a useful tool in stereotactic surgery. *Stereotact Funct Neurosurg* 1993;60:168–174.

112. Suhm N, Gotz MH, Fischer JP, et al. Ablation of neural tissues by short-pulsed lasers: a technical report. *Acta Neurochir* 1996;138:346–349.

113. Richardson DE. Deep bain stimulation for the relief of chronic pain. *Neurosurg Clin North Am* 1995;6:135–144.

114. Andy OJ. Thalamic stimulation for control of movement disorders. *Appl Neurophysiol* 1983;46:107–111.

115. Brice J, McLellan L. Suppression of intention tremor by contingent deep-brain stimulation. *Lancet* 1980;1:1221—1222.

116. Mundinger F. New stereotactic treatment of spasmodic torticollis with a brain stimulation system [in German]. *Med Klin* 1977,18:1982–1986.

117. Benabid AL, Pollak P, Louveau A, et al. Combined (thalamotomy and stimulation) stereotactic surgery of the VIM thalamic nucleus for bilateral Parkinson disease. *Appl Neurophysiol* 1987;50:344–346.

118. Benabid AL, Pollak P, Gervason C, et al. Long-term suppression of tremor by chronic stimulation of the ventral intermediate thalamic nucleus. *Lancet* 1991;337:403–406.

119. Siegfried J. Therapeutic stereotactic procedures on the thalamus for motor movement disorders. *Acta Neurochir* 1993;124:14–18.

120. Siegfried J, Lippitz B. Chronic electrical stimulation of the VL-VPL complex and of the pallidum in the treatment of movement disorders: personal experience since 1982. *Stereotact Funct Neurosurg* 1994;62:71–75.

121. Starr PA, Vitek JL, Bakay RAE. Ablative surgery and deep brain stimulation for Parkinson's disease. *Neurosurgery* 1998;43:989–1015.

122. Tronnier VM, Fogel W, Kronenbuerger M, et al. Is the medial globus pallidus a site for stimulation or lesioning in the treatment of Parkinson's disease? *Stereotact Funct Neurosurg* 1997;69:62–68.

123. Schuurman PR, Bosch DA, Bossuyt PMM, et al. A comparison of continuous thalamic stimulation and thalamotomy for suppression of severe tremor. *N Engl J Med* 2000;342:461–468.

124. Gross C, Rougier A, Guehl D, et al. High-frequency stimulation of the globus pallidus internalis in Parkinson's disease: a study of seven cases. *J Neurosurg* 1997;87:491–498.

125. Burchiel KJ, Anderson VC, Favre J, et al. Comparison of pallidal and subthalamic nucleus deep brain stimulation for advanced Parkinson's disease: results of a randomized, blinded pilot study. *Neurosurgery* 1999;45:1375–1384.

126. Krauss JK, Pohle T, Weber S, et al. Bilateral deep brain stimulation of the globus pallidus internus for treatment of cervical dystonia. *Lancet* 1999;354:837–838.

127. Limousin P, Krack P, Pollak P, et al. Electrical stimulation of the subthalamic nucleus in advanced Parkinson's disease. *N Engl J Med* 1998;339:1105–1011.

128. Siebner HR, Ceballos-Baumann A, Standhardt H, et al. Changes in handwriting resulting from bilateral high-frequency stimulation of the subthalamic nucleus in Parkinson's disease. *Mov Disord* 1999;14:964–971.

129. Siegfried J, Lippitz B. Bilateral chronic electrostimulation of ventroposterolateral pallidum: a new therapeutic approach for alleviating all parkinsonian symptoms. *Neurosurgery* 1994;35:1126–1130.

130. Benabid AL, Pollak P, Gao D, et al. Chronic electrical stimulation of the ventralis intermedius nucleus of the thalamus as a treatment of movement disorders. *J Neurosurg* 1996;84:203–214.

131. Blond S, Caparros-Lefebvre D, Parker F, et al. Control of tremor and involuntary movement disorders by chronic stereotactic stimulation of the ventral intermediate thalamic nucleus. *J Neurosurg* 1992;77:62–68.

132. Hubble JP, Busenbark KL, Wilkinson S, et al. Deep brain stimulation for essential tremor. *Neurology* 1996;46:1150–1153.

133. Koller W, Pahwa R, Busenbark K, et al. High-frequency unilateral thalamic stimulation in the treatment of essential and parkinsonian tremor. *Ann Neurol* 1997;42:292–299.

134. Ondo W, Jankovic J, Schwartz K, et al. Unilateral thalamic deep brain stimulation for refractory essential tremor and Parkinson's disease tremor. *Neurology* 1998;51:1063–1069.

135. Nguyen JP, Degos JD. Thalamic stimulation and proximal tremor. *Arch Neurol* 1993;50:498–500.

136. Pahwa R, Wilkinson S, Smith D, et al. High-frequency stimulation of the globus pallidus for the treatment of Parkinson's disease. *Neurology* 1997;49:249–253.

137. Krauss JK, Simpson RK, Ondo WG, et al. Concepts and methods in chronic thalamic stimulation for treatment of tremor: technique and application. *Neurosurgery* 2001;68:535–541.

138. Krauss JK, Pohle T. Intraoperative test stimulation with a modified implantable pulse generator in deep brain stimulation. *Acta Neurochir* 2000;142:587–589.

139. Siegfried J, Blond S. Thalamic stimulation. In: Siegfried J, Blond S, eds. *The neurosurgical treatment of Parkinson's disease and other movement disorders.* London: Williams & Wilkins, 1997, 73-86.

140. Favre J, Taha JM, Steel T, et al. Anchoring of deep brain stimulation electrodes using a microplate: technical note. *J Neurosurg* 1996;85:1181–1183.

141. Hosobuchi Y. Subcortical stimulation for control of intractable pain in humans: report of 122 cases (1970–1984). *J Neurosurg* 1986;64:543–553.

142. Young RE. Intracranial procedures for pain management. In: Appuzo MLJ, ed. *Brain surgery: complication avoidance and management,* vol 2. New York: Churchill Livingstone, 1993:1497–1508.

143. Broggi G. Chronic deep brain stimulation: clinical results. In: Germano IM, ed. *Neurosurgical treatment of movement disorders.* Park Ridge, IL: American Association of Neurological, 1998.

144. Kumar R, Lozano AM, Montgomery E, et al. Pallidotomy and deep brain stimulation of the pallidum and subthalamic nucleus in advanced Parkinson's disease. *Mov Disord* 1998; 13[Suppl 1]:73–82.

145. Rodriguez MC, Obeso JA, Olanow CW. Subthalamic nucleus-mediated excitotoxicity in Parkinson's disease: a target for neuroprotection. *Ann Neurol* 1998;44[Suppl 1]:S175–188.

146. Limousin P, Greene J, Pollak P, et al. Changes in cerebral activity pattern due to subthalamic nucleus or internal pallidum stimulation in Parkinson's disease. *Ann Neurol* 1997;42:283–291.

147. Ashby P, Kim YJ, Kumar R, et al. Neurophysiological effects of stimulation through electrodes in the human subthalamic nucleus. *Brain* 1999;122:1919–1931.

148. Strafella A, Ashby P, Munz M, et al. Inhibition of voluntary activity by thalamic stimulation in humans: relevance for the control of tremor. *Mov Disord* 1997;12:727–737.

149. Caparros-Lefebvre D, Ruchoux MM, Blond S, et al. Long-term thalamic stimulation in Parkinson's disease: postmortem anatomoclinical study. *Neurology* 1994;44:1856–1860.

150. Haberler C, Alesch, F, Mazal PR, et al. No tissue damage by chronic deep grain stimulation in Parkinson's disease. *Ann Neurol* 2000; 48:372–376.

151. Tronnier VM, Staubert A, Hahnel S, et al. Magnetic resonance imaging with implanted neurostimulators: an *in vitro* and *in vivo* study. *Neurosurgery* 1999;44:118–125.

152. Rezai AR, Lozano AM, Crawley AP, et al. Thalamic stimulation and functional magnetic resonance imaging: localization of cortical and subcortical activation with implanted electrodes: technical note. *J Neurosurg* 1999;90:583–590.

Surgery for Parkinson's Disease and Movement Disorders,
edited by J.K. Krauss, J. Jankovic, and R.G. Grossman.
Lippincott Williams & Wilkins, Philadelphia © 2001.

6

TECHNIQUES OF MICROELECTRODE RECORDING IN MOVEMENT DISORDERS SURGERY

WILLIAM D. HUTCHINSON

The routine use of *microelectrode recording* for localizing subcortical targets for stereotactic brain surgery started in the 1950s and is generally attributed to Albe-Fessard and Guiot (1). The advances in brain imaging since then have contributed immensely to the development of stereotactic brain surgery, but there is still a need for the fine degree of localization provided by microelectrode recording. Research into the individual properties and population characteristics of neurons in the basal ganglia, thalamus, and subthalamic nucleus (STN) continues to give important insight into the pathophysiology of various movement disorders. Microelectrode techniques are also continuing to evolve for examining simultaneous recordings from multichannel electrode arrays to assess the spatiotemporal properties of neuronal assemblies (2). This approach has been capable of real-time remote control of a robotic arm by recordings from neuronal assemblies in rat motor cortex (3). Multichannel methods may also increase our knowledge of network-based neurophysiologic deficits leading to movement disorders, and they could give rise to neuronal "correction" therapies based on mathematic transformation of disordered neural signals that could drive electrical stimulation arrays to produce normal motor function.

Several reports of single-unit microelectrode techniques have been published, with a focus on thalamus (4,5), globus pallidus (GP) (6–9), and STN (10,11). The purpose of this chapter is to review the current methodology in use in our operating room and briefly outline the major neurophysiologic landmarks that need to be identified for target determination in each case.

TECHNOLOGY OF MICROELECTRODE RECORDING

Microelectrode Assembly

Some detail is required in a discussion of microelectrodes, because most problems with recording are the result of faulty or damaged electrodes. Microelectrode tips are obtained from a commercial source and are mounted on Kapton (polyimide, DuPont, Wilmington, DE) insulated stainless steel tubing to extend the length for use in the stereotactic guide tube. Tungsten wire electrodes insulated with Parylene-C (parachloroxylylene, Union Carbide, XXX, XX are subjected to a high-voltage spark to expose a small portion of the tip for recording from neurons. Tip exposures in the range of 15 to 40 μm are available, but a 15 or 25 μm exposure is the most useful for single-unit and occasionally multiunit recordings. Larger tip sizes pick up several neurons and make single-unit discrimination more difficult, and smaller tip sizes may record cells only in the immediate vicinity of the tip. Extensions to a length of approximately 24 cm are made for use in the stereotactic guide tube by stripping off the insulation, crimping the shank, and inserting the electrode into 25-gauge stainless steel tubing. The 22-gauge Kapton tubing insulation slides over the 25-gauge tubing, and epoxy glue is used to make a continuous seal between the two insulators. The insulation can be tested by inserting just the electrode tip and then the rest of the shank into saline while observing the impedance reading, which should remain constant if there is no breech. Another method is to apply 3 to 10 v DC to the electrode in saline to watch electrolytic bubble formation, which should only occur at the tip. The thin coating of Parylene-C on the electrode tip is particularly sensitive to scratching, so caution needs to be exercised during handling.

The tungsten electrodes are electroplated with platinum and gold to reduce the impedance from about 1.0 to 0.2 Mohm. The plating serves to increase the signal-to-noise properties and also makes the tip more resistant to

W.D. Hutchinson: Department of Neurosurgery, Division of Neurosurgery, Toronto Western Hospital; Department of Physiology, Faculty of Medicine, University of Toronto, Toronto, Ontario Canada M5S 1A8.

electrolytic erosion during repeated or long trains of microstimulation. If microstimulation is carried out with biphasic pulses instead of monophasic pulses, then there is no net charge transfer, and this also preserves the tip from electrolytic erosion (12). Plating is carried out with a low DC current supply (about 200 nA setting for 15 seconds) and is observed under a microscope to control the amount of metal deposited. Electrodes are best backloaded into 19-gauge tubing and secured with adhesive tape so the tip is protected inside the tube. Our method is usually gas sterilization with ethylene oxide. Some centers are moving away from this procedure because of the toxic hazards of ethylene oxide, and it is possible to sterilize electrodes in the autoclave for 3 to 10 minutes. Electrodes should be also compatible with the hydrogen peroxide–based systems such as Sterad. With any system of sterilization, it is good practice to keep the electrodes protected in the tubes to avoid damage to the tips during handling.

Instrumentation

Several companies have developed intraoperative systems for microelectrode recording in neurosurgical procedures. Axon Instruments (Foster City, CA) has designed and developed the Guideline System 3000, which is approved by the United States Food and Drug Administration, and details of the system are available at *http://www.axon.com/FN_GS3000.html.* Certain safety features are built into the system, such as the electrical isolation of the high-voltage rack instrumentation from contact with the patient. In addition, the stimulation circuit is monitored and will shut down the high-voltage power supply in the unlikely event of instrument failure.

The basic components of the system are shown in Fig. 6.1. The electrode is attached to a head stage amplifier with a driven-shield arrangement that feeds the output of the unity gain FET back to the shielding on the microelectrode leads. This prevents any stray current induced by surrounding electrical fields set up by other electronic equipment from being amplified and creating noise on the recordings. The main low-noise differential amplifier is mounted on the rack and has a variable gain of 1,000 to 10,000.

Filtering the Signal and Discriminating the Spikes

The high- and low-pass filters are included on the same panel and set the bandwidth of the recording to condition the signal to remove noise for spike display and discrimination. The Guideline System allows settings of the high-pass (low-cut) filter in the range of 10 to 300 Hz, and the low-pass filter ranges from 1 to 20 kHz. Typical filter settings of 200 Hz to 10 kHz bandpass allow observation of action potentials on a stable baseline for spike discrimination. For recording from the flash-evoked potential from optic tract during pallidotomy procedures, the low-cut filter should be "opened up" and set at 10 Hz. The spikes are discriminated using a software-based trigger that can be quickly set to any voltage level to count individual spikes and to display the counts in bins (0.1 to 1 second) in a firing rate histogram or "Chart Recorder."

Microstimulation Mapping

Electrical stimulation through the electrode tip ("microstimulation") during functional stereotactic procedures has the

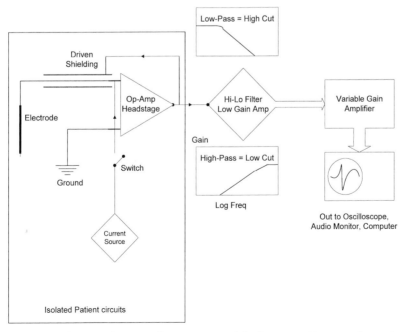

FIGURE 6.1. Schematic diagram of components of the intraoperative recording system.

advantage of being highly localized in current spread so a detailed map in the submillimeter range of resolution can be obtained. For example, paresthesias of small body parts, such as the fingertip, are often produced when stimulating in the tactile region of the ventral caudal nucleus, which correspond to the receptive fields of the cells recorded at that site. The Guideline System has a useful handheld remote control for setting the stimulation intensity that allows the patient to be closely monitored as the stimulation intensity is varied. The usual stimulation parameters are 1 to 100 μA and a 1-second train of pulses at 300 Hz with pulse widths of 200 μseconds. The stimulation parameters can be varied in frequency and pulse width.

Sources of Noise on Recordings and Other Practical Considerations

Probably the most common problem with noise and poor recordings results from faults with the electrode, because the tip is fragile and is easily damaged. Early recognition of the problem and simply replacing the microelectrode may be the fastest way to reduce bothersome noise. If the tip is bent or curled, it will still record small spikes from the neuron, but often more injury discharge is heard. Injury discharge is a high-frequency, decrementing amplitude and transient burst discharge of spikes as the neuronal membrane is torn and the cell depolarizes because of the large sodium influx. A hooked tip is suspected when the tip retains tissue when retracted from the brain. If the electrode tip has been eroded from repeated high intensity of electrical stimulation, it will show a high or off-scale impedance reading and poor, noisy, or absent recordings. The vibration of the stereotactic frame caused by the patient's talking may produce noise on recordings, as well as movements of the body, either voluntary or involuntary (tremor, dystonia, or dyskinesia). Another preventable measure is to ensure there are no metal-on-metal contacts that are moving such as the handles of retractors used on the bur holes against each other or the frame.

One source of noise that is bothersome even with the new instrumentation is monopolar cautery performed in an adjacent operating room. This interference from the high-voltage induction coils of the monopolar current source is difficult to eliminate entirely, but switching to bipolar cautery and changing to a lower impedance electrode may improve the situation enough to obtain noise-free recordings.

MICROELECTRODE RECORDING IN THALAMIC AND BASAL GANGLIA SURGERY

Surgical Technique

In the current stereotactic method used by Dr. Lozano, the target is calculated based on the anterior commissure (AC) and posterior commissure (PC) coordinates on magnetic res-

onance imaging (MRI) (8). Using local anesthesia, the surgeon applies a Leksell model G stereotactic frame to the patient's head, and a fiducial box is placed over the frame to obtain the coordinates of AC-PC in three dimensions relative to the frame (x, medial/lateral, y, anterior/posterior, and z, up/down). The frame coordinates of AC and PC are obtained from the MRI console software (GE-Signa 1.5-Tesla magnet), and these are entered into a computer program that modifies sagittal maps from the Schaltenbrand and Wahren atlas (13). In this way, a customized map is obtained for each patient.

Recordings During Pallidal Procedures

For pallidotomy recordings (6), different groups use slightly different techniques and place varying time and emphasis on the recording session. The following is a description of our method. The target is similar to that used by Leksell and published by Laitinen (14) in the ventral lateral portion of the internal segment of the GP (GPi), that is, 20 mm lateral to the midline, 3 to 6 mm inferior to the AC-PC line, and 2 to 3 mm anterior to the midcommissural point. Usually, the first cells encountered are those of external segment of the GP (GPe), because in our procedure the recording starts about 15 mm from the target in an anterosuperior position (Fig. 6.2).

Each region of the GP has characteristic cell types that are described later, but normally there is a range of firing rates and patterns of the neurons encountered requiring all the information from the tract to be integrated before assigning particular location to a group of cells (Table 6.1). After several of these tracts in the same plane have been obtained, it usually becomes clear what the discrepancy is between the physiologic location of the nuclear structures and the initial estimate of the target based on the stereotactic anatomic map.

The GPe has two "signature" types of neuron described based on recordings in normal monkeys (15). These are the low-frequency discharge with bursts (LFD-B) and the slow-frequency discharge with pauses (SFD-P). LFD-B neurons are not very common in GPe (about 11% of all neurons encountered) and may not be as useful an indicator of the region as the other type. LFD-B neurons have a low overall firing rate 5 to 10 Hz, and the short bursts occur at irregular time intervals that reach about 300 to 500 Hz (Fig. 6.2). SFD-P neurons have a higher spontaneous firing rate of approximately 20 to 50 Hz that is sporadically interrupted by pauses in firing lasting approximately 150 to 300 milliseconds (Fig. 6.2). We also find cells in GPe with higher firing rates of 50 to 70 Hz, and these may receive excitatory input from the STN, which is known to be hyperactive and has a prominent glutamatergic projection into GPe (16). The firing rate of cells in GPe may be modulated by active and passive movements of limbs.

Between GPe and GPi is a white matter lamina that is relatively quiet in the background level of noise on the recordings. Border cells are found in this region, and they

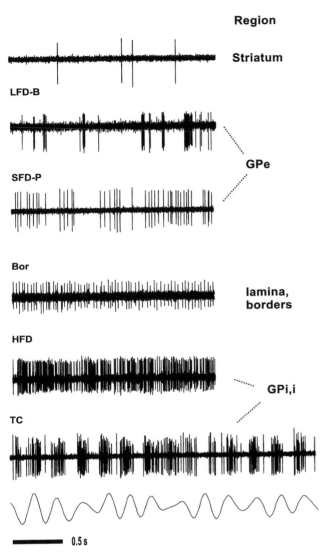

Region

Striatum

LFD-B

GPe

SFD-P

lamina, borders

Bor

HFD

GPi,i

TC

0.5 s

FIGURE 6.2. Typical recordings of "signature" cell types in segments of globus pallidus during microelectrode exploration. Bor, Border cell; HFD, high-frequency discharge; LFD-B, low-frequency discharge with bursts; SFD-P, slow-frequency discharge with pauses; TC, tremor cell. The trace below TC is the accelerometer attached to the dorsum of the contralateral hand.

have a longer afterhyperpolarization than pallidal cells that imparts a regular firing pattern because of the longer relative refractory period (Fig. 6.2). These unique electrophysiologic characteristics as well as immunoreactivity for acetylcholinesterase indicate that the cells are cholinergic and may be displaced cells of the nucleus basalis of Meynert that project in a medial and lateral pathway to the amygdala and large areas of the cerebral cortex (17). A sample of 17 border cells was found to have a mean firing rate of 35 Hz (18).

Further advancement of the electrode tip into GPi gives an increase in background noise and multiunit recordings. GPi neurons have spikes with a large amplitude, irregular discharge patterns, and higher firing rates than the other pallidal cells. The firing rates of GPi neurons are in the range of 60 to 80 Hz, and the most common interspike (modal) intervals for GPi neurons are in the range of 5 to 7 milliseconds. Passive and voluntary movements of limbs and orofacial structures modulate the firing rate of about 20% of GPi neurons. The neuronal responses to movements may be excitatory or inhibitory and may occur with movements of more than one joint or occasionally in a reciprocal fashion, that is, excitation to arm flexion and inhibition to arm extension. In some preliminary analyses of the data, there was no clear topographic organization of GPi neurons based on passive manipulation of individual body parts. Cells can be found in GPi with periodic oscillations in firing rate at the same frequency as the tremor (19,20). These tremor cells show periods of coherent oscillation with limb tremor and appear to be located in ventral and lateral portions of the GPi (21), a finding consistent with observations that lesions placed in a more ventral and lateral location appear to be associated with better control of tremor (22).

When the electrode passes ventral to GPi into white matter tracts of the ansa lenticularis, the background noise decreases, and border cells may also be recorded here. About 2 mm from the ventral border of GPi there may be a discernible increase in noise again as the electrode tip enters the optic tract. At this point, microstimulation (1-second

TABLE 6.1. CHARACTERISTIC FIRING RATES AND PATTERNS OF CELLULAR REGIONS ENCOUNTERED DURING STEREOTACTIC PROCEDURES FOR MOVEMENT DISORDERS

Procedure	Region	Rate s.d. (n)	Firing Pattern Index[a]
Pallidal surgery (posteroventral lateral GPi)	GPe	60 ± 36 (40)	2.7
	GPi dorsal	53 ± 27 (73)	2.8
	ventral	82 ± 32 (89)	2.3
	Border cells	35 ± 16 (17)	1.2
Subthalamic surgery	Anterior thalamus		
	Bursting	15 ± 19 (51)	29 (17–57)[b]
	Nonbursting	28 ± 19 (52)	2.1 (1.4–3.8)
	STN	37 ± 17 (248)	3.1 (2.2–4.8)
	SNr	71 ± 23 (56)	1.7 (1.3–2.1)

[a] Firing pattern index calculated as FPI = mean firing rate; 1/(modal interspike interval)
[b] Twenty-fifth and seventy-fifth percentiles given for STN data.
Gpe, globus pallidus pars externa; Gpi, globus pallidus pars interna; SNr, substantia nigra pars reticulata; STN, subthalamic nucleus.

train of biphasic pulses at 200 Hz and a pulse duration of 300 microseconds) almost always evokes phosphenes in the contralateral visual field at low current intensities (5 to 20 μA). Patients frequently report white or yellow flashes of light, stars, sparkles, or lightning-like patterns. This can occur in a wedge-shaped portion of the visual field that is reported to shift to a more dorsal portion of the visual field with more ventral stimulation sites in the optic tract, consistent with the rotation of the fibers in the tract at this level. In rare cases when patients do not report stimulation-evoked visual sensation, it is worthwhile also to carry out strobe-light–evoked potentials by opening up the high-pass filter and recording the slow-wave average (about 30 to 40 milliseconds at this site).

If the first pass with the microelectrode has identified GPe cells, the lamina between GPe and GPi with border

cells, high-frequency discharge neurons of GPi, and cells with movement-related activity including tremor cells, the ventral border of the GPi, and the optic tract below this, then the next trajectory should be made 3 mm posterior to identify the internal capsule. In posterior tracts, the cell-dense region usually ends higher up, a finding indicating that the posterior aspect of the GPi and the tip of the electrode will pass into the internal capsule. Recordings in the capsule are usually quiet, but an occasional unit or fiber is encountered. Microstimulation (up to 100 μA, 0.2-millisecond pulse width, 300 Hz, 1-second train) through the electrode may produce tetanic contraction of the contralateral body part or tremor reduction or tremor arrest.

A complete map usually comprises two or three electrode trajectories in which the optic tract and internal capsule have been unambiguously located (Fig. 6.3). The physiologic data

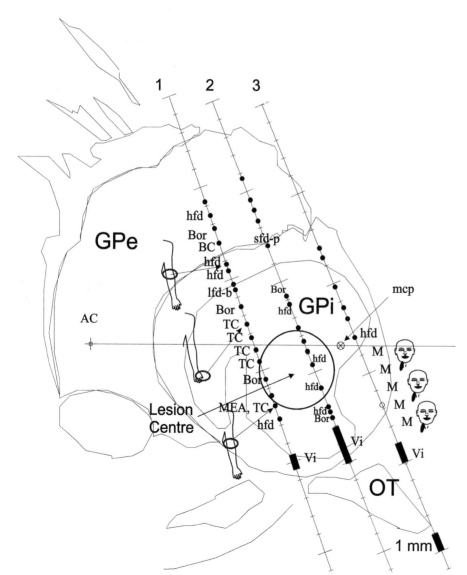

FIGURE 6.3. Completed functional map of the globus pallidus, showing identified neuronal types and responses of neurons to active and passive movements. Abbreviations are as in Fig. 6.2; AC and mcp, anterior commissure and midcommissural point; BC, bursting cell; MEA, movement-related activity; Vi and M, visual and motor responses to microstimulation; OT, optic tract. Arm figurines with *circles* indicate the location of cells with responses to movements about that joint.

should show a reasonably good spatial relation to the corresponding anatomic map. Lesions are made at least 3 mm distant from these eloquent structures in a cell-dense area that contains movement-related activity and tremor cells.

Recordings During Subthalamic Nucleus Procedures

Research with monkeys treated with 1-methyl-4-phenyl-1,2,3,6-tetrahydropyridine (MPTP) revealed that a remarkable reversal of Parkinson-like symptoms could be produced with electrolytic and cytotoxic lesions of the STN (23). These beneficial effects were also seen with continuous electrical stimulation of the STN in monkeys (24). Following closely on this work, Benabid et al. in Grenoble showed remarkable improvement of motor symptoms can occur in patients with Parkinson's disease during bilateral deep brain stimulation (DBS) of the STN (25,26). The small size and deep location of the STN as well as the absence of structures easily identified with microstimulation place an increased emphasis on good single-unit microelectrode recording to position the DBS electrodes accurately.

To identify the STN for the purposes of DBS implantation, the major landmarks to identify are (a) the anterior thalamus with bursting cells, (b) the superior and inferior borders of the STN, and (c) the dorsal border of the substantia nigra pars reticulata (SNr). The target for the initial electrode trajectory into the STN is in the center of the nucleus at about 10 to 12 mm lateral to the midline, 1 mm posterior to the midcommissural point, and 5 mm below the AC-PC line.

Depending on the trajectory angle in the sagittal plane, recording usually starts 10 mm above the target in the thalamic reticular nucleus or in the anterior thalamus ventralis oralis anterior or posterior (or lateropolaris if more lateral). Bursting cells are characteristic of this region, particularly in the thalamic reticular formation and have been reported previously (27,28). Table 6.1 lists the mean firing rates of thalamic bursting and nonbursting cells.

The region between the ventral border of thalamus and the dorsal border of the STN is generally quiet on recordings (cell sparse) and corresponds to the thalamic and lenticular fasciculi. A few cells may be recorded in the zona incerta between these tracts, and they may have a similar firing rate and response to movements (29).

The entry into the STN is apparent when high-amplitude spikes with firing rates of 25 to 45 Hz are found. STN neurons show clear modulation with active and passive movements of the limbs. Rapid passive movements most often increase the firing rate of STN cells, and tremor cells may be found with oscillation of the ongoing firing rate at the same frequency as the limb or orofacial tremor. If the electrode trajectory does not pass through the center of the structure, STN neurons may only be recorded over only a few millimeters. Typical STN neurons are shown in

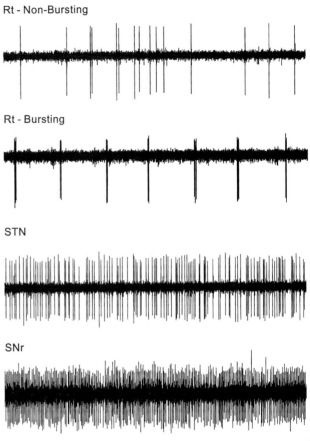

Rt - Non-Bursting

Rt - Bursting

STN

SNr

FIGURE 6.4. Typical spike recordings of cell types encountered in trajectories targeting the subthalamic nucleus. **Top** to **bottom:** Rt, thalamic reticular nucleus; STN, subthalamic nucleus; SNr, substantia nigra pars reticulata. The traces are 2 seconds in duration.

Fig. 6.4, and the firing rate and burst index are found in Table 6.1.

The SNr is usually the final neurophysiologic landmark to be identified at the end of the trajectory (Fig. 6.5). Cells in the SNr have a characteristic high firing rate (60 to 90 Hz) and a regular pattern of the spike train. There may be another group with lower rates of approximately 20 to 30 Hz, possibly reflecting functional differences within the nucleus (10,30,31). The different firing rates in SNr may depend on the portion of the reticulata that is explored, because motor regions are more laterally located in this nucleus (about 15 mm from the midline).

Microstimulation in these areas is not as useful as with pallidal or thalamic surgery but stimulation-induced tremor arrest or reduction from within STN has been observed. Paresthesias have been encountered in more ventral and posterior positions and may result from current spread to medial lemniscus or prelemniscal radiation. Motor responses may also be rarely observed in the ventral and anterior portion of tracts in the STN region, and these may result from activation of corticobulbar fiber tracts. If the plane of trajectories is medial, there may be activation of the oculomotor nerve

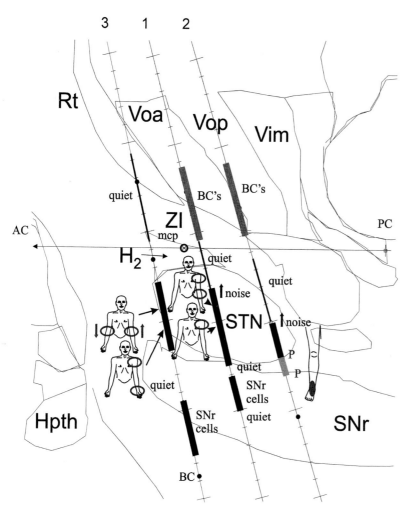

FIGURE 6.5. Completed functional map in the region of subthalamic nucleus (STN), showing identified neuronal types and responses of neurons to active and passive movements (body-part figurines with *circles*). The trajectory targeting the STN is superimposed on a 12-mm sagittal map of the Schaltenbrand and Wahren atlas. The map is reformatted to correspond to the length of this patient's anterior commissure-posterior commissure (AC-PC) line. H2, fields of Forel; Hpth, hypothalamus; IC, internal capsule; Rt, thalamic reticular nucleus; SNr, substantia nigra pars reticulata; Voa, ventralis oralis anterior; Vop, ventralis oralis posterior, Vim, ventralis intermedius; ZI, zona incerta.

and deviation of the orbit during stimulation. It is necessary to microstimulate at these ventral and medial sites in these trajectories because these may give rise to unwanted side effects of STN DBS therapy.

Recording and Microstimulation During Thalamic Procedures

Detailed methods for functional stereotactic thalamic procedures have been reviewed elsewhere (5,32,33) and a brief description is given here for the sake of completion. Thalamic surgery for treatment of movement disorders (essential, Parkinson's disease, cerebellar tremors) targets the ventralis intermedius (VIM) nucleus of the ventral tier thalamic nuclei, or VLp of Jones' terminology in which spinal afferents from deep kinesthetic and muscle spindle receptors and cerebellar afferents converge (34,35), and are relayed predominantly to the motor cortex.

The neurophysiologic landmarks to identify in the thalamic mapping session are (a) the kinesthetic zone with tremor cells, (b) the deep tactile zone, (c) the cutaneous tactile zone,

and (d) the ventral border of the tactile region. A summarized schematic of the results from a typical thalamic mapping session is illustrated in Fig. 6.6.

"Motor Thalamus"

Recordings at the top of trajectories may lie anterior to the VIM and are similar to those already described in thalamic areas slightly more medially. Bursting cells are frequently encountered as well as nonbursting cells. In the VIM proper, movement-related activity (kinesthetic responses) may be present, and some cells may respond to deep pressure or deep touch. In patients with tremor, tremor cells may be recorded in this region, and microstimulation produces tremor arrest or tremor reduction.

Ventralis Caudalis

Passing further down with the electrode, the spontaneous activity usually increases with entry into the thalamic tactile relay of the V.c. Cells in this region respond to a light stroke with a brush or cotton swab. There may also be

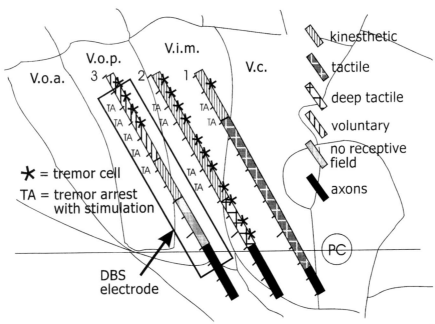

FIGURE 6.6. Summary of microelectrode mapping results for localization of thalamic nuclei on one side. Deep brain stimulation (DBS) electrodes were implanted bilaterally in the ventralis intermedius (V.i.m.). V.o.a., ventralis ordis anterior; V.o.p., ventralis ordis posterior; V.c., ventral caudal nucleus. Background outlines of the thalamic nuclei are drawn from the Schaltenbrand and Wahren stereotactic atlas 14.5 mm from the midline.

"spurious tremor cells" that are rhythmically activated by the skin brushing as the limb oscillates with tremor. The well-known somatotopic organization within the V.c. is used to advantage to guide the laterality of the given electrode tract. Laterality in the VIM therefore is largely determined with reference to V.c. somatotopy, with the leg indicating a more lateral location than the face and hand. Microstimulation within the V.c. produces focal paresthesia showing a somatotopic organization roughly corresponding to that obtained by recording the cellular responses to touch. Microstimulation in the ventral may elicit painful sensation. Ventral to the V.c. microstimulation may also elicit hemibody paresthesias resulting from lemniscal fiber activation.

Usually, several trajectories are made to define the anterior border of the V.c. and to map a large enough segment of the motor thalamus to find the focus and extent of sites of effective tremor suppression from microstimulation. Usually, lesions or DBS implantations are made 2 to 3 mm anterior to the V.c.-VIM border.

CONCLUSIONS

Microelectrode recording is useful for accurately delineating deep brain structures and subnuclei for various stereotactic targets. In addition, it yields additional information on the cellular pathophysiology of movement disorders and the rationales for development of surgical therapies for the treatment of movement disorders.

ACKNOWLEDGMENTS

The support of the Parkinson's Foundation of Canada and the University of Toronto Connaught Fund is gratefully acknowledged.

REFERENCES

1. Guiot G, Hardy J, Albe-Fessard D. Délimitation précise des structures sous-corticales et identification de noyaux thalamiques chez l'homme par l'électrophysiologie stéréotaxique. *Neurochirurgia (Stutt)* 1962;51:1–18.
2. Nicolelis MAL, ed. *Methods for neural ensemble recordings.* Boca Raton, FL: CRC, 1998.
3. Chapin JK, Moxon KA, Markowitz RS, et al. Real-time control of a robot arm using simultaneously recorded neurons in the motor cortex . *Nat Neurosci* 1999;2:664–670.
4. Lenz FA, Dostrovsky JO, Kwan HC, et al. Methods for microstimulation and recording of single neurons and evoked potentials in the human central nervous system. *J Neurosurg* 1988;68:630–634.
5. Tasker RR, Davis KD, Hutchison WD, et al. Subcortical and thalamic mapping in functional neurosurgery. In: Gildenberg PL, Tasker RR, eds. *Textbook of stereotactic and functional neurosurgery.* New York: McGraw-Hill, 1998:94-5–94-31.
6. Sterio D, Beric A, Dogali M, et al. Neurophysiological properties of pallidal neurons in Parkinson's disease. *Ann Neurol* 1994;35:586–591.
7. Vitek JL, Bakay RA, Hashimoto T, et al. Microelectrode-guided pallidotomy: technical approach and its application in medically intractable Parkinson's disease. *J Neurosurg* 1998;88:1027–1043.

8. Lozano AM, Hutchison WD, Kiss ZHT, et al. Methods for microelectrode-guided posteroventral pallidotomy. *J Neurosurg* 1996;84:194–202.

9. Hutchison WD. Microelectrode techniques and findings of globus pallidus. In: Krauss JK, Grossman RG, Jankovic J, eds. *Pallidal surgery for the treatment of Parkinson's disease and movement disorders.* Philadelphia: Lippincott–Raven; 1998:135–152.

10. Hutchison WD, Allan RJ, Opitz H, et al. Neurophysiologic identification of the subthalamic nucleus in surgery for Parkinson's disease. *Ann Neurol* 1998;44:622–628.

11. Starr PA, Vitek JL, Bakay RAE. Deep brain stimulation for movement disorders. *Neurosurg Clin North Am* 1998;XX: 381–402.

12. Millar J, Stamford JA. Extracellular single and multiple unit recording with microelectrodes. In: Millar J, Stamford JA, eds. *Monitoring neuronal activity: a practical approach.* New York: IRL Press at Oxford, 1992:1–27.

13. Schaltenbrand G, Wahren W. *Atlas for stereotaxy of the human brain.* Stuttgart: Thieme, 1977.

14. Laitinen LV, Bergenheim AT, Hariz MI. Leksell's posteroventral pallidotomy in the treatment of Parkinson's disease. *J Neurosurg* 1992;76:53–61.

15. DeLong MR. Activity of pallidal neurons during movement. *J Neurophysiol* 1971;34:414–427.

16. Smith Y, Bevan MD, Shink E, et al. Microcircuitry of the direct and indirect pathways of the basal ganglia. *Neuroscience* 1998;86:353–387.

17. Selden NR, Gitelman DR, Salamon-Murayama N, et al. Trajectories of cholinergic pathways within the cerebral hemispheres of the human brain. *Brain* 1998;121:2249–2257.

18. Hutchison WD, Lozano CA, Davis KD, et al. Differential neuronal activity in segments of globus pallidus in Parkinson's disease patients. *Neuroreport* 1994;5:1533–1537.

19. Hutchison WD, Lozano AM, Kiss ZHT, et al. Tremor-related activity (TRA) in globus pallidus of Parkinson's disease (PD) patients. *Soc Neurosci Abstr* 1994;20:783.

20. Hutchison WD, Lozano AM, Tasker RR, et al. Identification and characterisation of neurons with tremor-frequency activity in human globus pallidus. *Exp Brain Res* 1997;113:557–563.

21. Hutchison WD, Benko R, Dostrovsky JO, et al. Coherent relation of rest tremor and pallidal tremor cells in Parkinson's disease patients. *Mov Disord* 1998;13[Suppl 2]:204(abst).

22. Gross RE, Lombardi WJ, Lang AE, et al. Relationship of lesion location to clinical outcome following microelectrode-guided pallidotomy for Parkinson's disease. *Brain* 1999;122: 405–416.

23. Bergman H, Wichmann T, DeLong MR. Reversal of experimental parkinsonism by lesions of the subthalamic nucleus. *Science* 1990;249:1436–1438.

24. Benazzouz A, Boraud T, Féger J, et al. Alleviation of experimental hemiparkinsonism by high-frequency stimulation of the subthalamic nucleus in primates: a comparison with L-dopa treatment. *Mov Disord* 1996;11:627–632.

25. Pollak P, Benabid AL, Gross C, et al. Effets de la stimulation du noyau sousthalamique dans la maladie de Parkinson. *Rev Neurol* 1993;149:175–176.

26. Limousin P, Pollak P, Hoffmann D, et al. Abnormal involuntary movements induced by subthalamic nucleus stimulation in parkinsonian patients. *Mov Disord* 1996;11:231–235.

27. Raeva SN, Lukashev A. Unit activity in human thalamic reticularis neurons. II. Activity evoked by significant and non-significant verbal or sensory stimuli. *Electroencephalogr Clin Neurophysiol* 1993;86:110–122.

28. Raeva SN, Lukashev A, Lashin A. Unit activity in human thalamic reticular nucleus. I. Spontaneous activity. *Electroencephalogr Clin Neurophysiol* 1991;79:133–140.

29. Ma T. Saccade-related omnivectoral pause neurons in the primate zona incerta. *Neuroreport* 1996;7:2713–2716.

30. DeLong MR, Crutcher MD, Georgopoulos AP. Primate globus pallidus and subthalamic nucleus: functional organization. *J Neurophysiol* 1985;53:530–543.

31. DeLong MR, Crutcher MD, Georgopoulos AP. Relations between movement and single cell discharge in the substantia nigra of the behaving monkey. *J Neurosci* 1983;3:1599–606.

32. Tasker RR, Lenz FA, Dostrovsky JO, et al. The physiological basis of Vim thalamotomy for involuntary movement disorders. In: Struppler A, Weindl A, eds. *Clinical aspects of sensory motor integration.* Berlin: Springer, 1987:265–276.

33. Tasker RR, Dostrovsky JO, Hutchison WD. Microelectrode recording technology. *Tech Neurosurg* 1999;5:46–64.

34. Macchi G, Jones EG. Toward an agreement on terminology of nuclear and subnuclear divisions of the motor thalamus. *J Neurosurg* 1997;86:77–92.

35. Hirai T, Jones EG. A new parcellation of the human thalamus on the basis of histochemical staining. *Brain Res Rev* 1989;14:1–34.

Surgery for Parkinson's Disease and Movement Disorders,
edited by J.K. Krauss, J. Jankovic, and R.G. Grossman.
Lippincott Williams & Wilkins, Philadelphia © 2001.

7

FUNCTIONAL IMAGING IN THE EVALUATION OF STEREOTACTIC SURGERY OF MOVEMENT DISORDERS

CHRISTINE EDWARDS
VON PILLAI
DAVID EIDELBERG

Functional brain imaging techniques such as *positron emission tomography* (PET) and *single photon emission computed tomography* (SPECT) have contributed to our understanding of the pathophysiology of Parkinson's disease (PD) and other movement disorders. PET employs small amounts of positron emitting radioligands to produce quantitative measures of physiologic and biochemical processes in the brain and other organs. In a PET experiment, a subject is given a compound of biologic interest. The spatial and temporal distribution of the radiotracer is measured quantitatively in the course of the PET study, to provide a tomographic representation of regional radioactivity concentration. SPECT provides a more affordable way to perform some of the same applications as PET; however, it is less quantifiable and less accurate. In movement disorders, PET and SPECT have been applied in the investigation of striatal dopaminergic nerve terminals using [18F] fluorodopa (FDOPA) (1–4), dopamine transporter (DAT) ligands (5,6), and [11C] raclopride (RAC) (1,7). These neuroimaging techniques have also been used to study glucose metabolism using [18F]fluorodeoxyglucose (FDG) (3,8–11) as well as regional cerebral blood flow (rCBF) with [15O] H$_2$O/PET (12–14).

In this review, we focus on the potential application of functional imaging techniques such as PET and SPECT in the selection of suitable candidates for stereotactic surgical interventions such as pallidotomy, thalamotomy, deep brain stimulation (DBS), and fetal transplantation. We also examine the role of functional brain imaging in the assessment of these surgical interventions.

DOPAMINE SYSTEM IMAGING IN MOVEMENT DISORDERS

Presynaptic Dopaminergic Function

FDOPA is a commonly applied radiotracer for the study of striatal dopaminergic nerve terminals in PD and related movement disorders. PET studies with this tracer measure the rate of decarboxylation of FDOPA to [18F] fluorodopamine by dopa-decarboxylase acid and its subsequent storage in the striatal dopaminergic nerve terminals. The assessment of nigrostriatal dopaminergic function using FDOPA/PET yields quantitative parameters that correlate with independent disease severity measures and can discriminate patients with early-stage PD from neurologically normal control subjects (1,3,4,15). Investigators have shown that striatal FDOPA measurements conducted *in vivo* correlate with dopamine cell counts measured in postmortem specimens (16). Differential diagnosis is possible using FDOPA/PET. Atypical parkinsonian syndromes (APSs) are often difficult to distinguish from PD on clinical grounds alone. In patients with early-stage idiopathic PD, FDOPA uptake is relatively preserved in the caudate and anterior putamen early in the disease. By contrast, in patients with APSs such as multiple system atrophy, equivalent impairment of FDOPA uptake can be observed in the caudate and the putamen. However, this differential dopaminergic topography is often insufficient to discriminate idiopathic PD from multiple system atrophy at early clinical stages (10). Striatal FDOPA uptake has been noted to be diminished in other parkinsonian movement disorders such as striatonigral degeneration and progressive supranuclear palsy. Additionally, asymmetric parkinsonian syndromes such as hemiparkinson-hemiatrophy syndrome and corticobasal degeneration show relative reductions in basal ganglia FDOPA uptake contralateral to the affected side (17,18).

C. Edwards, V. Pillai, and D. Eidelberg: Functional Brain Imaging Laboratory, North Shore-Long Island Jewish Research Institute Manhasset, New York 11030.

Dopamine Transporter

The development of radiotracers that bind to the striatal DAT led to another means for directly measuring the nigrostriatal dopaminergic system with PET or SPECT. Cocaine analogs, such as 2-β-carbomethyl-3β-(4-iodophenyl) tropane (βCIT) and its fluoroalkyl esters (6), are the most extensively studied agents in this category. DAT is expressed on dopaminergic nigral terminals, and quantification of striatal DAT appears to be directly related to the extent of nigral cell degeneration (19).

SPECT studies have demonstrated the utility of DAT binding ligands as effective markers of nigrostriatal dopaminergic degeneration in parkinsonism (4,20). SPECT imaging with these tracers reliably differentiates patients with PD from neurologically normal volunteers, and the degree of striatal binding correlates with clinical measures of PD severity. In contrast to FDOPA/PET, both PET and SPECT measures of DAT binding decline with normal aging (4). Thus, the DAT binding agents may have utility in quantifying the attrition in nigrostriatal dopamine function that occurs in the course of the normal aging process. Nevertheless, this sensitivity may require the introduction of age corrections in longitudinal studies of disease progression in PD. A report from our laboratory noted that PET imaging with [^{18}F] fluoropropyl CIT can provide images with higher resolution and better quantification than SPECT images with the same ligand (6).

Postsynaptic Dopaminergic Function

Dopamine receptor–bearing neurons constitute approximately 80% of the neuronal population in the striatum (21,22). In the striatum, dopamine receptors are located mainly on γ-aminobutyric acid (GABA)-ergic neurons projecting to the globus pallidus. In neurologically normal persons, RAC/PET studies have demonstrated a decrement of dopamine D_2 receptor binding of approximately 0.6% per year, a finding suggesting that the striatal projection neurons may also progressively decline with normal aging (23). By contrast, in PD, the postsynaptic response to nigrostriatal deafferentation is likely to differ from that of normal aging. Investigators have suggested that loss of dopaminergic terminals in association with changes in postsynaptic dopamine receptors may underlie motor complications occurring in the course of treatment of PD (15). Relative dopamine D_2 receptor upregulation has also been demonstrated in the striatum of subjects with 1-methyl-4-phenyl-1,2,3,6-tetrahydropyridine (MPTP)–induced parkinsonism (24). However, the initial dopamine D_2 receptor upregulation in putamen may reverse with increasing disease severity, and binding values are in the range of control subjects or lower in patients with advanced PD (7,25). Because RAC and FDOPA changes are associated throughout the disease course, it is likely that dopamine D_2 receptor

changes result from the decline in presynaptic dopaminergic drive (1).

BRAIN METABOLISM AND REGIONAL BLOOD FLOW IN PARKINSON'S DISEASE

Measurements of regional rates of glucose utilization with FDG/PET in PD can be used to quantify the effect of nigrostriatal degeneration on brain regions functionally related to the dopaminergic system. Historically, FDG was used with PET in attempts to map focal areas of abnormal metabolism that could underlie the clinical manifestations of the movement disorders. Parallel efforts have employed [^{15}O] H$_2$O to identify pathologic abnormalities in regional oxygen consumption and rCBF as additional indices of localized functional pathologic processes in these diseases. In 1994, we reviewed the status of this approach in delineating the pathophysiology of PD and related disorders (26). Although early PET studies revealed that individual elements of the motor system could be abnormal in these diseases, the results were inconsistent. We attributed this situation to the differences in technical and data analytic approaches among PET laboratories. Indeed, this lack of methodologic standardization was particularly striking in the first decade after the introduction of PET. Another cause for these discrepancies was biologic. It is now accepted that although primary abnormalities may be well localized, focal neurodegeneration results in widespread functional alterations in brain regions spatially removed from the histologic or neurochemical locus of disease. For instance, nigral dopaminergic degeneration in PD can result in changes in the activity of the pallidum, thalamus, and motor cortex (27). Analogously, as discussed later, the degeneration of striatal D_2 projection neurons in Huntington's disease (HD) (28) is likely to cause changes in the activity of the thalamus and cerebellum. Therefore, the measurement of local rates of metabolism in isolation may not fully describe the complexities of the neural systems involved in neurodegenerative processes.

METABOLIC NETWORK MAPPING IN PARKINSON'S DISEASE

We developed and applied a statistical model of regional metabolic covariation to identify abnormal brain topographies in PD and related disorders (3,9–11,29). This algorithm, known as the *Scaled Subprofile Model* (SSM) (30–32), is a form of principal component analysis (PCA) and can be applied to identify patterns of regional covariation in brain metabolism data. Through modifications of the functional imaging data before performing the PCA, SSM analysis both characterizes the regional covariance structure of subject groups and measures the expression of the obtained regional covariance patterns in individual subjects (subject scores). In this way, SSM provides a means of comparing the expression of these patterns in different populations and of examining their relationship with independent clinical descriptors such as disease severity or subject age.

In patients with PD, SSM analysis revealed a reproducible pattern of regional metabolism characterized by increased lentiform and thalamic metabolism associated with reduced metabolism in the lateral frontal, paracentral, and parietooccipital areas (Fig. 7.1) (3,9–11,29). In addition, the degree of individual expression of this covariance pattern correlated with disease severity ratings and independent PET measurements of striatal FDOPA uptake in patients with PD (3,9, 10,29). These results agree with experimental animal models, in which parkinsonian signs are associated with excessive pallidofugal inhibitory outflow with concomitant suppression of brain function in primary and association motor cortical regions (27). A reduction of nigrostriatal dopaminergic activity leads to increased functional activity in the putamen and the subthalamic nucleus (STN) (33). Increased activity in the STN results in overactivity of the pallidothalamic pathway with concomitant suppression of thalamocortical excitatory inputs.

FDG/PET is also a powerful tool in the differential diagnosis of parkinsonism (9,18,25,29,34). APSs can account for up to 10% of patients with parkinsonism and are characterized clinically by progressive rigidity and minimal or absent response to dopaminergic therapy (35). A reliable clinical diagnosis of APS can be made only when patients present with a combination of parkinsonism, autonomic dysfunction, and cerebellar and pyramidal signs (35). The recognition of patients with possible APSs manifesting with predominant parkinsonism and only marginal atypical signs is a more challenging task. Although the presence of resting tremor or levodopa responsiveness is commonly considered to be diagnostic of classic PD, these signs have been recognized in parkinsonian patients ultimately found to have APSs at neuropathologic examination. Therefore, an adjunctive diagnostic test such as FDG/PET may be helpful in supporting the clinical suspicion of APS even in the presence of minimal atypical features. We reported FDG/PET data from a cohort of 43 patients suspected as having possible APSs based on the development of diminished levodopa responsiveness, orthostatic hypotension, or both (8). All patients had convincing levodopa responses without autonomic dysfunction or other atypical features at the time of original clinical presentation. We used 56 other patients without atypical features as a reference population with likely idiopathic PD. We found significant reductions in the striatum and in the thalamus of the patients suspected of having an APS relative to the group with likely PD. Indeed, a linear combination of caudate, lentiform, and thalamic metabolic values accurately discriminated between typical and atypical

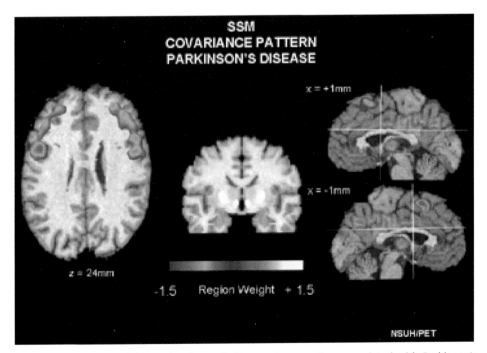

FIGURE 7.1. Display of the regional metabolic covariance pattern associated with Parkinson's disease (PD) identified using the Scaled Subprofile Model (SSM). Region weights for this PD-related pattern (PDRP) have been overlaid on standard Talairach transformed magnetic resonance imaging (MRI) sections. The pattern is characterized by relative lentiform and thalamic hypermetabolism *(yellow)* covarying negatively with bilateral metabolic reductions *(blue)* in motor and premotor regions and in the supplementary motor area (SMA). (See Color Figure 7.1.)

patients. This finding was reproduced in two independent APS and PD populations scanned on different PET cameras (8). These results indicate that FDG/PET can be a helpful adjunct to the clinical examination in differential diagnosis of parkinsonism. Indeed, this discrimination may be critical in the assessment of patients for possible surgical intervention.

METABOLIC NETWORK MAPPING IN HYPERKINETIC MOVEMENT DISORDERS

Idiopathic torsion dystonia (ITD) and *HD* are common hereditary movement disorders affecting the basal ganglia. Because ITD and HD are genetically mediated, these disorders provide a unique opportunity to assess the complex interrelationship between gene expression and brain network organization. The study of hyperkinetic movement disorders with functional brain imaging technology is complicated by several issues. First, it is not always clear whether the metabolic abnormalities discerned with PET are the cause or the effect of the abnormal movements. Additionally, network abnormalities may be genotype specific, thereby varying considerably in heterogeneous patient cohorts. Finally, it is unknown to what degree differences in phenotypic expression, such as somatic distribution, contribute to the variability in the network maps. To address these potential difficulties, we pursued several innovative experimental strategies. To identify pathologic network abnormalities in the absence of movement, we studied nonmanifesting carriers of abnormal disease-associated genotypes. This approach allowed for the delineation of abnormal functional networks in neurologically normal gene carriers, thereby eliminating the confounds of concurrent hyperkinesia and genotypic heterogeneity. Additionally, the abnormal hyperkinetic movements associated with these disorders often are suppressed in sleep. Thus, sleep induction can provide a useful experimental method to assess pathologic network architecture without the confound of movement.

Genotype-Related Networks in Dystonia

In our first ITD study (11), we identified an abnormal metabolic covariance pattern in patients with dystonia with predominantly right-sided signs. This pattern was characterized by relative bilateral lentiform hypermetabolism that was dissociated from metabolic activity in the thalamus. These changes were associated with covariate metabolic increases in primary motor and premotor regions including the supplementary motor area (SMA). Subject scores for this pattern correlated significantly with independent disability ratings for dystonia (36). We construed these results as evidence of resting overactivity of neural networks involving the lentiform nucleus and associative motor regions. Moreover, the dissociation between lentiform and thalamic metabolism in ITD suggested the possibility of a functional inhibition of

the internal segment of the globus pallidus (GPi), as has been postulated as a mechanism for hyperkinesia (37–39). We interpreted this metabolic dissociation as indicating an overactivity of direct inhibitory projections from the putamen to GPi releasing the ventral tier thalamic nuclei from pallidofugal inhibition (21,40). Indeed, the relative lentiform hypermetabolism noted by us may relate to an increase in GPi afferents through the direct striatopallidal pathway. These findings in the resting state are compatible with the results of motor activation studies of ITD (14,41), as well as with experimental animal models of dystonia (37,38).

Although most of the patients with ITD in the foregoing study had dystonia only on action (11) and therefore were not moving during the time of PET imaging (42), the possibility of contamination by concurrent motor activity could not be discounted. Moreover, the patients were selected with a variety of genotypes and considerable variability in clinical expression. To address the problem of concurrent movement during PET, as well as the genotypic and phenotypic variability inherent in our first study, we studied a cohort of nonmanifesting carriers of the DYT1 gene for ITD (43). To identify metabolic brain networks specifically associated with the DYT1 genotype, we performed SSM analysis on the combined metabolic data set for the gene carriers and the neurologically normal volunteers, blind to gene status. In this network analysis, we identified a significant covariance pattern that was topographically similar to that identified in our original ITD study. The DYT1-related pattern was characterized by bilateral lentiform hypermetabolism and thalamolentiform dissociation, associated with covarying increases in cerebellar and SMA metabolism (Fig. 7.2). Subject scores for this pattern were abnormally elevated in the nonmanifesting DYT1 carriers, a finding indicating a genotype-related increase in brain network expression in these clinically normal persons. Because this pattern was identified in clinically unaffected gene carriers in the resting state, we designated it as movement-free (MF). We next prospectively calculated the expression of the MF pattern in a separate cohort of *affected* DYT1 patients and found an abnormal increase in the expression of this network in the symptomatic patient cohort analogous to that found in the nonmanifesting gene carriers. These findings demonstrate that the functional abnormalities of corticostriatopallidothalamocortical (CSPTC) motor circuits are associated with the DYT1 genotype and are evident in independent gene-bearing cohorts with and without clinical manifestations of dystonia. Specifically, network-related metabolic overaction of the lentiform nuclei and motor association cortices may be evident in the resting state in both nonmanifesting and affected DYT1 carriers.

In a related set of experiments (43), we rescanned five affected patients with ITD and five neurologically normal volunteers after pharmacologic sleep induction. We found that in sleep, the DYT1-related MF pattern remained significantly elevated in the patients relative to the control subjects. These findings demonstrate that genotype-related network

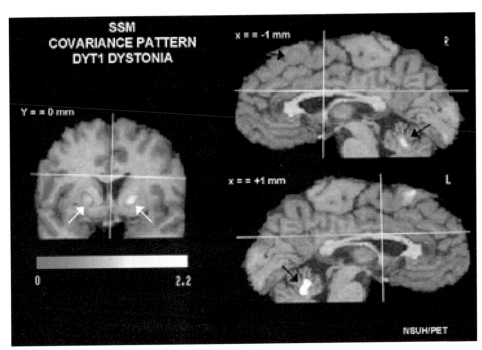

FIGURE 7.2. Display of the regional metabolic covariance pattern associated with DYT1 dystonia identified using the Scaled Subprofile Model (SSM). Region weights have been mapped on standardized Talairach magnetic resonance imaging sections. This pattern was characterized by relatively increased metabolism in the lentiform nucleus, supplementary motor area (SMA), and cerebellar hemispheres. (See Color Figure 7.2.)

abnormalities are not only present in nonmanifesting DYT1 carriers, but also persist in affected dystonia patients in whom movement has been suppressed. Whether analogous network abnormalities exist in the carriers of other dystonia mutations is a topic of ongoing investigation.

Overall, these findings lend credence to our analytic strategies for quantifying metabolic networks in hyperkinetic disorders and to the possibility of isolating disease-related networks that are not contaminated by involuntary movement at the time of PET. Our results suggest that definable abnormalities of CSPTC networks may be present *at rest* in clinically unaffected gene carriers. The behavioral concomitants of the resting state metabolic network abnormalities associated with the DYT1 genotype are unknown, although our preliminary psychophysical data suggest that motor learning may be abnormal in these persons. Indeed, PET imaging during the execution of motor tasks will be useful in delineating the relationship between altered network expression in the resting state and abnormal functional activation of motor circuits during the performance of specific motor tasks.

Genotype-Related Networks in Huntington's Disease

We extended this approach to the study of other hyperkinetic movement disorders. In a preliminary study (44), we found that HD is characterized by two discrete metabolic patterns, each associated with specific aspects of the disease process.

An MF pattern characterized by hypometabolism of caudate and putamen was expressed in preclinical gene carriers and to a greater extent in early symptomatic patients. A second pattern characterized by caudate hypometabolism covarying with relative metabolic increases in thalamus and cerebellum was expressed only in the symptomatic HD carriers (Fig. 7.3). We found that subject scores for this pattern correlated significantly with the product of trinucleotide (CAG) repeat length and patient age. This finding suggests the existence of a relationship between network expression and mutation load analogous to that described by us for striatal D_2-neuroceptor binding (8). Thus, quantifying the expression of these patterns in HD patients may provide insights into the functional topography of brain degeneration in this disorder.

Abnormal Brain Networks in Other Movement Disorders

Network imaging may be particularly useful in the investigation of movement disorders for which there is no known histopathologic, neurochemical, or genetic substrate. *Tourette's syndrome* (TS) is such a condition. In this disorder (40), we found that analogously to ITD, there is hyperexpression of a covariance pattern characterized by relative metabolic increases in the lateral premotor and supplementary motor regions. A second pattern, unique to TS, was characterized by a reduction in the activity of limbic basal

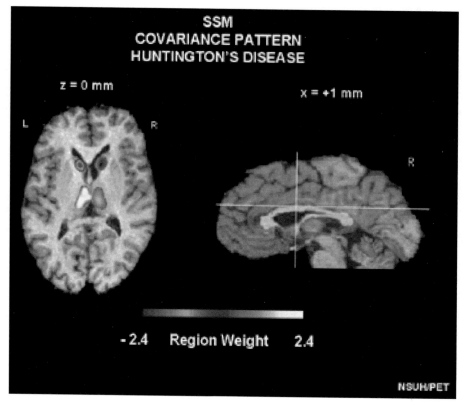

FIGURE 7.3. Display of the regional metabolic covariance pattern associated with Huntington's disease identified using the Scaled Subprofile Model (SSM). Region weights have been mapped on standardized Talairach magnetic resonance imaging sections. This pattern was characterized by caudate hypometabolism covarying with relative metabolic increases in the thalamus and cerebellum. (See Color Figure 7.3.)

ganglia–thalamocortical projection systems. Subject scores for this pattern correlated with Tourette Syndrome Global Scale (TSGS) ratings. Thus, in one respect, the hyperkinetic movement disorders may involve nonspecific abnormalities in the expression of certain motor system networks. In another respect, their phenomenologic signatures may be related to additional brain networks mediating the specific behavioral manifestations of each condition.

SURGICAL TREATMENT OF MOVEMENT DISORDERS

Pallidotomy or Thalamotomy for Parkinson's Disease

Posterolateral ventral pallidotomy has been shown to improve akinetic symptoms significantly in PD as well as to relieve dyskinesia associated with levodopa administration (45,46). The pathophysiology of pallidal ablation for the relief of parkinsonism is not completely understood. The ameliorative effects of pallidotomy have been attributed to the reduction of excessive inhibitory outflow from the GPi (47).

We originally reported eight patients with PD who were undergoing pallidotomy and who were scanned with FDG/PET preoperatively and 6 months postoperatively (48). We found that pallidotomy resulted in a metabolic decline in the thalamus that occurred in conjunction with a metabolic increase in primary and associative motor cortical regions. Indeed, the improvement in limb performance at 6 months postoperatively was significantly correlated with the operative metabolic decline in the thalamus and with the accompanying increases in lateral premotor cortex. To quantify potential modulations in the expression of motor networks by pallidotomy, we applied SSM/PCA to operative differences in regional glucose metabolism. We found that the topography identified in this analysis closely resembled the PD-related profile identified previously (3,11), and it was characterized by a postoperative decline in the lentiform and thalamic metabolism ipsilateral to the surgical side associated with bilateral increases in SMA metabolism (Fig. 7.4).

The individual expression of this pattern of metabolic operative change correlated significantly with improvements in both contralateral and ipsilateral limb performance (CAPIT: Core Assessment Protocol for Intracerebral Transplantation) (49) scores. These findings indicate that metabolic brain networks comprising functionally and anatomically

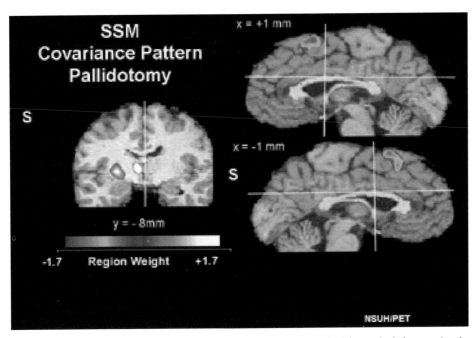

FIGURE 7.4. Display of the regional covariance pattern associated with surgical changes in glucose metabolism after pallidotomy identified using the Scaled Subprofile Model (SSM). Region weights have been overlaid on standardized Talairach transformed magnetic resonance imaging sections. This pattern was characterized by operative declines in lentiform metabolism covarying with bilateral metabolic increases in the supplementary motor area (SMA). (See Color Figure 7.4.)

interconnected brain regions remote from the lesion site may be modulated by unilateral pallidotomy, including motor cortical regions of the hemisphere contralateral to the surgery.

Because local rates of glucose are a reflection of net afferent synaptic activity (50), it is reasonable to expect a decline in thalamic metabolism subsequent to surgical interference with pallidofugal inhibitory projections to the thalamus. Similarly, the metabolic increases in motor cortical areas occurring with pallidotomy may be related to enhanced cortical afferent synaptic activity from the ventral thalamus after surgical reduction in pallidothalamic inhibitory output (21,27, 51,52). Indeed, we have shown that spontaneous GPi single-unit activity recorded intraoperatively during pallidotomy correlated significantly with preoperative measures of thalamic glucose utilization obtained in the same patients under comparable behavioral conditions (40). This physiologic-metabolic relationship was reproduced in the subgroups of patients scanned on different PET cameras. Moreover, we found that GPi firing rates were also significantly correlated with the expression of an SSM network related to the pallidum and its major efferent projections. It is therefore likely that pallidal ablation may exert its primary metabolic effect in spatially distributed projection fields lying in the ventral tier and intralaminar thalamic nuclei as well as in the brainstem.

PET activation studies using [^{15}O]H$_2$O have also supported the notion of pallidotomy-induced modulation

of the CSPTC motor circuit. Subtraction of resting state from task-specific data allows isolation of changes in rCBF relating to various motor tasks (53). In 1995, Grafton et al. reported postpallidotomy increases in rCBF in the ipsilateral premotor and in the SMA with movement (13). In another study employing network analysis of motor system connectivity, Grafton and colleagues in 1994 found significant postoperative reductions in the strength of interactions between the globus pallidus and thalamus and between the thalamus and mesial frontal motor area (12). These findings are consistent with the notion that pallidal ablation induces alterations in the normal functioning of CSPTC motor networks (47,51,54).

In addition to adding to our understanding of the network modulations occurring with pallidotomy, FDG/PET may be used to select optimal candidates for this procedure. In our original study of ten patients undergoing pallidotomy, we found that preoperative FDG/PET measurements of lentiform metabolism in the "off" state correlated with clinical outcome up to 6 months postoperatively (Fig. 7.5) (48). We subsequently studied an additional cohort of 22 patients with PD to assess the usefulness of preoperative FDG/PET, quantitative motor performance indices, and magnetic resonance imaging (MRI) measurements of lesion size and location as potential predictors of surgical outcome (55). We found that the pallidotomy lesions were comparable in location and size in all patients, and therefore they did not correlate with individual differences in surgical

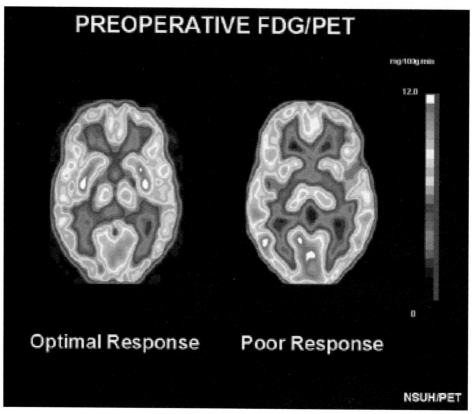

FIGURE 7.5. Preoperative [^{18}F] fluorodeoxyglucose (FDG) positron emission tomography images from two patients with idiopathic Parkinson's disease who underwent right unilateral pallidotomy. **Left:** A patient with preoperative lentiform glucose hypermetabolism had an optimal surgical outcome. **Right:** A patient with a lower rate of metabolism in the lentiform nucleus had no therapeutic response to surgery. Both pallidotomy lesions were comparable in size and location. (The *color stripe* represents regional rates of glucose metabolism in mg/min/100g.) (See Color Figure 7.5.)

outcome. Nonetheless, in this series we confirmed that preoperative measures of lentiform glucose metabolism offered an accurate prediction of ultimate surgical improvement.

The finding of a significant correlation between levodopa response and clinical outcome postoperatively suggests that the dynamic range of the CSPTC motor loop with pallidal suppression may be clinically estimated using a levodopa challenge. These findings have been supported by FDG/PET experiments in patients with PD showing reduction of pallidal hypermetabolism during levodopa infusion (16). To the extent that the severity of clinical manifestations is correlated with the expression of abnormal CSPTC metabolic networks, the measured clinical benefit with levodopa administration may provide a simple indicator of the dynamic range of network modulation that can occur with either pharmacologic or surgical pallidal suppression. Similarly, we found that preoperative measurements of lentiform metabolism with FDG/PET reproducibly predict approximately 50% of operative improvement in off-state CAPIT scores. The preoperative levodopa responsiveness index, although simpler to measure, predicted approximately 36% of individual differences in outcome. Together, however, both preoperative measures predicted approximately 70%

of the pallidotomy response. The combination of preoperative FDG/PET measurements of lentiform metabolism and clinicopharmacologic estimates of the patient's individual capacity for network modulation can provide useful and complementary criteria for patient selection for pallidotomy.

Stereotactic thalamotomy has been shown to improve drug-resistant tremor significantly in PD. The thalamic ventralis intermedius nucleus (VIM) is targeted in thalamotomy as it relays cerebellar and proprioceptive output to sensorimotor cortical areas. In 1997, using [^{15}O]H$_2$O/PET, Boecker et al. observed significant operative declines in sensorimotor, premotor, and parietal rCBF both at rest and during motor activation in two patients with PD who underwent thalamotomy for tremor (56). This finding supports the notion that parkinsonian tremor arises through the overaction of ventral thalamic projections to cortical motor regions (8). These findings indicate that in relieving PD tremor, thalamotomy may also alter functional input from the surgical target to sensorimotor cortical regions. Nevertheless, a comprehensive network modeling approach to define the mechanism of surgical improvement using imaging awaits future investigation.

Pallidotomy or Thalamotomy for Other Movement Disorders

Pallidotomy and thalamotomy may also provide symptom relief for *dystonia* (57,58). In 1998, Vitek et al. found marked improvement in motor functioning and dystonic symptoms after GPi pallidotomy in three patients with primary dystonia (59). Additionally, thalamotomy has been reported effective in relieving primary and secondary dystonia, although lesion location played a role in the degree of benefit (58, 60–63). In regard to neuroimaging studies, the effects of pallidotomy and thalamotomy in dystonia and other movement disorders remain a topic of future investigation.

Deep Brain Stimulation in Parkinson's Disease

High-frequency DBS has the advantage of avoiding permanent side effects of the ablative lesion, therefore inducing the possibility of a reversible amelioration of parkinsonian symptoms. In addition, this technique is adaptable because the stimulation frequency can be increased or decreased. Inhibitory DBS of the ventral portion of the thalamus, usually VIM, has been employed originally for the control of parkinsonian resting tremor. More recently, DBS has been applied to the GPi to improve rigidity and bradykinesia in PD (64) and to the STN to improve rigidity, akinesia, and tremor (65). In 1992, Parker et al. investigated the effect of thalamic stimulation (66). They observed that rCBF increased in the sensorimotor area, premotor area, SMA, caudate nucleus, and cerebellar vermis and hemisphere during the tremor period compared with the period of tremor arrest. In 1993, Deiber et al. observed that suppression of tremor induced by sufficient stimulation was specifically associated with the reduction of cerebellar rCBF, whereas the incomplete arrest of tremor induced by insufficient stimulation only reduced rCBF in frontal cortex. These investigators suggested that tremor suppression is mainly associated with a decrease of synaptic activity in the cerebellum (67).

In 1997, Davis et al. examined rCBF and parkinsonian symptoms in patients who had VIM DBS implants using [^{15}O]H$_2$O/PET. These investigators found a decrease in rCBF in the SMA, contralateral cerebellum, and cingulate motor area and in the ipsilateral sensory association areas during thalamic stimulation. An increase in rCBF was seen in bilateral frontal and ipsilateral occipital regions and in the dorsolateral prefrontal cortex (DLPFC) during VIM stimulation (68).

[^{15}O]H$_2$O/PET has also been used to study the mechanism of pallidal stimulation. In their study, Davis et al. measured the effects of GPi DBS on cerebral blood flow. They found an increase in rCBF in ipsilateral premotor areas during GPi stimulation, which clinically improved rigidity and bradykinesia (68). Comparable rCBF changes with GPi DBS were not evident in the joystick activation study

of Limousin et al. (69). We studied six patients with advanced PD who were undergoing pallidal stimulation (70). GPi stimulation during a kinematically controlled motor execution task resulted in significant rCBF increases in contralateral primary motor cortex and in premotor regions as well as in the cerebellar hemisphere ipsilateral to the moving hand. These findings are similar to our previous FDG/PET studies in pallidotomy and suggest that disrupting the excessive inhibitory GPi output to the thalamus reverses the symptoms of parkinsonism by activating areas involved in the initiation of movement.

STN is thought to be more effective than GPi stimulation for akinetic symptoms of PD. Limousin et al. investigated the effect of STN stimulation on rCBF during an activation task. Using [^{15}O]H$_2$O/PET, six patients with PD with STN DBS implants were scanned while they performed self-directed movements with a joystick. Results showed significant rCBF increases in the SMA, cingulate cortex, and DLPFC during effective STN stimulation. This finding suggests that STN DBS may play a role in potentiating nonprimary motor cortical areas, especially the DLPFC, which showed greater activation than in GPi during effective stimulation (69). High-frequency DBS has the potential of a useful experimental method to assess the modulation of structural and functional relationships during the successful treatment of PD. Nonetheless, the role of preoperative PET in patient selection for STN DBS in parkinsonism remains a topic of future investigation.

Deep Brain Stimulation for Other Movement Disorders

DBS may be used as an alternative to pallidotomy and thalamotomy in dystonia and essential tremor (71–74). The assessment of the preoperative and postoperative effects of DBS in dystonia and other movement disorders using PET is a topic of ongoing investigation.

Dopamine Cell Implantation Procedures in Parkinson's Disease

The *implantation of fetal mesencephalon* may prove useful in the treatment of PD (75,76). *In vivo* assessment of presynaptic nigrostriatal dopaminergic function with FDOPA/PET may be used to monitor graft survival and development after transplantation. To date, only a few patients have been studied with PET. One patient exhibited sustained postoperative increases in FDOPA uptake in the grafted putamen 33 months after transplantation (77). In 1992, Sawle et al. subsequently reported two patients with PD who underwent unilateral transplantation into the putamen and who had FDOPA/PET imaging before surgical treatment and 12 and 13 months postoperatively. These patients had substantial increases in FDOPA uptake in the grafted putamen and decreases in the nongrafted striatum, presumably associated with disease progression. In one of these patients, clinical improvement continued 3 years after transplantation and was accompanied by a further increase in FDOPA uptake in the grafted putamen. The other patient had no further increase in FDOPA uptake or improvement in clinical symptoms between 1 and 3 years after transplantation (78). In 1995, Remy et al. reported increases in FDOPA uptake in five patients with unilateral implantation in the putamen; changes in FDOPA uptake rate constant were significantly correlated with clinical improvement measures (79). In 1999, Hauser et al. reported six patients with advanced-stage PD who were treated with bilateral implantation in the putamen. These patients showed significant clinical improvement 1 year after transplantation, as well as appreciable bilateral increases in striatal FDOPA uptake (80). We reported similar results in a cohort of 19 patients with advanced PD who were undergoing fetal nigral implantation as part of a randomized blinded comparison with sham-operated controls (81) (Fig. 7.6).

Some caveats must be considered in the interpretation of these findings. FDOPA crosses the blood-brain barrier (BBB) in competition with other neutral amino acids (82, 83). Thus, any alteration of plasma amino acid content (including changes in peripheral levodopa levels) may alter FDOPA transport and can confound FDOPA/PET quantifiers of dopaminergic function. In addition, the assessment of graft survival and growth using FDOPA/PET may potentially be overestimated by postoperative increases in the net transport of FDOPA across the BBB (84). Indeed, evidence indicates that both permeability and surface area can increase after tissue transplantation.

Fluorescence histochemical measurements of monoamine uptake into central neurons suggest that the BBB to monoamines may not be fully developed in infant rats (85). The influx rate of amino acids is greater during the first weeks of life and falls subsequently to the level found in adult rats at 8 to 10 weeks of age (86). In 1989, Guttman et al. reported five patients who underwent adrenal medulla implantation and who had preoperative and postoperative FDOPA/PET scans. In two patients, increased permeability of the BBB was shown at the implanted sites using gallium ([^{68}Ga] ethylenediaminetetraacetic acid) and PET (87). Furthermore, Dusart et al. demonstrated two different types of angiogenesis in the thalamus after transplantation of dissociated fetal tissue. Although these authors observed mature angiogenesis in the grafted site, reactive angiogenesis may also induce significant increases in local FDOPA uptake without necessarily implicating reinnervation from the grafted tissues (88).

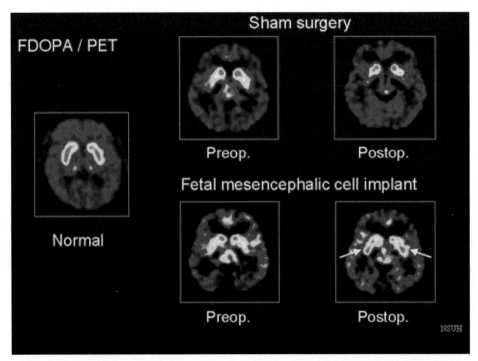

FIGURE 7.6. [^{15}F] fluorodopa (FDOPA) positron emission tomography (PET) images from a normal volunteer **(left)** and from two patients studied in the course of a blinded sham-controlled study of fetal nigral dopamine cell implantation for advanced Parkinson's disease **(right).** The **upper tier** represents baseline and 15 month follow-up FDOPA/PET scans from a patients with Parkinson's disease who was randomized to sham surgery. The **lower tier** represents baseline and 15-month postoperative scans from another patient who was randomized to bilateral implantation in the putamen. At baseline, both patients demonstrated bilateral increases in putamen FDOPA uptake compatible with engraftment *(arrows).* (See Color Figure 7.6.)

Postmortem results from two patients who underwent fetal mesencephalic implantation and postoperative FDOPA/PET have been reported. Kordower and colleagues reported one patient who showed substantial clinical improvement as well as an increase in FDOPA uptake in the grafted putamen (89). PET examination 18 months postoperatively (8 months before death) disclosed increased radiotracer uptake in the pericaudate area and in the putamen, sites where implantation had been performed. Necropsy revealed only gliosis and inflammatory response in these areas (90).

Further technologic development is required to optimize fetal implantation surgery as a therapeutic option in advanced parkinsonism. The safety and efficacy of these procedures is currently unknown and is a topic of several controlled clinical studies including investigations of porcine nigral cells (91). Whether or not changes in striatal FDOPA uptake accurately reflect graft survival is also the subject of ongoing investigation.

Neurotransplantation Procedures in Huntington's Disease

The *transplantation of fetal mesencephalon* as a treatment for HD is still in the experimental stage. To date, between 20 and 30 patients with HD have undergone fetal engraftment (92,93). MRI of three HD patients showed graft survival and growth after 1 year after transplantation (94).

Alternative dopaminergic imaging methods may afford a complementary tool for the assessment of outcome after fetal implantation. Specifically, adjunctive PET imaging of striatal DAT activity before and after implantation procedures, as well as the application of functional mapping methods with FDG and $[^{15}O]H_2O/PET$, may lead to a broader understanding of the effects of neural transplantation on the nigrostriatal dopaminergic system.

CONCLUSION

Reliable *in vivo* markers of neuronal activity are needed to assess surgical outcome. Currently available clinical scales are relatively insensitive and inherently variable, and they may not accurately reflect the extent of neuropathologic change. By contrast, quantitative functional brain imaging markers may be suitable as outcome measures for the surgical treatment of PD. Indeed, we have found that functional brain imaging may serve as a useful tool in predicting optimal candidates for certain surgical interventions.

ACKNOWLEDGMENT

This work is supported by National Institutes of Health grants RO1 32368, 35069, and 37564, as well as generous grants from the National Parkinson Foundation, the Parkinson Disease Foundation, and the American Parkinson Disease Association.

REFERENCES

1. Antonini A, Vontobel P, Psylla M, et al. Complementary positron emission tomographic studies of the striatal dopaminergic system in Parkinson's disease. *Arch Neurol* 1995;52:1183–1190.
2. Brooks DJ, Ibanez V, Sawle GV, et al. Differing patterns of striatal ^{18}F-dopa uptake in Parkinson's disease, multiple system atrophy, and progressive supranuclear palsy. *Ann Neurol* 1990;28:547–555.
3. Eidelberg D, Moeller JR, Dhawan V, et al. The metabolic anatomy of Parkinson's disease: complementary $[^{18}F]$fluorodeoxyglucose and $[^{18}F]$fluorodopa positron emission tomographic studies. *Mov Disord* 1990;5:203–213.
4. Ishikawa T, Dhawan V, Chaly T, et al. Clinical significance of striatal DOPA decarboxylase activity in Parkinson's disease. *J Nucl Med* 1996;37:216–222.
5. Assenbaum S, Brucke T, Pirker W, et al. Imaging of dopamine transporters with iodine-123-beta CIT and SPECT in Parkinson's disease. *J Nucl Med* 1997;38:1–6.
6. Chaly T, Dhawan V, Kazumata K, et al. Radiosynthesis of $[^{18}F]$ N-3-fluoropropyl-2-beta-carbomethoxy-3-beta-(4-iodophenyl) nortropane and the first human study with positron emission tomography. *Nucl Med Biol* 1996;23:999–1004.
7. Brooks D, Ibanez V, Sawle G, et al. Striatal D_2 receptor status in patients with Parkinson's disease, striatonigral degeneration, and progressive supranuclear palsy, measured with ^{11}C-raclopride and positron emission tomography. *Ann Neurol* 1992;31:184–192.
8. Antonini A, Kazumata K, Feigin A, et al. Differential diagnosis of parkinsonism with $[^{18}F]$fluorodeoxyglucose and PET. *Mov Disord* 1998;13:268–274.
9. Eidelberg D, Moeller JR, Ishikawa T, et al. Assessment of disease severity in parkinsonism with fluorine-18-fluorodeoxyglucose and PET. *J Nucl Med* 1995;36:378–383.
10. Eidelberg D, Moeller JR, Ishikawa T, et al. Early differential diagnosis of Parkinson's disease with ^{18}F-fluorodeoxyglucose and positron emission tomography. *Neurology* 1995;45:1995–2004.
11. Eidelberg D, Moeller JR, Ishikawa T, et al. The metabolic topography of idiopathic torsion dystonia. *Brain* 1995;118:1473–1484.
12. Grafton S, Sutton J, Couldwell W, et al. Network analysis of motor system connectivity in Parkinson's disease: modulation of thalamocortical interactions after pallidotomy. *Hum Brain Mapping* 1994;2:45–55.
13. Grafton S, Hazeltine E, Ivry R. Functional mapping of sequence learning in normal humans. *J Cogn Neurosci* 1995;7:497–510.
14. Ceballos-Baumann A, Passingham R, Warner T, et al. Overactive prefrontal and underactive motor cortical areas in idiopathic dystonia. *Ann Neurol* 1995;37:363–372.
15. Brooks D, Salmon E, Mathias C, et al. The relationship between locomotor disability, autonomic dysfunction, and the integrity of the striatal dopaminergic system in patients with multiple system atrophy, pure autonomic failure, and Parkinson's disease, studied with PET. *Brain* 1990;113:1539–1552.
16. Blesa R, Blin J, Miletich R. Levodopa-reduced glucose metabolism in striatopallido-thalamocortical circuit in Parkinson's disease. *Neurology* 1991;41[Suppl 1]:359.
17. Eidelberg D, Dhawan V, Moeller JR, et al. The metabolic landscape of cortico-basal ganglionic degeneration: regional asymmetries studied with positron emission tomography. *J Neurol Neurosurg Psychiatry* 1991;54:856–862.

18. Przedborski S, Giladi N, Takikawa S, et al. Metabolic topography of the hemiparkinsonism-hemiatrophy syndrome. *Neurology* 1994;44:1622–1628.

19. Wilson JM, Levey AI, Rajput A, et al. Differential changes in neurochemical markers of striatal dopamine nerve terminals in idiopathic Parkinson's disease. *Neurology* 1996;47:718–726.

20. Seibyl JP, Marek KL, Quinlan D, et al. Decreased single-photon emission computed tomographic [^{123}I]beta-CIT striatal uptake correlates with symptom severity in Parkinson's disease. *Ann Neurol* 1995;38:589–598.

21. Parent A, Hazrati LN. Functional anatomy of the basal ganglia. I. The cortico-basal ganglia-thalamo-cortical loop. *Brain Res Brain Res Rev* 1995;20:91–127.

22. Parent A, Hazrati L. Functional anatomy of the basal ganglia. II. The place of subthalamic nucleus and external pallidum in basal ganglia circuitry. *Brain Res Brain Res Rev* 1995;20:128–154.

23. Antonini A, Leenders KL. Dopamine D$_2$ receptors in normal human brain: effect of age measured by positron emission tomography (PET) and [^{11}C]-raclopride. *Ann NY Acad Sci* 1993;695:81–85.

24. Perlmutter J, Kilbourn M, Raichle M, et al. MPTP-induced up-regulation of *in vivo* dopaminergic radioligand-receptor binding in humans. *Neurology* 1987;37:1575–1579.

25. Antonini A, Schwarz J, Oertel W, et al. Long-term changes of striatal dopamine D$_2$ receptors in patients with Parkinson's disease: a study with positron emission tomography and [^{11}C]raclopride. *Mov Disord* 1997;12:33–38.

26. Takikawa S, Eidelberg D. Movement disorders. In: Kelley R, ed. Functional neuroimaging. Armonk, NY: Futura, 1994:247–262.

27. Alexander GE, Crutcher MD, DeLong MR. Basal ganglia-thalamocortical circuits: parallel substrates for motor, oculomotor, "prefrontal" and "limbic" functions. *Prog Brain Res* 1990;85:119–146.

28. Albin R, Young A, Penney J. The functional anatomy of basal ganglia disorders. *Trends Neurosci* 1989;12:366–375.

29. Eidelberg D, Moeller JR, Dhawan V, et al. The metabolic topography of parkinsonism. *J Cereb Blood Flow Metab* 1994;14:783–801.

30. Alexander G, Moeller J. Application of the scaled subprofile model to functional imaging in neuropsychiatric disorders: a principal component approach to modeling brain function in disease. *Hum Brain Mapping* 1994;2:1–16.

31. Moeller JR, Strother SC, Sidtis JJ, et al. Scaled subprofile model: a statistical approach to the analysis of functional patterns in positron emission tomographic data. *J Cereb Blood Flow Metab* 1987;7:649–658.

32. Moeller JR, Strother SC. A regional covariance approach to the analysis of functional patterns in positron emission tomographic data. *J Cereb Blood Flow Metab* 1991;11:A121–A135.

33. Wooten G, Collins R. Metabolic effects of unilateral lesions of the substantia nigra. *J Neurosci* 1981;1:285–291.

34. Eidelberg D, Takikawa S, Dhawan V, et al. Striatal ^{18}F-dopa uptake: absence of an aging effect. *J Cereb Blood Flow Metab* 1993;13:881–888.

35. Quinn N. Multiple system atrophy: the nature of the beast. *J Neurol Neurosurg Psychiatry* 1989;52:78–89.

36. Burke R, Fahn S, Marsden C, et al. Validity and reliability of a rating scale for the primary torsion dystonias. *Neurology* 1985;35:73–77.

37. Mitchell I, Luquin R, Boyce S, et al. Neural mechanisms of dystonia: evidence from a 2-deoxyglucose uptake study in a primate model of dopamine agonist-induced dystonia. *Mov Disord* 1990;5:49–54.

38. Crossman AR. A hypothesis on the pathophysiological mechanisms that underlie levodopa- or dopamine agonist–induced dyskinesia in Parkinson's disease: implications for future strategies in treatment. *Mov Disord* 1990;5:100–108.

39. Hallett M. Physiology of basal ganglia disorders: an overview. *Can J Neurol Sci* 1993;20:177–183.

40. Eidelberg D, Moeller JR, Kazumata K, et al. Metabolic correlates of pallidal neuronal activity in Parkinson's disease. *Brain* 1997;120:1315–1324.

41. Ceballos-Baumann A, Sheean G, Passingham R, et al. Botulinum toxin does not reverse the cortical dysfunction associated with writer's cramp: a PET study. *Brain* 1997;120:571–582.

42. Fahn S. Idiopathic torsion dystonia. In: Calne D, ed. *Neurodegenerative diseases.* Philadelphia: WB Saunders, 1994:705–715.

43. Eidelberg D. Functional brain networks in movement disorders. *Curr Opin Neurol* 1998;11:319–326.

44. Thut G, Antonini A, Spiegel R, et al. The metabolic topography of Huntington's disease. *Neurology* 1996;46[Suppl]:A258.

45. Baron MS, Vitek JL, Bakay RA, et al. Treatment of advanced Parkinson's disease by posterior GPi pallidotomy: 1-year results of a pilot study. *Ann Neurol* 1996;40:355–366.

46. Dogali M, Fazzini E, Kolodny E, et al. Stereotactic ventral pallidotomy for Parkinson's disease. *Neurology* 1995;45:753–761.

47. Marsden C, Obeso J. The functions of the basal ganglia and the paradox of stereotaxic surgery in Parkinson's disease. *Brain* 1994;117:877–897.

48. Eidelberg D, Moeller JR, Ishikawa T, et al. Regional metabolic correlates of surgical outcome following unilateral pallidotomy for Parkinson's disease. *Ann Neurol* 1996;39:450–459.

49. Langston J, Widner H, Goetz C, et al. Core assessment program for intracerebral transplantations (CAPIT). *Mov Disord* 1992;7:2–13.

50. Mata M, Fink D, Gainer H. Activity-dependent energy metabolism in rat posterior pituitary primarily reflect sodium pump activity. *J Neurochem* 1980;34:213–215.

51. DeLong MR. Primate models of movement disorders of basal ganglia origin. *Trends Neurosci* 1990;13:281–285.

52. Mitchell I, Boyce S, Sambrook M, et al. A 2-deoxyglucose study of the effects of dopamine agonists on the parkinsonian primate brain. *Brain* 1994;115:809–824.

53. Friston K, Holmes A, Worsley K, et al. Statistical parametric maps in functional imaging: a general linear approach. *Hum Brain Mapping* 1995;2:189–210.

54. Bathia K, Marsden C. The behavioral and motor consequences of focal lesions of the basal ganglia in man. *Brain* 1994;117:859–876.

55. Kazumata K, Antonini A, Dhawan V, et al. Preoperative indicators of clinical outcome following stereotaxic pallidotomy. *Neurology* 1997;49:1083–1090.

56. Boecker H, Wills AJ, Ceballos-Baumann A, et al. Stereotactic thalamotomy in tremor-dominant Parkinson's disease: an H$_2$(15)O PET motor activation study. *Ann Neurol* 1997;41:108–111.

57. Ondo W, Desaloms J, Jankovic J, et al. Pallidotomy for generalized dystonia. *Mov Disord* 1998;13:693–698.

58. Tasker R, Doorly T, Yamashiro K. Thalamotomy in generalized dystonia. *Adv Neurol* 1988;50:615–631.

59. Vitek J, Zhang J, Evatt M, et al. GPi pallidotomy for dystonia: clinical outcome and neuronal activity. *Adv Neurol* 1998;78:211–219.

60. Burzaco J. Stereotaxic pallidotomy in extrapyramidal disorders. *Appl Neurophysiol* 1985;48:283–287.

61. Cooper I. 20-year follow up study of the neurosurgical treatment of dystonia musculorum deformans. *Adv Neurol* 1976;14:423—452.

62. Andrew J, Fowler C, Harrison M. Stereotaxic thalamotomy in 55 cases of dystonia. *Brain* 1983;106:981–1000.

63. Cardoso F, Jankovic J, Grossman R, et al. Outcome after stereotaxic thalamotomy for dystonia and hemiballismus. *Neurosurgery* 1995;36:501–507.
64. Siegfried J, Lippitz B. Bilateral chronic electrostimulation of ventroposterolateral pallidum: a new therapeutic approach for alleviating all parkinsonian symptoms. *Neurosurgery* 1994;35:1126–1130.
65. Krack P, Pollak P, Limousin P, et al. Subthalamic nucleus or internal pallidal stimulation in young onset Parkinson's disease. *Brain* 1998;121:451–457.
66. Parker F, Tzourio N, Blond S, et al. Evidence for a common network of brain structures involved in parkinsonian tremor and voluntary repetitive movement. *Brain Res* 1992;584:11–17.
67. Deiber MP, Pollak P, Passingham R, et al. Thalamic stimulation and suppression of parkinsonian tremor: evidence of a cerebellar deactivation using positron emission tomography. *Brain* 1993;116:267–279.
68. Davis KD, Taub E, Houle S, et al. Globus pallidus stimulation activates the cortical motor system during alleviation of parkinsonian symptoms. *Nat Med* 1997;3:671–674.
69. Limousin P, Greene J, Pollak P, et al. Changes in cerebral activity pattern due to subthalamic nucleus or internal pallidum stimulation in Parkinson's disease. *Ann Neurol* 1997;42:283–291.
70. Eidelberg D, Nakamura T, Mentis M, et al. Brain activation responses with internal pallidal stimulation in Parkinson's disease. *Neurology* 1999;52:A176.
71. Blond S, Siegfried J. Thalamic stimulation for the treatment of tremor and other movement disorders. *Acta Neurochir* 1991;52:109–111.
72. Benabid A, Pollak P, Seigneuret E, et al. Chronic Vim thalamic stimulation in Parkinson's disease, essential tremor, and extra-pyramidal dyskinesias. *Acta Neurochir* 1993;58[Suppl]:39–44.
73. Sellal F, Hirsch E, Barth P, et al. A case of symptomatic hemidystonia improved by ventroposterolateral thalamic electrostimulation. *Mov Disord* 1993;8:515–518.
74. Benabid A, Pollak P, Gao D. Chronic electrical stimulation of the ventralis intermedius nucleus of the thalamus as a treatment of movement disorders. *J Neurosurg* 1996;84:203–214.
75. Bjorklund A. Reconstruction of the nigrostriatal dopamine pathway by intracerebral nigral transplants. *Brain Res* 1979;177:555–560.
76. Fahn S. Fetal-tissue transplants in Parkinson's disease [Editorial]. *N Engl J Med* 1992;327:1589–1590.
77. Freed C, Breeze R, Rosenberg N, et al. Survival of implanted fetal dopamine cells and neurologic improvement 12 to 46 months after transplantation for Parkinson's disease. *N Engl J Med* 1992;327:1549–1555.
78. Sawle G, Bloomfield P, Bjorklund A, et al. Transplantation of fetal dopamine neurons in Parkinson's disease: PET [^{18}F]6-L-fluorodopa studies in two patients with putaminal implants. *Ann Neurol* 1992;31:166–173.
79. Remy P, Samson Y, Hantraye P, et al. Clinical correlates of [^{18}F]fluorodopa uptake in five grafted parkinsonian patients. *Ann Neurol* 1995;38:580–588.
80. Hauser RA, Freeman TB, Snow BJ, et al. Long-term evaluation of bilateral fetal nigral transplantation in Parkinson disease. *Arch Neurol* 1999;56:179–187.
81. Dhawan V, Nakamura T, Margouleff C, et al. Double-blind controlled trial of human embryonic dopaminergic tissue transplants in advanced Parkinson's disease: fluorodopa PET imaging. *Neurology* 1999;52:A405.
82. Ishikawa T, Dhawan V, Chaly T, et al. Fluorodopa positron emission tomography with an inhibitor of catechol-O-methyltransferase: effect of the plasma 3-O-methyldopa fraction on data analysis. *J Cereb Blood Flow Metab* 1996;16:854–863.
83. Leenders K, Salmon E, Tyrrell P, et al. The nigrostriatal dopaminergic system assessed *in vivo* by positron emission tomography in healthy volunteer subjects and patients with Parkinson's disease. *Arch Neurol* 1990;47:1290–1298.
84. Martin WR, Stoessl AJ, Adam MJ, et al. Positron emission tomography in Parkinson's disease: glucose and DOPA metabolism. *Adv Neurol* 1987;45:95–98.
85. Loizou LA. Uptake of monoamines into central neurones and the blood-brain barrier in the infant rat. *Br J Pharmacol* 1970;40:800–813.
86. Banos G, Daniel PM, Pratt OE. The effect of age upon the entry of some amino acids into the brain, and their incorporation into cerebral protein. *Dev Med Child Neurol* 1978;20:335–346.
87. Guttman M, Burns RS, Martin WR, et al. PET studies of parkinsonian patients treated with autologous adrenal implants. *Can J Neurol Sci* 1989;16:305–309.
88. Dusart I, Nothias F, Roudier F, et al. Vascularization of fetal cell suspension grafts in the excitotoxically lesioned adult rat thalamus. *Brain Res Dev Brain Res* 1989;48:215–228.
89. Kordower J, Freeman T, Snow B, et al. Neuropathological evidence of graft survival and striatal reinnervation after the transplantation of fetal mesencephalic tissue in a patient with Parkinson's disease. *N Engl J Med* 1995;332:1118–1124.
90. Folkerth RD, Durso R. Survival and proliferation of nonneural tissues, with obstruction of cerebral ventricles, in a parkinsonian patient treated with fetal allografts. *Neurology* 1996;46:1219–1225.
91. Deacon T, Schumacher J, Dinsmore J, et al. Histological evidence of fetal pig neural cell survival after transplantation into a patient with Parkinson's disease. *Nat Med* 1997;3:350–353.
92. Bjorklund A, Lindvall O. Transplanted nerve cells survive and are functional for many years. *Lakartidningen* 1999;96:3407–3412.
93. Madrazo I, Franco-Bourland R, Castrejon H, et al. Fetal striatal homotransplantation for Huntington's disease: first two case reports. *Neurol Res* 1995;17:312–315.
94. Kopyov O, Jacques S, Lieberman A, et al. Safety of intrastriatal neurotransplantation for Huntington's disease patients. *Exp Neurol* 1998;149:97–108.

PARKINSON'S DISEASE

Surgery for Parkinson's Disease and Movement Disorders,
edited by J.K. Krauss, J. Jankovic, and R.G. Grossman.
Lippincott Williams & Wilkins, Philadelphia © 2001.

8

ROLE OF SURGERY IN THE MANAGEMENT OF PARKINSON'S DISEASE

JOSÉ A. OBESO
JORGE GURIDI
M.C. RODRIGUEZ-OROZ
L. ALVAREZ
R. MACIAS

The role of surgery in the management of Parkinson's disease (PD) has had very variable appreciation in different periods. Opinions about its value have ranged from such extremely opposite views as to consider it "curative" or "ineffective." Present interest in the surgical treatment of PD mainly results from the development in the 1980s of a pathophysiologic model of the basal ganglia that accurately predicted the effect of focal lesioning in the parkinsonian state (1,2). Studies in monkeys treated with 1-methyl-4-phenyl-1,2,3,6-tetrahydropyridine (MPTP) showed that lesioning of the subthalamic nucleus (STN) led to marked motor improvement and finally served to prove the paramount role of the STN-glutamatergic projections in the pathophysiology of PD (3–5). Investigators recognized that increased neuronal activity in the STN drives neurons of the internal segment of the globus pallidus (GPi), which, in turn increases inhibition of the thalamocortical motor projections (2). These findings set the scene for a revitalization of pallidotomy and subsequently led to the application of deep brain stimulation (DBS) of the STN and GPi (6). The resurgence and development of ablative surgery and DBS for PD occurred in parallel with substantial efforts to restore striatal dopamine deficiency by grafting fetal tissue as well as other, more sophisticated procedures (Table 8.1). Both approaches are complementary and are not necessarily exclusive. None, however, can be considered curative at present. Thus, surgery for PD currently consists of treatment to reduce symptoms.

Why is surgery rapidly gaining an important role in the management of PD? There are two main reasons. First, long-term treatment of PD is associated with various problems that are not controlled with available pharmacologic tools. The main complications may be summarized as motor fluctuations, dyskinesias, psychiatric manifestations, levodopa-resistant motor features such as freezing of gait, postural and equilibrium problems, and swallowing difficulties. It is crucially important to realize that although some of these complications may be related to levodopa therapy, others depend more on the evolution of the disease process and its extension beyond the limits of the basal ganglia. The latter complications are much less amenable to improvement by surgery of any kind. The second reason for the revitalization of functional neurosurgery for PD is the improvement of stereotactic techniques, particularly thanks to the refinement of neuroimaging techniques (computed tomography and magnetic resonance imaging) and software programs that allow more precise and rapid performance of surgery.

Any surgical therapy poses a risk. The decision to operate is based on a careful consideration and assessment of all potential benefits and risks. Surgery for PD has been mainly applied to patients with advanced disease, and its main aim is alleviating a severe and highly disabling motor state. The risk in this patient population is, however, higher than in younger subjects with less advanced disease process. The desired evolution of surgery for PD should be to change from the treatment of symptoms to a curative approach. Similarly, the indication for surgery should shift in the future toward earlier intervention with the hope of modifying the natural history of the disease process. This is the ultimate goal of surgical treatment of PD. Whether or not this is achievable within a relatively short period cannot be answered at present. In this chapter, we mainly discuss the current indications

J. Obeso and M.C. Rodriguez-Oroz: Department of Neurology and Neurosurgery, Division of Neuroscience, Clinica Universitaria and Medical School. Pamplona, Spain.

J. Guridi: Service of Neurosurgery, Hospital de Navarra, Pamplona, Spain.

L. Alvarez and R. Macias: Centro Internacional de Restauración Neurologica, Havana, Cuba.

TABLE 8.1. SUMMARY OF SURGICAL TREATMENT OF PARKINSON'S DISEASE

Method	Status	Presumed Evolution
Ablative procedures		
Thalamotomy	Well established	Minimal indication
Pallidotomy	Growing experience	Limited application
Subthalamotomy	Pending clinical trials	Promising future
Deep brain stimulation		
Ventralis intermedius nucleus	Established efficacy for tremor	Limited application
Globus pallidus pars interna	Growing experience and evidence of efficacy	Moderate application
Subthalamic nucleus	Growing experience and evidence of efficacy	Best present choice
Grafting		
Adrenal	Negative therapeutic profile	Out of use
Fetal	Double-blind studies under way	Limited application
Glomus	Experimental	Unknown
Gene therapy	Experimental	Highly promising
Stem cells	Experimental	Potentially very promising

for and limitations of surgery for the treatment of PD. The following chapters discuss in detail the methodologic and clinically relevant issues. Therefore, we concentrate on the most practical, but nevertheless, difficult task of deciding what type of surgical procedure is best indicated for specific problems arising in the management of PD.

ABLATIVE SURGERY

Thalamotomy

Clinical Efficacy

Lesioning of the ventralis intermedius (VIM) nucleus of the thalamus has been performed in thousands of patients for several decades. It is now well established that *thalamotomy* has a marked effect against resting tremor in PD. Published studies report a variable degree of efficacy, ranging from about 45% to 92%, in tremor resolution after a unilateral lesion (7). The more recent application of neurophysiologic recording and microstimulation intraoperatively has given greater consistency to the antitremor effect of thalamotomy, reaching 90% of complete resolution and 5% to 10% of partial resolution (8). The antitremor effect of thalamotomy is long lasting. Thus, if there is no relapse of tremor in the first few months, the efficacy persists throughout the duration of the disease. Lesioning of the VIM has no effect against any other cardinal feature of PD, nor does it abolish levodopa-induced dyskinesia. Conversely, a more anteriorly placed lesion encroaching on the ventrolateral nuclei is associated with some degree (about 40%) of improvement of rigidity and may stop levodopa-induced dyskinesia (9), but it has less predictable antitremor efficacy.

Complications

The highest risk is the 1% to 3% reported frequency of intracranial bleeding associated with the stereotactic tech-

nique. More directly related to thalamotomy are hemiparesis and facial weakness, which have been reported in up to 50% in some series (7). Paresthesias and numbness are also common, but they are usually transitory. The rate of these complications is directly associated with the lesion procedure and varies enormously from team to team, depending on the method employed and experience. Bilateral thalamotomy is associated with a high frequency (up to 20%) of speech problems.

Role in Parkinson's Disease

Thalamotomy is performed much more rarely nowadays, for three main reasons:

1. It is only indicated for very asymmetric, severe, medically intractable tremor in patients with no other major parkinsonian features (10). Very few patients with longstanding PD have such clinical characteristics.
2. The growing tendency in the neurologic and neurosurgical community in general is to use DBS rather than lesioning procedures.
3. The antitremor efficacy of surgery of the STN or GPi is similar to that of thalamotomy, and STN or GPi procedures have many other advantages (see later).

Pallidotomy

Clinical Efficacy

Since its reintroduction in 1992, *unilateral pallidotomy* has been performed in a few thousand patients around the world. Many pilot, open-labeled studies have been published (10), and a few case-controlled trials have been conducted. There has been no double-blind assessment. The published material has a limited follow-up. Most studies report follow-up to 1 year, and few studies have documented follow-up at 2 years postoperatively (11–13).

The goal of pallidotomy is to reduce the excessive inhibitory output to the motor thalamus and brainstem target neurons by lesioning the sensorimotor region of the posteroventral pallidum. Theoretically, it is desirable not to interrupt the associative and limbic connections. Not every team undertaking pallidotomy has adopted this conceptual framework or has implemented the necessary electrophysiologic techniques to achieve such precise location of the lesion. As a result, the available clinical results may be difficult to analyze in complete fairness to the therapeutic possibilities of this approach in terms of both efficacy and side effects.

In general, it is accepted that pallidotomy conveys a dramatic improvement (90% to 100%) in levodopa-induced dyskinesias (10,14). This finding is the most consistent outcome of pallidotomy. The antiparkinsonian effect is also important but more variable. This may be summarized as follows:

1. Reduction of about 30% to 40% in the Unified Parkinson's Disease Rating Scale (UPDRS) in "off."
2. In general, no significant change in the "on" score of the UPDRS. Improvement in the Activities of Daily Life (ADL) scale in both "on" and "off."
3. Moderate to no improvement in fine manual tasks but substantial effect against tremor (50% to 60%) and rigidity (50% to 70%). Improvement in gait, freezing episodes, and axial signs is variable and less predictable (15).

The motor effects of pallidotomy are predominantly contralateral to the lesion. Analysis of patients 3 to 5 years postoperatively indicates that the main effects, that is, improvement of dyskinesias and rigidity, persist on the operated side, but gait and axial problems return and, along with emerging signs in the nonoperated side, become important sources of disability in many patients (16).

Bilateral pallidotomy has not been undertaken routinely in many patients because of the fear of severe side effects. Moderate to marked additional antiparkinsonian effects were reported after bilateral GPi lesions in a single operation (13, 17). However, the experience of other groups suggests that speech and swallowing problems are common and overshadow the clinical benefit (10,16).

Complications

Pallidotomy has been associated with a mean of 2% frequency of hemorrhages, but the frequency has ranged from 0% to 15% (10,16). This unexpected high frequency of bleeding in some groups was first attributed to the use of microrecording techniques. It is now clear that the incidence of hemorrhages, the major complication of stereotactic surgery, is not higher for groups who routinely record intraoperatively (18,19). The major factor seems to be experience. Thus, major complications fall with time, in keeping with the general assumption of the learning curve associated with any

new technique. The estimated mortality of pallidotomy is 0.3% (10).

Other than intracranial bleeding, the major complications associated with pallidotomy are visual field defect and facial weakness. The latter is very frequently transitory. The incidence of both complications has dropped dramatically in the last few years, probably related to optimization of the lesioning procedure. Worsening of cognitive function has been encountered in some patients, but overall cognitive impairment is minimal (20). In our experience, this outcome is determined by the patient's baseline cognitive status. In some patients with very severe motor complications, mild signs of dementia may be overlooked or minimized in the attempt to improve motor function. In such patients as well as in those who are more than 65 years old, pallidotomy may induce moderate to severe cognitive deficits (16).

Role in Parkinson's Disease

Unilateral pallidotomy is particularly indicated in young patients with unilateral, severe levodopa-induced dyskinesias, in whom reduction of dopaminergic drugs (to avoid dyskinesias) is associated with unbearable worsening of parkinsonian features. This is not a frequent clinical situation. We currently carry out pallidotomy in fewer than 10% of surgical candidates. In patients with bilateral disease, unilateral pallidotomy is not recommended except for practical reasons, such as to reduce the cost associated with DBS (see later). In such cases, patients should be aware of the limited and focal antiparkinsonian effect of pallidotomy.

Subthalamotomy

Clinical Efficacy

Experimental work undertaken in MPTP-treated monkeys (3–5) showed that *lesioning of the STN* with kainic or ibotenic acid remarkably alleviated parkinsonian features with few or no dyskinesias. Such impressive and well-documented results should have naturally led to lesioning the STN in patients with PD. However, the fear of inducing hemiballism delayed the use of this approach until recently. As a result, only a few preliminary reports are available. We first presented a report of the effect of unilateral subthalamotomy in five patients in 1997 (21). That initial experience was positive and indicated that lesioning of the STN in patients with PD was not necessarily associated with dyskinesias. Gill and Heywood also presented data confirming our findings (22). We have now studied 11 patients with unilateral subthalamotomy followed-up for up to 36 months (23) and seven patients with bilateral subthalamotomy (one-staged procedure) assessed during a 6-month period. We observed a dramatic improvement in motor function after unilateral subthalamotomy. In most patients, this effect was present immediately after completion of the lesioning procedure. The effect on the UPDRS motor and ADL scores was maintained during the follow-up period. Dyskinesias were not elicited by the lesion, except in one patient, who developed a large infarction several days postoperatively. Improvement was more striking contralateral to the lesion side and also against gait freezing (23). Patients with very severe "off" episodes need bilateral surgery. Our initial experience suggests that bilateral subthalamotomy provides a very significant reduction in "off" UPDRS scores and improved ADL scores (24).

Complications

The risks of the surgical procedure are similar to those described earlier for pallidotomy and thalamotomy. We have not encountered any cognitive or speech complication associated with the bilateral lesion. Transient dyskinesias are common but self-limiting.

Role in Parkinson's Disease

The experience is still limited and preliminary. It is not yet possible to indicate a given practical role in the surgical approach of PD. A prospective, randomized trial to compare bilateral subthalomotomy with DBS of the STN is needed.

DEEP BRAIN STIMULATION

The use of *DBS* for PD was introduced by Benabid and colleagues (25) in Grenoble and by Siegfried in Zürich in the late 1980s with the intention of providing an alternative to thalamotomy. In the last few years, the application of DBS has been extended to the GPi and STN. The exact mechanism of action of DBS in PD is not precisely defined. Benabid and colleagues suggested that DBS works by producing chronic neuronal depolarization (26), and therefore, it may mimic the effect of lesioning but in a reversible mode. However, other physiologic possibilities are under scrutiny.

Ventralis Intermedius

Clinical Efficacy

The antitremor effect of DBS in the VIM was firmly established by several clinical trials (27–30). Two studies included blinded assessments (29,30). The overall impression is that DBS of the VIM is associated with marked amelioration of resting tremor. More than 80% of patients have marked attenuation or abolition of tremor (10). Tolerance was documented by the Grenoble group in a few patients (less than 5%). Otherwise, maintained efficacy in the large group of

patients followed in Grenoble and by others in Europe is known to be present up to 10 years after implantation (28). As with thalamotomy, there is no effect against other cardinal features of PD.

Complications

Surgical complications are similar to those mentioned for thalamotomy. Specific complications related to the device are infection of the lead and the battery, erosion of the subcutaneous tissue around the cable, and seroma at the battery site. A common adverse effect is paresthesia when the stimulator is turned on. In most patients, this is transient and not limiting. However, when the location of the electrode is not precise enough, other side effects may be seen. These include dysarthria, tonic contraction of the contralateral limbs from corticospinal stimulation, ataxia and dysequilibrium, and persistent and unbearable paresthesia. As expected, all these adverse effects disappear when the stimulator is turned off or when the parameters are adjusted. Dysarthria is more frequent in patients with bilateral chronic thalamic DBS. Device and battery failure may occur in about 5% to 10% of patients. The life of the battery is 3 to 5 years, depending on the voltage and on whether the stimulator is stopped at night.

Role in Parkinson's Disease

The indications for DBS of the VIM are similar to those for thalamotomy. As mentioned earlier, however, the proportion of patients with monosymptomatic tremor is minimal. DBS is the technique of choice when considering bilateral thalamic surgery to allow better control of complications associated with bilateral procedures.

Globus Pallidus Internal Segment

A recent survey of the American Academy of Neurology encountered 64 patients who underwent DBS of the GPi (10). About half these patients had bilateral or unilateral implantations. This assessment found benefit in all aspects of PD and marked attenuation of motor fluctuations. A recent analysis of the effect of GPi DBS in 38 patients followed for 6 months in a multicenter study showed a significant reduction in the "off" UPDRS motor scores induced by stimulation, improvement in the ADL scale, and moderate reduction of levodopa-induced dyskinesias (31). This study included a double-blind assessment at 3 months for the stimulation condition, and it also revealed a very significant antiparkinsonian effect of DBS of the GPi. All studies concur in the need to continue or even slightly increase the patient's daily levodopa dose. As predicted from the experience with pallidotomy, patients treated with unilateral

DBS of the GPi showed a predominantly contralateral effect (10).

Complications

DBS of the GPi is associated with the general technical, device-related adverse effects described earlier for DBS of the VIM. Specific to the GPi are the possibilities of inducing dyskinesias with the most dorsal electrode and blocking the levodopa response with the ventral electrode (32,33). In our experience, these are not very frequent complications, but they may cause problems in the management of affected patients. Bilateral surgery in one session implies a prolonged procedure. In elderly patients, cognitive deficit may be observed after bilateral surgical procedures.

Role in Parkinson's Disease

The indications are very similar to those for pallidotomy, but DBS of GPi has the advantage of allowing bilateral surgery in one stage. Patients with severe, generalized dyskinesias are the best candidates. The drawback of DBS of the GPi is that it generally does not allow one to reduce the patient's daily levodopa requirements. At present, only limited information comparing bilateral DBS of the GPi and STN is available. Until data from a properly designed trial are obtained, team preferences and experience with either approach will guide the choice of procedure. In general, we are more impressed with STN surgery in terms of easiness of programming, efficacy, and levodopa dose reduction, but some of our best clinical results have been obtained in patients with DBS of the GPi.

Subthalamic Nucleus

Clinical Efficacy

Reports of clinical results with DBS of the STN are still limited. However, this approach has rapidly evolved to become the most frequently selected DBS procedure worldwide. A recently analyzed multicenter clinical trial included 96 patients during a 6-month follow-up period (31).

There was a marked and very significant reduction in the motor UPDRS score in the "off-drugs" state and a large improvement in the ADL scale. The "on" score was also reduced, a finding indicating a synergistic effect between medication and DBS. This results in better control of some features such as gait freezing and instability, which are typically poorly controlled with dopaminergic drugs. A double-blind assessment for the stimulation condition at 3 months also showed a very significant effect of DBS. The daily dose of levodopa was reduced by about 30%. Our more recent experience (n = 8) not only confirmed these results but actually surpassed them, particularly because excellent clinical control was achieved

with a drastic reduction (about 90%) of levodopa requirements. The Grenoble group has followed a number of patients for up to 5 years, with excellent therapeutic control.

Complications

Risks and side effects are similar to those mentioned for the GPi. Dyskinesias are easily induced when the electrode is correctly located in the sensorimotor region of the STN, but they subside later with the reduction in levodopa dose and further adjustment of the stimulation parameters.

Role in Parkinson's Disease

Although definitive conclusions cannot be reached because of the lack of clinical data, DBS of the STN seems the procedure of choice in the treatment of severe motor complications in PD. Almost unique to the STN is the possibility of improving motor features that are not adequately controlled with medication, gait problems in particular, and the capacity to reduce levodopa dependence. Overall, DBS of the STN provides a striking improvement in quality of life, and some patients regain almost normal motor capacity. From this point of view, STN DBS has a degree of efficacy not seen with other available therapeutic tools.

ABLATIVE SURGERY OR DEEP BRAIN STIMULATION: DECIDING WHAT SURGERY FOR WHICH PATIENTS

Ablative surgery and DBS are the two currently available techniques in clinical practice. Grafting is still an experimental approach limited to a few centers worldwide and therefore is not considered here. Its potential role in the management of PD is discussed in other chapters.

Targets

The observation that surgery of the STN and the GPi also has a profound antitremor effect has led to a substantial reduction in thalamic surgical procedures in the last few years. Choosing between the STN and the GPi cannot be based on data because there is no large prospective, controlled study comparing both targets. We do not find any major technical difference in the actual performance of either approach. Clinically, the only well-established difference is that surgery of the STN may allow a drastic reduction in daily requirements of levodopa, whereas surgery of the GPi does not. Theoretically, the STN has a larger capacity than the GPi to influence neuronal activity at different levels of the basal ganglia, thalamus, and brainstem (34), but whether this is clinically relevant has not been ascertained. Our clinical impression is that surgery of the STN is superior to procedures performed on other targets used presently.

Techniques

The clinical efficacy of lesioning or implanting of electrodes in the thalamus, GPi, and STN seems almost identical, but, again, few data formally demonstrate this point. The major advantage of DBS is when considering bilateral surgery to avoid the potentially high rate of complications associated with bilateral lesions. Conversely, DBS imposes the extra cost of the device and is enormously labor consuming. It is also more hazardous than lesioning with regard to the occurrence of infections and problems with the lead and battery. For patients who live far away from a referral medical center, the practicalities associated with DBS may be enormously cumbersome.

The notion of making an irreversible lesion in a patient with progressive, neurodegenerative disease is conceptually problematic. However, almost half a century's experience with thalamotomy and pallidotomy has not provided any hint of specific long-term complications or aggravation of the disease process in patients treated with ablative surgery of the basal ganglia or thalamus. In this regard, the position of DBS is theoretically advantageous because there is no lesion associated with it (see later). However, the lack of precise definition of the mechanism of action of DBS and the relatively short period of follow-up in most patients treated with this technique reduce the strength of the argument. In general, our view is to choose DBS when bilateral surgery is clearly needed and pallidotomy or subthalamotomy when unilateral surgery is indicated.

Candidates for Surgery

Several clinical situations lead one to consider surgery to alleviate PD.

1. *Patients with complicated PD.* The most obvious candidate for surgery is a patient with bilateral, severe parkinsonian signs in whom available pharmacologic tools do not provide sufficient control. Typically, such patients have severe dyskinesias when mobile ("on") and suffer unbearable immobility when "off." It must be clearly understood that surgery of the basal ganglia will rarely provide better quantitative benefit than the administration of a sufficiently high dose of levodopa or apomorphine. In other words, surgery and drugs provide a very similar antiparkinsonian benefit. The difference is that surgery may improve so dramatically the "off" state as to eradicate motor fluctuations, and it may thus allow patients to enjoy relatively constant and complete autonomy. In addition, dyskinesias are much improved. Thus, surgical treatment of the GPi or STN is the only currently available treatment for PD that can improve the motor state while dramatically reducing dyskinesias. In advanced PD, freezing of gait is a frequent complaint with a large impact on quality of life. Recent results with DBS or subthalamotomy of the STN indicate a very significant improvement of gait postoperatively (23,24,31). This effect has persisted for up to 4 years of follow-up in our personal experience. Patients with advanced PD may have also developed cognitive deficits or may have associated cerebrovascular disease. In such instances, the decision to operate must be carefully weighed against the risk of inducing further cognitive deterioration.

2. *Asymmetric but very severe PD with dyskinesias.* About 5% of patients undergoing surgical treatment have severe signs in one hemibody and have developed dyskinesias on that side. Usually, surgery provides relief of dyskinesias and reduces daily levodopa requirements. In this subgroup of patients, one must take into consideration, when deciding on the target and technique, that surgical treatment of the contralateral side will probably be required a few years later.

3. *Severe levodopa-resistant tremor.* A few patients have a severe resting tremor that may respond on a short-term basis to levodopa or apomorphine but that becomes impossible to control with drugs on a long-term basis. In such cases, particularly when the tremor is unilateral, surgical treatment is an excellent option to control the tremor and to reduce the exposure to large doses of dopaminergic drugs, otherwise not needed.

4. *Drug-induced side effects.* This is a very rare clinical situation. Young, frequently very active persons, do not tolerate levodopa and other antiparkinsonian drugs.

In summary, most patients requiring surgical treatment have advanced, generalized PD. Surgery is therefore bilateral, and the procedure of choice currently is DBS of the STN or GPi. The possibility of bilateral subthalamotomy as an alternative still requires further evaluation. For patients with asymmetric PD, pallidotomy seems the best approach. Subthalamotomy is a growing option but is limited to very few surgical teams.

TRANSPLANTS

Cell grafting to replace dopamine deficit and ideally to restore nigrostriatal physiology is theoretically a more fundamental approach to treat PD. However, practical, ethical, and technical aspects have enormously limited the development and application of grafting for PD. Of all possible methods (Table 8.1), only fetal mesencephalic grafting is currently used in patients. Adrenal medullary transplantation has been virtually abandoned because of its poor therapeutic risk-to-benefit risk ratio (10). Newer possibilities such as genetically modified cells to produce dopamine (35), neural progenitor cells (36), or glomus jugulare cells to release dopamine (37) are still within the laboratory framework.

The experience with *grafting of fetal tissue* in patients with PD is now relatively large (38,39). Embryonic cells have been shown to survive in the host striatum (40), to form synaptic connections (41), and partially to restore dopamine deficiency (42). Open-labeled studies have shown substantial motor improvement (38,39). However, a double blind-study resulted in less striking benefits (43). A subpopulation of patients, those with disease onset when they were less than 45 years old, did show significant improvement compared with the placebo-treated group. Another double-blind study currently undertaken in the United States (by Olanow and Freeman) is anxiously awaited, to judge more precisely the impact of fetal transplantation in PD. However, even if the outcome is positive, we do not foresee embryonic cell grafting as adequate for restoring dopamine deficiency in PD. This approach involves a highly complex organization of experts, it is tremendously time consuming and costly, and it depends entirely upon the legal status of each country. In addition, ethical considerations make it unlikely to become a routine therapeutic option.

SURGERY AND THE NATURAL HISTORY OF PARKINSON'S DISEASE: FUTURE TRENDS

Surgical treatment of symptoms (i.e., ablative and DBS procedures) benefit patients with PD. The main reason that so few patients (about 10% per year) undergo surgery is the risk it carries. As technical aspects improve, the morbidity and mortality will be greatly reduced. It will then be possible to conceive of early intervention as a means to reduce the progressive disability of PD, particularly in young-onset PD.

Both surgical procedures to relieve symptoms and striatal grafting have the potential for modifying the natural history of PD. However, some provisos have to be considered. First, surgery may provide sufficient control of PD to avoid or minimize the need for dopaminergic drugs for a very long period. From this point of view, surgical treatment would reduce the incidence of motor complications and side effects associated with long-term levodopa therapy. Conversely, a modification in the pathologic process leading to progressive loss of nigra cells could be induced surgically only if the *excitotoxicity hypothesis* (or another similar mechanism) is truly important in PD (44).

The postulated mechanism of excitotoxicity (45) is based on two main findings:

1. Dopamine deficiency leads to overactivity of the STN, which is known to use glutamate as neurotransmitter. The STN projects to the GP, the substantia nigra pars reticulata, and the pedunculopontine nucleus. There is also a glutamatergic innervation of the substantia nigra pars compacta (SNc). STN firing induces neuronal bursting activity in the SNc. The generation of bursting neuronal firing is associated with massive entrance of calcium intracellularly (46).

2. In PD, complex I mitochondrial activity specific of SNc neurons is reduced (47). This leads to a deficit in energy production and increases the vulnerability to glutamatergic stimulation (48). It is therefore conceivable that increased STN activity in the parkinsonian state could produce further neuronal damage in the SNc and other basal ganglia structures innervated by the STN. If this is the case, early intervention to inhibit the overactive STN could reduce the progression of PD. Similarly, physiologic restoration of dopaminergic activity by striatal grafting, or theoretically with long-acting dopaminergic drugs (49), could also stabilize STN activity and reduce excitotoxicity.

Finally, the putative neuroprotective effect of surgery has to be viewed in the general context of the process of neuronal degeneration in PD. One theoretic possibility is that neuronal loss in the SNc is indeed the primary event. Extension of the pathologic process to other brain regions could be mediated by the pathophysiologic changes induced by dopamine depletion. In such an instance, early intervention could indeed be neuroprotective. Another possibility, perhaps more likely, is that PD begins at the level of the SNc but neuronal vulnerability is actually increased at several levels of the nervous system. As a result, spreading of the pathologic process is not directly related to the pathophysiologic changes occurring at the level of the basal ganglia. In this situation, restoring dopamine deficiency or eliminating STN abnormal activity would control the cardinal features of PD, perhaps for longer than currently achieved with dopaminergic agents, but it would not reduce complications such as dementia, loss of postural control, or swallowing difficulties, which complicate the long-term evolution of PD.

CONCLUSIONS

Surgery is gaining an increased role in the management of motor complications in PD. The STN has become the preferred option as a target, and DBS is becoming the most widely used method. However, appropriate clinical trials to demonstrate the advantages of the STN over the GPi have not been conducted. Surgery of the thalamus has lost favor, particularly because its antitremor effect is also obtained with surgery of the STN, which has additional clinical benefits. In the near future, the risk of these surgical approaches will be further reduced as methodologic advances take place. It will then be possible to extend the indications for surgery to patients with less advanced states of the disease process. In the more distant future is the hope of fully restoring the integrity of the nigrostriatal system in an efficacious and permanent way and to halt the extension of the degeneration process by delivering neurotrophic factors and other substances. This would be as near as one could hope to a cure for PD.

ACKNOWLEDGMENT

Dr. Obeso is partially supported by the National Parkinson Foundation, Miami. Charlotte Smith and Anabel Perez prepared the article for publication.

REFERENCES

1. Albin RL, Young AB, Penney JB. The functional anatomy of basal ganglia disorders. *Trends Neurosci* 1989;12:366–375.
2. DeLong MR. Primate models of movement disorders of basal ganglia origin. *Trends Neurosci* 190;13;281–285.
3. Bergman H, Wichamann T, DeLong MR. Reversal of experimental parkinsonism by lesions of the subthalamic nucleus. *Science* 1990;249:1436–1438.
4. Aziz TZ, Peggs D, Sambrook MA, et al. Lesion of subthalamic nucleus for the alleviation of MPTP-induced parkinsonism in the primate. *Mov Disord* 1991;6:288–293.
5. Guridi J, Herrero MT, Luquin MR, et al. Subthalamotomy in parkinsonian monkeys: behavioral and biochemical analysis. *Brain* 1996;119:1717–1727.
6. Obeso JA, Guridi J, DeLong MR. Surgery for Parkinson's disease. *J Neurol Neurosurg Psychiatry* 1997;62:2–8.
7. Jankovic J, Cardoso F, Grossman RG, et al. Outcome after stereotactic thalamotomy for parkinsonian, essential and other types of tremor. *Neurosurgery* 1995;45:1743–1746.
8. Ohye C, Narabayashi H. Physiological study of presumed ventralis intermedius neurons in the human thalamus. *J Neurosurg* 1979;50:290–297.
9. Narabayashi H, Yokochi F, Nakajima Y. Levodopa-induced dyskinesia and thalamotomy. *J Neurol Neurosurg Psychiatry* 1984;47:831–839.
10. Hallett M, Litvan I, and the Task Force on Surgery for Parkinson's disease. Evaluation of surgery for Parkinson's disease. *Neurology* 1999;53:1910–1921.
11. Fazzini E, Dogali M, Sterio D, et al. Stereotactic pallidotomy for Parkinson's disease: a long-term follow-up of unilateral pallidotomy. *Neurology* 1997;48:1273–1277.
12. Lang AE, Lozano AM, Montgomery E, et al. Posteroventral medial pallidotomy in advanced Parkinson's disease. *N Engl J Med* 1997;337:1036–1042.
13. Lai EC, Jankovic J, Krauss JK, et al. Short- and long-term efficacy of microelectrode-guided, posteroventral, unilateral and bilateral pallidotomy in the treament of Parkinson's disease. *Neurology* 2000;24:1218–1222.
14. Jankovic J, Lai E, Ben-Arie L, et al. Levodopa-induced dyskinesias treated by pallidotomy. *J Neurol Sci* 1999;167:62–67.
15. Jankovic J, Lai EC, Ondo WG, et al. Effects of pallidotomy on gait and balance. In: Ruzicka E, Jankovic J, Hallett M, eds. *Gait disorders.* Philadelphia: Lippincott Williams & Wilkins, 2000.
16. Bronstein JM, DeSalles A, DeLong MR. Stereotactic pallidotomy in the treatment of Parkinson's disease: an expert opinion. *Arch Neurol* 1999;56:1064–1069.
17. Iacono R, Shima F, Lonser RR, et al. The results, indications and physiology of posteroventral pallidotomy for patients with Parkinson's disease. *Neurosurgery* 1995;36:1118–1127.
18. Lang AE, Lozano AM. Parkinson's disease: second of two parts. *N Engl J Med* 1998;339:1044–1053.
19. Baron MS, Vitek JL, Bakay RAE, et al. Treatment of advanced Parkinson's disease by posterior pallidotomy: one-year results of a pilot study. *Ann Neurol* 1996;40:355–366.
20. Rettig GM, Lai EC, Krauss JK, et al. Neuropsychological evaluation of patients with Parkinson's disease before and after pallidal surgery. In: Krauss JK, Grossman RG, Jankovic, eds. *Pallidal surgery for the treatment of Parkinson's disease and movement disorders.* Philadelphia: Lippincott–Raven, 1998:211–231.
21. Obeso JA, Alvarez L, Macias J, et al. Lesions of the subthalamic nucleus (STN) in Parkinson's disease (PD). *Neurology* 1997;48[Suppl 3]:138A.
22. Gill SS, Heywood P. Bilateral dorsolateral nucleotomy can be accomplished safely. *Mov Disord* 1998;13[Suppl 2]:201.
23. Alvarez L, Macias R, Guridi J, et al. Dorsolateral subthalamotomy for Parkinson's disease. *Mov Disord* 2001;16:72–78.
24. Alvarez L, Macias R., Rodriguez-Oroz MC, et al. Bilateral subthalamotory in Parkinson's disease. *Neurology* 2001;56:404.
25. Benabid AL, Pollak P, Louveau A, et al. Combined (thalamotomy and stimulation) stereotactic surgery of the Vim thalamic nucleus for bilateral Parkinson's disease. *Appl Neurophysiol* 1987;50:344–346.
26. Benabid AL, Pollak P, Gao DM, et al. Chronic electrical stimulation of the ventralis intermedius nucleus of the thalamus as a treatment of movement disorders. *J Neurosurg* 1996;84:203–214.
27. Benabid AL, Pollak P, Gervason C, et al. Long-term suppression of tremor by chronic stimulation of the ventral intermediate thalamic nucleus. *Lancet* 1991;337:403–406.
28. Alesch F, Pinter MM, Helscher RJ, et al. Stimulation of the ventral intermediate thalamic nucleus in tremor dominant Parkinson's disease and essential tremor. *Acta Neurochir* 1995;136:75–81.
29. Koller W, Pahwa R, Busenbark K, et al. High-frequency unilateral thalamic stimulation in the treatment of essential and parkinsonian tremor. *Ann Neurol* 1997;42:292–299.
30. Ondo W, Jankovic J, Schwartz K, et al. Unilateral thalamic deep brain stimulation for refractory essential tremor and Parkinson's disease tremor. *Neurology* 1998;51:1063–1069.
31. Obeso JA, Olanow WL, Rodriguez MC, et al. Bilateral deep brain stimulation of the subthalamic nucleus or globus pallidus pars interna in patients with advanced Parkinson's disease: a prospective trial with a double blind cross-over evaluation. *N Engl J Med,* in press.
32. Bejjani B, Damier P, Arnulf I, et al. Pallidal stimulation for Parkinson's disease: two targets?. *Neurology* 1997;49:1564–1569.
33. Krack P, Pollak P, Limousin P, et al. Opposite motor effects of pallidal stimulation in Parkinson's disease. *Ann Neurol* 1998;43:180–192.
34. Obeso JA, Rodriguez MC, DeLong MR. Basal ganglia pathophysiology: a critical review. *Adv Neurol* 1997;74:3–18.
35. Gage FH, Kawafa MD, Fischer LJ. Genetically modified cells: applications for intracerebral grafting. *Trends Neurosci* 1991;14:328–333.
36. Gage FH. Survival and different of adult neuronal progenitor cells transplanted to the adult brain. *Proc Natl Acad Sci USA* 1995;92:11879–1883.
37. Luquin MR, Montoro RJ, Guillen J, et al. Recovery of chronic parkinsonian monkeys by autotransplants of carotid body cell aggregates into putamen. *Neuron* 1999;22:743–750.
38. Olanow CW, Freeman TB, Kordower JH. Neural transplantation as a therapy for Parkinson's disease. *Adv Neurol* 1997;74:249–270.
39. Lindvall O, Odin P. Clinical application of cell transplantation and neurotrophic factors in CNS disorders. *Curr Opin Neurobiol* 1994;4:752–757.
40. Lindvall O, Sawle G, Widner H, et al. Evidence for long-term survival and function of dopaminergic grafts in progressive Parkinson's disease. *Ann Neurol* 1994;35:172–180.
41. Kordower JH, Freeman TB, Snow BJ, et al. Neuropathological evidence of graft survival and striatal reinnervation after the transplantation of fetal mesencephalic tissue in a patient with Parkinson's disease. *N Engl J Med* 1995;332:1118–1124.

42. Remy P, Samson Y, Hantraye P, et al. Clinical correlates of (18-F) fluorodopa uptake in five grafted parkinsonian patients. *Ann Neurol* 1995;38:580–588.
43. Freed CR, Greene PE, Brueze RE, et al. Trasportation of embryonic dopamine neurons for severe Parkinson's disease. *N Engl J Med* 2001;344:710–719.
44. Albin RL, Greenmayre JT. Alternative excitotoxic hypotheses. *Neurology* 1992;42:733–738.
45. Rodriguez MC, Obeso JA, Olanow CW. Subthalamic nucleus-mediated excitotoxicity in Parkinson's disease: a target for neuroprotection. *Ann Neurol* 1998;44[Suppl 1]:175–188.
46. Michaels RL, Rothman SM. Glutamate neurotoxicity *in vitro,* antagonist pharmacology and intracellular calcium concentrations. *J Neurosci* 1990;10:283–292.
47. Schapira AHV, Cooper JM, Dexter D, et al. Mitochondrial complex deficiency in Parkinson's disease. *J Neurochem* 1990,54:823–827.
48. White RJ, Reynolds IJ. Mitochondrial depolarization in glutamate-stimulated neurons: an early signal to excitotoxin exposure. *J Neurosci* 1996;16:5688–5697.
49. Olanow CW, Obeso JA. Preventing dyskinesias in Parkinson's disease. *Ann Neurol* 2000;47:167–178.

Surgery for Parkinson's Disease and Movement Disorders,
edited by J.K. Krauss, J. Jankovic, and R.G. Grossman.
Lippincott Williams & Wilkins, Philadelphia © 2001.

9

THALAMOTOMY FOR TREATMENT OF PARKINSON'S DISEASE TREMOR

KNUT WESTER

Introduced in the late 1940s, *stereotactic ablative surgery* is the oldest neurosurgical procedure still offered to patients with Parkinson's disease. After Spiegel and Wycis performed their first operation ("stereoencephalotomy") in 1947 (1), interest in these operations increased over the next two decades, because they proved to be the only effective treatment one could offer patients with Parkinson's disease. *Thalamotomy,* as we know it today, was first introduced in 1952 (2), and for many years it remained the mainstay of neurosurgical treatment. When levodopa was introduced in the late 1960s, interest in thalamotomy declined dramatically throughout the world. However, as it gradually became evident that drugs did not alleviate all symptoms, the operation emerged again as a potent *symptomatic* treatment for drug-resistant parkinsonian symptoms in the 1970s, especially for tremor and rigidity (3–8). Readers with an interest in the history of functional stereotactic neurosurgery are referred to the reviews by Krauss and Grossman (9) and by Speelman and Bosch (10).

I am in the awkward position of not knowing whether the results of my intellectual exercise are of interest to anyone but medical historians. Having gloriously defended its role almost since neurosurgery's childhood, it may well be that thalamotomy now envisions its final defeat. When this chapter is read, the procedure may already have become obsolete, because deep brain stimulation appears to have taken over the field rapidly and completely. However, it is my *belief* that thalamotomy once again will prove its existence, but probably only in a few, selected patients.

There are elements of craftsmanship in every neurosurgical procedure. This is perhaps especially true for thalamotomy. For example, the target coordinates have, in many departments and also among departments, been passed on from master to apprentice through "generations" of neurosurgeons, without necessarily being evidence based when first chosen. Thus, it may remain obscure to the younger generation why they are taught a specific set of coordinates, but

no one questions them; these coordinates are not changed, because they apparently work well, although they may be different from those employed elsewhere (11). Similarly, numerous tricks of the trade are learned in a similar fashion, as part of a neurosurgical "subculture" not published in any article or textbook. The present chapter is therefore based not only on available scientific contributions, but also on personal, practical experience collected during more than 250 thalamotomy procedures, most of them in patients with Parkinson's disease.

INDICATIONS

Thalamotomy is not a cure for Parkinson's disease, but it is a treatment for the *symptoms* of the disease. The paradoxic aim of the procedure is to destroy presumably normal brain tissue in patients already suffering from substantial local and general loss of nerve cells. Consequently, only patients with disabling symptoms that are not alleviated by medication, or in whom effective medication is not tolerated, should be subjected to such ablative surgery. Only few patients are potential candidates for thalamic ablative neurosurgery.

Distal tremor, above all, hand and finger tremor, is generally regarded as the symptom most easily alleviated by thalamotomy, followed by rigidity, whereas bradykinesia responds poorly to the procedure (4,12). My personal experience, however, is that tremor *and* rigidity are equally well alleviated by thalamotomy. As discussed later, variations in target location and size may explain this discrepancy. Our lesions are oriented as a sheet parallel to and close to the internal capsule, with a considerable anteroposterior extension. The most anterior portion of our lesions extends into the ventrooralis posterior and ventrooralis anterior nuclei, where some investigators have found a better effect on rigidity (13,14). It is a common clinical experience that proximal and midline symptoms, such as head or neck tremor, are more resistant to the procedure than distal tremor and therefore may require a larger lesion, if the condition is alleviated at all. This correlates well with the anatomic observation that the proximal

K. Wester: Department of Neurosurgery, Haukeland University Hospital, N 5021 Bergen, Norway.

muscles' representation in the primate thalamus is weaker and more dispersed than that of the distal muscles (15).

Occasionally (1% to 2% of our patients), a patient with parkinsonism may have isolated limb pain as the most disabling symptom. We have successfully treated these patients with thalamotomies.

Because older age, surgery in the speech-dominant (usually left) hemisphere, and bilateral surgery predispose for complications (see later), the ideal patient for thalamotomy has traditionally been a young person with hand or finger tremor in the nondominant side as the main symptom.

TARGET: LOCATION AND LESION SIZE

Location

Many attempts have been made to provide theoretic explanations of the effects of thalamotomy, and many circuitry diagrams have been constructed through the years (16,17).

Targets for thalamotomy are usually located in the ventrolateral thalamic nuclear complex, the so-called "motor" thalamus. The exact location within that complex is probably not absolutely critical, because Laitinen found in his survey that the targets varied considerably from one department to another (11), presumably with equally good results. However, lesions involving the ventralis intermedius area appear especially effective in abolishing tremor (14, 18,19).

Direct visualization of the target nucleus with magnetic resonance imaging (MRI) is still suboptimal. Most departments therefore use the indirect method based on identification of internal landmarks, such as the anterior commissure (AC) and the posterior commissure (PC). An informal survey in connection with this chapter showed that computed tomography, MRI, and even ventriculography all are used for image-guided stereotactic target localization. Target coordinates are usually given as distances in relation to the intercommissural line between the AC and the PC.

When evaluating results and complications, one should bear in mind that they may vary from one department to another, depending on the exact location and spatial orientation of the target as well as the lesion size. Because some of our studies on cognition in patients who underwent thalamotomy are referred to later in this chapter, I include the target coordinates here: 2 mm behind the midcommissural plane, 2 to 3 mm above the intercommissural line, and 14 mm lateral from the midsagittal plane. The lesions were made with two electrodes (2-mm tips), 6 mm apart, oriented parallel to the internal capsule (Fig. 9.1), thus affecting the following nuclei: the ventrooralis anterior and posterior, the ventralis intermedius, and probably also the reticular nucleus (Fig. 9.2) (20).

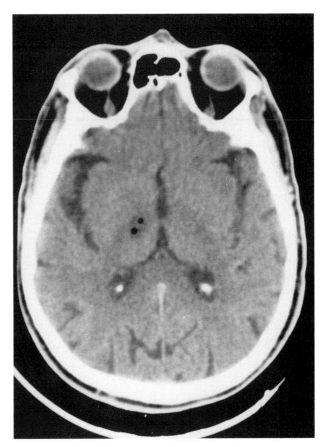

FIGURE 9.1. Postoperative computed tomography scan showing the lesion a few minutes after a right thalamotomy made with an original, standard Leksell generator. The two electrode trajectories can be seen as *black dots,* still filled with air that was forced down the hollow shafts by the thermosensors acting as pistons. Note the orientation of the electrodes close to and parallel to the internal capsule (see text).

As discussed in Chapter 5 and elsewhere (21), physiologic confirmation is of great help, not to say mandatory, in determining the final focus of the lesion. My colleagues and I have used low macrostimulation threshold intensities and a "microthalamotomy" effect caused by the mechanical insertion of the electrode (Fig. 9.3) as good prognostic indicators (22). Others use microelectrode recordings, and they have found that lesions should be placed very close to thalamic "tremor cells" (23).

Sometimes, the microthalamotomy effect poses a problem during the operation. It may temporarily abolish the tremor for the rest of the day and may make it impossible to use disappearance of tremor as an indicator of when to stop building up the lesion. In those cases, we take the microthalamotomy effect as an indication of optimal electrode placement and make a standard-sized lesion there in the usual staged manner, while watching carefully for unwanted side effects.

After the patient's skull is opened, an increasing distance between the dura and the cortical surface can be observed

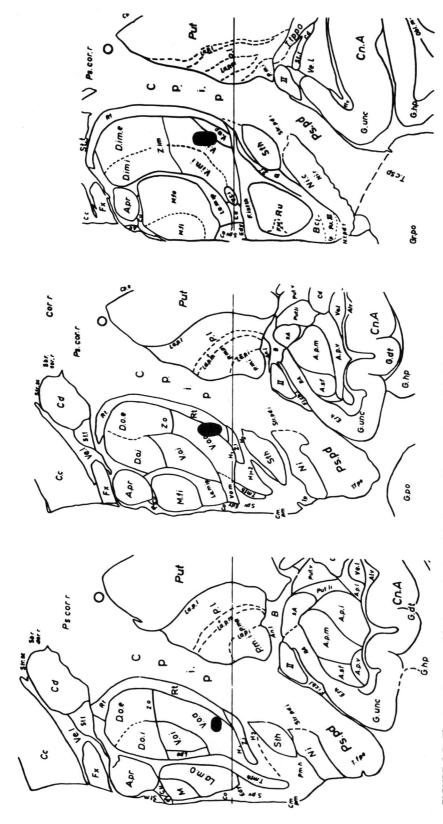

FIGURE 9.2. The target area and lesion center I used in Bergan, Norway, drawn (*black*) on three coronal sections from the Schaltenbrand and Wahren atlas. The nuclear subdivisions affected are the anterior and posterior ventrooralis nuclei (Voa and Vop), the ventralis intermedius nucleus (Vim), and the reticular (Rt) nucleus. To the **left**, the most anterior portion of the lesion; to the **right**, the most posterior portion. (Coronal sections from Schaltenbrand G, Wahren W. *Atlas for stereotaxy of the human brain*. Stuttgart: Thieme, 1977, with permission.)

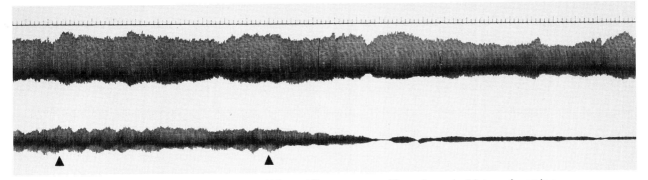

FIGURE 9.3. Polygraph recording of bilateral finger tremor with mechanoelectric transducers in a patient with Parkinson's disease. A "microthalamotomy" effect with marked reduction of tremor in the left index finger **(lower trace)** can be seen after insertion of the electrodes from the cortical surface *(left arrowhead)* into the target in the right thalamus *(right arrowhead)*. The gain in the lower trace is reduced fivefold because of the higher amplitude of the left-sided tremor compared with the right-sided tremor **(upper trace)**. **Far upper trace:** time (in seconds).

as the operation proceeds. Not only does the surface of the brain sink, but we have found that the thalamic target also sinks, approximately half the distance of the surface (unpublished observations). This observation has implications for the accuracy of the target localization: if the patient is operated on while in the supine position, the brain will move backward in the skull because of gravity (and relative to the stereotactic frame), and the electrode will inevitably miss the precalculated target and will end up in a more anterior position than intended. We have taken the consequences of this observation and operate all our patients while they are in the *sitting position.* If or when the brain sinks, one can always catch up with the sinking target simply by advancing the electrode another few millimeters vertically along the same trajectory.

Lesion Size

Figure 9.4 shows two typical thalamotomy lesions of different size in the acute and chronic stages. The final lesion size is usually the result of a staged procedure, during which the lesion is successively built up until the desired clinical effect is achieved. For each stage, the temperature and heating time are increased in a controlled fashion, first with the electrodes in one position, and, if necessary, the sequence is repeated with a new lesion center a few millimeters away. In my experience as well as that of others (6,23–25), relatively small, properly located lesions with calculated volumes of 50 to 70 mm^3, or even smaller, are sufficient to obtain good tremor control. It is also my experience that the lesions required to alleviate movement disorders other than Parkinson's disease are generally larger, except for essential tremor.

An excellent effect in the operating room does not necessarily guarantee long-term success. Neural elements in the lesion center are destroyed by the heat, whereas those in the periphery may only be temporarily impaired by nonlethal heat or the edema surrounding the lesion (Figs. 9.1 and

9.4). I therefore routinely carry the lesion a little beyond the point of tremor control and aim at slight temporary contralateral motor deficits in the acute stage, such as a facial hemiweakness revealed in the patient's spontaneous smile, or very brief periods (lasting fractions of a second) of tonus loss in an extended, elevated arm.

THALAMOTOMY BY STEREOTACTICALLY FOCUSED IRRADIATION

The issue of functional radiosurgery (26) is covered more extensively in Chapter 22. Leksell used the gamma knife for thalamotomy in a few patients with tremor between 1968 and 1970 (27). This technique was revived in the 1990s (28), and several centers published their experiences with thalamotomy or pallidotomy lesions produced by stereotactically focused irradiation (29–38). The number of reported patients is still low; only two publications (8,37) reported on more than ten thalamotomies in Parkinson's disease, with results that compare favorably (38) or less favorably (37) with reports on open thalamotomy procedures. The general impression one has from reading these reports is that gamma thalamotomy so far seems less effective, and one may encounter late complications (34,36). Stereotactic radiosurgery clearly has the advantage of saving the patient from the risks associated with an open stereotactic procedure. Conversely, the procedure allows the neurosurgeon no possibility to collect the physiologic feedback from the patient that is so important during an open, conventional procedure, information that may tell the surgeon that the electrode is in the right (or wrong) spot and when the lesion is large enough. During an open procedure, one may record thalamic cell activity, which has been shown to correlate well with good results (23), or one may stimulate the target area in the final search for an optimal location. In the latter case, one often experiences that the

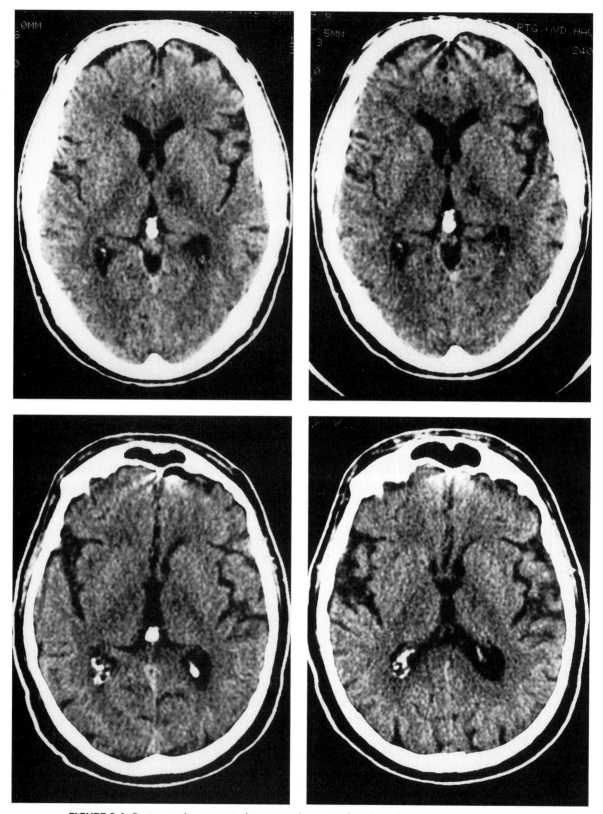

FIGURE 9.4. Postoperative computed tomography scans of a relatively large thalamotomy lesion **(upper)** and a small lesion **(lower)**, in the left thalamus, close to the internal capsule. Both lesions relieved tremor permanently. **Left:** Second postoperative day. **Right:** After 3 months.

effect on the tremor is better some distance away from the calculated target or that some unwanted side effects appear during the stimulation, observations that can be used to find a more optimal center of the lesion. In our department, we have the option of using the gamma knife for thalamotomy procedures, but we have declined to do so, because we find the intraoperative physiologic and clinical observations to be crucial in the final selection of location and extension of the lesion.

At present, gamma knife thalamotomy appears to be an attractive procedure for the few patients who are unsuited for open surgical treatment. In the future, imaging techniques could be envisioned that render a *closed* physiologic target confirmation possible and thus might enhance the efficacy and safety of functional stereotactic radiosurgery.

RESULTS AND COMPLICATIONS

Two aspects must be kept in mind when evaluating the results of thalamotomy for Parkinson's disease: (a) results cannot be transferred automatically from one department to another, because the location and size of the lesion may vary, and (b) eliminating the tremor does not necessarily improve the patient's quality of life. If a patient is no longer able to walk after thalamotomy, because the procedure also produced a loss of equilibrium or reduced contralateral muscle tonus, the patient is probably left in a worse situation postoperatively, even if the tremor is completely relieved. Moreover, the beneficial effects of thalamotomy are achieved by destroying normal brain tissue, and the entire operation is a balancing act between doing just enough and doing too much.

Results on Tremor

Moderate to complete tremor relief has consistently been reported to occur in 80% to 100% of patients since the revival of the procedure in the postlevodopa era (3,6,13,39,40). Patients often complain that the tremor ipsilateral to the site of the operation has increased after thalamotomy. This is probably an illusion that occurs when the patient becomes more aware of this tremor when the contralateral tremor, which was previously more pronounced, has disappeared. Jankovic et al. could not find any significant postoperative increase of the ipsilateral tremor (40).

Is tremor relief lifelong? This is certainly my general impression, supported by the findings of Diederich et al. (39), who, in a blinded evaluation, found good tremor relief in all patients after a mean follow-up period of 10.9 years. Conversely, Kelly and Gillingham found a considerable reduction of tremor relief, down from 90% after 2 years to 57% after 10 years (41).

Results on Quality of Life

Although this factor is a prerequisite for a good result, there is more to quality of life than just tremor relief. With tremor as the only recorded parameter, patients who undergo thalamotomy are either improved or unchanged, not worse. An appropriate evaluation of the procedure must therefore also include an assessment of a patient's total function, taking into account other factors than tremor relief. Very few recent studies have accomplished this goal (8,40).

Unwanted side effects are not at all uncommon as a consequence of thalamotomy procedures (see later). These range from temporary or permanent slight neurologic deficits, regarded as trivial by the patient, to the most severe complications, causing permanent invalid status. Thus, it is only natural that the success rate in terms of quality of life is slightly less impressive than when tremor relief is regarded exclusively, that is, about 80% (8,40). A moderate reduction of levodopa medication has been reported after thalamotomy (6,8,40), and this alone is perhaps a gain for the patient.

One of my own patients may serve as an example of how difficult it may be to evaluate the result of an operation. This woman underwent bilateral thalamotomies, 1 year apart. During and immediately after the second procedure, she suffered permanent dysarthria so severe that her speech was absolutely incomprehensible. We regarded this complication as the worst occurring in any of our patients, but this patient was of a different opinion. She was satisfied with the result, because she was no longer forced into social isolation by a disabling tremor. After the operation, she moved freely about without people staring at her, her handwriting became clear and legible, and her family somehow learned to understand her dysarthric speech.

Complications

Thalamotomy is a functional procedure that aims at improving the patient's life, but not curing the disease itself. The tolerance for disabling complications is therefore lower than for most other neurosurgical procedures.

We have reason to believe that refined recording, stimulation, and lesioning techniques have reduced complication rates and have enhanced the safety of the thalamotomy procedure. The absence in recent reports of the hyperkinetic complications of the earlier days, such as hemiballism, is only one indication of this altered complication situation. Because most of the reports dealing with complications are old, often published 20 to 30, or even 40 years ago, it is difficult to give an updated account of the complication rates (12). Few reports from the 1990s deal with complications of open thalamotomy. In our patients with Parkinson's disease (8), we found that three of 33 unilateral thalamotomies caused additional permanent disability (mental changes and speech disturbance), but in only one patient were these complications so severe that he was classified as worse postoperatively. Jankovic et al. observed a 58% rate of transient neurologic changes, but none of these resulted in increased disability (40). Conversely, more than 20% of their patients experienced "persistent complications," or "unwanted side effects" (see later).

Two categories of complications may be seen after a thalamotomy: (a) those infrequent complications (intracranial hematomas and infections) that may occur in any stereotactic operation and that are not specific for thalamotomies; and (b) those that are a direct consequence of the deliberate destruction of normal brain tissue in, or close to, the target area. The latter category constitutes the majority of complications.

The mortality after unilateral thalamotomy for Parkinson's disease is low, probably less than 1% (42); our department had no deaths in 195 consecutive patients. The mortality is probably higher in bilateral procedures, but again, most of the relevant information is from before the levodopa era (12).

As previously discussed, most thalamotomy complications are functional deficits that stem from the destruction of normal brain tissue during the procedure. Older age, surgery in the speech-dominant hemisphere, bilateral procedures, preexisting mental deterioration, and pronounced cerebral atrophy are the most common risk factors predisposing for these complications. Most of the deficits seen after thalamotomy are mild and hardly deserve the designation "complication." They do not result in any increased total disability, especially not when balanced against the beneficial effects on tremor; "unwanted side effect" is perhaps a better designation. There are gradual transitions, however, between these minor side effects and disabling complications.

Speech disturbances may occur as dysarthria or dysphasia, the latter infrequently and only after surgery in the speech-dominant hemisphere (8). Dysarthria appears to be a larger problem, especially in patients who already have a soft voice preoperatively, or in patients undergoing bilateral procedures (41).

Postoperative mental deterioration is more frequent in the elderly, in patients who already suffer from mental deterioration, and in patients with pronounced cerebral atrophy. Hauglie-Hanssen and I observed mental deterioration in three of our 33 patients, all elderly and operated on in the left hemisphere. In only one patient was this deterioration pronounced (8). Again, bilateral procedures carry a much greater risk, particularly if thalamotomy is combined with pallidotomy on the other side. The risk in bilateral thalamotomies has been reported to be 34.8%, and in the combined bilateral procedure it is 60.7% (43).

Hemiparesis may occur if the lesion encroaches on the internal capsule, which is situated only a few millimeters more laterally. With the small lesions of today and physio-logic confirmation of the target, this is probably an uncommon complication. We found no persistent paresis in our 33 patients (8), and neither did Jankovic et al. in their 42 patients (40).

According to Tasker (12), disabling hypotonia, either alone or in combination with dystonic inversion of the foot, occurs in 2% to 5% of patients, even if the lesion is properly sized and located.

Complication Avoidance

The main prerequisite for avoiding thalamotomy complications is to acknowledge their existence, and not to cease to be afraid that they will occur, during the next increase of the present lesion or during the next operation. Second, the thalamotomy procedure must include routines for detecting minor functional deficits before they manifest themselves as disabling complications. Such routines include a stepwise building up of the lesion until symptom relief is achieved, with a thorough examination of the patient during and between each extension of the lesion. To detect such deficits, my patients sit with elevated arms during the lesioning, they carry out rapid hand and finger movements (to detect beginning paresis), they count (for dysarthria), they answer questions (for impressive dysphasia), and my colleagues and I also test their memory functions. Foot dystonia is not so easily detected in the operating room, because this complication becomes apparent only after the patient has resumed walking.

THALAMOTOMY AND COGNITION

Impaired cognition, particularly memory impairment, is common in patients with Parkinson's disease (44–46). Preexisting deficits render these patients particularly susceptible to additional cognitive impairment after a thalamotomy lesion. The relay function of the thalamus in different neuronal networks involves areas such as sensation, language, attention, and memory. Any of these functions may therefore be affected by thalamotomy. Earlier studies showed adverse effects of thalamotomy on cognition (47–50), but these investigations may not be relevant any longer, because the lesions of today in general are smaller and are placed with better physiologic control. My colleagues and I investigated several cognitive functions in 53 consecutive patients with clinically successful thalamotomies before and after surgery: verbal memory, visuospatial functions, spatial perception and memory, executive function, attention shift, and set formation and maintenance. Preoperatively, they had, as expected, impaired cognition compared with healthy age-matched controls, but their cognitive capacity was not further reduced by the operation (51).

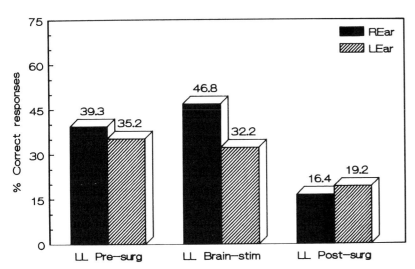

FIGURE 9.5. Performance in a dichotic listening task for parkinsonian patients, measured as percentages of correct responses. In this task, *different* acoustic stimuli (syllables) are simultaneously presented to the patient's two ears. The patient is asked to repeat the sounds that are perceived. Preoperatively, a slight (normal) superiority of the right ear was found **(left pair of columns)**. During stimulation of the left thalamus **(middle)**, this superiority of the right ear was significantly enhanced, indicating an increased attention toward the contralateral ear. Immediately after the thalamotomy **(right)**, the overall performance was impaired, and the normal right ear superiority disappeared, but both were restored in a test 3 months later. A similar effect could not be demonstrated for stimulation and lesions of the right thalamus. Results from Hugdahl K, Wester K, Asbjørnsen A. The role of the left and the right thalamus in language asymmetry: dichotic listening in Parkinson patients undergoing stereotactic thalamotomy. *Brain Lang* 1990;39:1–13. (From Academic Press, with permission.)

In another study (52), we demonstrated that stimulation of the left thalamus may enhance the attention toward the contralateral ear in an acoustic perception test, with a subsequent reduction after thalamotomy (Fig. 9.5). These findings indicate that thalamotomy may result in reduced attention or awareness toward the contralateral side of the body postoperatively (53).

ADVANTAGES AND DISADVANTAGES OF THALAMOTOMY VERSUS DEEP BRAIN STIMULATION

When comparing thalamotomy and deep brain stimulation, it is clear that both have advantages and disadvantages. Their capacity for relieving tremor is probably not significantly different (54,55). In thalamotomy's favor is simplicity. Once it is performed successfully, there is no need for the patient to come back for several adjustments of the pacemaker and replacement of the batteries. Deep brain stimulation, conversely, carries a smaller risk of the severe complications associated with destruction of normal brain tissue, but it is more expensive and time consuming, and the implanted equipment ties the patient very strongly to the treating physician. In our experience, this means that the patient has to return with an estimated frequency of once per year for the rest of his or her life. Even with a moderate practice, one will therefore build up a considerable pool of patients in a few years, and they will regularly require assistance. This has to be taken into account for future planning, because it requires additional capacity in the operating room and staffing. Finally, there are social, economic, and medicolegal aspects to discuss, such as who should pay for the expensive pacemaker equipment and how long it will be possible to con-

tinue with a procedure (thalamotomy) that carries a potential risk of severe complications when there are less risky procedures available, although they are more expensive and time consuming.

WHAT HAPPENS TO THE VENTRALIS INTERMEDIUS THALAMOTOMY FOR PARKINSON'S DISEASE?

The increasing popularity of deep brain stimulation makes it tempting to rephrase Tasker et al.'s title from 1983 (3). For this chapter, a survey on the practice from 1990 to 1998 was performed among 13 centers in Europe, Japan, and North America (Table 9.1). The findings were surprising. When one compares the first part of the 1990s with the second, there was a slight decline in thalamotomies, but the total number of lesioning procedures increased, mainly because of the growing popularity of pallidotomies. Looking at both lesioning and deep brain stimulation; there was a marked overall increase during the 1990s, a finding indicating that DBS has gained *in addition to,* and not instead of, lesioning procedures. There was sharp decline of both pallidotomies and thalamotomies in 1998 which may continue for the next few years. It is my *belief* that deep brain stimulation in the future will take over many of the indications for movement disorders surgery, but thalamotomy will still be a good treatment in selected patients.

ACKNOWLEDGMENT

Part of my research presented in this chapter was supported by the Norwegian Research Council.

TABLE 9.1 SURVEY ON FUNCTIONAL STEREOTACTIC SURGERY FOR MOVEMENT DISORDERS FROM 13 INTERNATIONAL CENTERS, 1990–1998 (GRAZ, AUSTRIA; TORONTO, CANADA; OULU, FINLAND; AMSTERDAM, NETHERLANDS; GUMMA, JAPAN; BERGEN AND OSLO, NORWAY; LUND AND UMEA, SWEDEN; BAYLOR COLLEGE OF MEDICINE-HOUSTON, EMORY-ATLANTA, JOHN HOPKINS BALTIMORE, MAYO CLINIC-ROCHESTER, USA)

| Year | Lesions | | Lesions Total | Deep Brain Stimulation | | | DBS Total |
	Thalamotomies	Pallidotomies		Unilateral Thalamus	Bilateral Thalamus	Pallidum	
1990	113	3	116	—	—	—	—
1991	126	—	126	—	—	—	—
1992	130	25	155	—	—	—	—
1993	180	83	263	13	2	—	15
1994	116	137	253	33	4	—	37
1995	107	208	315	43	11	2	56
1996	103	192	295	54	13	8	75
1997	120	232	352	134	21	16	171
1998	105	170	275	138	32	23	193

REFERENCES

1. Spiegel EA, Wycis HT. *Stereoencephalotomy (thalamotomy and related procedures). Part I. Methods and stereotaxic atlas of the human brain.* NewYork: Grune & Stratton, 1952:1–176.
2. Hassler R, Riechert T. Indikationen und Lokalisationsmethode der gezielten Hirnoperationen. *Nervenarzt* 1954;25:441–447.
3. Tasker RR, Siqueira J, Hawrylyshyn P, et al. What happened to VIM thalamotomy for Parkinson's disease? *Appl Neurophysiol* 1983;46:68–83.
4. Gildenberg PL. The present role of stereotactic surgery in the management of Parkinson's disease. *Adv Neurol* 1984;40:447–452.
5. van Manen J, Speelman JD, Tans RJJ. Indications for surgical treatment of Parkinson's disease after levodopa therapy. *Clin Neurol Neurosurg* 1984;86:207–212.
6. Nagaseki Y, Shibazaki T, Hirai T, et al. Long-term follow-up of selective VIM-thalamotomy. *J Neurosurg* 1986;65:296–302.
7. Broggi G, Giorgi C, Servello D. Stereotactic neurosurgery in the treatment of tremor. *Acta Neurochir Suppl (Wien)* 1987;39:73–76.
8. Wester K, Hauglie-Hanssen E. Stereotaxic thalamotomy: experiences from the levodopa era. *J Neurol Neurosurg Psychiatry* 1990;53:427–430.
9. Krauss JK, Grossman RG. Historical Review of pallidal surgery for treatment of Parkinsonises and other movement disorders. In: Krauss JK, Grossman RG, Jankovic J, eds. *Pallidal surgery for the treatment of Parkinson's disease and movement disorders.* Philadelphia: Lippincott-Raven, 1998:1–23.
10. Speelman JD, Bosch DA. Resurgence of functional neurosurgery for Parkinson's disease: a historical perspective. *Mov Disord* 1998;13:582–588.
11. Laitinen LV. Brain targets in surgery for Parkinson's disease: results of a survey of neurosurgeons. *J Neurosurg* 1985;62:349-351.
12. Tasker RR. Movement disorders. In: Apuzzo MLJ, ed. *Brain surgery: complications avoidance and management,* vol 2. New York: Churchill Livingstone, 1993:1509–1524.
13. Fox MW, Ahlskog JE, Kelly PJ. Stereotactic ventrolateralis thalamotomy for medically refractory tremor in post-levodopa era Parkinson's disease patients. *J Neurosurg* 1991;75:723–730.
14. Hassler R, Mundinger F, Reichert T. Correlations between clinical and autoptic findings in stereotaxic operations of parkinsonism. *Confin Neurol* 1965;26:282–290.
15. Vitek JL, Ashe J, deLong MR, et al. Physiologic properties and somatotopic organization of the primate motor thalamus. *J Neurophysiol* 1994;71:1498–1513.
16. Gildenberg PL. Surgical therapy of movement disorders. In: Wilkins RH, Rengachary SS, eds. *Neurosurgery,* vol 3. New York: McGraw-Hill, 1985:2507–2516.
17. Starr PA, Vitek JL, Bakay RAE. Ablative surgery and deep brain stimulation for Parkinson's disease. *Neurosurgery* 1998;43:989–1015.
18. Cooper IS, Bergmann LL, Caracalos A. Anatomic verification of the lesion which abolishes parkinsonian tremor and rigidity. *Neurology* 1963;13:779–787.
19. Pagni CA, Wildi E, Ettore G, et al. Anatomic verification of lesions which abolished tremor and rigor in parkinsonism. *Confin Neurol* 1965;26:291–294.
20. Schaltenbrand G, Wahren W. *Atlas for stereotaxy of the human brain.* Stuttgart: Thieme, 1977.
21. Linhares MN, Tasker RR. Microelectrode-guided thalamotomy for Parkinson's disease. *Neurosurgery* 2000;46:390–395.
22. Wester K, Hauglie-Hanssen E. The prognostic value of intra-operative observations during thalamotomy for parkinsonian tremor. *Clin Neurol Neurosurg* 1992;94:25–30.
23. Lenz FA, Normand SL, Kwan HC, et al. Statistical prediction of the optimal site for thalamotomy in parkinsonian tremor. *Mov Disord* 1995;10:318–328.
24. Ohye C, Narabayashi H. Physiological study of presumed ventralis intermedius neurons in the human thalamus. *J Neurosurg* 1979;50:290–297.
25. Hirai T, Miyazaki M, Nakajima H, et al. The correlation between tremor characteristics and the predicted volume of effective lesions in stereotaxic nucleus ventralis intermedius thalamotomy. *Brain* 1983;106:1001–1018.
26. Kondziolka D. Functional radiosurgery. *Neurosurgery* 1999;44:12–22.
27. Steiner L, Prasad D, Lindquist C, et al. Gamma knife surgery in vascular, neoplastic, and functional disorders of the nervous system. In: Schmidek HH, Sweet WH, eds. *Operative neurosurgical techniques: indications, methods, and results.* Philadelphia: WB Saunders, 1995:667–694.
28. Lindquist C, Kihlstrom L, Hellstrand E. Functional neurosurgery: a future for the gamma knife? *Stereotact Funct Neurosurg* 1991;57:72–81.
29. Rand RW, Jacques DB, Melbye RW, et al. Gamma knife thalamotomy and pallidotomy in patients with movements disorders:

preliminary results. *Stereotact Funct Neurosurg* 1993;61[Suppl 1]: 65–92.

30. Otsuki T, Jokura H, Takahashi K, et al. Stereotactic gamma-thalamotomy with a computerized brain atlas: technical case report. *Neurosurgery* 1994;35:764–767.

31. Hirato M, Ohye C, Shibazaki T, et al. Gamma knife thalamotomy for the treatment of functional disorders. *Stereotact Funct Neurosurg* 1995;64 Suppl 1:164–171.

32. Friehs GM, Ojakangas CL, Pachats P, et al. Thalamotomy and caudotomy with the gamma knife as a treatment for parkinsonism with a comment on lesion sizes. *Stereotact Funct Neurosurg* 1995;64[Suppl 1]:209–221.

33. Young RF. Functional neurosurgery with the Leksell gamma knife. *Stereotact Funct Neurosurg* 1996;66:19–23.

34. Pan L, Dai JZ, Wang BJ, et al. Stereotactic gamma thalamotomy for the treatment of parkinsonism. *Stereotact Funct Neurosurg* 1996;66[Suppl 1]:329–332.

35. Ohye C, Shibazaki T, Hirato M, et al. Gamma thalamotomy for parkinsonian and other kinds of tremor. *Stereotact Funct Neurosurg* 1996;66[Suppl 1]:333–342.

36. Bonnen JG, Iacono RP, Lulu B, et al. Gamma knife pallidotomy: case report. *Acta Neurochir (Wien)* 1997;139:442–445.

37. Duma CM, Jacques DB, Kopyov OV, et al. Gamma knife radiosurgery for thalamotomy in parkinsonian tremor: a five-year experience. *J Neurosurg* 1998;88:1044–1049.

38. Young RF, Shumway-Cook A, Vermeulen SS, et al. Gamma knife radiosurgery as a lesioning technique in movement disorder surgery. *J Neurosurg* 1998;89:183–193.

39. Diederich N, Goetz CG, Stebbins GT, et al. Blinded evaluation confirms long-term asymmetric effect of unilateral thalamotomy or subthalamotomy on tremor in Parkinson's disease. *Neurology* 1992;42:1311–1314.

40. Jankovic J, Cardoso F, Grossman R, et al. Outcome after stereotactic thalamotomy for parkinsonian, essential, and other types of tremor. *Neurosurgery* 1995;37:680–687.

41. Kelly PJ, Gillingham FJ. The long-term results of stereotaxic surgery and l-dopa thaerapy in patients with Parkinson's disease: a 10-year follow-up study. *J Neurosurg* 1980;53:332–337.

42. Mundinger F. Postoperative and long-term results of 1,561 stereotactic operations in parkinsonism. *Appl Neurophysiol* 1985;48:293.

43. Krayenbühl H, Wyss OAM, Yasargil MG. Bilateral thalamotomy and pallidotomy as treatment for bilateral parkinsonism. *J Neurosurg* 1961;18:429.

44. Boller F, Mizutani T, Roessmann U, et al. Parkinson's disease, dementia and Alzheimer disease. *Ann Neurol* 1980;7:329–335.

45. Riklan M, Reynolds CM, Stellar S. Correlates of memory in Parkinson's disease. *J Nerv Ment Dis* 1989;177:237–240.

46. Hugdahl K, AsbjФrnsen A, Wester K. Memory performance in Parkinson's disease. *Neuropsychiatry Neuropsychol Behav Neurol* 1993;6:170–176.

47. Selby G. Stereotactic surgery for the relief of Parkinson's disease. I. A critical review. *J Neurol Sci* 1967;5:315–342.

48. Selby G. Stereotactic surgery for the relief of Parkinson's disease. II. Analysis of the results of a series of 303 patients (413 operations). *J Neurol Sci* 1967;5: 343–375.

49. Almgren PE, Andersson AL, Kullberg G. Differences in verbally expressed cognition following left and right ventrolateral thalamotomy. *Scand J Psychol* 1969;10:243–249.

50. Vilkki J. Visual hemi-inattention after ventrolateral thalamotomy. *Neuropsychologia* 1984;22:399–408.

51. Lund-Johansen M, Hugdahl K, Wester K. Cognitive function in patients with Parkinson's disease undergoing stereotaxic thalamotomy. *J Neurol Neurosurg Psychiatry* 1996;60:564–571.

52. Hugdahl K, Wester K, Asbjørnsen A. The role of the left and the right thalamus in language asymmetry: dichotic listening in Parkinson patients undergoing stereotactic thalamotomy. *Brain Lang* 1990;39:1–13.

53. Hugdahl K, Wester K. Neurocognitive correlates of stereotactic thalamotomy and thalamic stimulation in Parkinsonian patients. *Brain Cogn* 2000;42:231–252.

54. Tasker RR, Munz M, Junn FSCK, et al. Deep brain stimulation and thalamotomy for tremor compared. *Acta Neurochir Suppl (Wien)* 1997;68:49–53.

55. Schuurman PR, Bosch DA, Bossuyt PM, et al. A comparison of continuous thalamic stimulation and thalamotomy for suppression of severe tumor. *N Engl J Med* 2000;342:461–468.

Surgery for Parkinson's Disease and Movement Disorders,
edited by J.K. Krauss, J. Jankovic, and R.G. Grossman.
Lippincott Williams & Wilkins, Philadelphia © 2001.

10

THALAMIC STIMULATION FOR TREATMENT OF PARKINSON'S DISEASE TREMOR

RICHARD K. SIMPSON, JR.
JOACHIM K. KRAUSS
WILLIAM G. ONDO

One of the hallmarks of the "shaking palsy," or paralysis agitans as initially described by James Parkinson in 1817, is *tremor* (1). Indeed, Parkinson stated that: "The tremulous motion of the limbs occur during sleep, and augment until they awaken the patient, and frequently with much agitation and alarm. The power of conveying the food to the mouth is at length so much impeded that he is obliged to consent to be fed by others.... As the debility increases and the influence of the will over the muscles fades away, the tremulous agitation becomes more vehement. It now seldom leaves him for a moment; but even when exhausted nature seizes a small portion of sleep, the motion becomes so violent as not only to shake the bed-hangings, but even the floor and the sashes of the room." Tremor can be a disabling and socially embarrassing feature for many patients suffering from Parkinson's disease. Effective management of tremor, among other features of Parkinson's disease, has been a major impetus for surgical intervention before and since the advent of helpful medications such as levodopa. Different types of surgical techniques have been developed and applied to patients over the last several decades in an attempt to control tremor. This chapter addresses the use of stereotactically placed electrodes in the thalamus for chronic, continuous stimulation to accomplish this objective.

In the 1970s, implantable deep brain stimulators were used for patients with chronic pain disorders. Richardson and Akil (2,3), Hosobuchi (4), and Mazars (5), among others, provided major contributions to our understanding of chronic deep brain stimulation using implantable devices. Likewise, early work by Bechtereva and colleagues

in 1975 revealed that thalamic stimulation could influence features of Parkinson's disease (6). These patients were monitored for up to 18 months and clearly demonstrated the beneficial effects of this approach to their disabilities. Despite the inherent limitations in the technology, these devices proved to be beneficial in a large number of patients.

It was not until the 1980s that deep brain stimulation for control of tremor became practical as the necessary technologic improvements in these devices occurred. The initial observations by Andy in 1983 revealed that patients who were to be treated by thalamotomy could have adequate control of their tremor by thalamic stimulation (7). Tasker and colleagues, in 1984, implanted a monopolar deep brain stimulator system in a patient with Parkinson's disease and tremor as a successful alternative to thalamotomy (8). Siegfried pioneered the use of thalamic deep brain stimulation in Europe since the early 1980s (9).

Benabid and his associates popularized the concept of chronic thalamic stimulation for control of tremor in patients suffering from Parkinson's disease (10). He and his colleagues carefully began to study the various parameters of frequency, intensity, pulse width, polarity, and duration of electrical impulses applied to the ventralis intermedius (VIM) nucleus of the thalamus to control tremor. In an early report, Benabid and colleagues studied the effects of VIM stimulation using a frequency of 100 Hz, a pulse width of 0.5 milliseconds, and an intensity of 1 to 2 v (10). The stereotactic coordinates chosen were at the anterior commissure–posterior commissure (AC-PC) level, the posterior quarter of the AC-PC line, and 13.5 mm from the midline. Of the six patients tested, three patients had a dramatic improvement in their tremor and were implanted with permanent impulse generators. The results were comparable to those in patients receiving a thalamotomy for their tremor.

By the early 1990s, many more patients with Parkinson's disease were treated with deep brain stimulation using

R.K. Simpson, Jr.: Department of Neurosurgery, Baylor College of Medicine, Houston, Texas 77030.

J.K. Krauss: Department of Neurosurgery, University Hospital, Klinikum Mannheim, Mannheim 68167, Germany.

W.G. Ondo: Department of Neurology, Baylor College of Medicine, Houston, Texas 77030.

stereotactically placed electrodes into the VIM nucleus of the thalamus. Benabid and colleagues, in 1991, reported the first large series of such patients treated in this manner (11). Of the 26 patients with Parkinson's disease and seven patients with essential tremor, 88% showed either complete relief or a major improvement in their tremor. Neurosurgeons began to consider deep brain stimulation for tremor as the primary mode of treatment, rather than classic thalamotomy. The intraoperative electrical parameters used to test for tremor control and postoperative programming paradigms continue to be refined. Likewise, improved clinical outcomes are currently reported and are discussed in detail later.

INDICATIONS

As with the application of any form of surgical or medical treatment, careful patient selection is paramount for a reasonable likelihood of an effective outcome (12–14). The importance of this issue cannot be overstressed. If tremor is the most disabling feature of a patient with Parkinson's disease, such patients are considered candidates for deep brain stimulation of the VIM nucleus of the thalamus. Either such patients should be intolerant of medications for tremor management or the medications are not sufficiently effective. These patients must exhibit the necessary cognitive ability to manage the device with magnets, and they must have adequate access to transportation for follow-up clinic visits and device reprogramming. Because many patients with Parkinson's disease have significant problems with rigidity, bradykinesia, freezing, gait disturbances, and associated cognitive features in addition to a pronounced and debilitating tremor, control of the tremor must make a reasonable impact on the patient's lifestyle, comfort, and overall well-being.

Patients with unilateral or bilateral tremor are candidates for this therapy (15). Patients who have had a thalamotomy in the opposite thalamus but who have tremor originating from the untreated side are candidates because of the possible complications of bilateral thalamotomy. This same approach can be applied to patients who may have suffered a thalamic infarct on the opposite side as well. Patients who have undergone pallidotomy but who have not experienced satisfactory tremor relief may be candidates for deep brain stimulation with the VIM as the target.

Other factors may need to be considered before a patient is considered for deep brain stimulation, such as the presence of a cardiac pacemaker or defibrillator and intracranial abnormalities such as the presence of a small thalamic infarct in the target area. Patients who may require periodic magnetic resonance imaging (MRI) for a variety of reasons may not be candidates, although the issue of MRI compatibility with the deep brain stimulator system is currently under debate (16). Preoperative MRI scans to rule out craniospinal abnormalities have been suggested, as have carotid Doppler studies

for stenotic carotid artery disease (17,18). The ultimate goal of this therapy is directed toward treating the tremor in the upper extremity and in particular the distal or hand tremor. Some patients may have unrealistic expectations about proximal upper extremity control as well as lower extremity, axial, head, and voice tremor control. Several recent studies, however, have demonstrated considerable improvement in the tremor at these other locations with the VIM as the target (19).

The degree of tremor, again if it is the most disabling feature of a patient's Parkinson's disease, is generally evaluated by standard Parkinson's disease rating schemes (20). The Unified Parkinson's Disease Rating Scale (UPDRS) was used during the North America Multi-Center Deep Brain Stimulation Trial protocol and is currently and preferentially used by many other centers to rate tremor. However, there are several inherent limitations to this tool as it pertains to tremor assessment. The UPDRS is made up of four subscales, and tremor assessment is addressed by only two of 18 items in subscale III. The degree of tremor is generally overshadowed by the other items. For this reason, several investigators have modified this portion of the UPDRS into a simple tremor severity scale from 0 or no tremor to 4 or severe tremor. For the North America Multi-Center Deep Brain Stimulation Trial protocol, a tremor severity of 3 or 4 at rest was required before patient was considered for surgery.

Several other useful methods to assess tremor have been used in patients with Parkinson's disease (21). These include 0 to 4 scales to quantify writing a sentence, drawing a spiral, and drawing a straight line between two parallel lines. Another common tool for tremor assessment is pouring water from one cup to another. Based on a 0 to 4 scale, this task involves quantifying the amount of water spilled: none, minimal (10%), up to 10% to 50%, and most (more than 50%). Patients may be screened as candidates for deep brain stimulation based on these criteria and others concerning the severity of tremor. Although scales and scores are helpful in the decision-making process, many factors are used in deciding the indications for surgery. Quantifying tremor in terms of its severity and disability is necessary to demonstrate the impact of various therapies, particularly within the contemporary economic environment. Ultimately, sound clinical judgment is the major prerequisite of a satisfactory outcome.

RESULTS

Deep brain stimulation of the thalamus has been shown to be highly successful in the management of tremor associated with Parkinson's disease, essential tremor, multiple sclerosis, and other neurologic conditions. The objective of this chapter is a discussion of the results of thalamic stimulation for Parkinson's disease tremor, although patients with other types of tremor may have been included in the reports discussed later. There have been several reports generated since the 1991 study by Benabid and colleagues that demonstrated the utility and high degree of success using VIM stimulation control or abate tremor associated with Parkinson's disease (11). Other sites for stimulation such as the internal segment of the globus pallidus and the subthalamic nucleus, have received considerable attention lately (12–14). Stimulation of these sites is effective in controlling rigidity, bradykinesia, gait disorders, and other features of Parkinson's disease, but also tremor to some degree.

The largest reported series of patients with Parkinson's disease is that of Benabid and colleagues, and it was reaffirmed in a more recent review of their experience (22,23). Their series included 80 patients with Parkinson's disease treated with VIM thalamic stimulation of whom 38 received bilaterally implanted devices. These patients were followed up to 8 years postoperatively. The effectiveness of stimulation was determined based on a five-point scale and included the following: 4, complete disappearance of tremor; 3, slight tremor reappearance after a stress event; 2, moderate benefit; 1, slight, definite benefit without improvement in activities of daily living; and 0, no benefit. Based on these criteria measured 3 months postoperatively, 88% of the thalamic stimulator systems were effective in reducing the contralateral tremor to levels 4 and 3. Approximately 11% of the systems reduced the contralateral tremor to scores of 2 and 1, whereas only 0.9% resulted in a score of 0. In addition to the benefits on tremor, 48.7% of patients decreased their dopamine medication 3 months postoperatively.

The Baylor experience, as reported by Ondo and colleagues, includes 67 patients with 3 months to 2 years of follow-up (24). Thirty-two of these patients were treated with VIM stimulation for Parkinson's disease–induced tremor. Other patients treated in this manner included 33 with essential tremor, one with cerebral palsy, and one with olivopontocerebellar degeneration. Of the patients with Parkinson's disease, 18 (56%) had excellent results, 12 (38%) demonstrated marked improvement, one had (3%) moderate improvement, and one (3%) had only mild improvement of their tremor. In a similar study by Krauss and Simpson, 27 patients were treated with deep brain stimulation of VIM for tremor (25). Of these patients, 14 had Parkinson's disease, and seven (50%) had excellent results, four (29%) had marked improvement, and three (21%) had moderate improvement of their tremor.

Another large series was reported by Siegfried and Lippitz (9). Forty patients out of a total of 73 patients received deep brain stimulation systems implanted into the VIM for Parkinson's disease–induced tremor. Of the 40 patients, 29 (72.5%) were described as having perfect control of their tremor. Most of these patients had previous thalamotomies on the opposite side.

Tasker's 1998 report of the Toronto Hospital series included 16 patients receiving deep brain stimulation for treatment of tremor associated with Parkinson's disease (18). Of these patients, 79% had either complete or nearly complete abolition of their tremor. Moreover, 49% of patients experienced a significant reduction in their rigidity, 68% of patients demonstrated improved manual dexterity, and 50% of patients had a reduction in L-dopa–induced dyskinesias. Approximately 11% of patients experienced a significant but incomplete reduction in their tremor, and 5% of patients experienced only a slight degree of tremor improvement. In one patient, the procedure had to be abandoned. A recurrence rate of 5% was seen in patients who were followed beyond 2 years. These results were an extension of an earlier report from the Toronto group in which the results from deep brain stimulation compared favorably to traditional thalamotomy.

Koller and associates studied 24 patients with Parkinson's disease and tremor, of whom 18 patients had bilateral symptoms (21). Approximately 58.3% of patients had complete abolition of their tremor, whereas 13% had moderate and 17% had mild improvement in their tremor. Only 8% had no tremor relief, and one patient (4%) had reported worsening of tremor. Likewise, in a preliminary study by Ondo and associates (20), the results of unilateral stimulation of 19 patients with Parkinson's disease revealed that 57.9% had complete cessation of their rest tremor, and 31.6% had resting, postural, and kinetic tremor relief at least 3 months postoperatively. All patients experienced some degree of tremor relief in this study. Most recently, a study by Taha and associates reviewed their experience with six patients with Parkinson's disease tremor (19). This study included the results of treatment of tremor associated with different diseases; however, the overall results showed that 96% of patients had significant tremor relief. Moreover, these results clearly showed that head and voice tremor could be significantly attenuated by deep brain stimulation of the VIM.

Other series include that of Blond and colleagues in a 1992 report (26). Thalamic stimulation (VIM) was undertaken in ten patients with Parkinson's disease, and eight patients (80%) reported significant tremor relief. Caparros-Lefebvre and colleagues reiterated these results in a separate 1993 report (27). Alesch and colleagues studied the benefits of deep brain stimulation in 23 patients with tremor from Parkinson's disease, of whom six patients had bilateral implants (17). Approximately 64% of these patients had complete arrest of their tremor, and 18% revealed a major degree of tremor reduction. More recently, Hubble and her associates reported that 100% of ten patients suffering from Parkinson's disease–induced tremor were tremor free 3 months postoperatively (28). Likewise, the multicenter European study of thalamic stimulation, as reported by Limousin and associates, confirmed and extended the earlier reports on tremor of Parkinson's disease (29). In

83% of 73 patients, a two-point reduction in tremor was achieved as assessed by the UPDRS subscore 12 months postoperatively.

BILATERAL STIMULATION

Two recent studies explored bilateral VIM stimulation in more detail (24,25). With regard to the Baylor experience, Ondo reported that of the 24 patients with bilateral deep brain stimulation implants, 11 of these procedures were for Parkinson's disease–induced tremor (24). Of these 11 patients, five (45%) demonstrated excellent control, five (45%) marked control, and one (10%) moderate control of their tremor. Similar findings were noted in a smaller study by Krauss and associates from Bern (25).

Most of the reports to date concerning deep brain stimulation of the thalamus (VIM) for tremor control do not clearly separate the outcome of patients treated for unilateral or bilateral tremor. The following discussion is based on the extrapolation of results of published studies describing the benefits of this technique whereby bilateral thalamic stimulation for control of bilateral tremor was used. This approach is partly justified, again, by the lack of published data distinguishing differences between unilateral or bilateral stimulation for contralateral tremor control but also by personal experience with this topic. Most authors describe their results in terms of the number of "sides" stimulated or the number of thalami tested. Adding some confusion to the issue is that some studies merge the results of deep brain stimulation on tremor originating from Parkinson's disease and essential tremor. However, based on the available data, it appears that bilateral stimulation is as effective on upper extremity tremor as is unilateral stimulation. Conversely, the issue of increased side effects from bilateral stimulation as compared with unilateral stimulation has gained considerable attention.

SIDE EFFECTS

Operative complications are to be distinguished from the side effects of the implantable thalamic stimulating devices once the current is turned on. The most common side effects expressed by patients while using the devices include dysarthria, paresthesias, dystonia, and disequilibrium. The largest series of reported long-term side effects from deep brain stimulation for tremor is from Benabid and associates (22). His 1996 report described 80 patients with Parkinson's disease, 38 of whom had bilateral implants, and 20 patients with essential tremor, 13 of whom had bilateral implants. Persistent paresthesias, those not induced by higher simulation intensity than necessary to control tremor, were experienced by one patient with Parkinson's disease who had

bilateral stimulation. Approximately 9% of all the patients experienced transient paresthesias that were modified by reprogramming of the device. Disequilibrium was seen in ten patients, including six with Parkinson's disease and four with essential tremor. Of this group, six (60%) had bilateral stimulation, and four (40%) had unilateral stimulation. Contralateral dystonia was seen in four patients with Parkinson's disease and two with essential tremor. Four (66.7%) patients had bilateral stimulation, and two (33.3%) had unilateral stimulation. Interestingly, 9% of all the patients experienced dystonia, primarily of the lower extremity and especially the foot, 1 year after the procedure. In general, reprogramming the device controlled this complication as well. This also has been the authors' personal experience in a single case of dystonia involving the contralateral foot. Bilateral stimulation did not induce neuropsychologic deficits, nor did patients complain of such disturbances. However, careful neuropsychologic testing did reveal that simulation of the left VIM produced a slight decrease in verbal performance, whereas stimulation of the right VIM produced a slight decrease in spatial performance.

Other series have reported similar types of side effects. Alesch and colleagues reported that of 27 patients who underwent deep brain stimulation, six had bilateral VIM implants, all in patients with Parkinson's disease (17). Approximately 50% of these patients with bilateral implants had dysarthria. Only 18% of patients with unilateral implants had dysarthria. Of the total patient group, 7% had paresthesias, 4% had disequilibrium, and none reported dystonias. Siegfried and Lippitz reported that in 40 patients with Parkinson's disease, 25% had dysarthria, 7% had persistent paresthesias, and 5% had disequilibrium (9). Most of these patients who had undergone deep brain stimulator placement had undergone thalamotomy on the other side. Blond and associates studied ten patients with Parkinson's disease and four patients with essential tremor, with no reports of long-term side effects (26). In general, all the reported side effects, as discussed earlier, were immediately abated once the device or devices had been turned off.

Taha and colleagues, in a recent series studying bilateral deep brain stimulation for head and voice tremor control as well as limb tremor control, found that of the 23 treated patients (six with Parkinson's disease, 15 with essential tremor, and two with multiple sclerosis), seven (30%) developed dysarthria, seven (30%) developed disequilibrium, and one (4.4%) had memory deficits (19).

Ondo and associates, discussing the early Baylor experience with unilateral stimulation, also found one patient each with headache, nausea, diplopia, or altered mental status; again, all these effects were modified by altering the output of the device (20). In a more recent report, complications specifically attributed to bilateral stimulation were described (24). Of the 11 patients with Parkinson's disease and tremor, five (45%) had disequilibrium, three (27%) had dysarthria, one (9%) had diplopia, and one (9%) had excessive salivation. These side effects were controlled by adjusting the output of the pulse generators.

ADVANTAGES AND DISADVANTAGES

Treatment of tremor and other symptoms that are a consequence of Parkinson's disease can be effectively done with medication. However, since the advent of levodopa therapy, many patients have exhibited refractory tremor as well as other disease symptoms. These patients are considered surgical candidates if they meet the general criteria discussed earlier and if they are considered reasonable candidates based on the overall clinical judgment of the attending physicians. Both procedures, thalamotomy and deep brain stimulation, are effective in managing tremor, and either procedure has a range of advantages and disadvantages over the other. Thalamotomy is discussed in detail in Chapter 9; however, a general comparison between thalamotomy and deep brain stimulation provides a meaningful effort to clarify and distinguish which operation is best for a particular patient.

Several studies have provided evidence that the results of thalamotomy and deep brain stimulation are comparable (12–14,18). The primary advantage of thalamotomy is that if it provides successful tremor relief, the ordeal for the patient is essentially over. In addition, the patient does not have to worry about equipment problems, revision of the pulse generator after battery depletion, or repeat clinic visits for programming. Again, these are advantages if the procedure has produced a long-term and significant reduction in the patient's tremor. Some surgeons advocate that older, less healthy patients may benefit more from thalamotomy because of issues of life expectancy, length of the procedure, and lack of potentially cumbersome postoperative follow-up. The incidence of infection is potentially reduced compared with deep brain stimulation secondary to the absence of an implanted foreign body. However, data to suggest that these latter points are accurate have not been clearly established.

Schuurman and colleagues have examined the effects of thalamotomy versus thalamic deep brain stimulation in a randomized prospective study in 68 patients including 45 with Parkinson's disease (30). In this study, thalamic stimulation and thalamotomy were equally effective for the suppression of tremor, but thalamic stimulation had fewer adverse effects and resulted in greater improvement in function.

Recurrence rates for tremor over extended periods are well established, yet a repeat thalamotomy in the same target region can be problematic (15,23). Some surgeons advise that the incidence of deep hemorrhage is higher for thalamotomy than for deep brain stimulation, although the data are unclear on this point at present (18). If tremor is present bilaterally, bilateral thalamotomy is associated with a relatively high percentage of neurologic deficits including dysarthria, gait disturbances, cognitive difficulties, and other conditions. The

thalamic target for other types of future surgical intervention, including deep brain stimulation or perhaps experimental therapies such as tissue implants or microdialysis catheters, has been essentially destroyed. Thalamotomy therefore poses serious limits on the treatment options for patients with an unsuccessful procedure.

Deep brain stimulation, if optimally placed, has several unique advantages over traditional thalamotomy (14,18,24). Although there is a degree of microtrauma that occurs as a result of insertion of the electrode, the procedure is largely reversible. If tremor recurs, the "lesion" can be adjusted. The lesion can be amplified by modifying the various output parameters of the device. The lesion can be moved by altering which contacts are made active and by changing the polarity of the active contacts. Likewise, if tremor recurs over time despite aggressive reprogramming of the device, other therapies including medical and surgical intervention (thalamotomy) may be undertaken because the thalamic target is preserved. Another unique advantage of the deep brain stimulation technique is that bilateral tremor can be controlled with fewer complications than bilateral thalamotomies. Although some patients may experience dysarthria, disequilibrium, or persistent paresthesias, these effects tend to be mild and reversible if either or both stimulator settings are modified.

A significant limiting factor regarding deep brain stimulation, especially in the contemporary economic environment, is the cost of the device. The cost of performing the operation, as with thalamotomy, ranges among institutions. However, the cost of the implantable devices is a relative constant over and above the cost of thalamotomy. In addition is the additional cost of replacing the pulse generator every few years and the cost of programming the devices, as well as the costs of equipment and personnel in the outpatient setting.

CONCLUSIONS

Thalamic deep brain stimulation is an effective method for controlling medically refractory upper extremity tremor in properly selected patients suffering from Parkinson's disease. The clinical outcomes and risks associated with the procedure are comparable to those of traditional thalamotomy. Several additional benefits can be realized by this neurosurgical approach including the following: (a) the procedure is reversible; (b) the "lesion" is adjustable; (c) the target for tremor control is not destroyed, thus allowing for other forms of future surgical intervention; and (d) the procedure can be performed bilaterally with fewer, controllable, and less severe side effects. Cost remains the primary disadvantage at this point.

The observation that chronic stimulation of the subthalamic nucleus and of the globus pallidus internus has a profound antitumor effect has resulted in a substantial reduction of thalamic surgery in Parkinson's disease in the last few years. In most patients other symptoms progress over the years which are not improved by thalamic stimulation. It is anticipated that few patients with Parkinson's disease will undergo thalamic VIM stimulation in the future.

REFERENCES

1. Parkinson J. *An essay on the shaking palsy.* London: Sherwood, Neely, and Jones, 1817:7–9.
2. Richardson DE, Akil H. Pain reduction by electrical brain stimulation in man. I. Acute administration in periaqueductal and periventricular sites. *J Neurosurg* 1977;47:178–183.
3. Richardson DE, Akil H. Pain reduction by electrical brain stimulation in man. II. Chronic self-administration in the periventricular gray matter. *J Neurosurg* 1977;47:184–194.
4. Hosobuchi Y. Combined electrical stimulation of the periaqueductal gray matter and sensory thalamus. *Appl Neurophysiol* 1983;46:112–115.
5. Mazars G. Intermittent stimulation of nucleus ventralis posterolateralis for intractable pain. *Surg Neurol* 1975;4:93–95.
6. Bechtereva NP, Bondartchuck AN, Smirnov VM. Method of electrostimulation of the deep brain struictures in treatment of some chronic diseases. *Confin Neurol* 1975;37:136–140.
7. Andy OJ. Thalamic stimulation for control of movement disorders. *Appl Neurophysiol* 1983;46:107–111.
8. Tasker RR, Lang AE, Lozano AM. Pallidal and thalamic surgery for Parkinson's disease. *Exp Neurol* 1997;144:35–40.
9. Siegfried J, Lippitz B. Chronic electrical stimulation of the VL-VPL complex and of the pallidum in the treatment of movement disorders: personal experience since 1982. *Stereotact Funct Neurosurg* 1994;62:71–75.
10. Benabid AL, Pollak P, Loueau A, et al. Combined (thalamotomy and stimulation) stereotactic surgery of the VIM thalamic nucleus for bilateral Parkinson disease. *Stereotact Funct Neurosurg* 1987;50:344–346.
11. Benabid AL, Pollak P, Gervason C, et al. Long-term suppression of tremor by chronic stimulation of the ventral intermediate thalamic nucleus. *Lancet* 1991;337:403–406.
12. Starr PA, Vitek JL, Bakay RAE. Ablative surgery and deep brain stimulation for Parkinson's disease. *Neurosurgery* 1998;43:989–1015.
13. Starr PA, Vitek JL, Bakay RAE. Deep brain stimulation for movement disorders. *Neurosurg Clin North Am* 1998;9:381–402.
14. Arle JE, Alterman RL. Surgical options in Parkinson's disease. *Med Clin North Am* 1999;83:483–498.
15. Benabid AL, Pollak P, Hoffmann D, et al. Chronic stimulation for Parkinson's disease and other movement disorders. In: Gildenburg PL, Tasker RR, eds. *Stereotactic and functional neurosurgery.* New York: McGraw-Hill, 1998:1199–1212.
16. Tronnier VM, Staubert A, Hahnel S, et al. Magnetic resonance imaging with implanted neurostimulators: an *in vitro* and *in vivo* study. *Neurosurgery* 1999;44:118–126.
17. Alesch F, Pinter MM, Helscher J, et al. Stimulation of the ventral intermediate thalamic nucleus in tremor dominated Parkinson's disease and essential tremor. *Acta Neurochir (Wien)* 1995;136:75–81.
18. Tasker RR. Deep brain stimulation is preferable to thalamotomy for tremor suppression. *Surg Neurol* 1998;49:145–154.
19. Taha JM, Janszen MA, Favre J. Thalamic deep brain stimulation for the treatment of head, voice, and bilateral limb tremor. *J Neurosurg* 1999;91:68–72.
20. Ondo W, Jankovic J, Schwartz K, et al. Unilateral thalamic deep brain stimulation for refractory essential tremor and Parkinson's disease tremor. *Neurology* 1998;51:1063–1069.
21. Koller W, Pahwa R, Busenbark K, et al. High-frequency unilateral thalamic stimulation in the treatment of essential tremor and Parkinsonian tremor. *Ann Neurol* 1997;42:292–299.
22. Benabid AL, Pollak P, Gao D, et al. Chronic electrical stimulation of the ventralis intermedius nucleus of the thalamus as a treatment of movement disorders. *J Neurosurg* 1996;84:203–214.
23. Benabid Al, Benazzouz A, Hoffmann D, et al. Long-term electrical inhibition of deep brain targets in movement disorders. *Mov Disord* 1998;13:119–125.
24. Ondo W, Almaguer M, Jankovic J, et al. Thalamic deep brain stimulation: comparison between unilateral and bilateral placement. *Arch Neurol* 2001;58:218–222.
25. Krauss JK, Simpson RK Jr., Ondo WG, et al. Concepts and methods in chromic thalamic stimulation for treatment of tremor: technique and application. *Neurosurgery* 2001;48:535–541.
26. Blond S, Caparros-Lefebvre D, Parker F, et al. Control of tremor and involuntary movement disorders by chronic sterotactic stimulation of the ventral intermediate thalamic nucleus. *J Neurosurg* 1992;77:62–68.
27. Caparros-Lefebvre D, Blond S, Vermersch P. Chronic thalamic stimulation improves tremor and levodopa induce dyskinesias in Parkinson's disease. *J Neurol Neurosurg Psychiatry* 1993;56:268–273.
28. Hubble JP, Busenbark KL, Wilkinson S, et al. Effects of thalamic deep brain stimulation based on tremor type and diagnosis. *Mov Disord* 1997;12:337–341.
29. Limousin P, Speelman JD, Gielen F, et al. Multicenter European study of thalamic stimulation in parkinsonian and essential tremors. *J Neurol Neurosurg Psychiatry* 1999;66:289–296.
30. Schuurman PR, Bosch DA, Bossuyt PM, et al. A comparison of continuous thalamic stimulation and thalamotomy for suppression of severe tremor. *N Engl J Med* 2000;342:461–468.

Surgery for Parkinson's Disease and Movement Disorders,
edited by J.K. Krauss, J. Jankovic, and R.G. Grossman.
Lippincott Williams & Wilkins, Philadelphia © 2001.

11

PALLIDOTOMY FOR TREATMENT
OF PARKINSON'S DISEASE

BRYAN R. PAYNE
ROY A.E. BAKAY
JERROLD K. VITEK

Surgical treatment of Parkinson's disease (PD) antedates effective medical therapy by more than 30 years. Before the 1960s, various surgical procedures were the only option in the treatment of PD. The corticospinal tract was the most common target before the introduction of stereotactic surgery (1–6). Results of these procedures were often good for reduction of tremor but at the high cost of varying degrees of hemiparesis and significant operative morbidity and mortality.

Meyers pioneered open ablative procedures of the basal ganglia (7–9). In a 1951 review, Meyers reported that pallidofugal sectioning and resection of the anterior two-thirds of the head of the caudate and anterior limb of the internal capsule to the genu provided the best results (10). Unacceptably high morbidity and mortality were associated with these open procedures targeting the basal ganglia and precluded their widespread application. Open procedures targeting the corticospinal tract remained popular. Ligation of the anterior choroidal artery was briefly popular for the treatment of PD (11,12).

Spiegel and Wycis introduced stereotaxy in 1947. This procedure allowed ablation of deep targets with significantly improved accuracy and reduced morbidity (13). Accumulated clinical data indicating that the globus pallidus (GP) was an effective target for ablation in the relief of parkinsonian symptoms, especially rigidity, made this a popular target, and an explosive increase in stereotactic surgical treatment of PD occurred (14). The work of Hassler, Riechert, and Mundinger in the 1950s and 1960s was instrumental in demonstrating the effectiveness of thalamotomy in the treatment of PD, particularly in the management of tremor (15–18).

The maturation of the posterior ventral GP as a target was largely based on the work of Leksell. A prospective analysis of various target points within the GP performed on 81 patients by Leksell was reported by Svennilson et al. in 1960 (19). The lesion of the posterior ventral internal segment of the GP (GPi) created in a subgroup of 20 patients was associated with relief of the cardinal symptoms of PD (rigidity, bradykinesia, and tremor) in 19 of the patients, with minimal adverse effects.

As the major effective targets of modern surgical management of PD were established, the introduction of L-dopa in 1967 (20) and of amantadine in 1969 (21) revolutionized medical management of the disease. However, it soon became evident that the dramatic response of the symptoms of PD to pharmacotherapy was neither permanent nor without adverse effects. Clinical improvement with L-dopa therapy begins to wane after several years. The patient's response to medications becomes less predictable, and motor fluctuations occur. Long-term use is associated with dyskinesias in 80% of patients (22). The therapeutic window in which medications are effective without causing dyskinesias narrows with time.

The modern era of surgery for PD differs from the pre–L-dopa era in several ways. Patients are generally very advanced in the course of their disease, which is poorly controlled medically. In the interval before the resurgence of surgical management and after the introduction of L-dopa, there were significant advances in the understanding of the anatomy and physiology of the basal ganglia and the pathophysiology of PD (23–26), improvement in imaging techniques, and refinement of methods for target localization and lesion placement (27,28). Although neurotransplantation with allografts and xenografts has been shown to be effective (29,30), the most frequent procedure performed over the past few years was posteroventral pallidotomy.

B.R. Payne and R.A.E. Bakay: Department of Neurosurgery, Rush Medical Center, Chicago, Illinois 60612.

J.K. Vitek: Department of Neurology, Emory University School of Medicine, Atlanta, Georgia 30322.

PALLIDUM AS A TARGET FOR TREATMENT OF PARKINSON'S DISEASE

The anatomy and physiology of the basal ganglia and the pathophysiology of PD are discussed elsewhere in this volume (Chapters 2–4). There are at least five basal ganglia–thalamocortical circuits (sensorimotor, occulomotor, limbic, and two prefrontal) (24,25). The primary symptoms of PD are related to dysfunction of the sensorimotor circuit. The posteroventral GPi is the final inhibitory relay in the thalamocortical sensorimotor loop. The involvement of the GP in the origin and maintenance of tremor in PD is less clear (31–40). Abnormal response to limb torque variations of the GPi of parkinsonian monkeys and the abnormal sensory receptive fields of GPi and thalamic cells of parkinsonian monkeys (33,34) and humans (27,35,36) support the theory that peripheral feedback mechanisms are involved with tremor genesis.

Oscillating cells are located within the GPi of parkinsonian patients. Population of cells with discharge rates of 5 to 7 Hz are seen in the GPi of patients who do have tremor (27,35,36). Evidence indicates that discharges from the GPi may stimulate the development of thalamic bursting activity responsible for parkinsonian tremor, and this activity is necessary for the development and maintenance of the pathophysiologic changes of the neural activity of the thalamus (41). Physiologic normalization of thalamic neuronal activity after pallidotomy subsequent to the loss of these GPi influences may take time, and this would explain the temporal delay in alleviation of tremor after surgical treatment (42).

The optimal target within the GP is the subject of debate (43–45). In early series, the anterior dorsal GPi was targeted and was located on the axial plane of the anterior commissure–posterior commissure (AC-PC) line, 0 to 5 mm posterior to the AC and lateral 15 to 17 mm. For a posteroventral GPi lesion, the target most commonly used is 0 to 4 mm anterior to the midpoint of the AC-PC line, 20 to 22 mm lateral and 4 mm ventral to it (45). Variability in individual anatomy makes it difficult to determine targets accurately based on predetermined targets and a fixed coordinate system.

Microelectrode recording allows exact identification of the targeted nucleus as well as its boundaries. Specific firing patterns of cells within the striatum and the GPi and external segment of the GP allow for physiologic mapping of the region and subsequent comparison to standard anatomic atlases (27,28). The posterior limb of the internal capsule defines the medial border of the posteroventral GPi. Corticospinal fibers to the mouth, face, and upper extremity are located in an anterior to posterior position. Inferior to the GPi and separated from it by pia and arachnoid is the optic tract. It is generally well seen on magnetic resonance imaging studies, but it is variable in location (Fig. 11.1).

The importance of accurate placement of the lesion cannot be overstated (Fig. 11.2). Microelectrode or macroelectrode stimulation is helpful in preventing lesioning too close to the optic tract or the internal capsule. However, this approach only decreases the risk of adverse effects and does not maximize benefit from the procedure. Transient and incomplete benefit from pallidotomy is associated with suboptimal lesion placement. Further sustained benefit can be achieved with reoperation and optimization of lesion placement and size (27,46). Pioneers such as Guiot and Spiegel and Wycis demonstrated that relesioning posterior to initial, ineffective lesions is associated with additional, sustained improvement (47). Studies comparing expected and actual lesion location based on preoperative and postoperative imaging studies show a significant improvement in target accuracy after microelectrode mapping of the GP (27, 48,49).

The optimal targeting method is still controversial (50). Advocates of microelectrode mapping of the GPi argue that this allows a definitive identification of the sensorimotor segment of the GPi (27,28,51,52). However, some groups use microelectrode identification of the GPi without detailed physiologic mapping and contend that verification of correct nuclear placement is adequate and provides similar clinical results (53–56). Still other centers use macrostimulation to avoid injury to the optic tract and internal capsule, but they make no effort to identify the target physiologically with microelectrode recording (57–62). The extreme approach is the use of radiosurgery, which relies only on image guidance both to identify the target and to avoid surrounding, vulnerable tracts. Lars Leksell abandoned the use of the gamma knife in functional disorders because of erratic results and unacceptable complication rates. Subsequent reports using gamma surgery had inconsistent outcomes. However, advances in imaging technology (computed tomography, magnetic resonance imaging) have led to an improvement in preoperative planning and a resurgence of gamma surgery for this indication (63). Most neurosurgeons agree that more information on which to base an ablative lesion is preferable to less. There is disagreement on whether the additional information obtained through microelectrode recording is worth the effort, time, and potential risks. The 2-year results of studies with microelectrode recording (51) and without microelectrode recording (57) suggest that the benefit may be more sustained after microelectrode recording. Although technically demanding, microelectrode recording can be performed safely and with little additional expenditure of time (27,28,49). Additionally, the use of multiple passes of the lesioning probe acting as a macrostimulator is itself time consuming. Complication rates reflect more the experience of the neurosurgeon than the specific technique. It remains to be proven which approach yields the best overall results.

RESULTS OF PALLIDOTOMY

Variations in methods of patient selection, assessment, outcome criteria, medical therapy, and surgical technique make

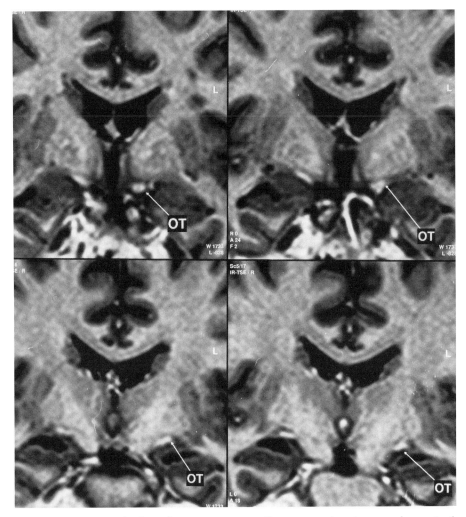

FIGURE 11.1. Preoperative inversion recovery magnetic resonance imaging scan demonstrating the variable position of the optic tract (OT) in relation to the internal segment of the globus pallidus (GPi). Note the difference in location from anterior to posterior and from side to side. The OT is in the ambient cistern, and the cerebrospinal fluid can conduct electrical current, thus increasing the difficulty of accurate localization.

comparison of results from various centers difficult at best and misleading at worst (Table 11.1). Patient selection criteria probably comprise the greatest source of variability in results among centers. Side-by-side comparison of results of retrospective series that differ in many of these variables and that use the treated patients as their own control is difficult at best. Reported various surgical techniques include not only differences in electrophysiology but also differences in target localization, size of the lesion, and postoperative lesion conformation studies. Results are reported for unilateral, bilateral staged, and bilateral simultaneous pallidotomies, further confusing comparison and analysis of results among centers. The quality of the clinical evaluation of patients before and after surgical procedures and the instruments used in these evaluations are also critical to any comparison of results among centers. With these variations in technique and reporting in mind, the results of pallidotomy for PD from

different studies are reviewed (Table 11.2). Blinded assessments by the evaluation of videotapes have confirmed the effects of pallidotomy on motor function (64). The results of an unpublished study sponsored by the National Institutes of Health (NIH) comparing outcome of pallidotomy versus best medical management for PD are also discussed (65).

Dyskinesias

In many patients, drug-induced *dyskinesias* are an embarrassing side effect of the medical treatment of PD. Dyskinesias develop in most patients with PD within 5 to 10 years of the institution of L-dopa therapy and can be the predominant clinical sign in the "on" state. Relief is usually dramatic after pallidotomy. No reported series has failed to show significant relief of contralateral limb dyskinesias after pallidotomy

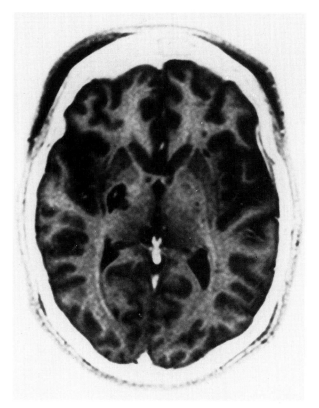

FIGURE 11.2. Postoperative inversion recovery magnetic resonance imaging scan obtained 6 hours after posteroventral pallidotomy demonstrates a well-demarcated lesion abutting the internal capsule medially and encompassing the internal segment of the globus pallidus (GPi). Note the edema in the pallidofugal tract.

(51–53,58–62,66). Complete relief of contralateral dyskinesias has been reported in most patients in most studies. Contralateral benefit was largely sustained when the patients of Samii et al. (59) and Lang et al. (51) were evaluated 2 years after pallidotomy. Significant relief of ipsilateral dyskinesias

is common but more modest than contralateral effects. Although most centers report loss of ipsilateral benefit by 1 to 2 years, the NIH randomized clinical trial observed extension of benefit to 2 years (65). Axial dyskinesias also improve after pallidotomy (42% to 50% improvement).

Tremor

Tremor was the primary indication for surgical intervention in the pre–L-dopa era. It remains a major indication in many instances and is a significant component of the clinical syndrome in patients with PD who undergo pallidotomy in more than 60% of cases (52, 60–62). As with dyskinesias, benefit is seen bilaterally but is sustained over time only on the contralateral side. The magnitude in reduction in the Unified Parkinson's Disease Rating Scale (UPDRS) (67) subscale for tremor varies widely in the literature. At 3 months postoperatively, reduction of contralateral "off" tremor scores ranged from 33% to 75% (52,53,56,57,68), at 6 months from 43% to 79% (51,52,56,57,60,68,69), and at 1 year from 53% to 93% (51,52,57,68,69). Data suggest that a more posterior lesion is most beneficial for alleviation of tremor (69). Thus, if lesion location or size varies among series, this would explain in part the differences in clinical improvement. Ipsilateral benefit in tremor control is seen in many instances. Reduction of up to 50% occurs after pallidotomy (57,59,69), but this ipsilateral benefit can be lost within 18 months of surgical treatment (59).

Rigidity

The benefit of pallidotomy for *rigidity* is generally high, but it varies among reports. Positive effects have been reported in both the "off" and "on" states, both contralateral and ipsilateral to the lesion. The benefits are most consistent on the contralateral side and most markedly in the

TABLE 11.1. ASSESSMENT FACTORS IN PALLIDOTOMY FOR PARKINSON'S DISEASE

Parameter	Laitinen et al. (73)	Iacono et al. (81)	Baron et al. (52)	Lai et al. (56)	Johansson et al. (61)	Kishore et al. (57)	Lang et al. (51)	Kondziolka et al. (58)	Vitek et al. (65)
No. of patients	32	126	15	89	22	20	39	58	36
Localization technique	CT	MRI Verticulography	MRI	CT	MRI	CT	MRI	MRI	MRI
Mapping technique	Macrostimulation	Macro-stimulation, micro-stimulation (n = 29)	Micro-electrode	Micro-electrode	Macro-stimulation	Macro-stimulation	Micro-electrode	Macro-stimulation	Micro-electrode
Assessment technique	Neurologic examination	UPDRS[a] Video	CAPIT	UPDRS Video	VAS UPDRS[a]	UPDRS	CAPIT	UPDRS Video	UPDRS
Mean age	60	62	57	62	64	61	59	67	58
Follow-up (mos)	2–71	1–12	12	12	12	6	6–24	9 months (mean)	6–24

[a]Modified.
CAPIT, Core Assessment Program for Intracerebral Transplantation; CT, computed tomography; MRI, magnetic resonance imaging; UPDRS, Unified Parkinson's Disease Rating Scale; VAS, Visual Analogue Scale.

TABLE 11.2. RESULTS OF PALLIDOTOMY FOR PARKINSON'S DISEASE

Parameter	Laitinen et al. (73)	Iacono et al. (81)	Baron et al. (52)	Johansson et al. (62)	Kishore et al. (57)	Lang et al. (51)	Kondziolka et al. (58)	Vitek et al. (65)	Lai et al. (56)
Tremor: contralateral	"Good or excellent" relief in 26/32	65% "off"	93% "off"	60% "off"	79% "off" 50% "on"	53% "off" (1 yr)	50% "off"	70% "off"	78% "off" (1 yr) 81% "on"
Tremor: ipsilateral			3 of 4 with improvement	33% worse "off"	57% "off" 68% worse "on"			67% "off"	55% "off" (1 yr) 11% "on"
Dyskinesia: contralateral			9/10–100%	33%-limb 42%-axial	76%	83% (1 yr) 0% (2 yr)	40%	75%	Duration 45% (1 yr) Disability 70%
Dyskinesia: ipsilateral			Unclear	33%-limb	41%	42% (1 yr) 0% (2 yr)		36%	Pain 87%
Rigidity: contralateral	"Good or excellent" relief in 35/38	70% "off"	Improved "off" No change "on"		55% "off" 38% "on"	54% "off" 29% "on"	38% "off"	55% "off"	55% "off" (1 yr) 71% "on"
Rigidity: ipsilateral			Unchanged		24% "off" 18% "on"			41% "off"	10% "off" (1 yr) 42% "on"
Bradykinesia: contralateral		61% "off"	Marked improvement "off"		43% "off" 18% "on"	41% "off" Unchanged "on"	24% "off"	39% "off"(UE) 27% "on"(UE) 41% "off"(LE)	47% "off" (1 yr) 57% "on"
Bradykinesia: ipsilateral			Moderate improvement "off"		32% "off" 7% "on"	19% "off" Unchanged "on"		27% "off"	25% "off" (1 yr) 29% "on"
Activities of Daily Living			26% "off" 14% "on" 69% S&E		25% "off"	30% "off" 30% "on" 67% S&E	6% "off" 6% "on" 10%-S&E	23% "off" 0% "on"	37% "off"(1 yr) 45% "on"

Improvement in percent (in general, according to UPDRS).

"off" state. Improvement in the UPDRS "off" score on the contralateral side ranged from 25% to 60% at 6 months (53,56,57,60,69), and it has been reported as high as 80% at 1 year (69). The effect during the "on" state is less significant, ranging from 25% to 38% at 6 months (53,56,69). Ipsilateral rigidity was not improved in one series in the "off" state (52), but it was reported to improve 22% to 40% at 3 to 6 months of follow-up by other investigators (53,69). Ipsilateral "on"-state effects are not commonly recorded in reports, but at 3 months they were improved 50% in one series (53).

Bradykinesia

As with rigidity, the effect of pallidotomy on *bradykinesia* is most significant on the contralateral side in the "off" state. Improvement in the UPDRS of 19% to 43% has been noted (51–53,56,57,60). Slight benefit has been reported in the "on" state by some authors, but it is minimal in general (51,56,57). Minimal to moderate ipsilateral improvement is reported in the "off" state in several reports (51,52); however, there is no or only little improvement in the "on" state (51,53). In a study of 41 patients with advanced PD, objective improvement of "off" bradykinesia contralateral to pallidotomy 3 months postoperatively was shown by significant improvement of both movement and reaction times (70).

Fluctuations and Percentages of "Off" State

Improvement in the amount of time spent by patients in the "on" state is reported by most authors after pallidotomy for PD. Fifteen of 20 patients reported decreased severity and depth of their "off" periods in the report of Dalvi et al. (68). This finding is similar to the report of Baron, in which there was significant improvement in the UPDRS Clinical Fluctuations mean scores (52). Patients also reported less recognizable "on-off" fluctuations. Although Johansson et al. did not report a decrease in the proportion of time spent in the "off" state, there was improvement in the quality of "on" time because of reduction of dyskinesias (61). Besides a direct benefit of pallidotomy on symptoms increasing the proportion of time in the "on" state, the reduction of drug-induced dyskinesias allows increased l-dopa therapy where appropriate. Both factors may be involved in improvement in proportion of "on" time and reduction of "off"-state severity.

Activities of Daily Living

There are various ways to evaluate a patient's quality of life. For evaluation of independent functioning in activities of daily living (ADLs), the ADL subscale of the UPDRS and the Schwab and England Scale of Functional Independence (S and E) are the most commonly reported methods. The

UPDRS ADL subscale is a rating of a patient's disability, whereas the S and E scale evaluates functional ability. After unilateral pallidotomy, there is an improvement in the scores in all reported series in the "off" state. Improvement in the "on" state is not as striking and is less likely to be sustained over time. Improvement in the "off" state measured by the UPDRS at 3 to 6 months was reported to be between 19% and 37% (51,52,57,60,62,68). The S and E scores improved between 42% and 73% (51,52,61). Although the gains in several studies were maintained at 1 year (52,53,57,68), the experience of Samii et al. was a return to preoperative functional performance at more than 3 months of follow-up (59). ADL performance while in the "on" state is more variable. There was no improvement postoperatively in some studies (53,58,68), significant improvement in others (51,57,60), and significant improvement that was subsequently lost within 1 year in others (52).

Overview of Results

The reason for the excellent response of dyskinesia relative to the cardinal signs of PD is unknown. However, in all reports, it has been the most consistently well-controlled aspect of the disease in nearly every patient suffering from it. The response of tremors can be nearly as striking, and the results are as long lasting as those for dyskinesias. However, the response is more variable across reports. The dyskinesias and tremors of contralateral limbs are those with the most marked and stable improvement. The benefit to the patient suffering with dyskinesias is usually immediate, but the benefit for tremors can take weeks to months to be fully appreciated. The benefit to the patient suffering from rigidity and bradykinesia is usually less pronounced but still significant, both statistically and functionally. Both these signs usually are improved immediately after lesioning. The outcome of gait disturbances was variable among different series. It is difficult to assess the functional benefit that a patient obtains after pallidotomy. Current methods generally emphasize the "off" state, so the overall improvements in the quality of a patient's life resulting from decreased motor fluctuations and increased functional capacities, both social and personal, are poorly reflected in these scores. What should not be lost in this review of results is that the randomized trial of unilateral pallidotomy demonstrated statistically significant improvement in all the cardinal symptoms of PD as well as drug-induced dyskinesias compared with best medical management (65).

Complications

Surgical *complications* can be broadly categorized as hemorrhage within the brain secondary to either passage of the lesioning electrode or recording electrode, hemorrhage sec-

ondary to creation of the lesion, neurologic deficits secondary to misplaced lesions, and medical complications associated with the procedure and hospitalization.

Among 303 patients who underwent unilateral pallidotomy reported in various series (excluding duplications) that noted surgical complications, there were four fatal intracerebral hemorrhages (1.3%) (51–53,56,58,60–62,68,71,72). There were also five nonfatal symptomatic hemorrhages (1.7%). Four of these nine hemorrhages were associated with the use of a sharp-tipped guide tube that is no longer employed. The incidence of asymptomatic hemorrhages is difficult to assess because few centers routinely obtain an imaging study in the immediate postoperative period. The incidence of hemiparesis was 2.6%, and the condition was permanent in 0.7% of cases. Facial weakness was seen in 7.0% of cases and was permanent in 1.3%. The incidence of visual field defects after pallidotomy reported in various series is highly dependent on whether formal visual field testing is routinely performed. If formal studies are performed only on symptomatic patients or on patients with hemianopsis discovered on confrontational visual field testing, the reported incidence is lower. Symptomatic permanent visual field defects occurred in 2.7% cases without formal visual field testing performed on all patients, excluding those of Laitinen et al. (73). However, in several studies with routine formal visual field testing, the incidence was higher (56,74). There was new or worsening dysarthria or dysphagia 5.6% of the time, and this was permanent in 2.6% of cases. Delayed infarction in the posterior internal capsule limb 10 to 117 days after pallidotomy was seen in patients suffering from previous cerebrovascular disease (75). This finding may indicate an increased risk in this subpopulation for ablative lesioning. This may be a relative indication for deep brain stimulation if these findings are confirmed and if the infarct results from the lesioning and not the passage of the electrodes.

Other uncommon complications reported include hiccups, contralateral hemihypotonia that resolved spontaneously within 12 hours, urinary incontinence, three instances of frontal lobe dysfunction (two attributable to technical problems with the introduction cannula acting as the electrical ground during radiofrequency lesioning) characterized by inappropriate sexual behavior, apathy, and disinhibition. Also noted in the perioperative period by various authors are wound infections and self-limited confusion, especially in elderly patients.

Although there are well-documented risks to language and memory function after thalamotomy, the risk of cognitive dysfunction after posterior ventral pallidotomy is less clear. Prospective trials report mixed findings, but none show severe or disabling neurocognitive changes (76). Multiple reports of neuropsychologic outcome after pallidotomy documented minimal changes in most patients (52,65,77, 78). Those changes that were observed were mild to moderate declines in frontal lobe functioning and memory. Trépanier et al. noted hemisphere specific changes in cognitive functioning after unilateral pallidotomy (79). Left-sided lesions were associated with impaired verbal learning and phonemic fluency, whereas right-sided lesions caused transient decreases in visuoconstructive abilities. Because of the associated improvement in proportion of time in the "on" state, there was associated improvement in allocation of attention resources. This translated into improvements in complex tasks, divided attention paradigms, and mental processing. The general consensus among authors is that only mild, if any, decline in neurocognitive functioning is seen after unilateral pallidotomy for PD in most patients.

Bilateral Pallidotomy

According to a nonexhaustive survey in 1996, 20% of patients who received a pallidotomy for PD underwent a *bilateral procedure,* of which 7% were staged and 13% were done simultaneously (80). However, this finding is not reflected in the published results of pallidotomy in which most reported cases are unilateral pallidotomies. The additional benefit of a second, contralateral pallidotomy is usually less than the initial procedure if the two procedures are staged (54), and the incidence of complications is higher. Although some authors belileve that bilateral pallidotomies can be performed without increased risk of speech and swallowing difficulties (73,81), this is not the experience of most investigators (80).

In a large series of bilateral pallidotomies, Iacono et al. did not report any clinical changes of this type (81). This report was limited in its description of prospective evaluation of neuropsychologic function, but it was noted by Ghika et al. as a complication in two of four patients treated (82).

Because of limited clinical improvement and two incidences of complete speech arrest during 12 staged attempted pallidotomies, Alterman and Kelly believed that bilateral procedures had little place in the treatment of PD (54). In a report of 12 unilateral and eight bilateral (simultaneous) posteroventral pallidotomies, Scott et al. noted significant declines in mean articulation rate and phonemic fluency scores only in the patients who received the procedure bilaterally (62). Concerns about hypophonia after bilateral procedures have led some centers to perform deep brain stimulation on one side and pallidotomy on the other or to place deep brain stimulators bilaterally (83). Ghika et al. described a case of a patient who had an acute reversible depressive state and dysarthria after placement of a pallidal deep brain stimulator contralateral to a previous pallidotomy. Through adjustments in the stimulator parameters, the syndrome was reversed while the patient maintained clinical improvement (82). The ability to adjust the effects of deep brain stimulation is a powerful rationale for its use.

CONCLUSIONS

Posteroventral pallidotomy for medication-resistant PD is an effective and safe palliative treatment for the disabling signs of the disease and of the dyskinesias associated with its pharmacologic therapy. The increasing use of deep brain stimulation will diminish the need for pallidotomy but will not completely replace it. In the future, it may be possible that transplantation procedures will allow restored function to patients with parkinsonism or that new medications will more effectively treat the symptoms with fewer side effects.

REFERENCES

1. Puusepp L. *Folia Neuropathol Estonia* 1930;10:62.
2. Bucy PC, Buchanon DN. Athetosis. *Brain* 1932;55:479.
3. Walker AE. Cerebral peduncuotomy for the relief of involuntary movements. *J Nerv Ment Dis* 1952;116:766–775.
4. Broager B. The surgical treatment of parkinsonism. *Acta Neurol Scand* 1963;39:181–187.
5. Putnam T. Treatment of unilateral paralysis agitans by section of the lateral pyramidal tract. *Arch Neurol* 1940;44:950–976.
6. Oliver LC. Surgery in Parkinson's disease: division of the lateral pyramidal tract for tremor. *Lancet* 1949;1:910–913.
7. Meyers R. Surgical procedure for postencephalic tremor, with notes on the physiology of the premotor fibres. *Arch Neurol Psychiatry* 1940;44:455–459.
8. Meyers R. Surgical interruption of the pallidofugal fibers: its effect on the syndrome of paralysis agitans and technical considerations in its application. *NY State J Med* 1942;42:317–325.
9. Meyers R. Surgical procedure for postencephalic tremor, with notes on the physiology of premotor fibers. *Arch Neurol* 1940;44:455–457.
10. Meyers R. Surgical experiments in the therapy of certain extrapyramidal diseases: a current evaluation. *Acta Psychiatr Neurol Scand Suppl* 1951;67:1–42.
11. Cooper IS. Ligation of the anterior choroidal artery for involuntary movements and parkinsonism. *Psychiatr Q* 1953;27:317–319.
12. Cooper IS. Surgical occlusion of the anterior choroidal artery in parkinsonism. *Surg Gynecol Obstet* 1954;99:207–219.
13. Spiegel EA, Wycis HT. Pallido-ansotomy: anatomic-physiological foundation and histopathologic control. In: Field WS, ed. *Pathogenesis and treatment of parkinsonism.* Springfield, IL: Charles C Thomas, 1958:86–105.
14. Krauss JK, Grossman RG. Historical review of pallidal surgery for treatment of parkinsonism and other movement disorders. In: Krauss JK, Grossman RG, Jankovic J, eds. *Pallidal surgery for the treatment of Parkinson's disease and movement disorders.* Philadelphia: Lippincott–Raven, 1998:1–23.
15. Hassler R. Die extrapyramidalen Rindensysteme und die zentrale Regelung der Motorik. *Dtsch Z Nervenheilk* 1956;175:233–258.
16. Hassler R, Riechert T. Indikationen und Lokalisationsmethode der gezielten Hirnoperationen. *Nervenarzt* 1954;25:441–447.
17. Hassler R, Mundinger F, Riechert T. Correlations between clinical and autopic findings in stereotaxic operations in parkinsonism. *Confin Neurol* 1965;26:282–290.
18. Hassler R, Riechert T, Mundinger F. Physiological observations in stereotaxic in extrapyramidal motor disturbances. *Brain* 1960;83:337–351.

19. Svennilson E, Torvik A, Lowe R. Treatment of parkinsonism by stereotactic thermolesions in the pallidal region: a clinical evaluation of 81 patients. *Acta Psychiatr Neurol Scand* 1960;35:358–377.

20. Cotzias GC, Van Woert MH, Schiffer LM. Aromatic amino acids and modification of parkinsonism. *N Engl J Med* 1967;276:374–379.

21. Schwab RS, England AC Jr, Poskanzer DC, et al. Amantadine in the treatment of Parkinson's disease. *JAMA* 1969;208:1168–1170.

22. Klawans HL, Topel JL, Bergen D. Deanol in the treatment of levodopa-induced dyskinesias. *Neurology* 1975;25:290–293.

23. DeLong MR, Crutcher MD, Georgopoulos AP. Primate globus pallidus and subthalamic nucleus: functional organization. *J Neurophysiol* 1985;53:530–543.

24. Alexander GE, DeLong MR, Strick PL. Parallel organization of functionally segregated circuits linking basal ganglia and cortex. *Annu Rev Neurosci* 1986;9:357–381.

25. Alexander GE, Crutcher MD, DeLong MR. Basal ganglia-thalamocortical circuits: parallel substrates for motor, oculomotor, "prefrontal" and "limbic" functions. *Prog Brain Res* 1990;85:119–146.

26. Albin RL, Young AB, Penney JB. The functional anatomy of basal ganglia disorders. *Trends Neurosci* 1989;12:366.

27. Vitek JL, Bakay RA, Hashimoto T, et al. Microelectrode-guided pallidotomy: technical approach and its application in medically intractable Parkinson's disease. *J Neurosurg* 1998;88:1027–1043.

28. Lozano A, Hutchison W, Kiss Z, et al. Methods for microelectrode-guided posteroventral pallidotomy. *J Neurosurg* 1996;84:194–202.

29. Bakay RAE, Sladek JR. Fetal tissue grafting into the central nervous system: yesterday, today and tomorrow. *Neurosurgery* 1993;33:645–647.

30. Watts RL, Subramanian T, Freeman A, et al. Effect of stereotaxic intrastriatal cografts of autologous adrenal medulla and peripheral nerve in Parkinson's disease: 2-year follow-up study. *Exp Neurol* 1997;147:510–517.

31. Schnider S, Kwong R, Kwan H, et al. Detection of feedback in the central nervous system of parkinsonian patients. *Trans IEEE Decision Control* 1986;25:291–294.

32. Tatton WG, Lee RG. Evidence for abnormal long-loop reflexes in rigid parkinsonian patients. *Brain Res* 1975;100:671–676.

33. Filion M, Tremblay L, Bedard PJ. Abnormal influences of passive limb movement on the activity of globus pallidus neurons in parkinsonian monkeys. *Brain Res* 1988;444:165–176.

34. Miller WC, DeLong MR. Altered tonic activity of neurons in the globus pallidus and subthalamic nucleus in the primate MPTP model of parkinsonism. In: Carpenter M, Jayaraman A, eds. *Basal ganglia: structure and fuction. II.* New York: Plenum, 1987:415–427.

35. Sterio D, Beric A, Dogali M, et al. Neurophysiological properties of pallidal neurons in Parkinson's disease. *Ann Neurol* 1994;35:586–591.

36. Taha JM, Favre J, Baumann TK, et al. Characteristics and somatotopic organization of kinesthetic cells in the globus pallidus of patients with Parkinson's disease. *J Neurosurg* 1996;85:1005–1012.

37. Pollack LT, Davis L. Muscle tone in parkinsonian states. *Arch Neurol Psychiatry* 1930;23:303–319.

38. Llinas RR. Rebound excitation as the physiologic basis for tremor: a biophysical study of the oscillatory properties of mammilian central neurones *in vitro*. In: Findley LJ, Capildea R, eds. *Movement disorders: tremor.* London: Macmillan, 1984:165–182.

39. Jahnsen H, Llinas R. Electrophysiological properties of guinea-pig thalamic neurons: an *in vitro* study. *J Physiol (Lond)* 1984;349:205–226.

40. Schell GR, Strick PL. The origin of thalamic inputs to the arcuate premotor and supplementary motor areas. *J Neurosci* 1984;4:539–560.

41. Pare D, Curro'Dossi R, Steriade M. Neuronal basis of the parkinsonian resting tremor: a hypothesis and its implications for treatment. *Neuroscience* 1990;35:217–226.

42. Giroux ML, Vitek JL. Pallidotomy: a treatment for Parkinsonian tremor? In: Krauss JK, Grossman RG, Jankovic J, eds. *Pallidal surgery for the treatment of Parkinson's disease and movement disorders.* Philadelphia: Lippincott–Raven, 1998:179–190.

43. Krauss JK, Grossman RG. Optimal target of pallidotomy: a controversy. In: Krauss JK, Grossman RG, Jankovic J, eds. *Pallidal surgery for the treatment of Parkinson's disease and movement disorders.* Philadelphia: Lippincott–Raven, 1998:291–296.

44. Laitinen LV. Optimal target of pallidotomy: a controversy. In: Krauss JK, Grossman RG, Jankovic J, eds. *Pallidal surgery for the treatment of Parkinson's disease and movement disorders.* Philadelphia: Lippincott–Raven, 1998:285–289.

45. Bakay RAE, Starr PA. Optimal target of pallidotomy: a controversy. In: Krauss JK, Grossman RG, Jankovic J, eds. *Pallidal surgery for the treatment of Parkinson's disease and movement disorders.* Philadelphia: Lippincott–Raven, 1998:275–283.

46. Eskandar EN, Cosgrove GR, Shinobu LA, et al. The importance of accurate lesion placement in posteroventral pallidotomy: report of two cases. *J Neurosurg* 1998;89:630–634.

47. Guiot G. Le traitment des syndromes parkinsoniens par la destruction du pallidum interne. *Neurochirurgie* 1958;1:94–98.

48. Tsao K, Wilkinson S, Overman J, et al. Comparison of actual pallidotomy lesion location with expected stereotactic location. *Stereotact Funct Neurosurg* 1998;71:1–19.

49. Alterman RL, Sterio D, Beric A, et al. Microelectrode recording during posteroventral pallidotomy: impact on target selection and complications. *Neurosurgery* 1999;44:315–321; discussion 321–323.

50. Eskandar EN, Shinobu LA, Penney JB Jr, et al. Stereotactic pallidotomy performed without using microelectrode guidance in patients with Parkinson's disease: surgical technique and 2-year results. *J Neurosurg* 2000;92:375–383.

51. Lang AE, Lozano AM, Montgomery E, et al. Posteroventral medial pallidotomy in advanced Parkinson's disease. *N Engl J Med* 1997;337:1036–1042.

52. Baron MS, Vitek JL, Bakay RA, et al. Treatment of advanced Parkinson's disease by posterior GPi pallidotomy: 1-year results of a pilot study. *Ann Neurol* 1996;40:355–366.

53. Samuel M, Caputo E, Brooks DJ, et al. A study of medial pallidotomy for Parkinson's disease: clinical outcome, MRI location and complications. *Brain* 1998;121:59–75.

54. Alterman RL, Kelly PJ. Pallidotomy technique and results: the New York University experience. *Neurosurg Clin North Am* 1998;9:337–343.

55. Krauss JK, Desaloms M, Lai EC, et al. Microelectrode-guided posteroventral pallidotomy for treatment of Parkinson's disease: postoperative magnetic resonance imaging findings. *J Neurosurg* 1997;87:358–367.

56. Lai EC, Jankovic J, Krauss JK, et al. Long-term efficacy of posteroventral pallidotomy in the treatment of Parkinson's disease. *Neurology* 2000;55:1218–1222.

57. Kishore A, Turnbull IM, Snow BJ, et al. Efficacy, stability and predictors of outcome of pallidotomy for Parkinson's disease: six-month follow-up with additional 1-year observations. *Brain* 1997;120:729–737.

58. Kondziolka D, Bonaroti E, Baser S, et al. Outcomes after stereotactically guided pallidotomy for advanced Parkinson's disease. *J Neurosurg* 1999;90:197–202.

59. Samii A, Turnbull IM, Kishore A, et al. Reassessment of unilateral pallidotomy in Parkinson's disease: a 2-year follow-up study. *Brain* 1999;122:417–425.

60. Masterman D, DeSalles A, Baloh RW, et al. Motor, cognitive, and behavioral performance following unilateral ventroposterior pallidotomy for Parkinson disease. *Arch Neurol* 1998;55:1201–1208.

61. Johansson F, Malm J, Nordh E, et al. Usefulness of pallidotomy in advanced Parkinson's disease. *J Neurol Neurosurg Psychiatry* 1997;62:125–132.

62. Scott R, Gregory R, Hines N, et al. Neuropsychological, neurological and functional outcome following pallidotomy for Parkinson's disease: a consecutive series of eight simultaneous bilateral and twelve unilateral procedures. *Brain* 1998;121:659–675.

63. Young RF, Vermeulen S, Posewitz A, et al. Pallidotomy with the gamma knife: a positive experience. *Stereotact Funct Neurosurg* 1998;70[Suppl 1]:218–228.

64. Ondo WG, Jankovic J, Lai EC, et al. Assessment of motor function after stereotactic pallidotomy. *Neurology* 1998;50:266–270.

65. Vitek JL, Bakay RAE, Freeman A, et al. Randomized clinical trial of pallidotomy versus medical therapy for Parkinson's disease. *Ann Neurol* (submitted).

66. Jankovic J, Lai EC, Ben-Arie L, et al. Levodopa-induced dyskinesias treated by pallidotomy. *J Neurol Sci* 1999;167:62–67.

67. Fahn S, Elton RL. Unified Parkinson's Disease Rating Scale. In: Fahn S, Marsden CD, Calne DB, et al., eds. *Recent developments in Parkinson's disease*, vol 2. Florham Park, NJ: Macmillan Health Care Information, 1987:153–164.

68. Dalvi A, Winfield L, Yu Q, et al. Stereotactic posteroventral pallidotomy: clinical methods and results at 1-year follow up. *Mov Disord* 1999;14:256–261.

69. Gross RE, Lombardi WJ, Lang AE, et al. Relationship of lesion location to clinical outcome following microelectrode-guided pallidotomy for Parkinson's disease. *Brain* 1999;122:405–416.

70. Jankovic J, Ben-Arie L, Schwartz K, et al. Movement and reaction times and fine coordination tasks following pallidotomy. *Mov Disord* 1999;14:57–62.

71. Shannon KM, Penn RD, Kroin JS, et al. Stereotactic pallidotomy for the treatment of Parkinson's disease: efficacy and adverse effects at 6 months in 26 patients. *Neurology* 1998;50:434–438.

72. Uitti RJ, Wharen RE Jr, Turk MF, et al. Unilateral pallidotomy for Parkinson's disease: comparison of outcome in younger versus elderly patients. *Neurology* 1997;49:1072–1077.

73. Laitinen LV, Bergenheim AT, Hariz MI. Leksell's posteroventral pallidotomy in the treatment of Parkinson's disease. *J Neurosurg* 1992;76:53–61.

74. Biousse V, Newman NJ, Carroll C, et al. Visual fields in patients with posterior GPi pallidotomy. *Neurology* 1998;50:258–265.

75. Lim JY, De Salles AA, Bronstein J, et al. Delayed internal capsule infarctions following radiofrequency pallidotomy: report of three cases. *J Neurosurg* 1997;87:955–960.

76. York MK, Levin HS, Grossman RG, et al. Neuropsychological outcome following unilateral pallidotomy. *Brain* 1999;122:2209–2220.

77. Soukup VM, Ingram F, Schiess MC, et al. Cognitive sequelae of unilateral posteroventral pallidotomy. *Arch Neurol* 1997;54:947–950.

78. Perrine K, Dogali M, Fazzini E, et al. Cognitive functioning after pallidotomy for refractory Parkinson's disease. *J Neurol Neurosurg Psychiatry* 1998;65:150–154.

79. Trépanier LL, Saint-Cyr JA, Lozano AM, et al. Neuropsychological consequences of posteroventral pallidotomy for the treatment of Parkinson's disease. *Neurology* 1998;51:207–215.

80. Favre J, Taha JM, Nguyen TT, et al. Pallidotomy: a survey of current practice in North America. *Neurosurgery* 1996;39:883–890; discussion 890–892.

81. Iacono RP, Shima F, Lonser RR, et al. The results, indications, and physiology of posteroventral pallidotomy for patients with Parkinson's disease. *Neurosurgery* 1995;36:1118–1125; discussion 1125–1127.

82. Ghika J, Ghika-Schmid F, Fankhauser H, et al. Bilateral contemporaneous posteroventral pallidotomy for the treatment of Parkinson's disease: neuropsychological and neurological side effects. Report of four cases and review of the literature. *J Neurosurg* 1999;91:313–321.

83. Ghika J, Villemure JG, Fankhauser H, et al. Efficiency and safety of bilateral contemporaneous pallidal stimulation (deep brain stimulation) in levodopa-responsive patients with Parkinson's disease with severe motor fluctuations: a 2-year follow-up review. *J Neurosurg* 1998;89:713–718.

Surgery for Parkinson's Disease and Movement Disorders,
edited by J.K. Krauss, J. Jankovic, and R.G. Grossman.
Lippincott Williams & Wilkins, Philadelphia © 2001.

12

PALLIDAL STIMULATION FOR TREATMENT OF PARKINSON'S DISEASE

PETER PAHAPILL
ANDRES M. LOZANO
ANTHONY E. LANG

Surgery of the internal segment of the globus pallidus (GPi) improves the cardinal manifestations of Parkinson's disease (PD) including tremor, bradykinesia, rigidity, and gait and postural disturbances and has a striking effect on the involuntary movements (dyskinesias) induced by L-dopa. Two pallidal procedures are in current use: pallidotomy and pallidal stimulation. Although the experience with pallidal lesioning is extensive, to date there are only a few reports involving small number of patients treated with chronic pallidal electrical deep brain stimulation (DBS).

Because of the potentially serious complications and the irreversible nature of lesions of the nervous system from pallidotomy, there is some reluctance to use this surgical strategy, particularly for bilateral procedures. Neurosurgeons have sought alternatives that achieve the effectiveness of pallidotomy while reducing the risks of permanent adverse effects. In this chapter, we review the indications and selection of patients, clinical results, and complications of chronic pallidal stimulation DBS.

PATIENT SELECTION

The *indications* for pallidal DBS are evolving. Current indications resemble those for pallidotomy. Patients considered good candidates include those with a diagnosis of idiopathic PD who experience motor fluctuations and drug-related motor complications and who experience significant disability despite best available medical treatment. Patients with "Parkinson-plus" syndromes or dementia are probably not good surgical candidates. Although pallidal surgery has

bilateral effects, the improvements are predominantly contralateral. Those patients with asymmetric symptoms can be effectively treated with unilateral GPi DBS. Additional indications for GPi DBS include (a) surgery contralateral to a previous pallidotomy (Fig. 12.1) in patients with bilateral symptoms (1) and (b) *de novo* bilateral therapy for patients with significant bilateral symptoms.

TARGET SELECTION

Although most groups are using a similar target for pallidal stimulation and pallidotomy, the *optimal target* within the pallidal complex for either procedure is yet to be determined. Because DBS may act through a variety of mechanisms, the optimal DBS target may prove to be different from the lesioning target.

Part of the difficulty in identifying the optimal target stems from the anatomic and functional complexity of the GP. Increasing evidence indicates that, within the GP, different regions subserve specific parkinsonian symptoms. This finding is not surprising given the segregated nature of basal ganglia circuits and the neuroanatomic evidence that subterritories within GPi project through a thalamic relay to influence separate and distinct cortical fields. In primates (2), the dorsal motor GPi relates to the supplementary motor cortex, whereas the central portion of the motor GPi projects to primary motor cortex and the ventral motor GPi area relates to premotor cortex. The segregation of these circuits within GPi in humans is supported by the observation that pallidal lesions in patients with PD have differential effects based on their location within Gpi (3). Further, differential effects of pallidal stimulation are seen depending on the position of the stimulating electrode within GPi. With the caveat that in the described studies the location within GPi or perhaps even the external segment of the GP is uncertain, some

P. Pahapill and A.M. Lozano: Division of Neurosurgery, Toronto Western Hospital, Toronto, Ontario, Canada M5T 2S8.

A.E. Lang: Morton And Gloria Sthulman Movement Disorders Clinic, Toronto Western Hospital, Toronto, Ontario, Canada M5T 2S8.

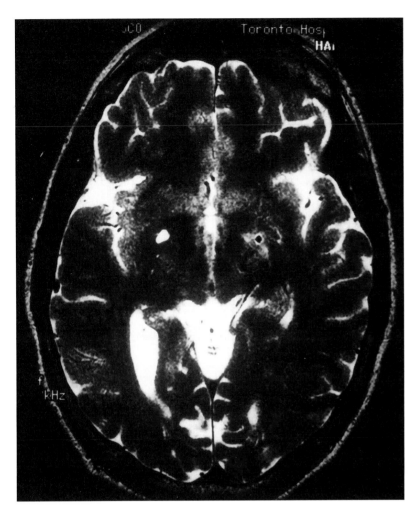

FIGURE 12.1. Axial magnetic resonance imaging scan showing a unilateral left internal segment of globus pallidus stimulating electrode contralateral to a previous right pallidotomy. (From Galvez-Jimenez N, Lozano A, Tasker R, et al. Pallidal stimulation in Parkinson's disease patients with a prior unilateral pallidotomy. *Can J Neurol Sci* 1998;25:300, with permission.)

investigators have reported an anti–L-dopa effect with respect to bradykinesia, but not rigidity, including the elimination of dyskinesias with the most ventral contacts of quadripolar electrodes and a prodyskinetic effect with improvements in parkinsonism (i.e., effects similar to those of L-dopa) when the dorsal contacts are used to deliver electrical stimulation (4,5).

Most published series report the use of microelectrode recording guidance for the selection of the pallidal stimulation targets. Bilateral GPi implants have been performed in one session or as staged procedures. All groups report high frequencies of stimulation for effective therapy (range, 130 to 185 Hz), with a range of pulse width of 50 to 200 microseconds.

CLINICAL RESULTS

Reports describing the effects of unilateral (73 patients) and bilateral (52 patients) chronic pallidal stimulation for PD are summarized in Table 12.1. Most reports were based on

a small number of patients with short follow-up. Fourteen series (reporting on a total of approximately 100 patients) presented results using standard Unified Parkinson's Disease Rating Scale (UPDRS) scores with a median follow-up of 6 months (Table 12.1). In nine studies, postoperative "nondrug" UPDRS scores were also reported. In four studies, blinded patient assessments were attempted (1,4–6).

Like pallidotomy, pallidal stimulation improves "off-drug" contralateral tremor, rigidity and bradykinesia, and "on-drug" dyskinesias. Improvements in "off-drug" UPDRS motor scores were reported in 11 of 13 studies and ranged from up to 50% with bilateral GPi DBS. In contrast, improvements in "on-drug" UPDRS motor scores were reported in only four of nine studies, with a mean improvement of 18%. Moreover, pallidal stimulation worsened some aspects of "on-drug" function in two studies (7,8), including increased freezing and akinetic episodes. Improvements in tremor were reported in ten of ten studies but only in the "off-drug" state (1,4–7,9–13). These results are very similar to those reported for unilateral pallidotomy, although increased "on-drug" freezing and akinetic episodes were not

TABLE 12.1. RESULTS OF CHRONIC PALLIDAL STIMULATION FOR PARKINSON'S DISEASE

Series (Ref.)	No. of Patients	Follow-up	Percentage of Decrease in UPDRS Motor, Off	Complications with Stimulator On
Siegfried and Lippitz, 1994 (9)	3 bilateral	6–12 mo	Not reported	None
Iacono et al., 1995 (20)	1 unilateral	6 mo	Not reported	None
Limousin et al., 1997 (24)	6 unilateral	Not reported	Mean, 40%	Not reported
Pahwa et al., 1997 (16)	3 bilateral; 2 unilateral	3 mo	Mean, 21%	1 facial dystonia, paresthesias requiring lead repositioning
Troster et al., 1997 (17)	9 unilateral	3–4 mo	Not reported	1 symptomatic basal ganglia hemorrhage
Bejjani et al., 1997 (4)	5 bilateral	10 d	Not reported; examiner blinded	Worsened akinesia and gait with ventral contact
Tronnier et al., 1997 (8)	6 bilateral	2–15 mo	No change	Increased freezing episodes
Gross et al., 1997 (10)	7 unilateral	12–36 mo	mean, 35%	None
Krack et al., 1998 (5)	5 bilateral; 3 unilateral	6 mo	mean, 32%; patient blinded	Worsening of speech, freezing, akinesia during on-drug state
Krack et al., 1998 (7)	5 bilateral	3–6 mo	mean, 40%	2 worsening of speech, 3 increased freezing
Kumar et al., 1998 (11)	4 bilateral; 4 unilateral	3–6 mo	mean, 27%	1 infection requiring lead removal
Galvez-Jimenez et al., 1998 (1)	5 unilateral	3–12 mo	mean, 33%; double-blinded	1 with a single seizure
Ghika et al., 1998 (12)	6 bilateral	24–30 mo	mean, 50%	3 with gait ignition failures; 1 lead repositioning for better effect
Volkmann et al., 1998 (13)	9 bilateral	5–17 mo	mean, 44%	1 infection; 2 skin erosions
Brown et al., 1999 (14)	6 bilateral	8 mo	mean, 42%	Not reported
Merello et al., 1999 (6)	6 unilateral	3 mo	mean, 30%	1 infraclavicular seroma
Vingerhoets et al., 1999 (15)	20 unilateral	3 mo	36%, mean total UPDRS	Not reported
Nieuwboer et al., 1998 (27)	5 unilateral	6–25 d	Not reported	Not reported

UPDRS, Unified Parkinson's Disease Rating Scale.

reported after pallidotomy. One study that reported worsening of these "on"-period symptoms as well as a lack of benefit in the "off" period failed to provide information about location of stimulated electrodes or stimulation parameters. It is possible that these results relate to the L-dopa–antagonizing effects of ventral electrode stimulation that were recognized subsequent to this report. As with pallidotomy, pallidal stimulation improved L-dopa–induced dyskinesias in all 16 published studies reporting this assessment (14,15). Improvements in "off-drug" activities of daily living (ADLs) of 25% to 30% were reported with pallidal stimulation in eight of eight studies (1,5–7,11–13,16), and improvements in "off-drug" axial symptoms (gait and instability) were reported in ten of ten studies (1,4,5,7,9–13,16). Improvements in "on-drug" ADLs were reported in only three of seven studies, mainly because of improvements in levodopa-induced dyskinesias (6,13,16). Again, these results are similar to those reported for unilateral pallidotomy. Although two groups reported a trend toward further improvement in scores with bilateral versus unilateral pallidal stimulation (5,16), this has not been shown consistently.

The percentage of the day spent "on" increased significantly in one study (16); it did not change in another (12). In three studies, the percentage of the day spent "off" decreased (12,13,16). As with pallidotomy, there were no re-

ports of significant changes in dosages of medications after pallidal stimulation.

Two groups reported that pallidal stimulation caused improvements in anxiety with "improved vigor" and reduced depression (13,17). However, these observations were limited to nine patients and at only 3- to 4-month follow-up in one group (17), and they did not approach significance in the other (13). "Off-drug" dystonia disappeared with pallidal stimulation in one study (7). There was no detectable difference in therapeutic results when comparing groups using microelectrode recordings and those using macrostimulation techniques.

Although the clinical effects of pallidal stimulation appear to be comparable to those of unilateral pallidotomy, the results are preliminary and more variable. Published pallidal stimulation studies (Table 12.1) suffer from a limited number of patients, often with unilateral and bilateral procedures mixed together from numerous groups using different surgical techniques, different targets, and various methods of patient assessment with short follow-up periods. Only one study was conducted in a randomized, prospective manner in which patients received either Gpi DBS or pallidotomy (6), and four studies were blinded (Table 12.1). Clearly, increased numbers of patients with longer follow-up periods are required to assess the effects of pallidal stimulation better.

COMPLICATIONS

Surgical Complications

Reported complications with pallidal DBS therapy have been minimal. There have been no operative deaths in 125 reported patients (177 implanted electrodes). One group reported a single symptomatic intraoperative subcortical hemorrhage (17), and another group noted a single seizure in the first postoperative week in a patient who was then treated with 3 months of antiseizure medications with no seizure recurrence or permanent sequelae (1). Transient confusion lasting up to 1 week has been reported, especially with bilateral procedures (5,7,13). There have been no reports of hemiparesis or visual field cuts, deficits that have occasionally been reported with pallidotomy. However, investigators have reported two infections (11,13), two skin erosions (13), one infraclavicular seroma (6), and two cases of intolerable side effects requiring lead repositioning (12,16).

Acute Adverse Effects of Stimulation

All groups commonly reported some short-term side effects with pallidal stimulation. These included the following:

1. Motor side effects such as eyelid closure (5,7), dysarthria (5,7,12), dyskinesias (1,5,7), limb and facial contractions (5,7,13), "dystonic posturing" (in some cases this may have been caused by capsular stimulation-induced tonic contraction rather than dystonia) (5,7,13,16), and freezing episodes (4,8).
2. Visual flashes (1,11–13).
3. Paresthesias (1,5,7,16).
4. Nonspecific sensations such as anxiety, panic, palpitations, nausea, and strange indescribable feelings (5,7,13,16). These sensations were voltage dependent and typically abated with chronic stimulation.

Chronic Adverse Effects of Stimulation

Ghika et al. reported intermittent gait ignition failure or increased freezing in three of six patients with bilateral pallidal stimulation persistent after 1 year after implantation (12). Another group reported worsening of "off-drug" akinesia in three patients and worsening of "on-drug" hypophonia with bilateral stimulation (7). Because of long-term side effects, two groups reported repositioning of electrode leads for better therapeutic effects (12,16). The efficacy of repositioning was not reported by either group. Long-term weight gain was reported in six of nine patients (13), as has been reported for pallidotomy (18). Two groups reported some loss of stimulation efficacy with time. One patient had a trend toward loss of therapeutic effect starting after 1 year (12). Another patient had appreciably decreased effects of stimulation at 1 year that were even more so at 2 years (10). This situa-

tion may have been the result of simple progression of the disease.

Psychologic Complications

In a series of nine patients with unilateral stimulation who were subjected to detailed neuropsychologic testing, statistically significant decrements were observed in only two tests, verbal fluency and Dementia Rating Scale (DRS) construction scores (17). In another series of 20 patients with unilateral pallidal stimulation, six patients experienced significant cognitive decline (15). These six patients were older (mean age of 62 years) and were taking higher preoperative daily levodopa doses (mean of 910 mg) versus the other 14 patients in the study with no postoperative cognitive decline (mean age of 52 years and daily levodopa dose of 660 mg). Decreased verbal fluency has been shown to occur with unilateral pallidotomy, and especially left pallidotomy (19). Two other groups reported subtle decreases in verbal fluency scores with bilateral procedures (12,13). This was uncommon and was not evident to the patients themselves. No such changes were reported for six other patients treated with bilateral pallidal stimulation (8). These studies support the relative cognitive safety of unilateral and especially bilateral pallidal therapeutic DBS procedures in contrast to bilateral pallidotomies (18). To this end, pallidal stimulation contralateral to a previous pallidotomy has not resulted in cognitive complications associated with bilateral pallidotomy (1). This finding remains to be confirmed in clinical trials.

ADVANTAGES AND DISADVANTAGES

Pallidal Deep Brain Stimulation Versus Pallidotomy

Preliminary results (summarized in Table 12.1) suggest that pallidal DBS provides therapeutic results similar to those of pallidotomy, and this finding is supported by a recent prospective, randomized comparison of unilateral pallidotomy with pallidal DBS in a small group of patients (6). Thus, similar results can be achieved without lesioning the brain, the integrity of which is preserved for any potential future therapies. Pallidal DBS represents an attractive alternative for patients who refuse lesioning. It may also be considered potential therapy for those patients who are cognitively challenged and who would therefore be excluded from a lesioning procedure, although the relative safety of DBS in this group of patients is not known, and these patients may have difficulty coping with the demands of the programming period. Inherent to DBS therapy is its adjustability, allowing for fine tuning of the system to minimize side effects, to maximize benefit, and to accommodate for titrations of medications and progression of the disease. In addition, different combinations of contacts (i.e., ventral versus dorsal contacts) can be chosen to tailor the therapy potentially to the unique symptom profiles of individual patients. The potential need for a repeat procedure, as is sometimes required with lesions, may be avoided by recapturing therapeutic effects by selecting different electrodes to stimulate or adjust the stimulation parameters. Of course, these advantages are offset by the disadvantages of having costly implanted metal hardware and its associated potential complications such as seeding of infection, extrusion, equipment failure, and the need for battery replacements, as well as the extensive use of medical staff resources to complete the many hours of programming and adjustments required to optimize the results.

Bilateral Surgery

Because unilateral pallidal procedures primarily treat contralateral symptoms, bilateral surgery is desirable for parkinsonian surgical candidates who typically suffer from bilateral limb symptoms as well as axial problems such as gait and balance dysfunction. Bilateral pallidotomy, although advocated by some groups (20–22), remains controversial because of a risk of postsurgical decline of cognitive function, change in personality, or bulbar symptoms (1,12,18,21). Thus, most surgeons believe that the additional benefits observed after bilateral pallidotomy do not justify the increased risk of side effects. Bilateral pallidal DBS was pioneered by Siegfried and Lippitz (9). There have been 11 reports of bilateral pallidal DBS in 52 patients and one report of pallidal DBS contralateral to a previous pallidotomy in four patients (Table 12.1). The key observation is that both bilateral pallidal DBS and pallidal DBS contralateral to a previous pallidotomy, in contrast to bilateral pallidal lesioning, have been well tolerated, at least in the short term (1,7,8,12,13), with minimal or only subtle cognitive side effects. The preliminary results suggest that bilateral pallidal DBS provides further benefits for axial symptoms such as gait and balance disturbances. Thus, bilateral pallidal DBS or pallidal DBS contralateral to a previous contralateral pallidotomy may provide a therapeutic advantage to bilateral pallidotomy for an appropriate subset of patients with parkinsonism. The potential benefits of bilateral pallidal stimulation have to be considered in light of other alternatives, including bilateral subthalamic nucleus (STN) stimulation.

Pallidal Versus Subthalamic Nucleus Deep Brain Stimulation

Three preliminary reports attempted to compare the effectiveness of STN and GPi stimulation in small samples of patients (7,11,14). Although clinical outcomes were comparable, greater reduction of antiparkinsonian medication coupled with lower stimulation amplitudes (resulting in longer battery life) in the STN group in these studies pointed to a possible practical advantage when stimulating the STN. The clinical differences observed were also reflected in differences in the pattern of cortical activation produced by STN and pallidal DBS in functional imaging studies (23,24).

Deep Brain Stimulation as a Research Tool

Altering brain function with reversible DBS provides numerous avenues of research in the human central nervous system. Magnetic resonance imaging visualization of electrode contacts is useful in correlating clinical effects with various electrode positions. The ability to turn the simulator on and off combined with functional imaging (including functional magnetic resonance imaging, positron emission tomography, magnetoencephalography) and electrophysiologic studies may allow additional insight into basal ganglia physiology and disease pathophysiology (23–26), as well as possible mechanisms of DBS. Such a line of investigation was used by Davis et al. (23), who showed that GPi stimulation in patients with PD activated supplementary motor areas. In this respect, GPi stimulation and pallidotomy appear to have similar effects on cortical motor fields. This observation, combined with the similar degree of clinical improvement observed with either lesions or stimulation in GPi, suggests that pallidal stimulation produces a net effect that is functionally similar to lesioning GPi. This finding suggests the possibility that GPi DBS may act as a reversible electrical blockade of the disrupted pallidal output that occurs in PD.

REFERENCES

1. Galvez-Jimenez N, Lozano A, Tasker R, et al. Pallidal stimulation in Parkinson's disease patients with a prior unilateral pallidotomy. *Can J Neurol Sci* 1998;25:300.
2. Hoover JE, Strick PL, et al. Multiple output channels in the basal ganglia. *Science* 1993;259:819–821.
3. Gross RE, Lombardi WJ, Lang AE, et al. Relationship of lesion location to clinical outcome following microelectrode-guided pallidotomy for Parkinson's disease. *Brain* 1999;122:405–416.
4. Bejjani B, Damier P, Arnulf I, et al. Pallidal stimulation for Parkinson's disease. Two targets? *Neurology* 1997;49:1564–1569.
5. Krack P, Pollak P, Limousin P, et al. Opposite motor effects of pallidal stimulation in Parkinson's disease. *Ann Neurol* 1998;43:180–192.
6. Merello M, Nouzeilles MI, Kuzis G, et al. Unilateral radiofrequency lesion versus electrostimulation of posteroventral pallidum: a prospective randomized comparison. *Mov Disord* 1999;14:50–56.
7. Krack P, Pollak P, Limousin P, et al. Subthalamic nucleus or internal pallidal stimulation in young onset Parkinson's disease. *Brain* 1998;121:451–457.
8. Tronnier VM, Fogel W, Kronenbuerger M, et al. Pallidal stimulation: an alternative to pallidotomy? *J Neurosurg* 1997;87:700–705.
9. Siegfried J, Lippitz B. Bilateral chronic electrostimulation of ventroposterolateral pallidum: a new therapeutic approach for alleviating all parkinsonian symptoms. *Neurosurgery* 1994;35:1126–1130.

10. Gross C, Rougier A, Guehl D, et al. High-frequency stimulation of the globus pallidus internalis in Parkinson's disease: a study of seven cases. *J Neurosurg* 1997;87:491–498.
11. Kumar R, Lozano AM, Montgomery E, et al. Pallidotomy and deep brain stimulation of the pallidum and subthalamic nucleus in advanced Parkinson's disease. *Mov Disord* 1998;13[Suppl 1]:73–82.
12. Ghika J, Villemure JG, Fankhauser H, et al. Efficiency and safety of bilateral contemporaneous pallidal stimulation (deep brain stimulation) in levodopa-responsive patients with Parkinson's disease with severe motor fluctuations: a 2-year follow-up review. *J Neurosurg* 1998;89:713–718.
13. Volkmann J, Sturm V, Weiss P, et al. Bilateral high-frequency stimulation of the internal globus pallidus in advanced Parkinson's disease. *Ann Neurol* 1998;44:953–961.
14. Brown RG, Dowsey PL, Brown P, et al. Impact of deep brain stimulation on upper limb akinesia in Parkinson's disease. *Ann Neurol* 1999;45:473–488.
15. Vingerhoets G, van der Linden C, Lannoo E, et al. Cognitive outcome after unilateral pallidal stimulation in Parkinson's disease. *J Neurol Neurosurg Psychiatry* 1999;66:297–304.
16. Pahwa R, Wilkinson S, Smith D, et al. High-frequency stimulation of the globus pallidus for the treatment of Parkinson's disease. *Neurology* 1997;49:249–253.
17. Troster AI, Fields JA, Wilkinson SB, et al. Unilateral pallidal stimulation for Parkinson's disease: neurobehavioral functioning before and 3 months after electrode implantation. *Neurology* 1997;49:1078–1083.
18. Lang AE, Lozano AM, Montgomery E, et al. Posteroventral medial pallidotomy in advanced Parkinson's disease. *N Engl J Med* 1997;337:1036–1042.
19. Rilling LM, Filoteo JV, Roberts JW, et al. Neuropsychological functioning in patients with Parkinson's disease pre- and post-pallidotomy. *Arch Clin Neuropsychol* 1996;11:442(abst).
20. Iacono RP, Lonser RR, Maeda G, et al. Chronic anterior pallidal stimulation for Parkinson's disease. *Acta Neurochir* 1995;137:106–112.
21. Scott R, Gregory R, Hines N, et al. Neuropsychological, neurological and functional outcome following pallidotomy for Parkinson's disease: a consecutive series of eight simultaneous bilateral and twelve unilateral procedures. *Brain* 1998;121:659–675.
22. Schuurman PR, de BRM, Speelman JD, et al. Bilateral posteroventral pallidotomy in advanced Parkinson's disease in three patients. *Mov Disord* 1997;12:752–755.
23. Davis KD, Taub E, Houle S, et al. Globus pallidus stimulation activates the cortical motor system during alleviation of parkinsonian symptoms. *Nat Med* 1997;3:671–674.
24. Limousin P, Greene J, Pollak P, et al. Changes in cerebral activity pattern due to subthalamic nucleus or internal pallidum stimulation in Parkinson's disease. *Ann Neurol* 1997;42:283–291.
25. Rezai AR, Lozano AM, Crawley AP, et al. Thalamic stimulation and functional magnetic resonance imaging: localization of cortical and subcortical activation with implanted electrodes. Technical note. *J Neurosurg* 1999;90:583–590.
26. Ashby P, Strafella A, Dostrovsky JO, et al. Immediate motor effects of stimulation through electrodes implanted in the human globus pallidus. *Stereotact Funct Neurosurg* 1998;70:1–18.
27. Nieuwboer A, De Weerdt W, Dom R, et al. Walking ability after implantation of a pallidal stimulator: analysis of plantar force distribution in patients with Parkinson's disease. *Parkinsonian Rel Disord* 1998;4:189–199.

ELECTRICAL INHIBITION OF THE SUBTHALAMIC NUCLEUS FOR TREATMENT OF PARKINSON'S DISEASE

ALIM LOUIS BENABID
PIERRE POLLAK
ADNAN KOUDSIE
ABDELHAMID BENAZZOUZ
JEAN-FRANÇOIS LEBAS

Three targets are currently used for surgical inhibition by lesioning or by high-frequency stimulation (HFS) in the treatment of advanced stages of Parkinson's disease (PD):

1. A thalamic target in the ventralis intermedius nucleus (VIM) and additionally in the centromedian/parafascicular nucleus (1).
2. The internal pallidum or internal segment of the globus pallidus (GPi), which was reintroduced as a target by Lauri Laitinen and Marwan Hariz (2), after it had been carefully evaluated by Leksell (3).
3. The subthalamic nucleus (STN), which has been our target since 1993.

Coming from surgical practice and from basic experimental research, we have long known the pivotal role in controlling various nuclei of the basal ganglia motor circuitry. During stereotactic lesioning of the thalamus for PD-related tremor of rest and for essential tremor, investigators have observed that stimulation at the site of the lesion can induce either an increase of the tremor or a diminution of the amplitude of the tremor. We established in 1987 that this duality of responses was related to the frequency of the stimulation (4–6). Low-frequency stimulation increased the tremor, and high-frequency stimulation (HFS) greater than 100 Hz resulted in complete abolition of the tremor during intraoperative test stimulation.

Although thalamic VIM stimulation is very efficient for treatment of tremor, it soon became clear that this approach

appeared to relieve only this symptom, without any significant improvement of the other parkinsonian symptoms, as has been already known from thalamotomy (7–23). Therefore, the evolution of the disease in these patients, who developed further rigidity and akinesia in addition to their initial tremor, made VIM stimulation ultimately useless (24). There was no solution for these highly disabling symptoms in advanced stages, except pallidotomy or, more exceptionally, neural tissue grafting, which was not and still is not useful at the therapeutic level (25). The data obtained by physiologists in rodents and monkeys showed that the STN played a key role in the organization of the basal ganglia (26–32), and this finding allowed us in 1993 to extend to it the concept of electrical neuroinhibition and to use it as a therapeutic target in human patients (33–36). This approach has proved one of the most effective neurosurgical procedures in patients with PD who are severely disabled by the natural evolution of the disease as well as by levodopa-induced motor complications.

In this chapter, we describe the application of electrical inhibition of the STN by chronic HFS to a consecutive series of 120 patients, and we discuss the mechanisms of action. Animal experiments (32) and our preliminary findings (33–41), as well as our current data, demonstrate that STN HFS actually inhibits the hyperactivity of the STN.

SPECIFIC INDICATIONS FOR STN HIGH-FREQUENCY STIMULATION

Indications

The current *indications* for STN HFS are advanced forms of PD, selected on the basis of the existence of "on-off" periods, involuntary abnormal movements, and periods of severe

Surgery for Parkinson's Disease and Movement Disorders, edited by J.K. Krauss, J. Jankovic, and R.G. Grossman. Lippincott Williams & Wilkins, Philadelphia © 2001.

A.L. Benabid, P. Pollack, A. Koudsie, A. Benazzouz, and J-F. LeBas: Department of Clinical and Biological Neurosciences, INSERM Preclinical Neurobiology U-318, Joseph Fourier University of Grenoble, Hôpital A. Michallon, F-38043 Grenoble, France.

akinesia despite high daily doses of levodopa. In the first hundred of our patients, indications were restricted to patients who had exhausted all benefits from medical treatment, after a mean duration of the illness of approximately 15 ± 5 years. Their mean Hoehn and Yahr stage was 4.4 ± 0.7 in the "off" motor condition and 2.4 ± 0.5 in the "on" motor condition. Most of these patients had lost their jobs and their autonomy in activities of daily life, they all needed assistance, and they could have lost their spouses. The argument in favor of operating only on patients with advanced disease was justified by the necessity during the evaluation period of the method to observe the real benefits and the incidence of side effects. Since this was confirmed, the current tendency is to operate patients at an earlier stage of their illness, when the initial evolution has demonstrated that they belong to the category of patients who will be rapidly disabled. These patients should be operated on before they reach a stage that is no longer compatible with professional activities, social relationships, and a satisfying personal life. They must respond to levodopa even if the duration of the pharmacologic effect is no longer functionally beneficial. The level of improvement at the "best-on" score during a dopa challenge is strongly predictive of the postoperative outcome. The presence of levodopa-induced dyskinesias (LIDs), which was formerly a typical indication for inhibition (by HFS or lesioning) of the GPi, is an additional indication for STN HFS because the significant lowering of drug dosage secondary to improvement of the patient's symptoms results, in turn, in the reduction of the dyskinesias. Tremor, which was the elective indication for thalamic VIM HFS, is even more dramatically improved by STN HFS, which we use now even when the patient has only tremor, because when the disease evolves, the other symptoms will not be controlled by the thalamic target. Therefore, when surgery is considered in the treatment sequence for a patient, STN is currently our unique target, because of its effectiveness in treating akinesia, rigidity, and tremor, as well as its indirect effect on the dyskinesias.

Of the 120 patients with parkinsonism who were operated on by STN stimulation, two suffered from parkinsonism and dementia, two had multiple system atrophy, and one had postanoxic parkinsonism. The benefit they received from surgical treatment was moderate or nil. Surgery did not prevent the subsequent worsening of nonmotor impairment and did not eventually justify its inherent risk. Patients who tend to fall spontaneously during their "best-on" motor periods (pull test greater than or equal to 3/4) should not undergo surgical treatment. Actually, only "off" motor symptoms responded to STN stimulation, proportionally to their presurgical response to levodopa. The age of onset of PD mainly affects the response to levodopa therapy, because it may increase the prevalence of nondopaminergic lesions of the brain (42). Therefore, a young age of onset of PD and a relatively young age at the time of levodopa-induced motor complications and a parallel young age at the time of surgery should favorably influence the outcome of STN stimulation.

Exclusion criteria are as follows: unstable angina pectoris; severe cerebral macroangiopathy; uncontrolled arterial hypertension; cancer or other life-threatening conditions; severe heart, pulmonary, renal, or hepatic failure; anticoagulant or antiplatelet therapy (aspirin and other nonsteroidal antiinflammatory drugs); and immunocompromise. Previous surgical treatment of for PD can be accepted, except if severe brain lesions resulted from the procedure. As a rule, one may consider that the failure of a previous operation, by definition, resulted from failing to involve the appropriate structure, which therefore may be targeted again. We have reoperated on several patients who were referred to us because their electrodes were not correctly placed, and repositioning led to satisfactory improvement of the symptoms. This finding stresses the importance of proper placement of the electrode at the target.

Patients with dementia who had a Mini-Mental Status Examination lower than 24/30 and a Mattis Dementia Scale lower than 130/144 were excluded. Patients with a Mattis Dementia Scale score between 120 and 130 must be considered on an individual basis after the completion of a neuropsychologic test battery to evaluate frontal lobe dysfunction. At the time of surgery, we exclude patients with hallucinations or psychosis, even minimal, and patients with severe depression in the "on-drug" condition, as assessed by the Beck scale or the Montgomery Asberg Depression Rating Scale.

Patients and Methods

From January 1993 to June 2000, we operated on 125 patients with PD (82 men, 43 women; age: 55.8 ± 9.25 years, minimum, 34 years and maximum, 77 years; age of onset: 36.0 ± 12.3, minimum, 27 years and maximum, 58 years), all of whom gave informed consent. We implanted 224 electrodes, in the last 123 patients during the same session. Implantation was bilaterally performed in the STN in 120 patients for bradykinesia and rigidity and unilaterally performed for predominant tremor in four patients. In one patient, STN implantation was contralateral to GPi implantation. This protocol received the approval of the Grenoble University Hospital and INSERM ethical committees.

All patients were treated by levodopa combined with a peripheral dopa decarboxylase inhibitor (mean daily levodopa dose $1,110 \pm 560$ mg), 73% were treated with an oral dopamine agonist, and 26% used subcutaneous apomorphine.

Clinical evaluations were based on the Core Assessment for Intracerebral Transplantation (CAPIT) (43). Videotaped evaluations were completed twice preoperatively and postoperatively at 3 and 12 months and then yearly. The resulting disability was assessed using the Unified Parkinson's Disease Rating Scale (UPDRS), the Hoehn and Yahr scale, a patient diary to evaluate the duration of akinetic periods over a 24-hour period, and video recording, while taking into account CAPIT recommendations. The motor examination of the UPDRS (part III) (44) was assessed in "off-drug" and "on-drug" conditions preoperatively and in four different conditions postoperatively: off-drug/off-stimulation, off-drug/on-stimulation, on-drug/off-stimulation, and on-drug/on-stimulation. Neuropsychologic evaluation was systematically performed for each patient preoperatively and each year postoperatively. The battery of tests included the Mattis Dementia Rating Scale (maximal score, 144) (45) for global cognitive assessment and a scale to assess frontal function adapted from Pillon et al. (maximal score, 50) (46) (including verbal fluency, two series of motor sequences, two series of graphic writing sequences, and the Wisconsin card sorting test) (47).

CONSIDERATIONS ON THE CHOICE OF DIFFERENT TARGET POINTS

Rigidity and akinesia are the symptoms that respond best to levodopa, and patients with severe akinetic-hypertonic forms of PD therefore depend most on medical treatment. Long-term levodopa therapy induces motor fluctuations and different patterns of dyskinesias that result in highly disabling "on-off" fluctuations, which constitute an important therapeutic challenge requiring alternative therapeutic strategies, such as surgical procedures. The VIM target has not proven to be able to reduce these symptoms significantly, either by lesioning or by stimulation. The observed effects of VIM stimulation on LIDs (48–50) may be related to involvement of adjacent structures such as the centromedian/parafascicular nucleus or the paralemniscal radiation (1). The reintroduction of the GPi as a surgical target has been very successful. Long-term follow-up of pallidotomies (3,51,52) and of pallidal stimulation (53,54) has shown that the effects are spectacular in LIDs but are less consistent in other symptoms, in that these procedures do not allow the decrease of drug dosage and may even require an increase (55–57). STN HFS has been proposed on the basis of previous extensive experimental investigation of the basal ganglia and the resulting concept of their functional connectivity (29,27). In parkinsonian monkeys, dopaminergic deafferentation induces hyperactivity in STN (30–32), and destruction (28,30) or HFS (29) of the STN suppresses rigidity and akinesia. This finding encouraged us to perform STN HFS in human patients, in whom we also observed the alleviation of akinesia and rigidity in the operating room (33–40). In our opinion, lesioning of the STN in human patients should not be considered, because of the high risk of inducing hemiballism, although there are reports of STN ablative procedures with mild or no complications (58). These apparently good results without complications are, in fact, related to very careful procedures producing very small targets, but the effects

may not be long lasting, and procedures may need to be repeated.

At this point of our practice, the targeting appears to be simple. Coordinates based on ventriculographic and magnetic resonance imaging (MRI) landmarks provide satisfactory preliminary pretargeting, which may be adapted to the individual patient by image fusion, to avoid magnetic distortion. The intraoperative neurophysiologic investigation (at least stimulation) using several 2-mm spaced tracts will correct the individual variations in such a way that we have not missed an STN nucleus in 244 operated sides. There are still improvements to be made, such as a better understanding of the functional somatotopy of this nucleus, mainly with regard to speech and facial expression.

SPECIFIC TECHNICAL OPERATIVE DETAILS

To ensure precise localization of the ideal target and to avoid too long a procedure for the patient, we divided the surgical procedure for thalamic implantation of electrodes into three sessions on different days and applied it to STN electrode implantation (24).

- Step I. Stereotactic ventriculography or MRI and implantation of titanium skull screws for repositioning.
- Step II. Implantation of electrodes into the STN.
- Step III. Implantation of the programmable stimulator.

Over our 7 years' experience, we have found it more convenient for the patient to be under general anesthesia during the first and third steps and to be awake, with local anesthesia, for the introduction of electrodes, when we need full patient cooperation. The surgical team may then easily plan the various steps. Stereotactic imaging, in particular, MRI, can also be scheduled more easily with this approach.

During step I, while the patient is under general anesthesia, titanium screws are implanted into the skull. Stereotactic positive contrast ventriculography under teleradiologic conditions with the patient in supine and prone positions provides a very precise delineation of the structures of the third ventricle, which are used to calculate the coordinates initially derived from the stereotactic atlases of Schaltenbrandt and Wahren and of Talairach et al. (59,60) (Table 13.1 and Fig. 13.1). Stereotactic MRI (1.5-Tesla Philips Gyroscan) is performed between steps I and II.

Step II, the stereotactic implantation of the electrodes under local anesthesia, is performed after 12 hours of drug withdrawal. Because of individual variations, the final target can be significantly different from the preliminary target, and it will be defined by the combination of the data obtained by (a) ventriculography using Guiot's scheme based on the anterior commissure–posterior commissure (AC-PC) line (21,61–63), (b) the MRI data, and (c) the results of electrophysiologic studies.

TABLE 13.1. COORDINATES OF THE SUBTHALAMIC NUCLEUS TARGET, (AVERAGE OF THE COORDINATES OF THE CONTACTS PROVIDING THE BEST CLINICAL RESULTS), EXPRESSED IN VALUES NORMALIZED TO AC-PC LENGTH AND TO THE HEIGHT OF THE THALAMUS (GUIOT'S SCHEME AND IN MILLIMETERS)

Coordinates of the Target		Laterality from Midline	Anterior to PC	Verticality to AC-PC
Normalized	Mean		5.17	−1.30
	SD		0.74	0.86
In mm with	Mean	11.63	12.19	−2.85
AC-PC = 25.66	SD	2.99	1.58	1.88
HT = 17.54				

AC, anterior commissure; HT, height; PC, posterior commissure.

Ventriculography provides a statistical estimation of the position of the STN. On the sagittal view, the nucleus is situated in the middle third of the AC-PC line, 0 to 6 mm below this plane, and at 10 to 15 mm from the midline (Fig. 13.1).

MRI, using T1-weighted sagittal images (IR-TSE), and T2-weighted coronal sections, provides the coordinates for the small, almond-shaped STN, which is 1 to 2 mm anterior to the red nucleus, 2 to 3 mm superior and slightly lateral to the substantia nigra, with the internal capsule at its lateral aspect, and the mamillary bodies at its posterior aspect.

Electrophysiologic testing helps to identify the STN. During STN HFS, continuous monitoring of rigidity of the patient's wrist reveals changes related to efficient stimulation. Microelectrode recordings show an increased neuronal firing rate in the STN as compared with the surrounding area, at the site where the best effects on rigidity and akinesia are obtained. STN cells produce large, asymmetric spikes with a firing rate of 35.2 ± 8.8 Hz and biphasic spikes at a lower rate (11.1 ± 2.3 Hz) that are responsive to passive movements and to tremor. Below the level of the STN, larger

spikes unresponsive to all types of stimuli can be recorded in the substantia nigra pars reticulata.

Two hundred forty-four STN quadripolar electrodes were implanted in 125 patients, parallel to the midsagittal plane (102 electrodes) or along a double oblique path (142 electrodes). These electrodes were fixed to the skull by a suture and dental cement.

During the postoperative period, the patient has a control MRI scan and undergoes the same series of tests as before the surgical procedure, with and without HFS. Internalization of the stimulators in the subclavicular area is performed within a week while the patient is under general anesthesia (step III). After implantation of the Itrel stimulators, patients are kept in the hospital for at least 3 weeks for evaluation of the effects of HFS and other symptoms.

Electrical Settings

The parameters for electrical stimulation are programmed after step III of the surgical procedure and at each follow-up visit. The parameters are set at a 60-microsecond pulse

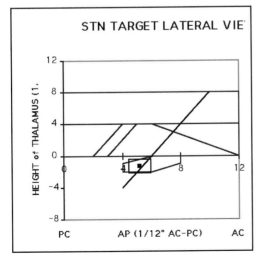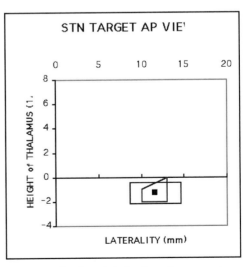

FIGURE 13.1. Schematic representation of the average target for the subthalamic nucleus according to Guiot's scheme *(black square and standard deviation rectangle)* and the trajectory of the electrode on lateral and coronal views.

width, 130 to 185 Hz, and 0.5 to 3.6 v, depending on the clinical effects and according to the needs of each patient. The effect of different electrical parameters is first studied in the "off-drug" state, with each contact successively selected as cathode with the pulse generator case as anode (monopolar stimulation). Beneficial effects on rigidity, akinesia, and tremor and adverse effects are evaluated. The contact that yields improvement of parkinsonian symptoms with the lowest voltage and without adverse effects is selected for chronic stimulation. The amplitude of the chronic stimulation is progressively increased over the first few postsurgical days. In the "on-drug" condition, the effect of the stimulation on dyskinesias is checked. Bipolar stimulation, at least one contact selected as cathode and one selected as anode, is used when the effect is better than that of monopolar stimulation. This has occurred, especially in patients with disabling dyskinesias during the postoperative period.

REVIEW OF THE CLINICAL RESULTS AND SIDE EFFECTS

Mortality, Morbidity, and Side Effects

The average follow-up of the 125 patients was 30 ± 21.0 months (minimum, 1; maximum, 123). We have analyzed the mortality and morbidity of 110 patients operated on since 1993, with a mean follow-up of 29.8 ± 18.9 months (minimum: 1; maximum: 83.6). The long-term follow-up on the benefits of STN HFS was evaluated in a series of 57 patients. There was no operative mortality. Seven patients died of various nonneurologic diseases at 3, 6, 7, 10, 11, 23, and 116 months postoperatively. Because of the long-distance referral of most of these patients, postmortem pathologic examinations were not available.

Three patients had symptomatic intracerebral hematomas (one patient from injury to a pericallosal artery branch by the exploratory electrode, and this patient died 3 years later; one patient from cortical bleeding; and one patient from thalamic hemorrhage, above the STN). Eight patients had asymptomatic intraventricular hematomas related to the transventricular approach or hematomas along the electrode trajectories on postoperative systematic MRI scans. One patient had a secondary scalp ulceration located in front of the electrode-to-extension connection.

Permanent hemiballism was not observed during clinical follow-up. However, acute and transient hemiballism, resolving within 24 hours, was observed in one patient at the moment of insertion of the permanent 3389 electrode. In several cases, advancement of recording electrodes and, in five cases, final insertion of chronic electrodes induced various degrees of peripheral limb dyskinesias and involuntary movements, which we considered symptoms of STN penetration. In three cases, a lesioning DC current leak from a defective test generator was responsible for hemiballism,

transient in all instances. One of these patients has continued to experience a major resolution of PD symptoms 6 months after surgery, thus making stimulation unnecessary so far. Seven patients were confused and disoriented for a few days to 3 months, and this was related to the clinical state and the age of the patients. Patients with this complication have not had any permanent sequelae.

Twenty percent of the patients exhibited transient eyelid-opening apraxia, and 30% of those patients needed botulinum toxin injection into the eyelids. Eyelid-opening apraxia is known to occur in patients with parkinsonism, but its pathophysiology is unknown. It could be related to the proximity of the substantia nigra pars reticulata, which projects onto the colliculus superior, which is itself related to vertical eye movements through the third cranial nerve, including extrinsic motor supply to the eyelids.

Hypophonia was also observed in about 20% of the patients. It must not be considered a complication of surgery because it may respond to increased doses of levodopa or even to stimulation. However, in these patients, the reduction in voice volume may be disabling because the patient is sometimes barely understandable. The current hypothesis to explain this phenomenon refers to the somatotopic organization of the STN: the present method of functional targeting is actually based on the rigidity assessed by passive mobilization of the wrist. It may be, then, that if midline functions such as motor control of facial expression and phonation are located in a different part of the STN, we may consistently miss it with the method employed. Therefore, when the patient, during chronic stimulation, enjoys marked improvement of rigidity and akinesia of the limbs, while the levodopa is reduced, it may be that there is insufficient therapeutic control of hypophonia. First, hypophonia is not surgically controlled because the electrode is not located in the STN area corresponding to voice control, and, second, it is no longer controlled medically because the levodopa dosage has been significantly reduced. This finding must be confirmed, but it suggests the need for intraoperative methods to explore phonation that would allow better targeting of hypophonia.

Worsening of motor performance is extremely rare and may be related more to the occurrence of HFS-induced dyskinesias, which are similar, than to LIDs. Fortunately, these conditions usually are observed when one uses voltages higher than those needed for improvement of motor symptoms. Most of the patients had weight gain related to recovery of normal behavior and loss of dyskinesias and not related to similar hypothalamic disturbances, as has also been observed after pallidotomy (64).

Clinical Benefits

STN HFS reduces tremor, rigidity, and akinesia. The clinical changes and the improvements in quantitative test results were strongly and rapidly evident when HFS was in use. The continuous follow-up of these patients (33,35) showed an increasing improvement of about 60% of all symptoms, evaluated on the corresponding scales, and a decrease in drug dosage of about 70% on average, which was responsible for the disappearance of LIDs, as long as drug dosages were progressively decreased. Thirty percent of the patients were free of levodopa medication at the time of the last follow-up. In all patients who had tremor, STN suppressed it in a way similar to that observed with VIM HFS, during the surgical procedure as well as during chronic HFS. As a general rule, it may be said that STN HFS provided the patient with a permanent level of improvement equal to the "best-on" status, and all dopa-sensitive parkinsonian symptoms were similarly improved. A detailed analysis of our first 24 patients who were followed-up for a period of at least 12 months showed that all items of the UPDRS scale were significantly improved, and this improvement was maintained over time for the majority of the patients (35).

UPDRS III Total and Subscores

Fifty-one surgical patients were followed-up for 1 year, 30 for 2 years, 16 for 3 years, nine for 4 years, and four for 5 years.

Off-Drug/On-Stimulation Condition

In the off-drug condition, stimulation greatly improved the UPDRS III total score in all groups of patients and at all follow-up periods in comparison with the preoperative evaluation. The improvement was more than 60% at the 1 to 3-year follow-up evaluations ($p < .0001$) and was maintained in the long term ($p < .005$ after 3 and 4 years). Whereas speech was not significantly modified, the scores for akinesia, rigidity, and tremor were greatly improved in the off-medication/on-stimulation condition in comparison with the preoperative off-drug condition, and this improvement was sustained in the long term. The degree of tremor improvement was the greatest, ranging between 63% and 100%. The rigidity score decreased from 50% to 76%. Akinesia was improved between 43% and 69%. The postural stability score significantly improved for all groups during the first years of follow-up. However, this improvement was no longer significant after 3 to 5 years. Gait significantly improved (between 52% and 70%). However after 5 years, the improvement decreased to 29%.

On-Drug/On-Stimulation Condition

In the on-drug condition, stimulation did not statistically change the UPDRS III total score in comparison with the preoperative evaluation. However, the patients followed-up for 5 years presented a clear deterioration essentially because

of two of the four patients. Speech was not significantly modified but tended to worsen at the 4- and 5-year follow-up. The postural stability score improved for groups 1, 2, and 3 ($p < .005$ only in group 2). In group 4 and 5, it was initially improved during the first 2 years of follow-up and then deteriorated after 3, 4, and 5 years ($p < .005$ after 5 years in group 5).

Off-Drug/Off-Stimulation Condition

In the off-drug/off-stimulation condition, the UPDRS III total score decreased from 7% to 22% in all groups and at all periods of follow-up in comparison with the preoperative off-drug condition. However, these differences were not significant. Speech tended to worsen in the long term. Akinesia did not significantly change. The tremor score tended to decrease, but this was not significant. The postural stability and gait scores were significantly improved in groups 1 and 2. In group 5, there was a progressive deterioration of postural stability after an initial improvement.

Axial Score

In the off-drug condition, the axial score greatly improved under stimulation. This improvement ranged from 55% to 77% and was statistically significant after 1 year, it was 55% after 2 to 4 years, and then it decreased to 37% at 5 years.

UPDRS II Total Score and Schwab and England Score for Global Activities of Daily Living

In the off-drug condition, the UPDRS II decreased in all groups and at all follow-up periods. After 1 year, the score decreased by 58% to 64% in all groups ($p < .0001$ for groups 1 to 4). This improvement was maintained at the longest follow-up (decreased by 51% to 61%). The Schwab and England score improved by more than 100% for all groups and at all follow-up periods. In the on-drug condition, the UPDRS II and Schwab and England scores did not change.

ADVANTAGES AND DISADVANTAGES

Advantages

Possible Neuroprotection

The observation of the STN glutamatergic output shutdown led us to expect a beneficial effect of HFS on the degenerative process underlying PD. Preliminary experiments indeed demonstrated that STN destruction prevents the nigral degeneration of dopaminergic cells after injection of

6-hydroxydopamine (6-OHDA) into the caudate nucleus (65). As shown earlier, in the off-drug/off-stimulation condition, the UPDRS III total score decreased, but not significantly, in all groups and at all periods of follow-up in comparison with the preoperative off-drug condition. The overall conclusion of this nonrandomized, nonblinded, noncontrolled study cannot provide arguments to address this important hypothesis, which we raised on the basis of the shutdown of STN activity after HFS, which could suggest that the glutamate output of STN neurons was suppressed or diminished. Experimental data from our laboratory tend to support this hypothesis. The proof could come from the observation of significant stability or, even better, an improvement, of the off-drug/off-stimulation scores, but the discomfort of the patients in this condition was so intense that it was not possible to observe the scores after a sufficiently long period to avoid long-lasting effects of stimulation or of drugs. We have to take into account that most of our patients, especially in the first 75 cases, had reached a far advanced stage of the disease in which the dopaminergic damage is extremely important. However, the present results are still consistent, as shown earlier, with this hypothesis because they tend to show an average stability of the scores related to so-called dopamine-sensitive symptoms, and they warrant a controlled study in patients with a shorter duration of illness, a lower degree of severity, and the use of non–drug-dependent parameters for evaluation, such as positron emission tomography and single photon emission computed tomography studies.

Comparison with Other Surgical Methods

Pallidotomy and High-Frequency Stimulation Globus Pallidus Internal Segment

The present data, although preliminary, are already significant enough to demonstrate that STN HFS relieves parkinsonian tremor, rigidity, akinesia, and LIDs, and it has no inherent complications, such as hemiballism, and no specific side effects. Ventroposterolateral pallidotomy has been recently reintroduced and is under investigation in several centers (64,66–70). The results reported in some studies were similar to those of STN HFS, but bilateral procedures have been reported to produce cognitive dysfunction. Moreover, the growing experience acquired by several teams with pallidal HFS (51–54,56,71) tends to suggests that the pallidal inhibitions could be done by HFS rather than by destruction, at least because bilateral procedures cause less morbidity using HFS methods. However, our experience with GPi HFS allowed us to compare the merits of the two methods in two matched series of patients with young-onset parkinsonism (Fig. 13.2), and our conclusions favor STN HFS, which has become our preferred method for treatment of akinetic-rigid and tremor-associated PD (53,54,56).

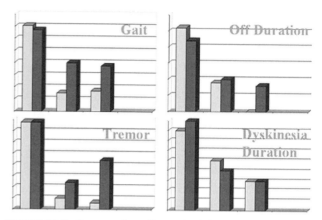

FIGURE 13.2. Comparative effects of subthalamic nucleus high-frequency stimulation (HFS) *(white columns)* and HFS of the internal segment of the globus pallidus *(black columns)* in two comparable series of bilaterally implanted patients with young-onset parkinsonism. Four items (gait, duration of "off" stage, dyskinesias, and tremor) were compared at the preoperative stage (OFF medication), at 6 and 36 months postoperatively (OFF medication, ON stimulation).

Neural Grafts

In our opinion, the indications for STN HFS are the same as those for neural grafts. Considering the ethical and technical problems raised by neural grafts that are still not resolved and the only moderate improvement reported so far, STN HFS can be offered as a reasonable alternative that leaves the future open, as long as neural grafting has not yielded significantly better results. (25)

Disadvantages

Costs

This method is obviously more expensive than thalamotomy or pallidotomy. In addition to the stereotactic procedure, which is almost the same in both methods, STN HFS requires electrodes, extension leads, and stimulators. Because of the high frequency at which they are used (130 to 185 Hz), battery life could be expected to be relatively short. However, in this series, so far we have changed only one Itrel II, after 74 months. The value of HFS STN is difficult to evaluate because there is currently no alternative procedure with which to compare it, given that ventroposterolateral pallidotomy is still under evaluation. However, the significant decrease in drug dosage we have observed in our patients who underwent HFS STN translates to a reduction in the cost of the procedure that must be evaluated further and seems already to be competitive with medical treatment. A French multicenter study is addressing this specific issue and is taking into account not only the drug dosage reduction but also the changes in needs for caregivers, medical visits, and accessories such as wheelchairs and the benefits in quality of life that are difficult to quantify, especially when loss of professional activity is concerned.

Targeting and Long-Term Stimulation

Targeting of STN is not difficult, provided good functional stereotactic practice rules are observed. It is not more difficult than targeting of the GPi. The STN is a smaller target, but the GPi is apparently composed of several subtargets with differential effects (53,55,56), and this configuration therefore requires a more precise positioning within the larger anatomoradiologic definition of this nucleus. The necessity of having in the operating room a team of neurosurgeons, neurophysiologists, and neurologists is not a drawback, but rather it is the consequence of the evolution of surgical concepts to meet all conditions necessary for the success of the procedure. Cardiac surgery has already reached this conclusion; neurosurgery has to do so.

Increased workload for neurologists has been reported as a drawback of the method: one must keep in mind that the patients involved by this method require a frequent and difficult, and still often unsatisfactory, follow-up by neurologists. Moreover, when the targeting is correct, the clinical improvement, as shown here, is rather long lasting and one follow-up per year is often sufficient.

Changing the generator is not a real drawback. This is usually done with local anesthesia as for cardiac pacemakers, and apparently it is required no more than every 5 years, perhaps even longer with the new double-chamber Kinetra (Medtronic. Minneapolis).

Infection is the neurosurgical consequence of an inadequate procedure and must be avoided. Late infection can be prevented by careful observation of the quality of the skin and placement of the leads and connectors under the periosteum, as well as by designing a flatter connector, which is actually under evaluation.

BILATERAL SURGERY

In our experience (34) and that of others (72), bilateral STN DBS improves the symptoms of parkinsonism considerably more than unilateral STN DBS. Bilateral simultaneous electrode implantation may be the most appropriate surgical option for most patients with bilateral as well as asymmetric symptoms. Because STN stimulation allows a major decrease in levodopa dose (34,36), parkinsonism may become unmasked on the nonoperated side. Unilateral STN DBS results in major improvement in contralateral tremor (37,38), and it can be advocated in some patients with highly asymmetric tremor-dominant PD.

Immediate postoperative morbidity has been observed to be higher in patients who undergo STN procedures than in those who have VIM procedures. The reason may be that the patient populations are different, although the STN-implanted patients are not significantly older (55.8 ± 9.2 years; n = 125). However, patients who undergo STN electrode implantation are in a more advanced stage of disease than patients of similar age (59.3 ± 11.4 years; n = 118) who undergo bilateral VIM electrode implantation and who most often are disabled only by their tremor and who have a better general clinical status. This higher morbidity could also result from the target itself and the difference in the stereotactic approach. The target itself does not seem to be responsible for the observed side effects because these were not always present. The tract, however, is closer to the midline, and it may involve at the upper level the white matter of the supplementary motor area or the thalamocortical frontal projections. In our last 69 patients in this series, we slightly modified the tract, using a 25-mm laterality entry point, which creates a double obliquity.

Nevertheless, the very low morbidity in this series stresses the good level of tolerance for bilateral STN surgery, as compared with the known high morbidity of bilateral ablative surgery in the thalamus (73) or in the GP (70). This finding also stresses the risks of ablative surgery in the STN, which may lead to a high percentage of severe hemiballism, even if one is careful, with lower morbidity but also with unstable results (58).

MECHANISMS OF HIGH-FREQUENCY STIMULATION

No currently available models can readily provide an explanation for the effect of STN HFS or VIM HFS on tremor. The Alexander diagram (27) provides a theoretic basis for explaining bradykinesia but not a clear-cut model for tremor, neither with regard to the role of the VIM nucleus nor with regard to the STN. In both cases, the response curve demonstrates the key importance of frequency. VIM HFS does not suppress tremor by means of an excitatory effect because thalamotomy or VIM inactivation by lidocaine injection produces the same effect. The mechanism of tremor suppression by VIM HFS could involve jamming of the neuronal network processing proprioceptive inputs from the spinal cord to the cortex, where a reflex response is elicited and is conducted to the anterior horn, which triggers a muscular contraction, inducing, in turn, a proprioceptive input. Feeding the system with artificial neural noise could deactivate this cyclic phenomenon and could stop the tremor, by making the network unable to recognize meaningful inputs. This hypothesis is supported by the existence of cells synchronous to tremor in the VIM (2,16,17,22,74–76) as well as in the STN.

It may be easier to understand the mechanism of action of STN HFS on akinesia and rigidity, which have been related in animals to the overactivity of STN cells increasing the inhibitory function of GPi (27,31). It could cause global hyperpolarization of the cell membrane resulting in a loss of excitability, or it could cause jamming of a neuronal loop, as we already suggested in the case of the VIM. Involvement of γ-aminobutyric acid (GABA)-ergic terminals resulting from the higher sensitivity of large myelinated fibers (77) could also be a possibility leading to local inhibition of STN neurons. Actually, little is known about long-term HFS of neural structures, and extensive experimental work remains to be done. However, we have reported experimental evidence in rats that HFS of STN induces an inhibition in the entopeduncular nucleus (equivalent in rat to the human GPi), in the nucleus reticularis thalami, and in the substantia nigra pars reticulata and an excitation in the GP (equivalent in rat to the human external GP segment or GPe) and in the ventrolateral nucleus of the thalamus (41). The mechanism could result from a local shutdown of the glutamatergic output of STN cells, as well as retrograde activation of GPe, which would therefore exert a strong inhibitory influence on both STN and GPi. However, recent data in our laboratory show that GP lesioning in rats does not induce hyperactivity in STN cells, nor does it prevent the effects of STN HFS on its efferent targets (78). The observation of the STN glutamatergic output shutdown led us to expect a beneficial effect of this HFS on the degenerative process underlying PD. Preliminary experiments have indeed demonstrated that STN destruction prevents the nigral degeneration of dopaminergic cells after 6-OHDA injection into the caudate nucleus (65,79).

Induction of laughter (80) or of transient acute depression (81) may occur at higher voltages and in lower contacts than those involved in production of beneficial effects. Therefore, one must be very careful before ascribing any observed effect directly to STN inhibition, and one should also consider the possible involvement of neighboring structures at higher amplitudes of stimulation.

CONCLUSIONS

In our experience, STN HFS is a remarkable tool and one of the most effective therapies for treating all symptoms of PD. Currently, it appears to be the method of first choice when the evolution of the disease and the failure of medical treatment suggest a surgical approach. The lack of permanent side effects and, moreover, the possibility of performing bilateral implantation in one session without significant permanent neuropsychologic side effects are the most important arguments in support of this method. The main features of this surgical approach are reversibility (particularly of side effects in case of misplacement of the electrode, which can even be changed or replaced), adaptability of the parameters to fit the patient's clinical status and even to follow the evolution of the underlying disease), and the possibility of performing bilateral implantation in one session without significant permanent neuropsychologic side effects (which is most often needed and was not easily possible to achieve by lesioning methods, such as thalamotomy or pallidotomy). Further-

more, levodopa doses can be reduced, and this subsequently decreases LIDs. Ultimately, the potential neuroprotection effect has to be mentioned. The relatively low percentage of permanent adverse effects makes the risk-to-benefit of this procedure highly favorable. Although randomized comparative studies between STN stimulation and other surgical procedures have not been published, long-term results of pallidotomy or pallidal stimulation appear not to be as favorable (2,51,54,67–71,82–91). Reports of STN lesioning are rare, and this procedure does not seem to be an alternative to HFS (58,92,93). The cost of the procedure of STN HFS has to be taken into consideration, but it is compensated for by the drug dosage reduction, the decrease in fluctuations of symptoms, the absence of severe complications, and the possibility that the patient may resume a normal and sometimes professional life. The mechanism of action is still unknown, and if the hypothesis of a high-frequency induced inhibition or jamming should account for the observed effects, a precise explanation is still needed. Moreover, this procedure does not exclude the patient from consideration of another type of treatment, such as fetal transplantation in the future.

Finally, STN HFS provides a privileged experimental opportunity, because of its reversibility and adaptability, to study and understand the mechanisms of PD as well as of normal motor control in human patients.

ACKNOWLEDGMENTS

This work was supported by grants from INSERM, MRT, CNAMTS, the Rhône-Alpes Region, the France Parkinson Association, the Fondation pour la Recherche Médicale, the Fondation de l'Avenir, ARSEP, CNEP, and the Joseph Fourier University of Grenoble.

REFERENCES

1. Caparros-Lefebvre D, Blond S, Feltin MP, et al. Improvement of levodopa induced dyskinesias by thalamic deep brain stimulation is related to slight variation in electrode placement: possible involvement of the centre median and parafascicularis complex. *J Neurol Neurosurg Psychiatry* 1999;67:306–314.
2. Laitinen L, Bergenheim AT, Hariz MI. Leksell's posteroventral pallidotomy in the treatment of Parkinson's disease. *J Neurosurg* 1992;76:53–61.
3. Svennilson E, Torvik A, Lowe R, et al. Treatment of parkinsonism by stereotactic thermolesions in the pallidal region: a clinical evaluation of 81 cases. *Acta Psychiatr Neurol Scand* 1960;35:358–377.
4. Benabid AL, Pollak P, Louveau A, et al. Combined (thalamotomy and stimulation) stereotactic surgery of the Vim thalamic nucleus for bilateral Parkinson disease. *Appl Neurophysiol* 1987;50:344–346.
5. Benabid AL, Pollak P, Gervason C, et al. Long-term suppression of tremor by chronic stimulation of the ventral intermediate thalamic nucleus. *Lancet* 1991;337:403–406.
6. Benabid AL, Pollak P, Gao DM, et al. Long-term suppression of tremor by chronic electrical stimulation of the ventralis

intermedius nucleus of the thalamus as a treatment of movement disorders. *J Neurosurg* 1996;84:203–214.

7. Derôme PJ, Jedynak CP, Visot A, et al. Traitement des mouvements anormaux par lésions thalamiques. *Rev Neurol (Paris)* 1986;142:391–397.

8. Fox MW, Ahlskog JE, Kelly PJ. Stereotactic ventrolateralis thalamotomy for medically refractory tremor in post-levodopa era Parkinson's disease patients. *J Neurosurg* 1991;75:723–730.

9. Goldman MS, Ahlskog JE, Kelly PJ. The symptomatic and functional outcome of stereotactic thalamotomy for medically intractable essential tremor. *J Neurosurg* 1992;76:924–928.

10. Hirai T, Miyazaki M, Nakajima H, et al. The correlation between tremor characteristics and the predicted volume of effective lesions in stereotaxic nucleus ventralis intermedius thalamotomy. *Brain* 1983;106:1001–1018.

11. Kelly P, Derome P, Guiot G. Thalamic spatial variability and the surgical results of lesions placed with neurophysiologic control. *Surg Neurol* 1978;9:307–315.

12. Matsumoto K, Asano T, Baba T, et al. Long-term follow-up review of cases of Parkinson's disease after unilateral or bilateral thalamotomy. *Appl Neurophysiol* 1976–1977;39:257–260.

13. Matsumoto K, Shichijo F, Fukami T. Long-term follow-up review of cases of Parkinson's disease after unilateral or bilateral thalamotomy. *J Neurosurg* 1984;60:1033–1044.

14. Nagaseki Y, Shibazaki T, Hirai T, et al. Long term follow-up of selective Vim-thalamotomy. *J Neurosurg* 1986;65:296–302.

15. Narabayashi H. Stereotaxic Vim thalamotomy for treatment of tremor. *Eur Neurol* 1989;29:29–32.

16. Ohye C, Maeda T, Narabayashi H. Physiologically defined Vim nucleus: its special reference to control of tremor. *Appl Neurophysiol* 1977;39:285–295.

17. Ohye C, Hirai T, Miyazaki M, et al. VIM thalamotomy for the treatment of various kinds of tremor. *Appl Neurophysiol* 1982;45:275–280.

18. Ohye C. Rôle des noyaux thalamiques dans l'hypertonie et le tremblement de la maladie de Parkinson. *Rev Neurol (Paris)* 1986;142:362–367.

19. Stellar S, Cooper IS. Mortality and morbidity in cryothalamectomy for Parkinson's disease: a statistical study of 2868 consecutive operations. *J Neurosurg* 1968;28:459–467.

20. Talairach J, Hecaen H, David M, et al. Recherches sur la coagulation thérapeutique des structures sous-corticales chez l'homme. *Rev Neurol (Paris)* 1949;81:4–24.

21. Taren J, Guiot G, Derome P, et al. Hazards of stereotaxic thalamotomy: added safety factors in corroborating X-ray target localization with neurophysiological methods. *J Neurosurg* 1968;29:173–182.

22. Tasker RR, Organ LW, Hawrylyshyn PA. Investigation of the surgical target for alleviation of involuntary movement disorders. *Appl Neurophysiol* 1982;45:261–274.

23. Tasker RR, Siquiera J, Hawrylyshyn P, et al. What happened to Vim thalamotomy for Parkinson's disease? *Appl Neurophysiol* 1983;46:68–83.

24. Benabid AL, Benazzouz A, Hoffmann D, et al. Chronic electrical stimulation of the ventralis intermedius nucleus of the thalamus and of other nuclei as a treatment for Parkinson's disease. *Tech Neurosurg* 1999;5:5–30.

25. Kordower JH, Freeman TB, Chen EY, et al. Fetal nigral grafts survive and mediate clinical benefit in a patient with Parkinson's disease. *Mov Disord* 1998;13:383–393.

26. Albin RL, Young AB, Penney JB. The functional anatomy of basal ganglia disorders. *Trends Neurosci* 1989;12:365–375.

27. Alexander GE, Crutcher MD. Functional architecture of basal ganglia circuits: neural substrates of parallel processing. *Trends Neurosci* 1990;13:266–271.

28. Aziz TZ, Peggs D, Sambrook MA, et al. Lesion of the subthalamic nucleus for the alleviation of 1-methyl-4-phenyl-1,2,3,6-tetrahydro-pyridine (MPTP)–induced parkinsonism in the primate. *Mov Disord* 1991;6:288–292.

29. Benazzouz A, Gross C, Feger J, et al. Reversal of rigidity and improvement in motor performance by subthalamic high-frequency stimulation in MPTP-treated monkeys. *Eur J Neurosci* 1993;5:382–389.

30. Bergman H, Wichmann T, DeLong MR. Reversal of experimental parkinsonism by lesions of the subthalamic nucleus. *Science* 1990;249:1346–1348.

31. DeLong M. Primate models of movement disorders of basal ganglia origin. *Trends Neurosci* 1990;13:281–285.

32. Feger J, Robledo P. The effects of activation or inhibition of the subthalamic nucleus on the metabolic and electrophysiological activities within the pallidal complex and substantia nigra in the rat. *Eur J Neurosci* 1991;3:947–952.

33. Limousin P, Pollak P, Benazzouz A, et al. Effect on parkinsonian signs and symptoms of bilateral subthalamic nucleus stimulation. *Lancet* 1995;345:91–95.

34. Limousin P, Pollak P, Benazzouz A, et al. Bilateral subthalamic nucleus stimulation for severe Parkinson's disease. *Mov Disord* 1995;10:672–674.

35. Limousin P, Krack P, Pollak P, et al. Electrical stimulation of the subthalamic nucleus in advanced Parkinson's disease. *N Engl J Med* 1998;339:1105–1111.

36. Pollak P, Benabid AL, Gross C, et al. Effets de la stimulation du noyau sous-thalamique dans la maladie de Parkinson. *Rev Neurol (Paris)* 1993;149:175–176.

37. Krack P, Benazzouz A, Pollak P, et al. Treatment of tremor in Parkinson's disease by subthalamic nucleus stimulation. *Mov Disord* 1998;13:907–914.

38. Krack P, Pollak P, Limousin P, et al. Stimulation of the subthalamic nucleus alleviates tremor in Parkinson's disease. *Lancet* 1997;350:1675.

39. Krack P, Limousin P, Benabid AL, et al. Chronic stimulation of the subthalamic nucleus improves levodopa-induced dyskinesias in Parkinson's disease. *Lancet* 1997;350:1676.

40. Krack P, Pollak P, Limousin P, et al. From off-period dystonia to peak-dose chorea: the clinical spectrum of varying subthalamic nucleus activity. *Brain* 1999;122:1133–1146.

41. Benazzouz A, Piallat B, Pollak P, et al. Responses of substantia nigra reticulata and globus pallidus complex to high frequency stimulation of the subthalamic nucleus in rats: electrophysiological data. *Neurosci Lett* 1995;189:77–80.

42. Blin J, Dubois B, Bonnet AM, et al. Does ageing aggravate parkinsonian disability? *J Neurol Neurosurg Psychiatry* 1991;54:780–782.

43. Langston JW, Widner H, Goetz CG, et al. Core assessment program for intracerebral transplantations (CAPIT). *Mov Disord* 1992;7:2–13.

44. Fahn S, Elton R. Unified Parkinson's Disease Rating Scale. In: Fahn S, Marsden CD, Calne D, et al., eds. *Recent developments in Parkinson's disease,* vol 2. Florham Park, NJ: MacMillan Healthcare Information, 1987:153–163.

45. Mattis S. Mental status examination for organic mental syndrome in the elderly patient. In: Bellak L, Karatsu TE, eds. *Geriatric psychiatry.* New York: Grune & Stratton, 1976:77–121.

46. Pillon B, Dubois B, Lhermitte F, et al. Heterogeneity of cognitive impairment in progressive supranuclear palsy, Parkinson's disease and Alzheimer disease. *Neurology* 1986;36:1179–1185.

47. Nelson HE. A modified card sorting test sensitive to frontal lobe defect. *Cortex* 1976;12:313–324.

48. Caparros-Lefebvre D, Blond S, Pecheux N, et al. Evaluation neuropsychologique avant et apràs stimulation thalamique chez 9 malades parkinsoniens. *Rev Neurol (Paris)* 1992;148:117–122.

49. Caparros-Lefebvre D, Blond S, Vermersch P, et al. Chronic thalamic stimulation improves tremor and levodopa induced dyskinesias in Parkinson's disease. *J Neurol Neurosurg Psychiatry* 1993;56:268–273.

50. Blond S, Caparros-Lefebvre D, Parker F, et al. Control of tremor and involuntary movement disorders by chronic stereotactic stimulation of the ventral intermediate thalamic nucleus. *J Neurosurg* 1992;77:62–68.

51. Lozano A, Lang AE, Galvez-Jimenez N, et al. Effect of GPi pallidotomy on motor function in Parkinson's disease. *Lancet* 1995;346:1383–1387.

52. Volkmann J, Sturm V, Weiss P, et al. Bilateral high-frequency stimulation of the internal globus pallidus in advanced Parkinson's disease. *Ann Neurol* 1998;44:953–961.

53. Krack P, Pollak P, Limousin P, et al. Opposite effects of pallidal stimulation in Parkinson's disease. *Ann Neurol* 1998;43:180–192.

54. Krack P, Pollak P, Limousin P, et al. Subthalamic nucleus of internal pallidal stimulation in young onset Parkinson's disease. *Brain* 1998;121:451–457.

55. Bejjani P, Damier B, Arnulf P, et al. Deep brain stimulation in Parkinson's disease: opposite effects of stimulation in the pallidum. *Mov Disord* 1998:13:967–970.

56. Krack P, Pollak P, Limousin P, et al. Inhibition of levodopa effects by internal pallidal stimulation. *Mov Disord* 1998;13:648–652.

57. Verhagen L, Mouradian M, Chase T. Altered levodopa dose-response profile after pallidotomy. *Neurology* 1996;46:A416–A417(abst).

58. Gill SS, Heywood P. Bilateral dorsolateral subthalamotomy for advanced Parkinson's disease. *Lancet* 1997;350:1224.

59. Schaltenbrand G, Wahren W. *Atlas for stereotaxy of the human brain,* 2nd ed. Stuttgart: Thieme, 1977.

60. Talairach J, David M, Tournoux P, et al. *Atlas d'anatomie stéreotaxique des noyaux gris centraux.* Paris: Masson, 1957:1–294.

61. Guiot G, Derome P, Trigo JC. Le tremblement d'attitude: indication la meilleure de la chirurgie stéreotaxique. *Presse Med* 1967;75:2513–2518.

62. Guiot G, Arfel G. Derôme P. La chirurgie stéreotaxique des tremblements de repos et d'attitude. *Gaz Med Fr* 1968;75:4029–4056.

63. Guiot G, Derome P, Arfel G, et al. Electrophysiological recordings in stereotaxic thalamotomy for parkinsonism. *Prog Neurol Surg* 1973;5:189–221.

64. Lang AE, Lozano A, Tasker R, et al. Neuropsychological and behavioral changes and weight gain after medial pallidotomy. *Ann Neurol* 1997;41:834–836.

65. Piallat B, Benazzouz A, Benabid AL. Subthalamic nucleus lesion in rat prevents dopaminergic nigral neuron degeneration after striatal 6-OHDA injection: behavioral and immunohistochemical studies. *Eur J Neurosci* 1996;8:1408–1414.

66. Eskandar EN, Cosgrove GR, Shinobu LA, et al. The importance of accurate lesion placement in psoteroventral pallidotomy. *J Neurosurg* 1998;89:630–634.

67. Lang AE, Lozano AM, Montgomery E, et al. Posteroventral medial pallidotomy in advanced Parkinson's disease. *N Engl J Med* 1997;337:1036–1042.

68. Dogali M, Fazzini E, Kolodny E, et al. Stereotactic ventral pallidotomy for Parkinson's disease. *Neurology* 1995;45:753–761.

69. Baron MS, Vitek JL, Bakay RA, et al. Treatment of advanced Parkinson's disease by posterior GPi pallidotomy: 1-year results of a pilot study. *Ann Neurol* 1996;40:355–366.

70. Tronnier VM, Fogel W, Kronenbuerger M, et al. Pallidal stimulation: an alternative to pallidotomy? *J Neurosurg* 1997;87:700–705.

71. Siegfried J, Lippitz B. Bilateral chronic electrostimulation of ventroposterolateral pallidum: a new therapeutic approach for alleviating all parkinsonian symptoms. *J Neurosurg* 1994;35:1126–1130.

72. Kumar R, Lozano AM, Sime E, et al. Comparative effects of unilateral and bilateral subthalamic nucleus deep brain stimulation. *Neurology* 1999;53:561–566.

73. Speelman JD. *Parkinson's disease and stereotaxic neurosurgery.* Thesis, Rodopi, Amsterdam, 1991:1–218.

74. Albe-Fessard D, Arfel G, Guiot G, et al. Identification et délimitation précise de certaines structures sous-corticales de l'homme par l'électrophysiologie: son interêt dans la chirurgie stéreotaxique des dyskinesies. *C R Acad Sci Paris* 1961;253:2412–2414.

75. Albe-Fessard D, Arfel G, Guiot G, et al. Dérivations d'activités spontanées et évoquées dans les structures cérébrales profondes de l'homme. *Rev Neurol (Paris)* 1962;106:89–105.

76. Albe-Fessard D, Arfel G, Guiot G. Activités électriques caractéristiques de quelques structures cérébrales chez l'homme. *Ann Chir* 1963;17:1185–1214.

77. Holsheimer J, Dijkstra EA, Demeulemeester H, et al. Chronaxie calculated from current-duration and voltage-duration data. *J Neurosci Methods* 2000;97:45–50.

78. Benazzouz A, Gao O, Ni Z, et al. High frequency stimulation of the STN influences the activity of dopamine neurons in the rat. *Neuroreport* 2000;11:1593–1596.

79. Piallat B, Benazzouz A, Benabid A. Neuroprotective effect of chronic inactivation of the subthalamic nucleus in a rat model of Parkinson's disease. *J Neural Transm* 1999;55[Suppl]:71–77.

80. Kumar R, Pollak P, Krack P. Laughter induced by subthalamic nucleus deep brain stimulation [Letter]. *N Engl J Med* 1999;341(13):1003–1004.

81. Bejjani BP, Damier P, Arnulf I, et al. Transient acute depression induced by high-frequency deep-brain stimulation. *N Engl J Med* 1999;340:1476–1480.

82. Golbe LI. Pallidotomy for Parkinson's disease: hitting the target ? *Lancet* 1998;351:998–999.

83. Galvez-Jimenez N, Lozano AM, Duff J, et al. Bilateral pallidotomy pronounced amelioration of incapacitating levodopa-induced dyskinesias but accompanying cognitive decline. *Mov Disord* 1996;11:242.

84. Samii A, Turnbull IM, Kishore A, et al. Reassessment of unilateral pallidotomy in Parkinson's disease: a 2-year folow-up study. *Brain* 1999;122:417–425.

85. Fazzini E, Dogali M, Sterio D, et al. Stereotactic pallidotomy for Parkinson's disease: a long-term follow-up of unilateral pallidotomy. *Neurology* 1997;48:1273–1277.

86. Kondziolka D, Bonaroti E, Baser S, et al. Outcomes after stereotactically guided pallidotomy for advanced Parkinson's disease. *J Neurosurg* 1999;90:197–202.

87. Samuel M, Caputo E, Brooks DJ, et al. A study of medial pallidotomy for Parkinson's disease: clinical outcome, MRI location and complications. *Brain* 1998;121:59–75.

88. Schrag A, Samuel M, Caputo E, et al. Unilateral pallidotomy for Parkinson's disease: results after more than 1 year. *J Neurol Neurosurg Psychiatry* 1999;67:511–517.

89. Pahwa R, Wilkinson S, Smith D, et al. High-frequency stimulation of the globus pallidus for the treatment of Parkinson's disease. *Neurology* 1997;49:249–253.

90. Gross C, Rougier A, Guehl D, et al. High frequency stimulation of the globus pallidus internalis in Parkinson's disease: a study of seven cases. *J Neurosurg* 1997;87:471–498.

91. Limousin P, Greene J, Pollak P, et al. Changes in cerebral activity

pattern due to subthalamic nucleus or internal pallidum stimulation in Parkinson's Disease. *Ann Neurol* 1997;42:283–291.

92. Guridi J, Obeso JA. The role of the subthalamic nucleus in the origin of hemiballism and parkinsonism: new surgical perspectives.

In: Obeso JA, DeLong MR, Ohye C, et al., eds. The basal ganglia and new surgical approaches for Parkinson's disease. *Adv Neurol* 1997;74:235–247.

93. Gill SS, Heywood P. Bilateral subthalamic nucleotomy can be accomplished safely. *Mov Disord* 1998;13[Suppl 2]:201(abst).

Surgery for Parkinson's Disease and Movement Disorders,
edited by J.K. Krauss, J. Jankovic, and R.G. Grossman.
Lippincott Williams & Wilkins, Philadelphia © 2001.

14

SUBTHALAMIC NUCLEUS LESIONING IN ADVANCED PARKINSON'S DISEASE

STEVEN S. GILL
PETER HEYWOOD

There was a resurgence of interest in functional neurosurgery for Parkinson's disease (PD) in the early 1990s with the demonstration by Laitinen et al. of the beneficial effect of pallidotomy in advanced PD (1). Most centers initiating programs in PD surgery advocated pallidotomy, unilateral or bilateral, but Benabid et al. showed more benefit with apparently fewer side effects from bilateral deep brain stimulation (DBS) of the subthalamic nucleus (STN) (2–4). As a result of the work by Benabid et al., many centers are changing target to STN. Lesions are less costly in time and equipment than DBS, but can lesions of STN be performed as safely and as effectively as DBS?

Some centers across the world have embarked on making lesions in STN. Results are few and preliminary and are reviewed in the following chapter. We emphasize that making STN lesions should be regarded as an experimental procedure, a technique that is in development rather than established, and not a technique that should be embarked on by teams without considerable experience in functional surgery for PD.

DEVELOPMENT OF THE SUBTHALAMIC NUCLEUS AS A SURGICAL TARGET

Strokes affecting the STN are known to cause hemiballism (5), but there are also reports of patients with PD who have improved after spontaneous hemorrhage into the STN (6,7). In recent years, surgeons have been reluctant to use the STN as a target for surgical lesions for fear of causing intractable hemiballism or biballism.

Pallidotomy and thalamotomy were first used successfully to treat advanced PD in the 1950s. Some surgeons attempted to improve their results with smaller lesions targeted at pal-

lidofugal fibers. These fibers pass through a small area within the H field of Forel that lies dorsal to the anterior STN. Lesions targeting this area (the procedure was sometimes called campotomy) were relatively common; Mundinger, for example, reported 500 cases (8). These lesions may well have involved the STN to a greater or lesser extent (9). Spiegel et al. reported campotomy in 25 patients with benefit and without major side effects (10). Andy et al. reported the results of lesioning in 58 patients (11). Their preferred target was the posterior subthalamus including the field of Forel and the zona incerta. Although they provoked transient hemiballism in five patients, in no case was it prolonged. The lesions were reported to be otherwise safe. Thus, although confirmation of target accuracy in the era before magnetic resonance imaging (MRI) was questionable, it is a misapprehension that surgical lesioning of the STN is new.

Surgical treatment for patients with hemiballism is sometimes used, and it is intriguing that an effective target is a lesion involving pallidofugal fibers and the zona incerta (12). These fibers lie immediately dorsal to the STN. Because it is likely that lesions or DBS of the STN will involve the zona incerta and pallidofugal fibers, it may be that damage to these areas is counteracting any prodyskinetic effect of the STN lesion itself.

The availability of an animal model of PD—the MPTP (1-methyl-4-phenyl-1,2,3,6-tetrahydropyridine)-lesioned monkey—by the mid 1980s resulted in greater understanding of basal ganglia function. In particular, the direct/indirect pathway model led to understanding of the pivotal role of the STN (13). Evidence from microelectrode recordings in MPTP-lesioned monkeys indicated that the STN becomes continuously overactive with a sustained increase in firing rates (14). Microelectrode recordings in patients undergoing surgical treatment for PD also demonstrated STN overactivity (15). Lesions of the STN in MPTP-lesioned monkeys have been shown to alleviate many parkinsonian symptoms (16–19). Bergman et al. lesioned the STN in two monkeys, and one of them had persisting

S.S. Gill: Department of Neurosurgery, Frenchay Hospital, Bristol, B516 1LE, United Kingdom.

P. Heywood: Department of Neurology, Frenchay Hospital, Bristol, B516 1LE, United Kingdom.

hemichorea at sacrifice. Subsequently, Aziz et al. lesioned the STN in six monkeys, three of which developed hemichorea persisting for up to 8 weeks. Benazzouz et al. reported on two monkeys who developed no hemichorea after STN lesions. Finally, Guridi and Obeso reported on eight monkeys of which three had hemichorea and one hemiballism after STN lesioning. Although the STN appeared to be a rational target for functional surgery in PD, the possibility of hemiballism has made surgeons reluctant in recent years to make lesions.

Benabid et al. observed that DBS in the ventralis intermedius nucleus (VIM) of the thalamus had the same beneficial effect as a lesion (20). They concluded that if side effects occurred with stimulation, these were reversible by turning off the stimulator. With the hope that any involuntary movements that would be caused would be reversible, these workers inserted quadripolar electrodes bilaterally into the STN (4). Benabid et al. demonstrated 60% improvement in most aspects of "off"-state parkinsonism, including improvement in gait and axial symptoms, that have even been reported to deteriorate with pallidotomy or pallidal stimulation (21). Unlike pallidotomy, STN stimulation allows reduction of L-dopa intake by approximately 50%, and consequently dyskinesia is significantly reduced (22). Thalamic lesioning or stimulation reduces tremor, but investigators have demonstrated that even in tremor-predominant PD, STN stimulation is as effective (23), and it is preferable because it will counter other PD symptoms not dealt with by thalamotomy. Therefore, the STN may well be the optimal target for any patients requiring surgical treatment of PD.

Implantable pulse generators are bulky and can be uncomfortable for the patient; they require regular adjustment, especially in the early months after insertion. Furthermore, they need to be replaced every 3 to 5 years. DBS has specific complications including electrode migration, electrode wire fracture, and electrical and mechanical problems with the pulse generator. There is the potential problem of induction by external electromagnetic fields, and as with any implanted device, there is a risk of infection. Lesions do not have these problems, but unlike electrodes, side effects may not be reversible, nor can lesions be adjusted, should their beneficial effect begin to wane. Most important, placement and maintenance of bilateral stimulators are expensive options both financially and in the time a neurologist will need to spend adjusting the parameters postoperatively. These problems make it inconceivable that the implantation of bilateral DBS electrodes into the STN could be a viable option for any but a few of the millions of patients worldwide who suffer from advanced PD.

In the late 1990s, unilateral STN lesions were reported in 11 patients by Alvarez, Guridi, Obeso, and their colleagues (24–27). The results obtained by this group, together with those of our group in Bristol, United Kingdom, are discussed.

We select the dorsolateral portion of the STN to place lesions, because this is recognized as the sensorimotor portion of the STN, it receives important cortical afferents capable of upregulating STN by 120%, and it also has efferents to the internal segment of the globus pallidus, the major outflow from the basal ganglia.

PATIENT SELECTION FOR SUBTHALAMIC NUCLEOTOMY

In general, indications and contraindications for subthalamic nucleotomy appear to be similar to those for other functional stereotactic procedures for treatment of advanced PD. The patient should be able to function at a reasonable level of independence for at least some part of the average day; our impression is that patients who are bed bound with end-stage disease do less well with surgical treatment. Age is not an absolute selection criterion, although analysis suggests that older patients do less well (28,29).

As described earlier, the evidence from bilateral DBS of STN from Limousin et al. suggests that STN rather than the internal segment of the pallidum is the preferred target for any patient with PD who requires functional neurosurgery, no matter what the predominant symptoms are (4). Even the patient with tremor-predominant disease who appears to be relatively little troubled by bradykinesia and rigidity will nevertheless progress to advanced disease; therefore, such a patient should be considered also for STN surgery. We can hope that as further evidence allowing comparison of outcomes in various patient groups emerges, it will be clearer whether this view is correct.

If it is decided for a given patient that STN is the appropriate target, then the issue of whether a lesion should be placed or stimulators should be implanted remains to be determined. Most patients with PD have bilateral symptoms and require bilateral procedures. Procedures that may be safe unilaterally may have significant morbidity when they are carried out bilaterally. The evidence is now clear that bilateral thalamotomy has significant risk of postoperative dysarthria and other problems (30–32), so most centers do not now contemplate bilateral thalamotomy. The evidence that bilateral pallidotomy carries significant risk is not clear cut. Some authors report few significant postoperative complications after bilateral pallidotomy (33); others regard bilateral pallidotomy as carrying too significant a risk to speech or cognitive function for it to be a surgical option for most patients (28,34). The Grenoble group reported no significant neuropsychologic deficit after bilateral implantation of deep brain stimulators into the STN (4), although some patients experienced hypophonia (Benabid, personal communication). The complications of unilateral and bilateral STN lesions remain to be determined—we discuss available results subsequently.

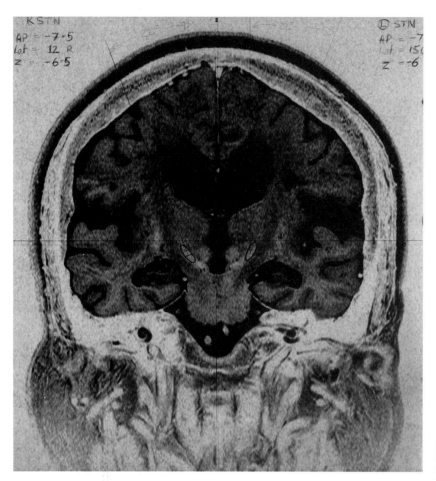

FIGURE 14.1. Coronal magnetic resonance imaging (inverted T2-weighted image) planning scan with subthalamic nuclei outlined.

PREOPERATIVE AND POSTOPERATIVE ASSESSMENT

Subthalamic lesioning is still at a developmental stage, and therefore patients must be rigorously assessed preoperatively and at intervals postoperatively. Members of the Bristol group assess all patients with the following protocols preoperatively and at least annually postoperatively: Unified Parkinson's Disease Rating Scale (UPDRS), Core Assessment Program for Intracerebral Transplantation (35), neuropsychometry, quality-of-life questionnaires, speech ssessment.

SURGICAL TECHNIQUE

No general agreement exists among neurosurgeons about the best and safest way to locate the target nucleus in functional PD surgery (34). The following procedure is adopted in Bristol. The STN is localized with high-resolution MRI T2-weighted scan sequences (1.5-Tesla TR 2,500, TE 150, TSE 11, NSA 12) and perioperative macrostimulation. While the patient is under general anesthesia, a modified Leksell stereotactic frame is fitted parallel to the orbitomeatal plane. The

anterior-posterior commissural (AC-PC) plane is identified on a midsagittal planning scan. Axial images, 2 mm thick, are obtained parallel to the AC-PC plane, and coronal images orthogonal to these are then obtained. We have found that these sequences give optimum delineation of the STN and related structures.

By using magnified hard copies of the MRI scans and after comparison to the Schaltenbrand and Bailey atlas (36), the boundaries of the STN are identified. The boundary of the STN is coregistered on the coronal and axial scans to give optimum three-dimensional target definition (Fig. 14.1). Stereotactic coordinates of the target, the dorsolateral portion of the STN, are recorded, and a trajectory is planned.

During the surgical procedure, patients are awake and in an "off" state, antiparkinsonian medications having been stopped 24 hours previously. A 1.24-mm diameter electrode with a 2-mm exposed tip (Radionics, Inc. Burlington, Ma.) is guided to the dorsolateral STN. The target is stimulated at 100 Hz and a 1-millisecond pulse width with an amplitude between 0.75 and 2 v, during which changes in tremor, rigidity, and bradykinesia are monitored. Because the procedure is relatively short, and patients are awake in the operating room for 1 to 2 hours, they are not so fatigued as

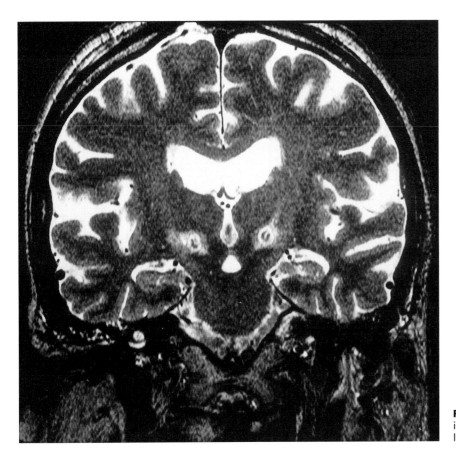

FIGURE 14.2. Postoperative T2-weighted image showing bilateral subthalamic nucleus lesions.

to be unable to cooperate with repeated clinical examination. Probe position is adjusted to gain maximal clinical improvement in the observed parameters without the development of side effects. At the optimal position, one or two radiofrequency lesions are made, typically at 80°C for 60 seconds.

The patient undergoes a postoperative high-resolution MRI scan to confirm lesion position (Fig. 14.2). Antiparkinsonian medication is reintroduced as required.

CLINICAL RESULTS OF SUBTHALAMIC NUCLEOTOMY

Three centers published their results of STN ablative surgery: Havana (24,25,27,37,38) and Bristol (39,40) and Ankari (41).

The Cuban group reported 11 patients who underwent unilateral subthalamic lesioning, in which the STN was localized with computed tomography and semimicroelectrode recording. These investigators reported improvement in axial motor tasks, facial expression, and all parkinsonian signs on the side contralateral to the lesion. The improvements were maintained for up to 24 months.

Hemiballism occurred in one patient 7 days postoperatively and was associated with an infarction of the whole subthalamic region and part of the thalamus. No other patients had hemiballism after the surgical procedure.

The Bristol group performed 54 STN lesions thus far in a total of 39 patients. Twenty-eight patients had unilateral lesions, 11 patients had 22 bilateral lesions. Seven patients had lesions on one side, with a deep brain stimulator placed on the other side.

We had two patients with major complications. One patient had an intracerebral hemorrhage superficially, not directly related to the STN; she had hemiparesis consequent to this hemorrhage and was rehabilitating well and mobilizing, but 2 months later she died of pulmonary embolism. Another patient had a seizure on the operating table. He has had no further seizures since then. Importantly, we have seen no major persistent complications directly related to STN as the surgical target. One patient had significant postoperative hemiballism on the contralateral side to an STN lesion, and it persisted for approximately 3 weeks. It gradually resolved without active treatment. Two other patients had minor choreiform involuntary movement after STN lesions that settled down quickly in the postoperative period. None had blepharospasm. One had significant confusion that settled after 3 months. One patient had worsening of his preexisting dysarthria.

All our patients after STN lesions showed improvement in contralateral tremor, rigidity, and bradykinesia. Patients still needed to take L-dopa; overall, their L-dopa intake was approximately halved, and with this was a reduction in dyskinesia by approximately 70%. Their activities of daily living scores in the subscale II of UPDRS improved in all cases. Total daily "on" time, without significant dyskinesia, more than doubled.

CONCLUSIONS

Preliminary results of STN lesioning demonstrate that this procedure can be carried out relatively safely and with good therapeutic effect. Despite this finding, STN lesioning should be regarded as an experimental procedure, not yet at the stage to be undertaken routinely by neurosurgical centers. As more data accumulate regarding the safety and efficacy of STN lesions, this approach may prove to be a viable alternative to bilateral DBS of the STN.

REFERENCES

1. Laitinen LV, Bergenheim AT, Hariz MI. Ventroposterolateral pallidotomy can abolish all parkinsonian symptoms. *Stereotact Funct Neurosurg* 1992;58:14–21.
2. Benabid AL, Pollak P, Gross C, et al. Acute and long-term effects of subthalamic nucleus stimulation in Parkinson's disease. *Stereotact Funct Neurosurg* 1994;62:76–84.
3. Limousin P, Pollak P, Benazzouz A, et al. Bilateral subthalamic nucleus stimulation for severe Parkinson's disease. *Mov Disord* 1995;10:672–674.
4. Limousin P, Krack P, Pollak P, et al. Electrical stimulation of the subthalamic nucleus in advanced Parkinson's disease. *N Engl J Med* 1998;339:1105–1111.
5. Shannon KM. Ballism. In: Jankovic J, Tolosa E, eds. *Parkinson's disease and movement disorders.* Baltimore: Williams & Wilkins, 1998:365–376.
6. Sellal F, Hirsch E, Lisovoski F, et al. Contralateral disappearance of parkinsonian signs after subthalamic hematoma. *Neurology* 1992;42:255–256.
7. Vidakovic A, Dragasevic N, Kostic VS. Hemiballism: report of 25 cases. *J Neurol Neurosurg Psychiatry* 1994;57:945–949.
8. Mundinger F. Results of 500 subthalamotomies in the region of the zona incerta. In: *Third symposium on Parkinson's disease.* Edinburgh: Livingstone, 1968.
9. Fager CA. Evaluation of thalamic and subthalamic surgical lesions in the alleviation of Parkinson's disease. *J Neurosurg* 1968;28:145–149.
10. Spiegel EA, Wycis HT, Szekely EG, et al. Campotomy in various extrapyramidal disorders. *J Neurosurg* 1963;20:871–881.
11. Andy OJ, Jurko MF, Sias FR. Subthalamotomy in treatment of parkinsonian tremor. *J Neurosurg* 1963;20:860–870.
12. Krauss JK, Mundinger F. Functional stereotactic surgery for hemiballism. *J Neurosurg* 1996;85:278–286.
13. Albin RL, Young AB, Penney JB. The functional anatomy of basal ganglia disorders. *Trends Neurosci* 1989;12:366–375.
14. Bergman H, Wichmann T, Karmon B, et al. The primate subthalamic nucleus. II. Neuronal activity in the MPTP model of parkinsonism. *J Neurophysiol* 1994;72:507–520.
15. Hutchison WD, Allan RJ, Opitz H, et al. Neurophysiological

16. Bergman H, Wichmann T, DeLong MR. Reversal of experimental parkinsonism by lesions of the subthalamic nucleus. *Science* 1990;249:1436–1438.
17. Aziz TZ, Peggs D, Sambrook MA, et al. Lesion of the subthalamic nucleus for the alleviation of 1-methyl-4-phenyl-1,2,3,6-tetrahydropyridine (MPTP)-induced parkinsonism in the primate. *Mov Disord* 1991;6:288–292.
18. Aziz TZ, Peggs D, Agarwal E, et al. Subthalamic nucleotomy alleviates parkinsonism in the 1-methyl-4-phenyl-1,2,3,6-tetrahydropyridine (MPTP)-exposed primate. *Br J Neurosurg* 1992;6:575–582.
19. Benazzouz A, Gross C, Feger J, et al. Reversal of rigidity and improvement in motor performance by subthalamic high-frequency stimulation in MPTP-treated monkeys. *Eur J Neurosci* 1993;5:382–389.
20. Benabid AL, Pollak P, Gao D, et al. Chronic electrical stimulation of the ventralis intermedius nucleus of the thalamus as a treatment of movement disorders. *J Neurosurg* 1996;84:203–214.
21. Bejjani B, Damier P, Arnulf I, et al. Pallidal stimulation for Parkinson's disease: two targets? *Neurology* 1997;49:1564–1569.
22. Krack P, Pollak P, Limousin P, et al. Subthalamic nucleus or internal pallidal stimulation in young onset Parkinson's disease. *Brain* 1998;121:451–457.
23. Krack P, Benazzouz A, Pollak P, et al. Treatment of tremor in Parkinson's disease by subthalamic nucleus stimulation. *Mov Disord* 1998;13:907–914.
24. Alvarez A, Macias J, Guridi J, et al. Unilateral dorsal subthalamotomy for Parkinson's disease. *Mov Disord* 1998;13:S266.
25. Obeso JA, Alvarez LM, Macias RJ, et al. Lesion of the subthalamic nucleus in Parkinson's disease. *Neurology* 1997;48:A138.
26. Guridi J, Obeso JA. The role of the subthalamic nucleus in the origin of hemiballism and parkinsonism: new surgical perspectives. *Adv Neurol* 1997;74:235–247.
27. Alvarez Gonzalez L, Macias J, Guridi J, et al. Lesion of the subthalamic nucleus in Parkinson's disease: long-term follow-up. *Ann Neurol* 1999;46:492.
28. Lozano AM, Lang AE. Pallidotomy for Parkinson's disease. *Neurosurg Clin North Am* 1998;9:325–336.
29. Baron MS, Virek JL, Bakay RAE, et al. Treatment of advanced Parkinson's disease by posterior GPi pallidotomy: 1-year results of a pilot study. *Ann Neurol* 1996;40:355–366.
30. Blumetti AE, Modesti LM. Long term cognitive effects of stereotactic thalamotomy on non-parkinsonian dyskinetic patients. *Appl Neurophysiol* 1980;43:259–262.
31. Kocher U, Siegfried J, Perret E. Verbal and nonverbal learning ability of Parkinson patients before and after unilateral ventrolateral thalamotomy. *Appl Neurophysiol* 1982;45:311–316.
32. Krayenbuhl H, Wyss OAM, Yasargil MG. Bilateral thalamotomy and pallidotomy as treatment for bilateral parkinsonism. *J Neurosurg* 1961;18:429.
33. Iacono RP, Shima F, Lonser RR, et al. The results, indications, and physiology of posteroventral pallidotomy for patients with Parkinson's disease. *Neurosurgery* 1995;36:1118–1125;discussion 1125–1127.
34. Scott R, Gregory R, Hines N, et al. Neuropsychological, neurological and functional outcome following pallidotomy for Parkinson's disease: a consecutive series of eight simultaneous bilateral and twelve unilateral procedures. *Brain* 1998;121:659–675.
35. Langston JW, Widner H, Goetz CG, et al. Core assessment program for intracerebral transplantations (CAPIT). *Mov Disord* 1992;7:2–13.
36. Schaltenbrand G, Bailey P. *Einführung in die Stereotaktischen*

Operationen mit einem Atlas des menschlichen Gehirns. Stuttgart: Thieme, 1959.

37. Obeso JA, Guridi J, Alvarez L, et al. Ablative surgery for Parkinson's disease. In: Jankovic J, Tolosa E, eds. *Parkinson's disease and movement disorders.* Baltimore: Williams & Wilkins, 1998:1049–1064.

38. Alvarez L, Macias R, Guridi J, et al. Dorsal Subthalamotomy for Parkinson's disease. *Mov Disord* 2001;16:72–78.

39. Gill SS, Heywood P. Subthalamotomy can be performed safely. *Mov Disord* 1998;13:201.

40. Gill SS, Heywood P. Bilateral dorsolateral subthalamotomy for advanced Parkinson's disease. *Lancet* 1997;350:1224.

41. Barlas O, Hanagasi HA, Imer M, et al. Do unilateral ablative tesions of the subthalamic nucleus in Parkinsonian patients lead to hemiballism? *Mov Disord* 2001;16:300–310

Surgery for Parkinson's Disease and Movement Disorders,
edited by J.K. Krauss, J. Jankovic, and R.G. Grossman.
Lippincott Williams & Wilkins, Philadelphia © 2001.

15

RATIONALES AND STRATEGIES OF FETAL NEURAL TRANSPLANTATION IN PARKINSON'S DISEASE

OLLE LINDVALL

The basic principle underlying neural transplantation as a new therapeutic strategy is very simple: functional restoration in the diseased human brain is achieved by replacement of dead neurons with implanted healthy neurons. There are three major reasons that this strategy is particularly suitable to explore for treatment of Parkinson's disease (PD). First is a definite need for new therapeutic approaches in PD. Many patients with PD become severely incapacitated after years of successful L-dopa treatment. Second, the main pathologic feature in this disorder is a selective degeneration of the nigrostriatal dopamine (DA) system, that is, of a specific neuronal population within a restricted area of the brain that leads to a major reduction of DA levels in the striatum. The dopaminergic deficit in PD should be easier to correct by transplantation as compared with, for example, the more widespread loss of many different cell types in Alzheimer's disease. Third, as described in detail later, studies in animal models of PD have shown that grafted embryonic DA neurons, taken from the ventral mesencephalon and implanted into the DA-denervated striatum in rodents and nonhuman primates, reinnervate the striatum, release DA, and improve motor function, including the cardinal symptoms of human PD.

The objectives of this chapter are fourfold: first, to summarize the knowledge obtained from grafting experiments in animals of particular relevance for the clinical application of neural transplantation in PD; second, to describe the indications for neural transplantation in patients; third, to discuss specific issues related to the transplantation procedure such as amount and age of donor tissue, placement of grafts, immunosuppression, tissue storage, and assessment of graft survival and function; and fourth, to discuss some ethical aspects regarding the use of human embryonic brain tissue for transplantation in patients with PD.

HISTORY OF NEURAL TRANSPLANTATION AND DEVELOPMENT

The clinical application of neural transplantation in patients with PD was first suggested in the late 1970s. In 1979, parallel studies by Perlow et al. (1) and Björklund and Stenevi (2) demonstrated that rotational asymmetry caused by unilateral neurotoxic lesions of the nigrostriatal DA system in rats was alleviated by transplants of embryonic mesencephalic DA-rich tissue placed in the denervated striatum. Subsequently, such grafts were also shown to reverse other deficits in hemiparkinsonian rats, such as in sensorimotor integration (3). However, the first clinical trials with cell transplantation in PD were carried out in 1982 to 1985 using stereotactic implantation of the patient's own adrenal medulla, mainly to avoid the ethical and immunologic problems linked to the use of human embryonic tissue. The application in patients was based on the findings by Freed et al. that intraventricular grafts of catecholamine-secreting adrenal medulla from rat donors could reduce drug-induced rotational asymmetry in hemiparkinsonian rats (4). Only minor and transient improvements, lasting for a couple of months, were seen after unilateral grafting to either the caudate nucleus or the putamen in four patients with PD (5,6). The major interest in this approach arose from the study by Madrazo and coworkers (7), in which they reported successful adrenal medulla autotransplantation in two young patients with PD. Instead of a stereotactic approach, the authors used open microsurgical techniques and implanted pieces of adrenal medulla tissue into a cavity prepared in the head of the caudate nucleus on one side. Over the next couple of years, hundreds of patients with PD were subjected to adrenal medulla autotransplantation. However, only modest symptomatic relief was observed (8), most likely because of poor graft survival.

In parallel, three scientific developments had brought neural transplantation to the forefront when it seemed justified to apply this approach clinically. Data obtained

O. Lindvall: Section of Restorative Neurology, Wallenberg Neuroscience Center, University Hospital, S-221 85 Lund, Sweden.

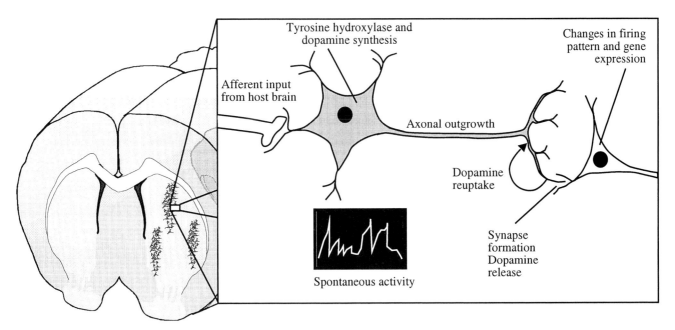

FIGURE 15.1. Grafted embryonic dopamine (DA) neurons exhibit several of the morphologic and physiologic features of normal DA neurons: they display electric activity and release DA spontaneously, form synaptic contacts with host striatal neurons, and induce changes in their pattern and gene expression and they receive afferents from the host.

from studies in rodent models of PD had demonstrated that grafted embryonic mesencephalic DA neurons exhibit several of the morphologic and physiologic features of normal DA neurons (see later; Fig. 15.1). Bakay, Redmond, Sladek, and their collaborators had shown that embryonic mesencephalic DA-rich grafts could survive and could also improve motor function in parkinsonian nonhuman primates (9–11). Finally, grafts of mesencephalic tissue from human embryos implanted in the rat PD model had been found to survive and to reinnervate the denervated rat striatum, release DA, and reverse behavioral deficits (12–15).

The first clinical trials with transplantation of human embryonic mesencephalic tissue to the striatum of patients with PD were performed in 1987 and 1988 in Mexico, the United States, Sweden, Cuba, and England (Fig. 15.2). The initial studies showed only modest symptomatic relief after transplantation, and there was no clear demonstration of graft survival. In 1990, Lindvall and collaborators provided the first evidence of survival of dopaminergic neurons in the grafts by showing increased uptake of [^{18}F]dopa, as measured by positron emission tomography (PET), associated with substantial clinical improvement (16). Similar findings were subsequently reported from clinical trials performed by Peschanski et al. (17) and by Freeman et al. (18). Definite proof of graft survival and dopaminergic reinnervation of the striatum was provided by Kordower et al. (19–21).

In a series of presentations and a recent publication, the results of the first double-blind placebo-controlled trial of fetal graft transplantation for advanced PD were summa-

rized (21a). Forty patients, stratified by age into younger than and older than 60 years of age, with mean history of 14 years of PD symptoms, were randomized to receive either cultured mesencephalic tissue from four embryos delivered through two needle passes to the left and two passes to the right putamen or a sham operation (four drill holes to the forehead without dural penetration). After 1 year, the "sham" patients were given the option to undergo implantation and were then followed in an open-label manner; a total of 33 patients received an implant. Overall, there was no statistically significant difference between the implanted and the "sham" patients with respect to the primary outcome variable, a global rating by the patients (from 3−, PD markedly worse, to 3+, PD markedly improved). There was, however, a significant improvement in bradykinesia and rigidity, but only in the younger (less than 60 years old) patients. No improvement was noted in freezing or motor fluctuations, and gait actually deteriorated. Although there were more adverse events in the implanted group, these events were not considered directly related to the surgical procedure. Of the 19 patients who underwent implantation, 12 had fluorodopa PET scans. No correlation was seen between the PET results and the Unified Parkinson's Disease Rating Scale (UPDRS). Four patients experienced dyskinesias even during "off" periods (presumably as a result of release of DA from the fetal implant). There was a marked placebo effect, sometimes lasting a year, and four patients in the "sham" group had a 15-point improvement in the UPDRS.

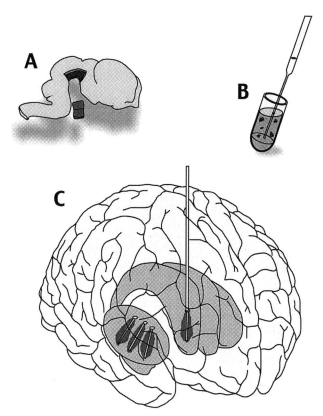

FIGURE 15.2. Schematic illustration of the most commonly used procedure for transplantation of human embryonic mesencephalic tissue into the striatum in patients with Parkinson's disease. Ventral mesencephalic dopamine-rich tissue **(A)** from human embryos aged 5.5 to 8 weeks after conception is dissociated **(B)** and then is implanted unilaterally or bilaterally using stereotactic surgery into the caudate nucleus or the putamen, or both **(C)**.

EXPERIENCE FROM LABORATORY STUDIES

Animal Models Used for Graft Studies

Two widely used models of PD, created by administration of 6-hydroxydopamine (6-OHDA) or 1-methyl-4-phenyl-1,2,3,6-tetrahydropyridine (MPTP), reproduce many of the pathologic, biochemical, and behavioral features of the disease. However, in these models, exposure to the neurotoxin stopped before transplantation. In contrast, patients with PD have an ongoing disease process, and the mechanisms of DA neuronal death are not known. Therefore, the degree and duration of functional recovery induced by transplants may be quite different in patients with PD as compared with experimental settings. This variation will occur if (a) the pattern of pathologic changes caused by the disease in the patient's brain differs from that in the animal models, (b) the disease process also destroys the grafted neurons, and (c) the ongoing degeneration outside the striatum leads to a rapid decline of the response to the graft.

Injection of 6-OHDA in the nigrostriatal pathway leads to extensive degeneration of mesencephalic dopaminergic

neurons and reduction of striatal DA levels by more than 95% (22). Bilateral 6-OHDA lesions in rats induce a debilitating syndrome with akinesia, adipsia and aphagia, and impairment of the initiation of spontaneous and goal-directed movements (23). Animals with unilateral lesions have provided the most useful model in which to study the morphology, growth, and function of grafted DA neurons. Such animals display a spontaneous postural bias to the damaged side, toward which they turn in circles. The circling behavior is amplified by the administration of the DA-releasing agent amphetamine, whereas the DA receptor agonist apomorphine causes rotational behavior in the opposite direction by stimulating supersensitive DA receptors in the denervated striatum (24). This rotational asymmetry can easily be quantified (25). Rats with unilateral lesions also exhibit disruption of motor responses to sensory stimuli on the side opposite the lesion ("sensory neglect") (26) and impairment of skilled limb use on this side (27). Small primates, such as marmosets, with unilateral 6-OHDA lesions exhibit a behavioral syndrome that includes several of the features observed in rats (28).

The MPTP-treated nonhuman primate (29) is advantageous for studies on the morphologic and functional characteristics of grafts in higher species. MPTP is administered either systemically to induce bilateral lesions or into a carotid artery (30) to induce unilateral lesions. It causes selective destruction of substantia nigra DA neurons and severe DA depletion in the striatum that lead to the development of the cardinal symptoms of human PD.

Anatomic and Biochemical Characteristics of Grafts

Embryonic mesencephalic tissue has been implanted into the rat brain as solid pieces in the lateral ventricle or into a cavity prepared in the neocortex adjacent to the striatum. In most studies, the donor tissue has been dissociated before grafting and has been implanted, in the form of a cell suspension, into one or several striatal sites by stereotactic surgery. The donor tissue has to be embryonic or fetal for the grafted DA neurons to survive.

Despite their surviving well in most sites in the rat brain, grafted DA neurons extend numerous axons only when they are implanted close to or directly into their normal target area. In the denervated rat striatum, mesencephalic grafts can give rise to dopaminergic innervation having about 50% of its normal density in the immediate vicinity of the graft and tapering off to approximately 20% at a distance of 1.0 mm from the graft (31). Using a microtransplantation approach with multiple small deposits along several tracts (32,33), the dopaminergic innervation can be restored to between 45% and 80% of normal in the caudate and putamen and to between 30% and 70% in the nucleus accumbens of rats (34). Electron microscopic studies have shown that the DA fibers also form synapses with host striatal cells, and dendrites from grafted cells make synaptic contact with axons of presumed host origin (35–37). Serotonergic fibers originating in the host raphe and corticostriatal fibers coming from the host frontal cortex innervate parts of the mesencephalic grafts. However, the innervation from the host striatum, a region that normally heavily innervates the substantia nigra, is sparse. Electric stimulation of the cortex, raphe, and striatum of the host leads to changes in the activity of cells in the grafts (38). Thus, even in their ectopic location in the striatum instead of in the substantia nigra, the grafted DA neurons receive a regulatory input from the host brain.

Embryonic mesencephalic grafts can restore DA levels in a completely denervated rat striatum to a mean of 6% to 30% of normal levels (39). Furthermore, there is a 50% to 200% increase in the ratio of dihydroxyphenylacetic acid to DA, a finding indicating a higher DA turnover in the grafts than in the normal nigrostriatal DA system (39). Spontaneously active DA neurons have been detected in the grafts by electrophysiologic methods, and, in agreement, *in vivo* microdialysis studies have shown that DA is released spontaneously from graft-derived terminals. Like normal neurons, the grafts respond to amphetamine administration with a severalfold increase of DA release, their DA reuptake system is blocked by nomifensine, and they exhibit autoregulatory features because their DA release is decreased by the receptor against apomorphine. In the host striatum, the graft-derived innervation causes upregulated postsynaptic DA binding sites to return to normal density (39). In agreement with the incomplete behavioral recovery (see later), the grafted DA neurons appear to influence different populations of neurons differentially in the denervated striatum. The lesion-induced upregulation of proenkephalin mRNA expression in the striatopallidal projection neurons is completely reversed throughout large parts of the caudate and putamen, whereas the downregulation of substance P and dynorphin expression in the striatonigral projection neurons are only partly normalized and only within the area close to the transplant (40–44).

Behavioral Effects of Grafts

Grafts of embryonic DA neurons are able to reverse several components of the 6-OHDA–induced hemiparkinsonian syndrome in rats. The pattern of functional recovery depends on the striatal region reinnervated by the grafts (Fig. 15.3A). Grafts innervating the dorsal striatum reverse rotational asymmetry but do not affect deficits in sensorimotor orientation (45,46). Conversely, grafts reinnervating the ventrolateral striatum reverse the latter impairment (3), but they leave rotational asymmetry unchanged. When grafts are implanted into the denervated nucleus accumbens, they can restore normal amphetamine-induced locomotor activity (47).

Animal studies have provided evidence of a role of DA released from dendrites of substantia nigra neurons into the pars reticulata in the regulation of basal ganglia output pathways. Intranigral grafts of embryonic mesencephalic tissue in rats with unilateral 6-OHDA lesions induce recovery in DA agonist–induced rotational asymmetry and in some tests of sensorimotor behavior (forelimb akinesia and balance test) (34,48–50), but not in a more complex motor task, that is, skilled forelimb use (49). These findings raise the possibility that combined grafts involving both the striatum and the substantia nigra may lead to more complete functional recovery than grafts placed in the striatum alone. However, in the experiments performed so far, intranigral mesencephalic grafts have not provided any additional recovery beyond that seen with intrastriatal grafts (34,49). Winkler et al. recently reported that intranigral grafts of embryonic striatal tissue improved coordinated forelimb use and that combined transplantation of DA neurons into the striatum and γ-aminobutyric acid (GABA)-rich striatal neurons into the substantia nigra produced additive effects on forelimb akinesia (34). These findings suggest that intranigral striatal transplants, possibly by suppressing the overactivity of host substantia nigra projection neurons, can be used to improve the functional efficacy of intrastriatal mesencephalic grafts.

Although many symptoms in animals with experimental parkinsonism can be alleviated or even abolished by intrastriatal grafts of embryonic mesencephalic tissue, others cannot. For example, DA-rich grafts induce limited improvement in several complex motor and sensorimotor tasks. These include, for example, deficits in so-called "disengage" behavior (51) and in the use of the contralateral forelimb for discrete skilled movements caused by unilateral lesions (27) or the aphagia and adipsia caused by bilateral 6-OHDA lesions (52). Even with grafts providing extensive dopaminergic reinnervation of the striatum, the recovery of skilled paw use and of disengage behavior is incomplete (49,53). The differential sensitivity of symptoms to graft-induced recovery in 6-OHDA–lesioned rats could have important clinical correlates: thus, mesencephalic grafts may alleviate some, but not all, symptoms of PD in humans.

Embryonic mesencephalic grafts also have functional effects after implantation into the striatum in primates (Fig. 15.3B). Grafts implanted into the caudate nucleus can improve parkinsonian signs in MPTP-treated monkeys (54). This effect was not observed after sham grafts (55). Other studies assessed specific deficits and described increased locomotion (56), reduced rotational asymmetry (57–59), and improved ability to use the hand and arm (58,59) after transplantation to the caudate nucleus or putamen. From the clinical perspective, it is highly important that Annett and co-workers also demonstrated a topographic organization of the graft-derived recovery in primates (58,59) (Fig. 15.3B). These investigators used marmosets with unilateral 6-OHDA lesions of the nigrostriatal DA pathway and implanted embryonic mesencephalic tissue into either the caudate nucleus or the putamen, or both. Grafts in the caudate

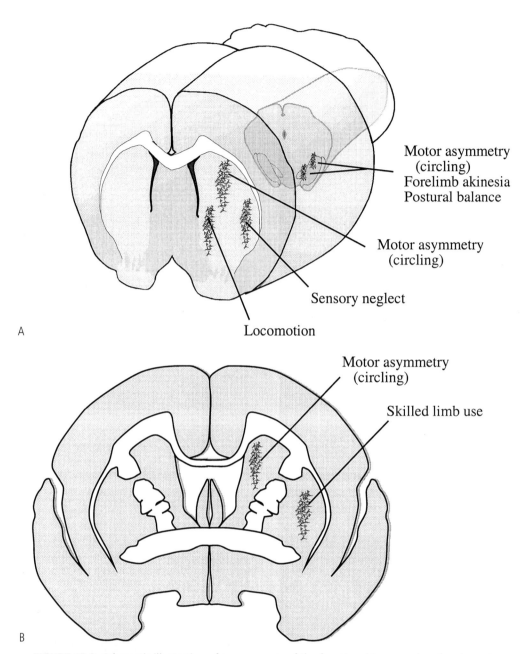

FIGURE 15.3. Schematic illustration of some aspects of the functional topography of embryonic dopamine-rich mesencephalic grafts in animal models of Parkinson's disease. In hemiparkinsonian rats **(A)**, grafts reinnervating the dorsal caudate-putamen reverse motor asymmetry (circling), grafts innervating the ventrolateral caudate-putamen reduce sensory neglect, implants located in the nucleus accumbens increase locomotion, and grafts placed in the substantia nigra improve rotational asymmetry, forelimb akinesia, and postural balance. In hemiparkinsonian nonhuman primates (marmosets) **(B)**, grafts in caudate nucleus reverse rotational asymmetry, whereas grafts in putamen improve the ability to use the contralateral hand and arm.

nucleus reversed rotational asymmetry, whereas grafts in the putamen alleviated deficits in skilled use of the contralateral hand. Multiple grafts in both structures produced additive recovery of both deficits. As in rats, functional recovery after transplantation was incomplete, and neither graft abolished the contralateral sensory neglect induced by the lesions.

Mechanisms of Improvement

The effects of transplantation on rotational asymmetry in animals depend on the DA neuron component in the transplants and disappear if the grafts are destroyed (39). Thus, long-lasting improvements require the continuous presence of the graft. There is no evidence that trophic actions exerted by the graft would lead to sprouting of the animal's own DA system to a degree that would explain major relief of symptoms. It is therefore conceivable that the functional changes after transplantation result from striatal reinnervation from DA neurons in the grafts.

The function of the grafts probably surpasses that of a simple DA delivery system. Functional integration of the grafted neurons into the host brain seems to be necessary to produce optimum functional recovery. In both rat and marmoset PD models, the development of the capacity for DA synthesis and storage in the grafts precedes the more gradual improvements in complex sensorimotor behavior by several months (34,59). The establishment of a new DA-storing terminal network in the host striatum is closely correlated to the onset of graft-derived DA release (60), as well as reversal of DA receptor supersensitivity in the rat PD model (27,34). These early effects may all be mediated by tonic, nonregulated release of DA from spontaneously active grafted neurons. However, the later development of more pronounced functional effects suggests a continued further maturation of the transplants or their synaptic connections with neuronal elements in the host. Fisher et al. showed that embryonic DA neurons grafted to the striatum in rats retained immature electrophysiologic features at 4 to 5 months postoperatively, and these neurons continued to mature over the subsequent months (61). This finding indicates that graft maturation may be a slow and protracted process that continues many months after the initial formation of the graft-derived DA-containing fiber projections (15).

Substantia nigra neurons *in situ* exert their functions in the striatum not only through tonic DA release but also by phasic changes in activity controlled by regulatory afferent inputs. In the study of Fisher et al. (61), a large proportion of the grafted DA neurons received functional afferent inputs from the host cortex and thalamus. Burst firing, which is a critical feature of the phasic type of DA release that depends, at least in part, on cortical afferents, developed in some of the grafted neurons. This finding suggests that functional integration into the host corticostriatal circuitry may be important for the full expression of the functional capacity of the grafted DA neurons.

SPECIFIC INDICATIONS

Diagnosis

Although the information is limited, available data indicate that only patients with idiopathic PD should undergo grafting. Thus, two patients with possible multiple system atrophy and atypical PD with dementia, respectively, showed poor functional outcome despite good graft survival, as indicated by [18F]dopa PET (62). It is reasonable to assume that maximum symptomatic relief after transplantation of embryonic DA neurons is obtained in patients with a selective loss of these neurons. In contrast, degeneration of other neuronal populations and, in particular, the outflow systems from the striatum will most likely attenuate or block the graft-derived improvement.

Symptom Profile

Based on the functional outcome observed in reported clinical trials, patients with the following characteristics should be primarily selected for neural transplantation: (a) no dementia; (b) "on-off" fluctuations with good "on" periods; (c) clear L-dopa response; (d) severe hypokinesia and rigidity during "off" phases, particularly in the arms; and (e) no major tremor. It is yet unclear to what extent intrastriatal dopaminergic grafts can improve axial features, balance, gait, and dyskinesias. Our knowledge of how to reverse a particular symptom in a parkinsonian patient, such as with respect to graft placement and dosage, is also limited. Probably, only symptoms caused by dopaminergic denervation in the striatum can be improved by intrastriatal implants of DA neurons. Symptoms derived from dopaminergic denervation outside the caudate and putamen or from other brain disease would probably not be reversed by these grafts. Such "resistant" symptoms may include postural and autonomic dysfunction, depression, cognitive deficits, and sensory symptoms.

Age of Patient

In the studies performed so far, no conclusive data have appeared indicating that the age of the patient with PD will significantly influence the functional outcome after grafting. The tissue implantation, which can be carried out with local anesthesia, is not a major neurosurgical procedure. At present, an upper age limit (approximately 60 to 65 years) seems justified because of the scientific character of the transplantation program (involving numerous assessments and repeated PET scans over several years) and the immunosuppressive regimen.

Duration of the Disease

Most patients have been in an advanced stage of PD at the time of transplantation, mainly because this approach is regarded as an experimental procedure. These patients have greater risks of perioperative and postoperative complications. It is conceivable that patients earlier in the disease course would exhibit a more marked response to a graft. At this early stage, both dopaminergic denervation and the possible degeneration of other neuron systems are less pronounced. However, there is no evidence that embryonic mesencephalic grafts will retard the rate of degeneration of the patient's own DA neurons. There has been a concern for graft viability in patients with advanced PD, who cannot reduce or withdraw antiparkinsonian drug treatment until symptomatic relief after transplantation is substantial. However, most studies in animals as well as the clinical trials in patients with PD indicate that continuing L-dopa treatment does not compromise graft survival (62–64).

Neural Transplantation Compared with Other Therapeutic Strategies

Several options now exist for the treatment of patients with advanced PD. Neural transplantation is still under development. The major advantage with grafting is that it is a restorative therapy that aims at correcting the actual deficit of brain function caused by the disease. Ideally, both immunosuppression and L-dopa treatment can be withdrawn, and, up to at least 10 years postoperatively, the grafts do not seem to be affected by the disease process. The adverse effects are only minor, and the patient can still undergo all other types of treatment. The problems with neural transplantation are mainly related to the use of human embryonic brain tissue and the low yield of surviving DA neurons after implantation. The need for tissue from several donors for each patient with PD severely restricts the usefulness of this approach. As discussed in detail later, it seems highly likely that these problems will be solved. In our own transplantation program, we include primarily younger patients who have to live with their disease for many years.

SPECIFIC OPERATIVE CONSIDERATIONS

Donor Tissue

The donor age is of crucial importance for the survival of DA neurons after transplantation of embryonic mesencephalic tissue (Fig. 15.4). The optimal donor age occurs after the DA neurons have developed in the ventral mesen-

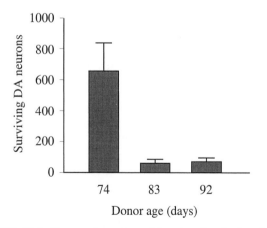

FIGURE 15.4. The number of surviving tyrosine hydroxylase–immunoreactive, presumed dopamine (DA) neurons in the caudate nucleus of three groups of marmosets implanted with mesencephalic tissue from embryonic donors of various ages. The graph illustrates a clear upper donor age limit for survival of DA neurons after transplantation. (Data from Annett LE, Torres EM, Clarke DJ, et al. Survival of nigral grafts within the striatum of marmosets with 6-OHDA lesions depends critically on donor embryo age. *Cell Transplant* 1997;6:557–569.)

cephalon but before they have extended neuritic processes. After this time, the survival of grafted DA neurons drops dramatically, probably because of axotomy during the dissection. The age of human donors should be between 5.5 and 8 weeks after conception for suspension grafts, whereas if small tissue pieces are implanted, the optimal donor age is extended up to 9 weeks after conception. Before or after this interval, transplantation into immunosuppressed rats revealed poor graft survival (65). In clinical trials, surviving dopaminergic grafts were observed only in patients with PD who received tissue from 5.5- to 9-week-old donors. Hitchcock and co-workers found few dopaminergic neurons in patients with grafts from fetuses older than 12 weeks (66). The grafted neurons were atrophic, did not reinnervate the striatum, and contained large amounts of neuromelanin. In contrast, the histopathologic studies of Kordower et al. demonstrated good graft survival and extensive dopaminergic fiber outgrowth, into the host striatum in two patients with PD who were implanted with tissue from 6.5- to 9-week-old donors (19–21).

It is well established from studies in animals that only the specific part of the embryonic ventral mesencephalon containing the dopaminergic neurons should be implanted, and the meninges have to be meticulously removed. The dissection technique is standardized but requires some training in microsurgery. In patients with PD, the consequences of grafting without taking into account the neurobiology of neural transplantation and without proper dissection are well illustrated in the report by Folkerth and Durso (67). They described autopsy findings in a patient with PD who had received intraventricular infusion of "diencephalic/mesencephalic region cells" from an early (5- to 6-week) human embryo. At 23 months after grafting, there were no surviving DA neurons, but marked overgrowth of nonneuronal tissues.

Site of Implantation

The main pathologic process in PD is degeneration of nigrostriatal dopaminergic neurons, and for a cell replacement strategy it seems most appropriate to place the grafted neurons in the substantia nigra region. However, animal studies have shown that although grafts placed in the substantia nigra will survive, they will not extend their axons along the nigrostriatal pathway (68). Various attempts have been made to reconstruct the nigrostriatal system in adult rats by creating a more favorable environment for the growth of the dopaminergic axons. Although promising data have been reported (69–71), clinical trials using such approaches seem distant.

In patients with PD, the embryonic mesencephalic grafts have to be placed in the projection area of the nigrostriatal system. Putamen should be the primary target for implantation. The DA depletion is most severe in this structure (72), which is also more closely related to primary motor circuitry as compared with the caudate nucleus (73). In the studies of Freeman, Kordower, Hauser, and their collaborators (18–21,74), tissue was implanted only in the postcommissural putamen, which seems to be both anatomically and functionally distinct from the anterior putamen and the caudate nucleus. However, grafts in both caudate and putamen are probably necessary for optimum functional recovery. In marmosets, grafts in the caudate nucleus had distinct effects on motor function as compared with implants in the putamen (59). In the clinical trials with neural transplantation performed so far, it is unclear whether the grafts in caudate nucleus have survived and which effects on parkinsonian symptoms they have induced.

Not only dopaminergic neurons innervating caudate and putamen but also those projecting to other forebrain regions, such as frontal, limbic and motor cortical areas, globus pallidus, and nucleus accumbens, degenerate in PD (75). It is conceivable that some of the motor or sensorimotor deficits that are not improved by grafts in the caudate or putamen are caused by these pathologic changes. The ventral striatum seems to be an attractive target region for dopaminergic grafts outside the caudate and putamen. In rats, grafts in the nucleus accumbens are important for amplitude of locomotion (47). Patients with disturbances in the locomotor component of movement may therefore need grafts in the nucleus accumbens for functional recovery. In addition, dopaminergic grafts in the ventral striatum could be important for correct switching of motor plan when environmental conditions change (76). However, in patients subjected to grafting in the ventral striatum, a preoperative PET scan has actually demonstrated a significant decrease of fluorodopa uptake in this region.

Unilateral and Bilateral Implants

Studies in patients with PD have shown that unilateral intrastriatal grafts give rise to bilateral effects (Fig. 15.5) (16,62,77,78). The improvements have been most pronounced in the limbs contralateral to the graft, but ipsilateral amelioration of parkinsonian symptoms and reduction of the duration and number of "off" periods (when patients have bilateral symptoms) have also been observed. The most likely explanation for the symptomatic relief on both sides is that a major output from the striatum is, through the pallidum and thalamus, directed to the supplementary motor area, which has bilateral connections. Piccini et al. recently showed, using PET, that well-developed dopaminergic grafts in patients restored the impaired activation of the supplementary motor area (79), which is believed to play an important role in the pathophysiology of akinesia in PD. Unilateral dopaminergic grafts could therefore reduce motor symptoms bilaterally by restoring the functional integrity of the ipsilateral corticostriatothalamocortical loop and activating the supplementary motor area, which controls both sides of the body.

Unilateral grafts can give rise to substantial clinical improvement and, in some cases, dramatic symptomatic relief allowing withdrawal of L-dopa treatment (Fig. 15.6) (16,62,77,78). However, for maximum and long-lasting functional recovery, implants should be bilateral. This conclusion is based on two main observations. First, Hagell et al. reported from a series of patients who underwent transplantation sequentially on both sides that when a second intraputaminal graft was added contralateral to the first one, the functional effect was enhanced (Fig. 15.5) (80). The magnitude of improvement induced by the second graft was less pronounced than that after the first implant. Second, after transplantation, a progressive degeneration of the patient's own DA neurons occurs, and this will lead to a gradual increase in functional impairment, predominantly on the side of the body contralateral to the nongrafted striatum (62,78).

Number of Donors and Implantation Sites

Each substantia nigra in the human brain contains 550,000 dopaminergic neurons (81). Approximately 250,000 of these neurons have been estimated to innervate the putamen, and a similar number project to the caudate nucleus. Grafting of dissociated human embryonic mesencephalic tissue into immunosuppressed parkinsonian rats results in about 40,000 surviving DA neurons from each donor (aged 6 to 8 weeks after conception) (82). Thus, fewer than 4% of human DA neurons survive grafting into rats, and similar findings (5% to 10% survival) have been reported after transplantation to patients (19–21). The low yield of surviving DA neurons after transplantation, which is also observed with animal tissue, is a major obstacle for the application of this procedure in a large number of patients. Using currently available procedures, mesencephalic tissue from at least three to four human embryos (giving rise to about 100,000 to 150,000 surviving grafted DA neurons) probably needs to be implanted per side in each patient to induce a substantial clinical improvement and a consistently significant increase of fluorodopa uptake.

Studies in animals indicate that the massive death of grafted embryonic dopaminergic neurons occurs during the first week after transplantation (83). Most of these cells probably die through an apoptotic mechanism, although necrosis is also likely to underlie some neuronal loss. Brundin and co-workers distinguished four main events that cause DA neuronal death in transplantation: (a) hypoxic or hypoglycemic insult from the removal of the embryo from its maternal blood supply, (b) axotomy and other damage during dissection and mechanical dissociation and hypoxia before implantation, (c) implantation and the first 1 to 3 days thereafter in the new environment, and (d) lack of appropriate neurotrophic support at a later stage during maturation (83). Several improvements of basic transplantation methods to increase DA neuron survival have been described. These include, for example, change of the medium for preparation, dissociation, and storage of the tissue (84,85) and less

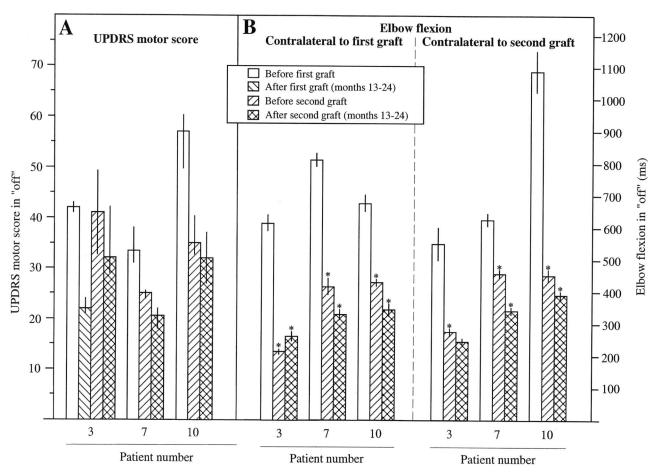

FIGURE 15.5. Illustration that (i) unilateral grafts have bilateral but predominantly contralateral effects, (ii) a second, contralateral graft implanted 10 to 56 months after the first one gives rise to additional symptomatic relief, and (iii) the magnitude of improvement induced by the second graft in these patients is less pronounced than that after the first implant. **(A):** Scores from the motor examination part of the Unified Parkinson's Disease Rating Scale in the practically defined "off" phase. Data are from assessments performed during the 6 months before each transplantation and during the second year after the second graft. Because of the long interval between the transplantations in patient 3 (56 months), data from the second postoperative year after the first graft are also included for this patient. Data are median +25th percentile. **(B):** Performance of elbow flexion contralateral to the first and second grafts, as assessed neurophysiologically. Data are mean +SEM. Statistical comparisons were made between the measurements before the first and the second graft and between the measurements before and after the second graft. *Asterisk, p< .05;* Student's *t*-test. Patient numbers refer to Lund-London series. (Data from Hagell P, Schrag A, Piccini P, et al. Sequential bilateral transplantation in Parkinson's disease: effects of the second graft. *Brain* 1999;122:1121–1132.)

extensive dissociation of the tissue with implantation of a mixture of cell aggregates and single cells (86,87). There is also evidence from studies using a microtransplantation technique in rats (32) that it is beneficial for graft survival to minimize the trauma in the host brain at the implantation site. In fact, Sinclair et al. recently reported that a delay of 1 to 3 hours between the insertion of the injection cannula and the ejection of the graft tissue improved DA neuron survival (88). This finding suggests that the damaged environment in the host brain may be particularly harmful to the grafted neurons during the acute postoperative period.

The survival of grafted dopaminergic neurons can also be improved by the administration of growth factors (89–97),

as well as by compounds that reduce oxidative stress (85,98–101) or inhibit caspases (102). Exposure of the graft to neurotrophic factors such as glial cell line–derived neurotrophic factor (GDNF) increases the survival of DA neurons at least twofold. Caspase inhibitors, which block apoptosis, can induce a greater than threefold increase of the number of surviving grafted DA neurons in rats. Whether these strategies also increase graft survival in patients with PD is unknown. The only compound that has been tested clinically is the lazaroid tirilazad mesylate, which inhibits lipid peroxidation. Administration of tirilazad mesylate supports a twofold increase of the number of surviving cultured rat mesencephalic DA neurons (101), as well as similar increases in

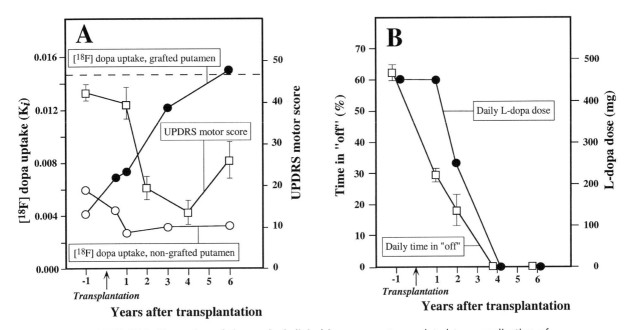

FIGURE 15.6. Illustration of the marked clinical improvement, correlated to normalization of [^{18}F]dopa uptake, in a patient with Parkinson's disease who underwent grafted unilaterally into the putamen with embryonic mesencephalic tissue from four human donors aged 6 to 8 weeks after conception. **(A):** [^{18}F]dopa uptake and score from the motor examination part of the Unified Parkinson's Disease Rating Scale (UPDRS) in the practically defined "off" phase. UPDRS scores are mean +95% confidence interval. The broken line depicts mean [^{18}F]dopa uptake in the putamen for a group of 17 healthy volunteers. **(B):** Percentage of the day spent in the "off" phase (mean +95% confidence interval) and daily L-dopa dose. (Data from Wenning GK, Odin P, Morrish P, et al. Short- and long-term survival and function of unilateral intrastriatal dopaminergic grafts in Parkinson's disease. *Ann Neurol* 1997;42:95–107.)

the survival of rat DA neurons grafted to the striatum anterior chamber of the eye (85). Furthermore, tirilazad mesylate significantly prolongs the time during which both rat and human embryonic mesencephalic cell suspensions displayed high viability when they were stored at room temperature (101). The clinical study of Brundin et al. provided evidence that tirilazad mesylate (administered to the graft tissue and intravenously to the patient) may improve survival of grafted DA neurons in patients with PD (103).

The volume of the striatum is about 200 times larger in the human brain than in the rat brain, and even with a large number of surviving DA neurons, the volume of the graft-derived innervation in a patient with PD could be insufficient. To what extent the striatum will be reinnervated depends not only on the total number of surviving grafted DA neurons but also on the number and location of implantations and the growth capacity of each DA neuron. Kordower and coworkers reported that the neuritic outgrowth from grafted human DA neurons in patients with PD extended up to approximately 7 mm within the putamen (19). They also found that with six tracts placed 5 mm apart, confluent reinnervation of 24% to 78% of the designated target area in the postcommissural putamen could be obtained, although in the patient with the densest reinnervation, the putamen was shrunken (21). Based on these findings and on our own experience, my colleagues and I estimate that covering most of the volume of the putamen with dopaminergic innerva-

tion of significant density (25% or more of normal) will require tissue implanted along six to seven tracts. Another approach to promote reinnervation is to stimulate axonal outgrowth by administration of a neurotrophic factor. Investigators showed that intrastriatal injections of GDNF (91) or implantation of polymer-encapsulated genetically modified GDNF-releasing cells (94) gave rise to increased DA fiber outgrowth from intrastriatal rat-to-rat grafts, a finding suggesting strategies that could be useful also in patients with PD.

For further details on the neurosurgical procedures for implantation of embryonic mesencephalic tissue in patients with PD, the reader is referred to, for example, Freeman et al. (18), Breeze et al. (104), and Rehncrona (105).

Immunosuppression

It is still not clear whether immunosuppression is needed in patients with PD who receive allografts of human embryonic mesencephalic tissue. The brain is an immunologically privileged site, and studies in animals demonstrated that allografts of embryonic mesencephalic tissue can show long-term survival without immunosuppression (106,107). The clinical data obtained so far clearly indicate that long-term immunosuppression is not necessary for graft survival, a finding that is important because the drugs used are expensive and may have severe side effects. In several studies, withdrawal of cyclosporine at 6 months to 3 years after transplantation did not interfere with graft survival, as assessed up to 3 years later using PET or histopathologic examination (17,19,62,74,78). However, the presence of microglia, macrophages, and T and B cells in the well-developed dopaminergic grafts in two patients with PD subjected to autopsy (108) indicated a potential for immune reactions.

The question remains whether short-term immunosuppression is necessary for graft survival. All patients with significant graft survival noted on PET have received immunosuppression at the time of transplantation and for at least 6 months thereafter. Conversely, immunologic rejection of the grafts has not been reported in any patient with PD.

In the clinical setting, regrafting may be important by allowing for multiple implant sites in both hemispheres, as well as for adding more tissue if a previous graft gives insufficient symptomatic relief. The rat data indicate that regrafting with allogeneic tissue can be performed without major risks of graft rejection, provided an atraumatic technique is used (107). Similar findings were reported in a group of five immunosuppressed patients who underwent regrafting to the contralateral striatum 10 to 56 months after the first implantation (80). The sequential transplantation in these patients did not compromise the survival and function of either the first or the second graft up to 2 years postoperatively (Fig. 15.7).

Monitoring Graft Survival and Function

For clinical studies of embryonic mesencephalic grafts in PD, the PET technique has several indications. First, [^{18}F]dopa uptake, that is, DA storage capacity, can be used as a measure of the survival of grafted DA neurons (Figs. 15.6 and 15.7), as well as of the denervation of the patient's own DA system. PET cameras with high resolution make it possible to reveal in detail the pattern of dopaminergic denervation preoperatively, which is highly recommended both for patient selection and to determine graft placements that will give rise to maximum improvements. Moreover, the distribution of graft-derived reinnervation can be correlated with the degree of symptomatic relief. Second, H$_2$^{15}O PET studies to monitor regional cerebral blood flow can demonstrate whether the grafts have restored the deficit in the movement-related activation of frontal cortical areas in the patients (79). This analysis seems to be a useful test to determine the degree of functional integration of the graft into the host brain. Third, the displacement of the binding to the DA receptor D$_2$ antagonist raclopride gives a measure of the occupancy of these receptors by the endogenous transmitter (109). DA release from the graft can be monitored *in vivo* using [^{11}C]raclopride PET both before and after amphetamine administration.

To avoid the problem with clinical data that could be compared among research groups, the Core Assessment Program

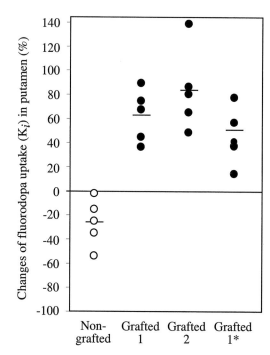

FIGURE 15.7. Survival of intrastriatal dopaminergic grafts after sequential implantation in the putamen in a group of five patients. Summary diagram showing the percentage of change of fluorodopa uptake (χ-value) compared with preoperative value in the nongrafted putamen ("Non-grafted") and grafted putamen ("Grafted 1"), at 8 to 12 months after the first transplantation and in the recently grafted putamen ("Grafted 2") and previously grafted putamen ("Grafted 1*") at 12 to 18 months after the second transplantation. There is no evidence that retransplantation compromises the survival of either the first or the second graft. (Data from Wenning GK, Odin P, Morrish P, et al. Short- and long-term survival and function of unilateral intrastriatal dopaminergic grafts in Parkinson's disease. *Ann Neurol* 1997;42:95–107; and Hagell P, Schrag A, Piccini P, et al. Sequential bilateral transplantation in Parkinson's disease: effects of the second graft. *Brain* 1999;122:1121–1132.)

for Intracerebral Transplantations (CAPIT) was developed (110). This has been revised and further developed (CAPSIT) (111). The CAPSIT contains guidelines on standardization of clinical trials of transplantation in PD, mainly with respect to inclusion criteria and methods of assessment.

Tissue Storage

There are several advantages with a tissue storage procedure that does not compromise the viability of the grafted DA neurons in patients with PD. First, donor tissue obtained from routine abortions over several days can be pooled. This approach is necessary in most cases because, at present, mesencephalic tissue from several human embryos is needed in each patient to achieve major symptomatic relief. Second, screening for infectious agents can be performed before implantation. Third, pretransplantation storage allows for preoperative manipulation of the graft tissue, such as addition of trophic factors, lazaroids, or caspase inhibitors.

Three main approaches for storage of embryonic DA neurons before transplantation have been explored, mainly in animal experiments: freezing, refrigeration above freezing ("hibernation"), and cell culture. Human embryonic tissue has been cryopreserved (112), or stored in culture for at least 1 week (113), before implantation in patients. However, with cryopreservation, the survival of DA neurons in the graft is markedly lower (114). In agreement, no obvious graft survival was demonstrated using PET in patients grafted with cryopreserved tissue (112). Similarly, storage in culture did not give rise to any detectable graft survival in a patient with PD (113). Currently, the most useful approach in clinical trials is to store the embryonic mesencephalic tissue at +4°C in a chemically defined "hibernation medium" (115). Human embryonic tissue can be stored in hibernation medium for up to 2 days, and it can be grafted into patients with PD with robust survival (19). Rat tissue can also be stored under such conditions, and then grafted, within 5 days, without significant morphologic and functional impairment compared with fresh tissue. My colleagues and I found that when the lazaroid tirilazad mesylate and GDNF are added to the medium, the tissue can be stored at least 8 days (Brundin et al., unpublished observations). This is now being tested in patients.

ETHICAL CONSIDERATIONS

The use of embryonic brain tissue from human donors for transplantation in patients is a controversial ethical issue. It is absolutely necessary that such use follows very clear, strict rules that are openly discussed. Furthermore, scientists should actively work to reduce the need for human embryonic tissue for each patient. Although several possible alternative tissues have been suggested, human embryonic mesencephalic tissue still represents the standard for implantation in patients with PD. An excellent and comprehensive analysis of the ethical aspects of neural transplantation was published by Boer (116). This article also discusses the ethical guidelines adopted by the Network of European CNS Transplantation and Restoration (NECTAR). NECTAR is composed of research groups from different European countries, and scientists from these groups have agreed to obey the following guidelines:

1. Tissue for transplantation or research may be obtained from dead embryos or fetuses, their death resulting from legally induced or spontaneous abortion. Death of an intact embryo or fetus is defined as absence of respiration and heartbeats.
2. It is not allowed to keep intact embryos or fetuses alive artificially for the purpose of removing usable material.
3. The decision to terminate pregnancy must under no circumstances be influenced by the possible or desired subsequent use of the embryo or fetus and must therefore precede any introduction of the possible use of the embryonic or fetal tissue. There should be no link between the donor and the recipient, nor should there be designation of the recipient by the donor.
4. The procedure of abortion, or the timing, must not be influenced by the requirements of the transplantation activity when this would be in conflict with the woman's interest or would increase embryonic or fetal distress.
5. No material can be used without informed consent of the woman involved. This informed consent should, whenever possible, be obtained before the abortion.
6. Screening of the woman for transmissible diseases requires informed consent.
7. Nervous tissue may be used for transplantation as suspended cell preparations or tissue fragments.
8. All members of the hospital or research staff directly involved in any of the procedures must be fully informed.
9. The procurement of embryos, fetuses, or their tissue must not involve profit or remuneration.
10. Every transplantation or research project involving the use of embryonic or fetal tissue must be approved by the local ethical committee.

CONCLUSIONS

Studies in animal models have provided a solid basis for the clinical application of neural transplantation, and in the 1990s, the basic principles of cell replacement were also shown to be valid in patients with PD. The available clinical data strongly support the concept that restorative strategies will become of value for the treatment of large numbers of patients with PD, although at present, neural transplantation is an experimental approach. Relief of symptoms should be increased by improved preoperative characterization of the dopaminergic denervation pattern in each patient and by more efficient reinnervation by the grafts. Moreover, the survival of DA neurons after transplantation has to be improved. The major obstacle to widespread application of this approach is that, at present, tissue from several human embryonic donors is necessary in each patient to induce a substantial clinical improvement. It is crucial that the use of human embryonic brain tissue for transplantation purposes be minimized by, for example, the development of xenograft approaches or engineering or expansion of DA-releasing neurons from stem cells or precursor cells.

ACKNOWLEDGMENTS

My own work was supported by grants from the Swedish Medical Research Council, the Kock, Wiberg and Söderberg Foundations, and the King Gustav V and Queen Victoria Foundation. I thank Peter Hagell for valuable discussions, Monica Olofsson for secretarial work, and Bengt Mattsson for illustrations.

REFERENCES

1. Perlow MJ, Freed WJ, Hoffer BJ, et al. Brain grafts reduce motor abnormalities produced by destruction of nigrostriatal dopamine system. *Science* 1979;204:643–647.
2. Björklund A, Stenevi U. Reconstruction of the nigrostriatal pathway by intracerebral nigral transplants. *Brain Res* 1979;177:555–560.
3. Dunnett SB, Björklund A, Stenevi U, et al. Grafts of embryonic substantia nigra reinnervating the ventrolateral striatum ameliorate sensorimotor impairments and akinesia in rats with 6-OHDA lesions of the nigrostriatal pathway. *Brain Res* 1981;229:209–217.
4. Freed WJ, Morihisa J, Spoor E, et al. Transplanted adrenal chromaffin cells in rat brain reduce lesion-induced rotational behaviour. *Nature* 1981;292:351–352.
5. Backlund EO, Granberg PO, Hamberger B, et al. Transplantation of adrenal medullary tissue to striatum in parkinsonism: first clinical trials. *J Neurosurg* 1985;62:169–173.
6. Lindvall O, Backlund EO, Farde L, et al. Transplantation in Parkinson's disease: two cases of adrenal medullary grafts to putamen. *Ann Neurol* 1987;22:457–468.
7. Madrazo I, Drucker-Colin R, Diaz V, et al. Open microsurgical autograft of adrenal medulla to the right caudate nucleus in two patients with intractable Parkinson's disease: *N Engl J Med* 1987;316:831–834.
8. Goetz CG, Stebbins GT III, Klawans HL, et al. United Parkinson Foundation Neurotransplantation Registry on adrenal medullary transplants: presurgical, and 1- and 2-year follow-up. *Neurology* 1994;41:1719–1722.
9. Bakay RAE, Fiandaca MS, Barrow DL, et al. Preliminary report on the use of fetal tissue transplantation to correct MPTP-induced parkinsonian-like syndrome in primates. *Appl Neurophysiol* 1985;48:358–361.
10. Redmond DE, Sladek JR Jr, Roth RH, et al. Fetal neuronal grafts in monkeys given methylphenyltetrahydropyridine. *Lancet* 1986;1:1125–1127.
11. Bakay RAE, Barrow DL, Fiandaca MS, et al. Biochemical and behavioural correction of MPTP parkinsonian-like syndrome by fetal cell transplantation. *Ann NY Acad Sci* 1987;495:623–640.
12. Brundin P, Nilsson OG, Strecker RE, et al. Behavioural effects of human fetal dopamine neurons grafted in a rat model of Parkinson's disease. *Exp Brain Res* 1986;65:235–240.
13. Strömberg I, Bygdeman M, Goldstein M, et al.. Human fetal substantia nigra grafted to the dopamine-denervated striatum of immunosuppressed rats: evidence for functional reinnervation. *Neurosci Lett* 1986;71:271–276.
14. Brundin P, Strecker RE, Widner H, et al. Human fetal dopamine neurons grafted in a rat model of Parkinson's disease: immunological aspects, spontaneous and drug-induced behaviour, and dopamine release. *Exp Brain Res* 1988;70:192–208.
15. Clarke DJ, Brundin P, Strecker RE, et al. Human fetal dopamine neurons grafted in a rat model of Parkinson's disease: ultrastructural evidence for synapse formation using tyrosine hydroxylase immunocytochemistry. *Exp Brain Res* 1988;73:115–126.
16. Lindvall O, Brundin P, Widner H, et al. Grafts of fetal dopamine neurons survive and improve motor function in Parkinson's disease. *Science* 1990;247:574–577.
17. Peschanski M, Defer G, N'Guyen JP, et al. Bilateral motor improvement and alteration of L-dopa effect in two patients with Parkinson's disease following intrastriatal transplantation of foetal ventral mesencephalon. *Brain* 1994;117:487–499.
18. Freeman TB, Olanow CW, Hauser RA, et al. Bilateral fetal nigral transplantation into the postcommissural putamen in Parkinson's disease. *Ann Neurol* 1995;38:379–388.

19. Kordower JH, Freeman TB, Snow BJ et al. Neuropathological evidence of graft survival and striatal reinnervation after the transplantation of fetal mesencephalic tissue in a patient with Parkinson's disease. *N Engl J Med* 1995;332:1118–1124.
20. Kordower JH, Rosenstein JM, Collier TJ, et al. Functional fetal nigral grafts in a patient with Parkinson's disease: chemoanatomic, ultrastructural, and metabolic studies. *J Comp Neurol* 1996;370:203–230.
21. Kordower JH, Freeman TB, Chen EY, et al. Fetal nigral grafts survive and mediate clinical benefit in a patient with Parkinson's disease. *Mov Disord* 1998;13:383–393.
21a. Freed CR, Greenc PE, Breeze RE, et al. Transplantation of embryonic dopamine neurons for severe Parkinson's disease. *N Eng J Med* 2001;344:710–719.
22. Ungerstedt U. 6-hydroxydopamine induced degeneration of central monoamine neurons. *Eur J Pharmacol* 1968;5:107–110.
23. Ungerstedt U. Aphagia and adipsia after 6-hydroxydopamine induced degeneration of the nigro-striatal dopamine system. *Acta Physiol Scand Suppl* 1971;367:95–122.
24. Ungerstedt U. Post-synaptic supersensitivity after 6-hydroxydopamine induced degeneration of the nigro-striatal dopamine system. *Acta Physiol Scand Suppl* 1971;367:49–68.
25. Ungerstedt U, Arbuthnott GW. Quantitative recording of rotational behavior in rats after 6-hydroxy-dopamine lesions of the nigrostriatal dopamine system. *Brain Res* 1970;24:485–493.
26. Marshall JF, Berrios N, Sawyer S. Neostriatal dopamine and sensory inattention. *J Comp Physiol Psychol* 1980;94:833–846.
27. Dunnett SB, Whishaw IQ, Rogers DC, et al. Dopamine-rich grafts ameliorate whole body motor asymmetry and sensory neglect but not independent limb use in rats with 6-hydroxydopamine lesions. *Brain Res* 1987;415:63–78.
28. Annett LE, Rogers DC, Hernandez TD, et al. Behavioural analysis of unilateral monoamine depletion in the marmoset. *Brain* 1992;115:825–856.
29. Burns RS, Chiueh CC, Markey SP, et al. A primate model of parkinsonism: selective destruction of dopaminergic neurons in the pars compacta of the substantia nigra by N-methyl-4-phenyl-1,2,3,6-tetrahydropyridine. *Proc Natl Acad Sci USA* 1983;80:4546–4550.
30. Bankiewicz KS, Oldfield EH, Chiueh CC, et al. Hemiparkinsonism in monkeys after unilateral internal carotid artery infusion of 1-methyl-4-phenyl-1,2,3,6-tetrahydropyridine (MPTP). *Life Sci* 1986;39:7–16.
31. Doucet G, Brundin P, Descarries L, et al. Effect of prior dopamine denervation on survival and fiber outgrowth from intrastriatal fetal mesencephalic grafts. *Eur J Neurosci* 1990;2:279–290.
32. Nikkah G, Cunningham MG, Jodicke A, et al. Improved graft survival and striatal reinnervation by microtransplantation of fetal nigral cell suspensions in the rat Parkinson model. *Brain Res* 1994;7:133–143.
33. Nikkah G, Olsson M, Eberhard J, et al. A microtransplantation approach for cell suspension grafting in the rat Parkinson model: a detailed account of the methodology. *Neuroscience* 1994;63:57–72.
34. Winkler C, Bentlage C, Nikkah G, et al. Intranigral transplants of GABA-rich striatal tissue induce behavioral recovery in the rat Parkinson model and promote the effects obtained by intrastriatal dopaminergic transplants. *Exp Neurol* 1999;155:165–186.
35. Freund TF, Bolam JP, Björklund A, et al. Efferent synaptic connections of grafted dopaminergic neurons reinnervating the host neostriatum: a tyrosine hydroxylase immunocytochemical study. *J Neurosci* 1985;5:603–616.
36. Mahalik TJ, Finger TE, Strömberg I, et al. Substantia nigra transplants into denervated striatum of the rat: ultrastructure of graft and host interconnections: *J Comp Neurol* 1985;240:60–70.

37. Bolam JP, Freund T, Björklund A, et al. Synaptic input and local output of dopaminergic neurons in grafts that functionally reinnervate the host neostriatum. *Exp Brain Res* 1987;68:131–146.

38. Arbuthnott G, Dunnett SB, MacLeod N. Electrophysological properties of single units in mesencephalic transplants in rat brain. *Neurosci Lett* 1985;57:205–210.

39. Brundin P, Duan WM, Sauer H. Functional effects of mesencephalic dopamine neurons and adrenal chromaffin cells grafted to the rodent striatum. In: Dunnett SB, Björklund A, eds. *Functional neural transplantation*. New York: Raven, 1994:9–46.

40. Manier M, Abrous DN, Feuerstein M, et al. Increase of striatal methionin enkephalin content following lesion of the nigrostriatal dopaminergic pathway in adult rats and reversal following the implantation of embryonic dopaminergic neurons: a quantitative immunohistochemical analysis. *Neuroscience* 1991;42:427–439.

41. Sirinathsinghji DJS, Dunnett SB. Increased proenkephalin mRNA levels in the rat neostriatum following lesion of the ipsilateral nigrostriatal dopamine pathway with 1-methyl-4-phenylpyridinium ion (MPP+): reversal by embryonic nigral dopamine grafts. *Mol Brain Res* 1991;9:263–269.

42. Mendez I, Naus CCG, Elisevitch K, et al. Normalization of striatal proenkephalin and preprotachykinin mRNA expression by fetal substantia nigra grafts. *Exp Neurol* 1993;119:1–10.

43. Bal A, Savasta M, Chritin M, et al. Transplantation of fetal nigral cells reverses the increase of preproenkephalin mRNA levels in the rat striatum caused by 6-OHDA lesions of the dopaminergic nigrostriatal pathway: a quantitative *in situ* hybridization study. *Mol Brain Res* 1993;18:221–227.

44. Cenci MA, Campbell K, and Björklund A. Neuropeptide messenger RNA expression in the 6-hydroxydopamine–lesioned rat striatum reinnervated by fetal dopaminergic transplants: differential effects of the grafts on preproenkephalin, preprotachykinin and prodynorphin messenger RNA levels. *Neuroscience* 1993;57:275–296.

45. Björklund A, Dunnett SB, Stenevi U, et al. Reinnervation of the denervated striatum by substantia nigra transplants: functional consequences as revealed by pharmacological and sensorimotor testing. *Brain Res* 1980;199:307–333.

46. Björklund A, Stenevi U, Dunnett SB, et al. Functional reactivation of the deafferented neostriatum by nigral transplants. *Nature* 1981;289:497–499.

47. Brundin P, Strecker RE, Londos E, et al. Dopamine neurons grafted unilaterally to the nucleus accumbens affect drug-induced circling and locomotion. *Exp Brain Res* 1987;69:183–194.

48. Nikkhah G, Bentlage C, Cunningham MG, et al.. Intranigral fetal dopamine grafts induce behavioral compensation in the rat Parkinson model. *J Neurosci* 1994;14:3449–3461.

49. Olsson M, Nikkhah G, Bentlage C, et al. Forelimb akinesia in the rat Parkinson model: differential effects of dopamine agonists and nigral transplants as assessed by a new stepping test. *J Neurosci* 1995;15:3863–3875.

50. Yurek DM. Intranigral transplants of fetal ventral mesencephalic tissue attenuate D$_1$-agonist-induced rotational behavior. *Exp Neurol* 1997;143:1–9.

51. Mandel RJ, Brundin P, Björklund A. The importance of graft placement and task complexity for transplant-induced recovery of simple and complex sensorimotor deficits in dopamine denervated rats. *Eur J Neurosci* 1990;2:888–894.

52. Dunnett SB, Björklund A, Schmidt RH, et al. Intracerebral grafting of neuronal cell suspensions. V. Behavioural recovery in rats with bilateral 6-OHDA lesions following implantation of nigral cell suspensions. *Acta Physiol Scand Suppl* 1983;522:39–47.

53. Nikkhah G, Duan WM, Knappe U, et al. Restoration of complex sensorimotor behavior and skilled forelimb use by a modified nigral cell suspension transplantation approach in the rat Parkinson model. *Neuroscience* 1993;56:33–43.

54. Taylor JR, Elsworth JD, Roth RH, et al. Grafting of fetal substantia nigra to striatum reverses behavioral deficits induced by MPTP in primates: a comparison with other types of grafts as controls. *Exp Brain Res* 1991;85:335–348.

55. Taylor JR, Elsworth JD, Sladek JR Jr, et al. Sham surgery does not ameliorate MPTP-induced behavioral deficits in monkeys. *Cell Transplant* 1995;4:13–26.

56. Fine A, Hunt SP, Oertel WH, et al. Transplantation of embryonic marmoset dopaminergic neurons to the corpus striatum of marmosets rendered parkinsonian by 1-methyl-4-phenyl-1,2,3,6-tetrahydropyridine. *Prog Brain Res* 1988;78:479–489.

57. Bankiewicz KS, Plunkett RJ, Jacobowitz DM, et al. The effect of fetal mesencephalon implants on primate MPTP-induced parkinsonism: histochemical and behavioral studies. *J Neurosurg* 1990;72:231–244.

58. Annett LE, Martel FL, Rogers DC, et al. Behavioural assessment of the effects of embryonic nigral grafts in marmosets with unilateral 6-OHDA lesions of the nigrostriatal pathway. *Exp Neurol* 1994;125:228–246.

59. Annett LE, Torres EM, Ridley RM, et al. A comparison of the behavioural effects of embryonic nigral grafts in the caudate nucleus and in the putamen of marmosets with unilateral 6-OHDA lesions. *Exp Brain Res* 1995;103:355–371.

60. Forni C, Brundin P, Strecker RE, et al. Time-course of recovery of dopamine neuron activity during reinnervation of the denervated striatum by fetal mesencephalic grafts as assessed by *in vivo* voltammetry. *Exp Brain Res* 1989;76:75–87.

61. Fisher LJ, Young SJ, Tepper JM, et al. Electrophysiological characteristics of cells within mesencephalon suspension grafts. *Neuroscience* 1991;40:109–122.

62. Wenning GK, Odin P, Morrish P, et al. Short- and long-term survival and function of unilateral intrastriatal dopaminergic grafts in Parkinson's disease. *Ann Neurol* 1997;42:95–107.

63. Blunt SB, Jenner P, Marsden CD. The effect of chronic L-DOPA treatment on the recovery of motor function in 6-hydroxydopamine–lesioned rats receiving ventral mesencephalic grafts. *Neuroscience* 1991;40:453–464.

64. Adams CE, Hoffman AF, Hudson JL, et al. Chronic treatment with levodopa and/or selegiline does not affect behavioral recovery induced by fetal ventral mesencephalic grafts in unilaterally 6-hydroxy-dopamine–lesioned rats. *Exp Neurol* 194;130:261–268.

65. Freeman TB, Sanberg PR, Nauert GM, et al. The influence of donor age on survival of solid and suspension, intraparenchymal human embryonic nigral grafts. *Cell Transplant* 1995;4:141–154.

66. Hitchcock EH, Whitwell HL, Sofroniew MV, et al. Survival of TH-positive and neuromelanin-containing cells in patients with Parkinson's disease after intrastriatal grafting of fetal ventral mesencephalon. *Exp Neurol* 1994;129:3(abst).

67. Folkerth RD, Durso R. Survival and proliferation of nonneural tissues, with obstruction of cerebral ventricles, in a parkinsonian patient treated with fetal allografts. *Neurology* 1996;46:1219–1225.

68. Björklund A, Dunnett SB, Nikkhah G. Nigral transplants in the rat Parkinson model. Functional limitations and strategies to enhance nigrostriatal reconstruction. In: Dunnett SB, Björklund A, eds. *Functional neural transplantation*. New York: Raven, 1994:47–69.

69. Brecknell JE, Haque NSK, Du JS, et al. Functional and anatomical reconstruction of the 6-hydroxydopamine lesioned nigrostriatal system of the adult rat. *Neuroscience* 1996;71:913–925.

70. Zhou FS, Chiang YH, Wang Y. Constructing a new nigrostriatal pathway in the parkinsonian model with bridged neural transplantation in substantia nigra. *J Neurosci* 1996,16:6965–6974.

71. Mendez I, Sadi D, Hong M. Reconstruction of the nigrostriatal pathway by simultaneous intrastriatal and intranigral dopaminergic transplants. *J Neurosci* 1996;16:7216–7227.

72. Kish SJ, Shannak K, Hornykiewicz O. Uneven pattern of dopamine loss in the striatum of patients with idiopathic Parkinson's disease: pathophysiologic and clinical implications. *N Engl J Med* 1988;318:876–880.

73. Alexander GE, Crutcher MD, DeLong MR. Basal ganglia-thalamocortical circuits: parallel substrates for motor, oculomotor, "prefrontal" and "limbic" functions. *Prog Brain Res* 1990;85:119–146.

74. Hauser RA, Freeman TB, Snow BJ, et al. Long-term evaluation of bilateral fetal nigral transplantation in Parkinson disease. *Arch Neurol* 1999;56:179–187.

75. Agid Y, Javoy-Agid F, Ruberg M. Biochemistry of neurotransmitter in PD. In: Marsden CD, Fahn S, eds. *Movement disorders 2*. London: Butterworth, 1987:166–230.

76. Reading PJ. Neural transplantation in the ventral striatum. In: Dunnett SB, Björklund A, eds. *Functional neural transplantation*. New York: Raven, 1994:197–216.

77. Lindvall O, Widner H, Rehncrona S, et al. Transplantation of fetal dopamine neurons in Parkinson's disease: 1-year clinical and neurophysiological observations in two patients with putaminal implants. *Ann Neurol* 1992;31:155–165.

78. Lindvall O, Sawle G, Widner H, et al. Evidence for long-term survival and function of dopaminergic grafts in progressive Parkinson's disease. *Ann Neurol* 1994;35:172–180.

79. Piccini P, Lindvall O, Björklund A, et al. Delayed recovery of movement-related cortical function in Parkinson's disease striatal dopaminergic grafts. *Ann Neurol* 2000;48:689–695.

80. Hagell P, Schrag A, Piccini P, et al. Sequential bilateral transplantation in Parkinson's disease: effects of the second graft. *Brain* 1999;122:1121–1132.

81. Pakkenberg B, Møller A, Gundersen HJG, et al. The absolute number of nerve cells in substantia nigra in normal subjects and in patients with Parkinson's disease estimated with an unbiased stereological method. *J Neurol Neurosurg Psychiatry* 1991;54:30–33.

82. Frodl EM, Duan WM, Sauer H, et al. Human embryonic dopamine neurons xenografted to the rat: effects of cryopreservation and varying regional source of donor cells on transplant survival, morphology and function. *Brain Res* 1994;647:286–298.

83. Brundin P, Karlsson J, Emgård M, et al.. Improving the survival of grafted dopaminergic neurons: a review over current approaches. *Cell Transplant* 2000;9:179–195.

84. Nikkhah G, Eberhard J, Olsson M, et al. Preservation of fetal ventral mesencephalic cells by cool storage: *in vitro* viability and TH-positive neuron survival after microtransplantation to the striatum. *Brain Res* 1995;687:22–34.

85. Björklund L, Spenger C, Strömberg I. Tirilazad mesylate increases dopaminergic neuronal survival in the *in oculo* grafting model. *Exp Neurol* 1997;148:324–333.

86. Barker RA, Fricker RA, Abrous DN, et al. A comparative study of preparation techniques for improving the viability of nigral grafts using vital stains, *in vitro* cultures, and *in vivo* grafts. *Cell Transplant* 1995;4:173–200.

87. Watts C, Hurelbrink C, Dunnett SB. The method of preparation of the donor tissue affects functional outcome in a rodent model of Parkinson's disease. *Soc Neurosci Abstr* 1998;223:1.

88. Sinclair SR, Fawcett JW, Dunnett SB. Delayed implantation of nigral grafts improves survival of dopamine neurons and rate of functional recovery. *Neuroreport* 1999;10:1263–1267.

89. Mayer E, Dunnett SB, Fawcett JW. Basic fibroblast growth factor promotes the survival of embryonic ventral mesencephalic dopaminergic neurons. II. Effects on nigral transplants *in vivo*. *Neuroscience* 1993;56:389–398.

90. Takayama H, Ray J, Raymon HK, et al. Basic fibroblast growth factor increases dopaminergic graft survival and function in a rat model of Parkinson's disease. *Nat Med* 1995;1:53–58.

91. Rosenblad C, Martinez-Serrano A, Björklund A. Glial cell-line derived neurotrophic factor increases survival, growth and function of intrastriatal fetal nigral dopaminergic grafts. *Neuroscience* 1996;75:979–985.

92. Sinclair SR, Svendsen CN, Torres EM, et al. GDNF enhances dopaminergic cell survival and fiber outgrowth in embryonic nigral grafts. *Neuroreport* 1996;7:2547–2552.

93. Zeng BY, Jenner P, Marsden CD. Altered motor function and graft survival produced by basic fibroblast growth factor in rats with 6-OHDA lesions and fetal ventral mesencephalic grafts are associated with glial proliferation. *Exp Neurol* 1996;139:214–226.

94. Sautter J, Tseng JL, Braguglia D, et al. Implants of polymer-encapsulated genetically modified cells releasing glial cell line–derived neurotrophic factor improve survival, growth and function of fetal dopaminergic grafts. *Exp Neurol* 1998;149:230–236.

95. Sullivan AM, Pohl J, Blunt SB. Growth/differentiation factor 5 and glial cell line–derived neurotrophic factor enhance survival and function of dopaminergic grafts in a rat model of Parkinson's disease. *Eur J Neurosci* 1998;10:3681–3688.

96. Yurek DM. Glial cell line-derived neurotrophic factor improves survival of dopaminergic neurons in transplants of fetal ventral mesencephalic tissue. *Exp Neurol* 1998;153:195–202.

97. Wilby MJ, Sinclair SR, Muir EM, et al. A glial-cell line–derived neurotrophic factor–secreting clone of the Schwann cell line SCTM41 enhances survival and fiber outgrowth from embryonic nigral neurons grafted to the striatum and to the lesioned substantia nigra. *J Neurosci* 1999;19:2301–2312.

98. Frodl EM, Nakao N, Brundin P. Lazaroids improve the survival of cultured rat embryonic mesencephalic neurones. *Neuroreport* 1994;5:2393–2396.

99. Nakao N, Frodl EM, Duan WM, et al. Lazaroids improve the survival of grafted rat embryonic dopamine neurons. *Proc Natl Acad Sci USA* 1994;91:12408–12412.

100. Grasbon-Frodl EM, Nakao N, Brundin P. Lazaroids improve the survival of embryonic mesencephalic donor tissue stored at 4°C and subsequently used for cultures or intracerebral transplantation. *Brain Res Bull* 1996;39:341–347.

101. Othberg A, Keep M, Brundin P, et al. Tirilazad mesylate improves survival of rat and human embryonic mesencephalic neurons *in vitro*. *Exp Neurol* 1997;147:498–502.

102. Schierle GS, Hansson O, Leist M, et al. Caspase inhibition reduces apoptosis and increases survival of nigral transplants. *Nat Med* 1999;5:97–100.

103. Brundin P, Pogarell O, Hagell P, et al. Bilateral caudate and putamen grafts of embryonic mesencephalic tissue treated with lazaroids in Parkinson's disease. *Brain* 2000;123:1380–1390.

104. Breeze RE, Wells TH Jr, Freed CR. Implantation of fetal tissue for the management of Parkinson's disease: a technical note. *Neurosurgery* 1995;36:1044–1048.

105. Rehncrona S. A critical review of the current status and possible developments in brain transplantation. *Adv Techn Stand Neurosurg* 1997;23:3–46.

106. Widner H, Brundin P. Sequential intracerebral transplantation of allogeneic and syngeneic fetal dopamine-rich neuronal tissue in adult rats: will the first graft be rejected? *Cell Transplant* 1993;2:307–317.

107. Duan WM, Widner H, Björklund A, et al. Sequential intrastriatal grafting of allogeneic embryonic dopamine-rich neuronal tissue in adult rats: will the second graft be rejected? *Neuroscience* 1993;57:261–274.

108. Kordower JII, Styren S, Clarke M, et al. Fetal grafting for Parkinson's disease: expression of immune markers in two patients with functional fetal nigral implants. *Cell Transplant* 1997;6: 213–219.

109. Piccini P, Brooks DJ, Björklund A, et al. Dopamine release from nigral transplants visualized *in vivo* in a Parkinson's patient. *Nature Neurosci* 1999;2:1137–1140.

110. Langston JW, Widner H, Brooks D, et al. Core assessment program for intracerebral transplantations (CAPIT). *Mov Disord* 1992;7:1–13.

111. Defer GL, Widner H, Marié RM, et al. Core assessment program for surgical interventional therapies in Parkinson's disease (CAPSIT). *Mov Disord* 1999;14:572–584.

112. Spencer DD, Robbins RJ, Naftolin F, et al. Unilateral transplantation of human fetal mesencephalic tissue into the caudate nucleus of patients with Parkinson's disease. *N Engl J Med* 1992;327:1541–1548.

113. Freed CR, Breeze RE, Rosenberg NL, et al. Survival of implanted fetal dopamine cells and neurologic improvement 12 to 46 months after transplantation for Parkinson's disease. *N Engl J Med* 1992;327:1549–1555.

114. Sauer H, Frodl EM, Kupsch A, tet al. Cryopreservation, survival and function of intrastriatal fetal mesencephalic grafts in a rat model of Parkinson's disease. *Exp Brain Res* 1992;90: 54–62.

115. Sauer H, Brundin P. Effects of cool storage on survival and function of intrastriatal ventral mesencephalic grafts. *Res Neurol Neurosci* 1991;2:123–135.

116. Boer GJ. Ethical guidelines for the use of human embryonic or fetal tissue for experimental and clinical neurotransplantation and research. *J Neurol* 1994;242:1–3.

117. Annett LE, Torres EM, Clarke DJ, et al. Survival of nigral grafts within the striatum of marmosets with 6-OHDA lesions depends critically on donor embryo age. *Cell Transplant* 1997;6: 557–569.

Surgery for Parkinson's Disease and Movement Disorders,
edited by J.K. Krauss, J. Jankovic, and R.G. Grossman.
Lippincott Williams & Wilkins, Philadelphia © 2001.

16

CLINICAL EXPERIENCE WITH FETAL NEURAL TRANSPLANTATION IN PARKINSON'S DISEASE

CURT R. FREED
EDWARD D. CLARKSON
MAUREEN A. LEEHEY
MICHAEL ZAWADA
LAETITIA L. THOMPSON
ROBERT E. BREEZE

As other chapters in this book describe, various neurosurgical procedures are used for the treatment of Parkinson's disease (PD) including lesions and deep brain stimulation of the thalamus, pallidum, and subthalamic nucleus (1–3). *Neurotransplantation* differs fundamentally from these strategies, because only neurotransplantation repairs the primary defect of PD, the loss of dopamine neurons. Neurotransplantation into human patients has depended on a rich background of experiments in animals, primarily rats. Nearly every principle established in the rat has proven applicable to humans. In the rat, embryonic dopamine neurons from a restricted period of development, 13 to 15 days after conception, are suitable for transplantation. For human transplantation, the equivalent stage of human embryonic development is 6 to 8 weeks after conception. All successful transplants of human embryonic tissue into human patients have come from tissue in this developmental window (4–19). Because the supply of human fetal tissue is limited and variable in quality, some researchers have transplanted chromaffin cells from the patient's own adrenal medulla (21–24), and others have transplanted fetal pig neural cells (25). Our recently completed double-blind placebo controlled trial provided the first data with a large enough group of carefully selected patients to draw statistically valid conclusions about outcome for a single transplant strategy (26–28).

EXPERIMENTAL DEVELOPMENT OF NEURAL TRANSPLANTATION IN PARKINSON'S DISEASE

Grafts of autologous adrenal chromaffin cells were put into the caudate nucleus of patients with parkinsonism (21), even though animal models showed that adrenal cells could not survive in brain without a source of nerve growth factor (29,30). Grafting of cells from the adrenal medulla was abandoned because of the lack of efficacy and the significant morbidity associated with the surgical procedure itself (31). Failure of the clinical trials of adrenal transplants after failed animal experiments highlights the finding that negative as well as positive animal data have been highly predictive of human transplant outcome. Xenografts of neural tissue offer immunologic challenges that have not been overcome. In the porcine graft, only a few hundred cells survived out of hundreds of thousands of dopamine neurons transplanted.

Key to the successful development of human neurotransplantation was the early development of the unilateral model of PD in the rat. In 1970, Ungerstedt and Arbuthnott showed that injection of the neurotoxin 6-hydroxydopamine (6-OHDA) into the medial forebrain bundle of rat brain produced unilateral destruction of dopamine neurons in the substantia nigra pars compacta and loss of dopamine nerve terminals in the striatum (32). Rats unilaterally lesioned with 6-OHDA turn toward their lesioned side when they are given methamphetamine. Dopamine released asymmetrically from the intact side of striatum drives the circling behavior. Conversely, the dopamine agonist apomorphine asymmetrically stimulates the supersensitive dopamine receptors

C.R. Freed, E.E. Clarkson, M.A. Leehey, M. Zawada, L.L. Thompson, and R.E. Breeze: Division of Clinical Pharmacology and Toxicology, University of Colorado Health Sciences Center, Denver, Colorado 80262.

in the denervated striatum and leads to circling in the direction contralateral to the lesion. In 1979, Björklund and Stenevi (33) and Perlow et al. (34) transplanted embryonic mesencephalic dopamine cells into the denervated side of striatum and showed that these grafts reduced drug-induced rotation. Histochemical staining demonstrated the presence of transplanted dopamine cells and neurite outgrowth.

Subsequent experiments showed that rat embryonic dopamine cells grafted into 6-OHDA–lesioned rats exhibited electrical firing patterns and responses to dopamine agonists and antagonists similar to dopamine cells recorded from the substantia nigra pars compacta of adult animals (35). Transplanted cells could synthesize and release dopamine (36). Fetal grafts have been shown to reinnervate up to two-thirds of the denervated striatum, and both host-to-graft and graft-to-host synapses are present in the host striatum (37). The behavioral effects of transplantation in rats are specific to mesencephalic dopamine cells. Rats transplanted with fetal tissue from mesencephalic raphe (which produces serotonin) or fetal tissue from striatum had no improvement in behavior (38).

A primate model of PD resulted when a group of persons addicted to narcotics inadvertently injected themselves with the neurotoxin 1-methyl-4-phenyl-1,2,3,6-tetrahydropyrine (MPTP) (39). From this striking misadventure came a nonhuman primate model of PD (40–43). Monkeys lesioned by MPTP showed signs such as bradykinesia, rigidity, and action tremor. Grafting fetal mesencephalic tissue significantly reduced the parkinsonian symptoms, provided the embryonic dopamine cells were obtained from early in embryogenesis at a stage equivalent to embryonic day 13 to 15 in the rat. Transplants into the monkey model of PD provided an important test of principle in a larger brain. Monkey experiments were most useful for showing that the principles established in rats also applied to the larger primate brain.

CLINICAL EXPERIENCE WITH FETAL NEURAL TRANSPLANTATION IN PARKINSON'S DISEASE

From the first published report in 1989 and continuing through 2000, clinical outcomes from a variety of transplant techniques have been published (4–19). Methods differ in the amount of tissue transplanted, the preparation of the tissue as suspensions or solid tissue fragments, the use of immunosuppression, the placement of tissue unilaterally or bilaterally, and the targeting of tissue into putamen, caudate, or both. Patients with parkinsonism provide additional variability. Age and sex may be important variables, as is the specific disease in the individual patient. To define patients as having idiopathic PD, most investigators have chosen patients who were responsive to L-dopa. Some investigators

have used fluorodopa positron emission tomography (PET) to image the characteristic pattern of dopamine depletion in putamen with relative sparing in the caudate nucleus. In an earlier review, we examined the effect of these different variables in 62 patients followed for at least 1 year to look for methodologic differences that would account for differences in clinical outcome (20). No single clinical rating score has been used by the different groups. Therefore, for purposes of our previous review, we characterized the clinical improvement as none, mild, or moderate. Somewhat more objective was the change in L-dopa dose. Thus, change in drug dosage may be a reasonable surrogate marker for successful transplant outcome.

In our double-blind placebo controlled trial, we found that 1 year after transplantation, patients showed improvements in bradykinesia and rigidity (26–28). Whereas tremor showed a trend for improvement, statistical significance was not reached. Transplants were detectable in 85% of patients by fluorodopa PET scan and grew equally well in younger and older patients. Patients less than 60 years of age were most likely to benefit, and changes in the Unified Parkinson's Disease Rating Scale (UPDRS) correlated with changes in PET signal. Patients older than 60 years showed significant improvement in rigidity, whereas gait worsened. Because some patients are now up to 5 years of posttransplant status, some long-term analysis is possible. By 3 years after transplantation, UPDRS "off" measurements improved (reduced) by 30% for both the younger and the older transplant groups. Although continuing changes were seen in younger and older patients, statistical significance was reached only in the transplant group as a whole and in the younger transplant recipients. The requirements for L-dopa and other drugs were reduced an average of 50%. The change in UPDRS scores reflected about 50% of the difference between the "off" scores and the "on" scores for patients preoperatively, Thus, at this stage of development, transplants replace half of the drug requirement and produce half of the clinical effect of dopaminergic agonists. These long-term changes are similar to what we first described in 1992 (8), and they are similar to what other groups have subsequently confirmed.

Long-term results have also included the appearance of dyskinesias in about 12% of transplant recipients (four of 34). These dyskinetic responses were present even after substantial reduction or even elimination of L-dopa and other dopamine agonist therapy. Although one patient with this complication had severe dyskinesias before the transplant, other patients had worse dyskinesias after transplantation than before. It appears that the transplantation of tissue from four embryos provided too much dopaminergic effect in these patients, particularly because all four had had remarkable resolution of their parkinsonian signs in the first year after the transplant. Because fluorodopa PET scans do not show supranormal concentrations of dopamine in these patients, it is possible that the dyskinetic response has its origin in other brain structures such as the subthalamic nucleus, the pallidum, or the pars reticulata of the substantia nigra. An imbalance between the restored dopamine innervation of putamen and the persistent denervation of substantia nigra pars compacta may be responsible for the dyskinetic responses. We reported a tendency toward dyskinetic movements in our first transplant recipient in 1990 (5), as well as in six of seven patients described in 1992 (8). In most of these patients, dyskinesias were controlled by reductions in drug doses.

Unilateral Versus Bilateral Transplantation

Unilateral transplantation of fetal tissue was used in the first clinical PD transplant trials (4–6,14). Typically, implants were made into the side of brain contralateral to the side of the body with the worse PD symptoms. In an attempt to provide more symmetric innervation and with the goal of improving axial functions such as walking, we and others began transplanting fetal tissue bilaterally in the early 1990s (8,12). Table 16.1 presents the change in motor performance and L-dopa dose in this patient group. Bilateral transplantation of fetal tissue led to a significantly greater reduction in the dose of L-dopa administered 1 year after transplantation (37%) when compared with the L-dopa dose administered to recipients of unilateral transplants (12%). Although bilateral recipients had a greater reduction in L-dopa administration, the overall benefit from transplantation was not different for the two groups; approximately 50% of patients in both groups demonstrated moderate improvement in motor skills. A moderate benefit was defined as a 35% drop in the UPDRS or Hoehn and Yahr scale (depending on which one the initial authors reported), with a mild benefit defined as a 5% to 34% drop in the UPDRS or Hoehn and Yahr scale. Because these scales are not strictly comparable, we did not perform statistical analysis on clinical benefit.

Solid Versus Suspension Graft

Fetal mesencephalic tissue can be transplanted either as a suspension of dissociated mesencephalon or as a solid graft. In some studies, human fetal tissue transplanted into immunosuppressed 6-OHDA–lesioned rats showed comparable

TABLE 16.1. OUTCOME AT 1 YEAR AFTER TRANSPLANT: UNILATERAL VERSUS BILATERAL

		Benefit			% Change in[a]
	N	None	Mild	Moderate	L-dopa at 1 Yr
Unilateral	15	7%	40%	53%	−12 ± 5
Bilateral	39	28%	26%	46%	−37 ± 5[b]

[a]All data represent the mean ± SEM.
[b]*p* < .005 by unpaired *t* test; changes in L-dopa dose based on 35 of the 54 patients.

TABLE 16.2. OUTCOME AT 1 YEAR AFTER TRANSPLANT: SOLID VERSUS SUSPENSION

		Benefit			% Change in[a]
	N	None	Mild	Moderate	L-dopa at 1 Yr
Suspension	21	24%	24%	42%	−8 ± 5
Solid	33	21%	33%	45%	−38 ± 5[b]

[a]All data represent the mean ± SEM.
[b]*p* < .001 by unpaired *t* test; changes in L-dopa dose based on 35 of the 54 patients.

survival of both solid and suspension grafts (45). However, our studies showed that rat mesencephalon transplanted in the form of a strand (made by extruding mesencephalic tissue through a tapered glass cannula with a 0.2-mm bore) into 6-OHDA–lesioned rats produced greater behavioral improvement and better dopamine neuron survival than transplants of dissociated mesencephalon (46).

Table 16.2 contrasts transplant outcome in patients receiving solid grafts or cell suspensions of mesencephalon. Recipients of solid tissue grafts had similar improvements in their motor skills but were able to reduce their L-dopa dose more than the cell suspension group (38% versus 8%, *p* < .001). These results suggest that patient outcome may be better after grafting of solid tissue fragments.

Gender and Transplant Outcome

Table 16.3 examines the outcome of transplants by patient gender. Clinical outcome appeared to be better in men than in women, with a larger fraction of men having a "moderate response" (56% men versus 33% women) and more women having no response (17% men; 33% women). Conversely, women had a significantly larger reduction in L-dopa dose than men (−42% versus −20%). Women were underrepresented in these early studies, making up only 33% of the total. In our double-blind study, women were represented about equally with men (19 women, 21 men).

Age as a Predictor of Transplant Outcome

Although PD is primarily a disease of elderly persons, some researchers have been hesitant to perform transplantation in

TABLE 16.3. OUTCOME AT 1 YEAR AFTER TRANSPLANT: MALE VERSUS FEMALE

		Benefit			% Change in[a]
	N	None	Mild	Moderate	L-dopa at 1 Yr
Male	36	17%	28%	56%	−20 ± 4
Female	18	33%	33%	33%	−42 ± 11[b]

[a]All data represent the mean ± SEM.
[b]*p* < .05 by unpaired *t* test; changes in L-dopa dose based on 35 of the 54 patients.

TABLE 16.4. CLINICAL BENEFIT VERSUS PATIENT AGE AT TRANSPLANT

	N	None	Mild	Moderate
< Age 54	27	11%	33%	56%
≥ Age 54	27	33%	26%	41%

TABLE 16.5. CLINICAL BENEFIT VERSUS NUMBER OF DONORS

Donors	N	None	Mild	Moderate
1–3	26	19%	23%	58%
4–8	28	25%	36%	39%

older patients with PD because of the potentially increased risk of complications. In the pool of transplant recipients we reviewed, the average age at the time of transplantation was 54 years, with disease duration of about 13 years. Because in PD the average age of onset is 55 years, and the average patient with PD is estimated to be 67 years old, it is clear that clinical trials have favored selecting young patients with PD.

Table 16.4 presents clinical outcome data as a function of age. The median age was 54 years. Younger patients were more likely to have a moderate response and were less likely to have no response than older patients. Our recently concluded double-blind study showed that transplants grow well in patients regardless of age, but older patients are less likely to have positive clinical benefit than patients less than 60 years old. Before the surgical procedure, the older patients had a lesser response to drugs as measured by the change in UPDRS "off" scores to "on" scores: 75% in age 60 years or younger; 59% in patients more than 60 years old. In the aging brain, the symptoms of PD are likely to be one manifestation of a more global neuropathologic process.

Number of Donors

The number of surviving dopaminergic neurons needed to improve motor function significantly in a patient with PD is unknown. The normal adult human substantia nigra contains approximately 500,000 dopamine-producing neurons (47). Unfortunately, about 95% of dopamine neurons die after transplantation of rat or human tissue. In human patients, no more than 20,000 to 25,000 dopamine cells survive from each embryo transplanted (15,31,48–50). Some investigators have argued that such a high rate of cell death requires that tissue from six or more donors be transplanted into each putamen to restore a complete complement of dopamine-producing neurons. Studies examining the ideal volume of grafted tissue in patients with PD are limited (51), and the issue is still widely debated (44). Because the symptoms of PD develop only after a 50% loss of nigral neurons and a 60% to 80% reduction in striatal dopamine (52,53), complete replacement of dopamine-producing neurons may not be required to improve motor skills and to reduce L-dopa dosage significantly (9).

Table 16.5 shows the relationship between clinical benefit and the number of donor embryos. Patients receiving cells from one to three embryos had a greater likelihood of a moderate clinical response than patients receiving four

to eight embryos. Ultimately, the optimal number of tissue donors will have to be established by a controlled clinical trial. For our double-blind study, tissue from four embryos was used for all patients. Because this dose produced dyskinetic responses in about 12% of patients, it is likely that the optimum number of cells will be derived from two to four embryos per patient.

Other variables in fetal tissue transplantation include the time and method of storage of fetal tissue before grafting, the postgestational age of the donor tissue, the location of graft sites, and the number of transplant tracts made. These parameters differed widely in the patients described in this chapter and may account for some of the variability in clinical outcome.

ALTERNATIVE TRANSPLANT STRATEGIES

In addition to the scientific controversies about techniques for transplantation of human fetal tissue, there remain ethical concerns about using human fetal tissue. There are also logistical problems of supplying tissue. With the demonstration that fetal pig neural cells can survive transplantation into a patient with PD (25), xenografts may be a potential alternative to human cell transplants, although the immunologic hurdles are enormous and unresolved. We reported that cloned transgenic animal embryos could be a useful source of fetal tissue for transplantation (54). Immortalized cell lines that do not generate tumors can reduce dopaminergic deficits and may offer an additional alternative to human fetal tissue (55). Because xenograft rejection remains an unsolved problem, aggressive immunosuppression is required for transplantation of all nonhuman tissue. Efforts to blunt the immune response by methods such as using fragments of a monoclonal antibody to major histocompatibility complex class I (56) or class II antigens may reduce xenograft rejection. Encapsulating dopamine-producing xenografts may also prevent rejection, although such anatomically isolated grafts have no capacity to reinnervate the host brain (57). Xenografts carry the potential risk of animal virus transmission to humans. With the concern about Creutzfeldt-Jakob disease, special efforts to monitor and control this risk are required. Although cloned animal embryos offer perhaps the best opportunity to manage this risk (54), another alternative source of tissue is the use of stem cells (58,59). Although studies have shown stem cells undergoing neuronal differentiation and migration within the brain, these studies are not as advanced as the studies applying xenotransplantation for the treatment of PD (58,59).

Interest has also focused on the delivery of neurotrophic factors to help reduce the number of dopamine neurons that die after transplantation. Cotransplantation of fibroblasts infected to produce basic fibroblast growth factor with mesencephalic grafts increased the number of dopamine neurons in these transplants (60). Treating embryonic dopamine neurons with growth factors such as basic fibroblast growth factor, insulinlike growth factor I, and glial cell line–derived neurotrophic factor also reduced apoptosis in the transplant (49,61,62). By inhibiting interleukin-converting enzyme in preparations of dissociated rat fetal tissue, dopamine cell survival was significantly increased in transplanted hemiparkinsonian rats (63).

PROSPECTS OF FETAL NEURAL TRANSPLANTATION

In summary, many patients with parkinsonism who have received human fetal tissue transplants have shown improvements in motor skills and have had reduced requirements for L-dopa. Solid grafts have produced better results than dispersed preparations. Nonetheless, clinical outcome is variable because of differences in transplant survival and in pathologic features in individual patients. Although some groups claim that mesencephalic tissue from six to eight embryos must be transplanted for maximal clinical benefit, there is no evidence supporting this position. Long-term results in our double-blind study showed that about 12% of patients receiving transplants showed signs of excess dopamine effect in the years after transplantation of tissue from four embryos. Age is also an important variable. Although transplants grow in patients regardless of age, clinical benefit appears to be more likely in younger patients. Because we have seen successful transplant survival with no immunosuppression, it is unlikely that immunosuppression plays a critical role in transplant outcome. Only a large clinical trial will establish the true benefit of immunosuppression.

Where shall human transplant research go from here? Open clinical trials of small numbers of patients have shown the feasibility of transplantation but have not answered any of the critical questions for the field. Only well-controlled double-blind studies, which we proposed and have carried out, can answer critical questions. Because of the limited clinical benefit of transplants even with substantial cell survival, we are obliged to consider new targets for transplantation. Because the region of dopamine cell loss, the substantia nigra pars compacta, has important regional connections with the pars reticulata, the subthalamic nucleus, and the pallidum, the substantia nigra should be the next target for transplantation. Although restoring the complete anatomic integrity of the nigrostriatal dopamine system is a daunting challenge, neurotransplantation has already demonstrated successful repair of the human parkinsonian brain. Refining methods to produce a transplant "cure" for PD appears possible.

CONCLUSIONS

Since 1988, neurotransplantation with embryonic dopamine cells has been tried as a treatment for patients with advanced PD. Although transplant methods have differed substantially among centers, most reports have found some efficacy to tissue implants made into caudate and putamen. Reduction of L-dopa dose requirements is frequently reported. Several principles have emerged. Mesencephalic tissue must be from early in embryonic development, typically 7 to 8 weeks after conception. Bilateral transplantation into putamen can be done safely during a single operation. Unilateral transplantation leads to asymmetric transplant effects. Although the clinical benefit in individual patients has made drug elimination possible, there is substantial variability in outcome. Contributing to this variability are differences in pathologic processes in individual patients and in dopamine neuron survival and outgrowth. In a recently completed double-blind placebo-controlled surgical trial, transplants have been shown to improve bradykinesia and rigidity, two of the principal motor impairments of PD. In about 12% of patients, worsening dyskinesias complicated transplantation, despite substantial reduction of L-dopa doses.

REFERENCES

1. Tasker RR, Lang AE, Lozano AM. Pallidal and thalamic surgery for Parkinson's disease. *Exp Neurol* 1997;144:35–40.
2. Koller WC, Wilkinson S, Pahwa R, et al. Surgical treatment options in Parkinson's disease. *Neurosurg Clin North Am* 1998;9:295–306.
3. Starr PA, Vitek JL, Bakay RA. Ablative surgery and deep brain stimulation for Parkinson's disease. *Neurosurg Clin North Am* 1998;9:381–402.
4. Lindvall O, Rehncrona S, Brundin P, et al. Human fetal dopamine neurons grafted into the striatum in two patients with severe Parkinson's disease. *Arch Neurol* 1989;46:615–631.
5. Freed CR, Breeze RE, Rosenberg NL, et al. Transplantation of human fetal dopamine cells for Parkinson's disease. *Arch Neurol* 1990;47:505–512.
6. Lindvall O, Brundin P, Widner H, et al. Grafts of fetal dopamine neurons survive and improve motor function in Parkinson's disease. *Science* 1990;247:574–577.
7. Henderson BT, Clough CG, Hughes RC, et al. Implantation of human fetal ventral mesencephalon to the right caudate nucleus in advanced Parkinson's disease. *Arch Neurol* 1991;48:822–827.
8. Freed CR, Breeze RE, Rosenberg NL, et al. Survival of implanted fetal dopamine cells and neurologic improvement 12 to 46 months after transplantation for Parkinson's disease. *N Engl J Med* 1992;327:1549–1555.
9. Freed CR, Breeze RE, Rosenberg NL, et al. Embryonic dopamine cell implants as a treatment for the second phase of Parkinson's disease: replacing failed nerve terminals. *Adv Neurol* 1992;XX:721–728.

10. Lindvall O, Widner H, Rehncrona S, et al. Transplantation of fetal dopamine neurons in Parkinson's disease: one year clinical and neurophysiological observations in two patients. *Ann Neurol* 1992;31:155–165.

11. Spencer DD, Robbins RJ, Naftolin F, et al. Unilateral transplantation of human fetal mesencephalic tissue into the caudate nucleus of patients with Parkinson's disease. *N Engl J Med* 1992;327:1541–1548.

12. Widner H, Tetrud J, Rehncrona S, et al. Bilateral fetal mesencephalic grafting in two patients with Parkinsonism induced by 1-methyl-4-phenyl-1,2,3,6-tetrahydropyridine (MPTP). *N Engl J Med* 1992;327:1556–1563.

13. Peschanski M, Defer G, N'Guyen JP, et al. Bilateral motor improvement and lateralization of L-dopa effect in two patients with Parkinson's disease following intrastriatal transplantation of foetal ventral mesencephalon. *Brain* 1994;117:487–499.

14. Defer GL, Geny C, Ricolfi F, et al. Long-term outcome of unilaterally transplanted parkinsonian patients. I. Clinical approach. *Brain* 1996;119:41–50.

15. Kordower JH, Freeman TB, Snow BJ, et al. Neuropathological evidence of graft survival and striatal reinnervation after the transplantation of fetal mesencephalic tissue in a patient with Parkinson's disease. *N Engl J Med* 1995;332:1118–1124.

16. Freeman TB, Olanow CW, Hauser RA, et al. Bilateral fetal nigral transplantation into the postcommissural putamen in Parkinson's disease. *Ann Neurol* 1995;38:379–388.

17. Freed CR, Breeze RE, Schneck SA, et al. Fetal neural transplantation for Parkinson's disease. In: Rich RR, ed. *Clinical immunology: principles and practice.* St. Louis: Mosby–Year Book, 1995:1677–1687.

18. Kopyov OV, Jacques D, Lieberman A, et al. Clinical study of fetal mesencephalic intracerebral transplants for the treatment of Parkinson's disease. *Cell Transplant* 1996;5:327–337.

19. Wenning GK, Odin P, Morrish P, et al. Short- and long-term survival and function of unilateral intrastriatal dopaminergic grafts in Parkinson's disease. *Ann Neurol* 1997;42:95–107.

20. Clarkson ED, Freed CR. Minireview: development of fetal neural transplantation as a treatment for Parkinson's disease. *Life Sci* 1999;65:2427–2437.

21. Lindvall O, Backlund EO, Farde L, et al. Transplantation in Parkinson's disease: two cases of adrenal medullary grafts to the putamen. *Ann Neurol* 1987;22:457–468.

22. Madrazo I, Drucker-Colin T, Daiz V, et al. Open micro-surgical autograft of adrenal medulla to the right caudate nucleus in two patients with intractable Parkinson's disease. *N Engl J Med* 1987;316:831–833.

23. Goetz CG, Olanow CW, Koller WC, et al. Multicenter study of autologous adrenal medullary transplantation to the corpus striatum in patients with advanced Parkinson's disease. *N Engl J Med* 1989;320:337–341.

24. Olanow CW, Koller WC, Goetz CG, et al. Autologous transplantation of adrenal medulla in Parkinson's disease: 18-month results. *Arch Neurol* 1990;47:1286–1289.

25. Deacon T, Schumacher J, Dinsmore J, et al. Histological evidence of fetal pig neural cell survival after transplantation into a patient with Parkinson's disease. *Nat Med* 1997;3:350–353.

26. Freed CR, Breeze RE, Greene PE, et al. Double-blind controlled trial of human embryonic dopamine cell transplants in advanced Parkinson's disease: study design, surgical strategy, patient demographics and pathological outcome. *Neurology* 1999;52 [Suppl 2]:A272(abst).

27. Greene PE, Fahn S, Tsai WY, et al. Double-blind controlled trial of human embryonic dopamine tissue transplants in advanced Parkinson's disease: long-term unblinded follow-up phase. *Mov Disord* 1999.

28. Freed CR, Greene PE, Breeze RE, et al. Transplantation of embryonic dopamine neurons for severe Parkinson's disease. *N Engl J Med* 2001;344:710–719.

29. Stromberg I, Herrera-Marachitz M, Ungerstedt U, et al. Chronic implants of chromaffin tissue into the dopamine-denervated striatum: effects of NGF on graft survival, fiber growth, and rotational behavior. *Exp Brain Res* 1985;60:335–349.

30. Kordower JH, Fiandaca MS, Notter MF, et al. NGF-like trophic support from peripheral nerve for grafted rhesus adrenal chromaffin cells. *J Neurosurg* 1990;73:418–428.

31. Kordower JH, Goetz CG, Freeman TB, et al. Dopaminergic transplants in patients with Parkinson's disease neuroanatomical correlates of clinical recovery. *Exp Neurol* 1997;144:41–46.

32. Ungerstedt U, Arbuthnott GW. Quantitative recording of rotational behavior in rats after 6-hydroxy-dopamine lesions of the nigrostriatal dopamine system. *Brain Res* 1970;24:485–493.

33. Björklund A, Steveni U. Reconstruction of the nigrostriatal dopamine pathway by intracerebral nigral transplants. *Brain Res* 1979;177:555–560.

34. Perlow MJ, Freed WJ, Hoffer BJ, et al. Brain grafts reduce motor abnormalities produced by destruction of nigrostriatal dopamine system. *Science* 1979;204:555–560.

35. Wuerthele SM, Freed WJ, Olson L, et al. Effect of dopamine agonists and antagonists on the electrical activity of substantia nigra neurons transplanted into the lateral ventricle of the rat. *Exp Brain Res* 1981;44:1–10.

36. Schmidt RH, Ingvar M, Lindvall O, et al. Functional activity of substantia nigra grafts reinnervating the striatum: neurotransmitter metabolism and (^{14}C)2-deoxy-D-glucose autoradiography. *J Neurochem* 1982;38:737–748.

37. Mahalik TJ, Finger TE, Stromberg I, et al. Substantia nigra transplants into denervated striatum of the rat ultrastructure of graft and host interconnections. *J Comp Neurol* 1985;240:60–70.

38. Dunnett SB, Hernandez TD, Summerfield A, et al. Graft-derived recovery from 6-OHDA lesions: specificity of ventral mesencephalic graft tissues *Exp Brain Res* 1988;71:411–424.

39. Langston JW, Ballard P, Tetrud JW, et al. Chronic parkinsonism in humans due to a produce of meperidine-analog synthesis. *Science* 1983;219:979–980.

40. Bakay RAE, Fiandaca MS, Barrow DL, et al. Preliminary report of the use of fetal tissue transplantation to correct MPTP-induced Parkinson-like symptoms in primates. *Appl Neurophysiol* 1985;48:358–361.

41. Freed CR, Richards JB, Sabol KE, et al. In: Beart PM, Woodruff G, Jackson DM, eds, *Pharmacology and functional regulation of dopaminergic neurons.* London: Macmillan, 1988:353–360.

42. Sladek, Jr JR, Collier TJ, Haber SN, et al. Reversal of parkinsonism by fetal nerve cell transplants in primate brain. *Ann NY Acad Sci* 1987;495:641–657.

43. Taylor JR, Elsworth JD, Roth RH, et al. Grafting of fetal substantia nigra to striatum reverses behavioral deficits induced by MPTP in primates: a comparison with other type of grafts as controls. *Exp Brain Res* 1991;85:335–348.

44. Olanow CW, Kordower JH, Freeman TB. Fetal nigral transplantation as a therapy for Parkinson's disease. *Trends Neurosci* 1996;19:102–109.

45. Freeman TB, Sanberg PR, Nauert GM, et al. The influence of donor age on the survival of solid and suspension intraparenchymal human embryonic nigral cells. *Cell Transplant* 1995;4:141–154.

46. Clarkson ED, Zawada WM, Adams FS, et al. Strands of embryonic mesencephalic tissue show greater dopamine neuron survival and better behavioral improvement than cell suspensions after transplantation in parkinsonian rats. *Brain Res* 1998;806:60–68.

47. Pakkenberg B, Moller A, Gundersen HJ, et al. The absolute number of nerve cells in substantia nigra in normal subjects

and in patients with Parkinson's disease estimated with unbiased stereological method. *J Neurol Neurosurg Psychiatry* 1991;54:30–33.

48. Brundin P, Barbin G, Isacson O, et al. Survival of intracerebrally grafted rat dopamine neurons previously cultured *in vitro. Neurosci. Lett* 1985;61:79–84.

49. Zawada WM, Zastrow DJ, Clarkson ED, et al. Growth factors improve immediate survival of embryonic dopamine neurons after transplantation into rats. *Brain Res* 1998;786:96–103.

50. Freed CR, Trojanowski JQ, Galvin JE, et al. Embryonic dopamine cells cultured as strands show long term survival without immunosuppression in a patient with advanced Parkinson's disease. *Soc Neurosci Abstr* 1997;23:1682.

51. Kopyov OV, Jacques DS, Lieberman A, et al. Outcome following intrastriatal fetal mesencephalic grafts for Parkinson's patients is directly related to the volume of grafted tissue. *Exp Neurol* 1997;146:536–545.

52. Bernheimer H, Birkmayer W, Hornykiewicz O, et al. Brain dopamine and the syndromes of Parkinson and Huntington's: clinical, morphological and neurochemical correlations. *J Neurol Sci* 1973;20:415–455.

53. Kish SJ, Shannak K, Hornykiewicz O. Uneven pattern of dopamine loss in the striatum of patients with idiopathic Parkinson's disease. *N Engl J Med* 1988;318:876–880.

54. Zawada WM, Cibelli JB, Choi PK, et al. Somatic cell cloned transgenic bovine neurons for transplantation in parkinsonian rats. *Nat Med* 1998;4:569–574.

55. Clarkson ED, La Rosa FG, Edwards-Prasad J, et al. Improvement of neurological deficits in 6-hydroxydopamine-lesioned rats after transplantation with allogeneic simian virus 40 large tumor antigen gene-induced immortalized dopamine cells. *Proc Natl Acad Sci USA* 1998;95:1256–1270.

56. Palzaban P, Deacon TW, Burns LH, et al. A novel mode of immunoprotection of neural xenotransplants: masking of donor major histocompatibility complex class I enhances transplant survival in the central nervous system. *Neuroscience* 1995;65:983–996.

57. Emerich DF, Winn SR, Christenson L, et al. A novel approach to neural transplantation in Parkinson's disease: use of polymer-encapsulated cell therapy. *Neurosci Biobehav Rev* 1992;16:437–447.

58. Reynolds BA, Weiss D. Generation of neurons and astrocytes from isolated cells of the mammalian central nervous system. *Science* 1992;255:1707–1710.

59. Lee SH, Lumelsky N, Studer L, et al. Efficient generation of midbrian and hindbrain neurons from mouse embryonic stem cells. *Nat Biotechnol* 2000;18:675–679.

60. Takayama H, Ray J, Raymon HK, et al. Basic fibroblasts growth factor increases dopaminergic graft survival and function in a rat model of Parkinson's disease. *Nat Med* 1995;1:53–58.

61. Clarkson ED, Zawada WM, Freed CR. GDNF reduces apoptosis in dopaminergic neurons *in vitro. Neuroreport* 1995;7:145–149.

62. Zawada WM, Kirschman DL, Cohen JJ, et al. Growth factors rescue embryonic dopamine neurons from programmed cell death. *Exp Neurol* 1996:140:60–67.

63. Schierle GS, Hansson O, Leist M, et al. Caspase inhibition reduces apoptosis and increases survival of nigral transplants. *Nat Med* 1999;5:97–100.

Surgery for Parkinson's Disease and Movement Disorders,
edited by J.K. Krauss, J. Jankovic, and R.G. Grossman.
Lippincott Williams & Wilkins, Philadelphia © 2001.

17

NEURAL TRANSPLANTATION WITH CELL SOURCES OTHER THAN HUMAN FETAL TISSUE

J. STEPHEN FINK

The adult mammalian central nervous system (CNS) has a limited capacity to generate new nerve cells. This limited capacity of the CNS for self-repair remains the most fundamental obstacle to treatment of neurodegenerative and other diseases of the CNS. The success of human fetal tissue transplants in Parkinson's disease (PD) has established as viable the principle of cell replacement therapy for diseases of the CNS. Human fetal transplants are reviewed in Chapters 15 and 16. The results of human fetal transplants for treatment of PD serve as lessons that are instructive for other cell therapies that are under development for treatment of diseases of the CNS, including PD. In this chapter, the status of new cell sources, other than human fetal tissue, which may be used as cell replacement therapy for the CNS will be reviewed, with particular reference to neurodegenerative diseases such as PD and also Huntington's disease (HD).

EXPERIENCE WITH HUMAN FETAL TRANSPLANTS

The first demonstration of that neuronal cells could be transplanted, survive, and repair motor deficits in the adult mammalian CNS was published in 1979 (1,2). Since the initial reports of human fetal transplantation in 1988 (3,4), there have been more than 300 human fetal transplant procedures performed in patients with PD. Although the outcome of only a small number of these patients has been reported in detail in the peer-reviewed literature (5–11), several conclusions can be made, as follows:

1. *Human fetal dopaminergic nerves are able to survive and grow when they are transplanted into patients with PD.* The results of imaging with ^{18}F-DOPA positron emission tomography (PET) and neuropathologic analysis of several

autopsies have demonstrated that transplanted human fetal dopaminergic neurons appear to be capable of differentiation and progressive fiber outgrowth accompanied by dopamine synthesis and release (10–14). Animal studies suggest the formation of reciprocal connections with host brain and regulated release of the neurotransmitter dopamine (15,16). Growth and differentiation of transplanted fetal neurons appear to be tightly regulated; when unregulated growth has occurred, it appears to be explained by deviation from standard dissection or surgical procedures (17,18).

2. *Long-term graft survival is possible.* Striatal ^{18}F-DOPA PET signal can be normalized by the graft (5,10,13), and in the longest reported case, graft survival and regulated release were demonstrated 10 years after transplantation (13).

3. *Sustained clinical improvement is possible, but the degree of improvement is variable.* In all reported studies, clinical improvement was observed in many patients, and some patients were able to stop taking antiparkinson medication, but there has been a broad range of clinical improvement (5–11). Additional results from human fetal transplants conducted in controlled, blinded clinical trials (in which placebo effect and observer bias are minimized) (19) will be required to determine accurately the quantitative improvement in clinical status after transplantation. The results of the first double-blind trial of human fetal transplants in PD showed modest quantitative improvement (20). Somewhat unexpectedly, there was an apparent age dependence in the degree of clinical improvement, and several patients developed spontaneous, disabling dyskinesias ("off"-medication) more than 1 year after neural transplantation (20). The factors that are responsible for the variability in clinical response remain to be determined.

4. *Long-term immunosuppression may not be necessary for fetal allograft survival.* Allograft survival was observed using a variety of immunosuppression protocols (5–11). Robust graft survival was observed with short-term, mild ("low-dose") cyclosporine, although at autopsy there was clear evidence of immune response at the site of surviving graft

J.S. Fink: Department of Neurology, Boston Medical Center, Boston University School of Medicine, Boston, Massachusetts 02118.

(22) 18 months after transplantation (7,11), as well as 1 year after immunosuppression had stopped. The significance of this observation for long-term graft viability is not known.

NEED FOR OTHER CELL SOURCES FOR PARKINSON'S DISEASE

Because of practical, ethical, and legal obstacles, it is likely that the use of human fetal cells for CNS transplantation will remain an experimental therapy. The inefficiency of fetal dopaminergic cell survival after transplantation (5% to 20%) and the need to acquire three to four usable fetuses over a 2-day period for transplantation of one hemisphere in a patient with PD make human fetal neural tissue an impractical cell source for neurotransplantation. There has therefore been great interest in finding an alternative cell source that could be used more routinely for transplantation in the CNS (Table 17.1). Adrenal medullary tissue has the capacity to synthesize dopamine and was the first cell source to be used in transplantation protocols for PD. In autologous adrenal transplant protocols, poor cell survival, modest clinical benefit, and significant morbidity led to the abandonment of this approach (23).

XENOGENEIC FETAL MAMMALIAN TISSUE

Based on the success of transplantation of human fetal mesencephalic cells in patients with PD, the use of xenogeneic fetal donor tissue has been considered. The practical advantage of a xenogeneic source of tissue is, theoretically, the unlimited supply of transplantable fetal neural tissue that could be available. The pig has been considered the most desirable source species of whole organs (24,25). Pigs provide a large litter size and optimally staged embryonic porcine tissue, and one can reliably dissect the developing brain areas. Screening of animals for bacterial and viral diseases is possible because animals can be raised under controlled, quarantined condi-

tions. Porcine tissue has been used in other medical applications such as heart valves, insulin replacement, pancreatic islet cell transplants, temporary skin for burn patients, and extracorporeal kidney and liver perfusion (26–29). Based on the promising results of transplantation of porcine fetal cells in animal models of PD and HD (30,31), pilot studies to assess the safety and efficacy of unilateral implantation embryonic porcine cells into the striatum of patients with PD have been initiated (32,33).

In phase I studies of porcine fetal neural cells grafted unilaterally into patients with PD, clinical improvement of 19% was observed in the Unified Parkinson's Disease Rating Scale "off"- state scores in ten patients with PD who were assessed 12 months after unilateral striatal transplantation of 12 million fetal porcine ventral mesencephalic cells. Several patients improved more than 30%. In a single autopsied patient with PD, porcine fetal ventral mesencephalic cells were observed to survive 7 months after transplantation (34), but the number of surviving porcine dopaminergic cells was small and not sufficient for reliable functional recovery. ^{18}F-DOPA PET scanning in this series of patients did not reveal increased dopamine synthesis capacity (32). Although the preliminary results from this phase I trial are encouraging, particularly from the safety perspective, the open design of this trial cannot eliminate the possible influence of observer bias and placebo effect (19) in the efficacy results. Therefore, the results of an ongoing, double-blind trial, which employs an "imitation" surgery control group and a larger number of transplanted porcine fetal cells, will be very informative.

In animal models of HD, transplanted embryonic striatal cells have been shown to integrate into the basal ganglia circuitry and to effect repair of some motor and cognitive deficits (31,35,36). Twelve patients with HD who underwent transplantation with fetal porcine cells derived from the lateral ganglionic eminence anlage of the striatum showed a favorable safety profile in a phase I trial (33). However, 1 year after unilateral striatal placement of up to 24 million fetal porcine striatal cells, there was slight worsening in their Total Functional Capacity score (33), a finding consistent with the natural history of the disease (37).

The major challenges to the successful use of xenogeneic fetal neuronal cells in neurodegenerative diseases appear to be management of the risk of xenotic infections (transmission of pathogens outside the normal host range and in the setting of xenotransplantation) and minimizing immune-mediated rejection. With transplantation of tissue across species, there is a risk of transmission of infectious pathogens from the animal source (38). Two sets of pig retroviruses (PERV), which are capable of replication in some human cells lines *in vitro*, have been identified (39–42). There was no evidence of PERV DNA in patient samples taken from 6 to 24 months after implantation of porcine fetal ventral mesencephalic and lateral ganglionic eminence cells in the phase I trials of porcine fetal transplants for PD or HD (32,33). Similar negative results for PERV transmission to humans

TABLE 17.1. SOME CELL SOURCES FOR TRANSPLANTATION IN THE CENTRAL NERVOUS SYSTEM

Cell	Source	Disease	Trials
Adrenal medulla	Autologous	PD	Yes
Human fetal	Human fetal brain	PD, HD	Yes
Porcine fetal	Pig fetal brain	PD, HD	Yes
RPE cells	Human	PD	Yes
HNT cells	Human tumor	Stroke	Yes
Carotid body cells	Human	PD	No
Stem/progenitor cell	Human	PD, other	No

HNT, human teratocarcinoma-derived cells; HD, Huntington's disease; PD, Parkinson's disease; RPE, retinal pigmented epithelial cells.

were observed in a large series of patients who were exposed to living porcine tissue (43–45). This finding suggests that the propensity of PERV to establish a productive infection in humans, compared with other human pathogenic viruses, is low. However, the risk of transmission of other porcine pathogens (known and unknown) from transplanted tissue remains a concern. This is particularly true because, in the absence of effective cryopreservation techniques for mammalian fetal neural tissue, current isolation protocols do not permit complete results of pathogen screening of fresh cells to be available before transplantation. Nonetheless, long-term monitoring of all patients receiving transplanted fetal porcine tissue will be necessary to assess the risk of transmission of xenotic infections accurately.

Although the requirements for immunosuppression for a xenograft placed in the CNS are clearly less stringent than when the xenograft is placed outside the CNS, it is assumed that long-term immunosuppression is necessary for durable survival of CNS xenogeneic cell grafts. Unresolved, however, is the identification of an optimal and tolerable immunosuppression regimen for CNS xenografts. Advances in modulations of host immune function (46), including transplantation on microcarrier beads (47), may permit long-term xenogeneic graft survival in the CNS with tolerable side effects from immunosuppression regimens.

The use of xenogeneic fetal tissue remains a promising, but unproved, therapy for cellular repair in the nervous system.

NEURAL STEM CELLS

Biology

Neural stem cells have the potential to give rise to differentiated cell types of the mature brain *in vivo* (neurons, astrocytes, and oligodendroglia) and to self-renew in an undifferentiated state (48,49). Differences among cells termed *embryonic stem cells, multipotent stem cells,* and *neural progenitors* are based on their origin and the type of cells into which they have the capacity to develop (Fig. 17.1). Neural stem cells are found within the CNS *in vivo* or have the capacity to develop into neural cell types.

The isolation of neural stem cells was first accomplished using rat brain (50). Cells were isolated from the ependymal and subependymal regions of the ventricular margin adjacent to the striatum and from the hippocampus. Once isolated, these cells are able to proliferate and respond to differentiation cues to form neurons (48). Multipotential neural stem cells have also been isolated from adult primate and human brain. In patients with laryngeal cancer who

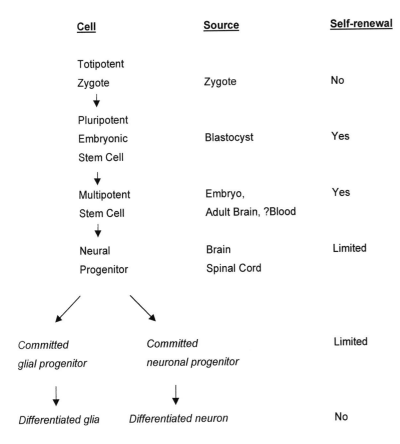

Sources of Neural Stem Cells

Cell	Source	Self-renewal
Totipotent Zygote	Zygote	No
Pluripotent Embryonic Stem Cell	Blastocyst	Yes
Multipotent Stem Cell	Embryo, Adult Brain, ?Blood	Yes
Neural Progenitor	Brain Spinal Cord	Limited
Committed glial progenitor / Committed neuronal progenitor		Limited
Differentiated glia / Differentiated neuron		No

FIGURE 17.1. Possible sources of neural progenitor cells that may be used for transplantation and their presumptive developmental relationships. (Adapted from Gage FH. Mammalian neural stem cells. *Science* 2000;287:1433–1438, with permission.)

were administered bromodeoxyuridine, postmortem analysis demonstrated that this mitotic marker was incorporated into neurons within the hippocampus (51), a finding indicating that neurogenesis occurs in the adult human brain. Cells with proliferative capacity have also been identified in surgical biopsy specimens of adult human brain (52). The ependymal cell layer and the subependymal region (53–55) have been proposed as the sites of origin of human neural stem cells that generate lineage-restricted precursor cells for neurons, astrocytes, and oligodendroglia.

These observations have several important implications for the neurobiology of CNS diseases. First, they raise the question of the role of neural stem cells in the functioning of the adult CNS. Is neurogenesis in the adult a vestige of evolution from lower organisms, or do neural stem cells function to contribute to plasticity of the adult CNS, perhaps in situations of injury or learning and memory? Indeed, investigators have demonstrated that the very small production of new neurons in the rodent hippocampus can be increased by mental activity, physical activity, and environmental enrichment (56–58). Second, the presence of neurogenesis in the CNS, which can be responsive to brain activity, raises the possibility that diffusible molecules could be identified that would induce neurogenesis in the mature mammalian CNS. Moreover, these inducers of neurogenesis could even be employed in a therapeutic context. The possible location of neural stem cells in the ependymal cell layer, directly adjacent to cerebrospinal fluid in the ventricular system, could support this function of neural stem cells. Investigators have demonstrated that basic fibroblast growth factor-2 or brain-derived neurotrophic factor will increase *in vivo* neurogenesis in the CNS (59,60). Taken together, these observations of regulatable neurogenesis in the adult CNS raise the possibility that, for some diseases of the CNS, the identification of appropriate stimuli and molecules may enable one to harness the brain's capacity for intrinsic self-repair.

Cells for Transplantation

From the perspective of cellular therapy, the most important implication of the identification of neural stem cells is that, by combining *ex vivo* expansion and intracerebral delivery, these neural progenitors could be used as a source of transplantable neural cells. Numerous laboratories have demonstrated that neural stem cells have the capacity to proliferate *in vitro* in an undifferentiated state and to retain some degree of ability to respond to differentiation signals. Fricker and co-workers expanded human neural stem cells in culture and transplanted them into the uninjured rat brain (61). These cells migrated and integrated into several brain areas. These animal experiments suggest that transplanted human neural stem cells have the capacity to survive (across species) and to respond to local environmental cues by

undergoing differentiation, migration, and integration into the host adult brain.

Neural stem cells can also be used as a source of glia. Two approaches have been demonstrated to have experimental utility in models of neurodegenerative disease. Zhang and co-workers isolated neural stem cells (62), expanded them *in vitro* with mitogens, and induced these expanded cells to differentiate into oligodendroglia precursors. Yandava and colleagues used an immortalized stem cell line derived from cerebellum (63). When these cells were transplanted into myelin-deficient rodents, there was evidence of migration and new myelin production. Taken together, these examples illustrate the potential for stem cells to serve as sources of neurons and glia in cell therapy paradigms.

There are several sources of neural progenitors (Fig. 17.1), and experimental approaches have used expanded progenitor cells for the production of transplantable dopaminergic neurons. Predifferentiated dopaminergic neuron progenitors, obtained from cultures of fetal rat mesencephalon, were expanded with fibroblast growth factor. Mitogen withdrawal, before implantation, led to modest dopaminergic differentiation (64). Progenitors have also been differentiated before implantation. In this approach, expanded lineage-restricted progenitors from rat mesencephalon were expanded (for months) in the presence of epidermal growth factor in "neurospheres." Differentiation before transplantation was achieved using cytokines and undefined differentiation signals from membrane fragments from midbrain and conditioned medium from striatum (65). An "immortalized" neural stem cell, induced toward a dopaminergic neuron phenotype by transfection of a transcription factor (Nurr1), underwent dopaminergic differentiation when it was exposed to the undefined differentiation factors contained in astrocyte-conditioned culture (66). After transplantation into the striatum of rodents, each approach yields survival and some degree of dopaminergic differentiation. However, survival of grafted neurons and, specifically, of dopaminergic neurons was low, even when differentiation *in vitro* into neurons expressing some dopaminergic neuron phenotypes was efficient. This finding suggests that differentiation of these precursors did not achieve full dopaminergic phenotype; it did not yield neurons with the ability to sustain differentiation or to achieve critical synaptic connections, or survival after transplantation of the differentiated dopaminergic cell was not complemented by other necessary neuronal or glial cell types.

PD has advantages and disadvantages as a target disease for stem-cell based cellular therapy. It is a disease with clinical symptoms largely secondary to the loss of a single, chemically defined neuronal phenotype. Thus, it appears that replacement with only one differentiated cell type needs to be achieved. There are also excellent primate and rodent neurochemical models of nigrostriatal deficiency. Successful correction of motor deficits in these models by stem cell–derived dopaminergic cell transplants is likely to be highly predictive of clinical efficacy in patients with PD.

However, the relative importance and effectiveness of region-specific signals in directing differentiation of transplanted progenitor cells are not fully understood, particularly when cells are placed outside the brain areas of ongoing neurogenesis. This issue may be of particular importance in cellular repair strategies employing neural stem cells in PD. When transplanted into the hippocampus or subventricular zones (areas of neurogenesis), neuronal progenitor cells will migrate, and a small percentage will differentiate into neurons and glia, a finding indicating the presence of local differentiation signals and the responsiveness of the progenitor cells to them (61,67,68). The likely target brain area for cell therapy in PD, the neostriatum, is not the normal site of dopaminergic cell generation, and it is not an area of active neurogenesis in the adult. Thus, if local (i.e., mesencephalic) signals are necessary to induce a stable dopaminergic phenotype fully, these differentiation signals may not be available if progenitor cells are implanted in the adult neostriatum. Region-specific differentiation signals in the adult brain may increase after injury, and they may direct differentiation of transplanted progenitors (69). However, it is not known whether sufficient instructions will be present in certain neurodegenerative diseases of the adult brain such as PD to direct specification of transplanted progenitors into the desired dopaminergic phenotype. The optimum stage of differentiation of the transplanted stem cell or precursor cell is also not known. Is it sufficient to transplant an uncommitted progenitor cell, or will it be more effective to "predifferentiate" the precursor cell toward a dopaminergic phenotype before transplantation? Finally, the process that regulates synaptogenesis and fiber outgrowth needs to be understood for stem cell–derived neurons. It appears that much is left to be learned about the process of stem cell differentiation, phenotype specification, integration, and establishment of synaptic connectivity before this source of transplantable dopaminergic neurons and other neural elements is ready for clinical application to PD and other neurodegenerative diseases.

OTHER SOURCES OF NEURONAL OR DOPAMINE-SECRETING CELLS

A transformed cell line that generates large numbers of differentiated, postmitotic neurons has been used as a cell source for transplantation. The *NT2 cell line* was established from human teratocarcinoma. These cells are capable of differentiating into postmitotic neurons after treatment with retinoic acid. After transplantation into rodent brain, a cell line (hNT, human teratocarcinoma-derived) derived form the original NT2 cell line displays features of a neuronal phenotype and integrates into host brain. Over a period of observation

(1 year), these transplanted hNT cells continued to survive and did not revert to the undifferentiated or neoplastic state. These cells produced some recovery of function in animal models of stroke, although the mechanism of this recovery is not entirely understood (70). These cells are currently in clinical trials in patients with stroke (71). hNT cells also have the capacity to differentiate into cells that express tyrosine hydroxylase under certain treatment conditions (72).

Neural cells for transplantation can be derived from other sources (Fig. 17.1). Rodent *embryonic stem (ES) cells* have been induced to differentiate into a population of cells enriched in oligodendroglia, which have been used as a cell source for transplantation in myelin-deficient animals (73). *Marrow cells* have also been reported to differentiate into cells of neural lineage (74). The ability of these sources to generate functional neurons and glia under controlled conditions needs to be established before these cells can be considered useful sources of transplantable neural cells.

The cell types discussed so far (embryonic, neural stem or progenitor, and retinoic acid–treated transformed cell lines) have the capacity to differentiate into cells of neural lineage and integrate into the host brain. Cells that would be useful for the treatment of PD may not need to be "functional" neurons (i.e., capable of activity-dependent release of dopamine and synaptic connectivity). It is possible that cells that simply secrete dopamine, or synthesize dopamine from its precursor, may be sufficient to achieve functional benefit in PD. In addition to adrenal chromaffin cells (discussed earlier), other cells in which dopamine secretion is the primary mechanism of benefit have been used in animal models of PD. Glomus cells from the carotid body (75), retinal pigmented epithelial cells (21) and nonneuronal cells that have been genetically engineered to produce high levels of dopamine or DOPA (76), and can ameliorate motor deficits and can reverse some of the neurochemical changes consequent to dopamine denervation in animal models of PD and, in pilot studies, in PD patients (21). To achieve maximum improvement of motor behavior in PD, it seems likely that other cellular functions subserved by dopaminergic neurons (reuptake and regulated release of dopamine) will be necessary characteristics of dopaminergic neurons derived from transplanted neural progenitors.

PROSPECTS FOR NEW CELL SOURCES

The lessons that have been learned from the use of fetal neural cells for transplantation will be instructive for the development of new cell therapies. Outcomes from the careful studies of human fetal transplants in PD and HD led by the pioneering work of several groups will be the standard against which new cell sources will initially be measured. Indeed, the accomplishments of human fetal transplants should not be minimized: attainment of approximate numbers of cells required for clinical efficacy in PD, long-term cell survival, apparent lack of need for long-term immunosuppression, normalization or innervation of significant areas of the grafted striatum, clinical benefit in PD sufficient in some cases to alter the natural progression of the disease, and functional integration into the complex motor circuitry of the CNS. The attainment of these biologic outcomes, however, took time. It was nearly one decade between the first successful fetal graft in experimental animals and the first human clinical trials in PD, and it was even longer before a protocol, which led to clinically meaningful results, was attained. It is likely that the lessons learned from human fetal transplants, and the greater knowledge of cellular neurobiology, may accelerate these developmental timelines for new cell therapies.

The challenge to generate reliably, from renewable neuronal precursor cells, mature neuronal elements capable of appropriate integration into the adult brain should not be underestimated. It is clear that additional knowledge must be gained about the identification of intrinsic and extrinsic signals that control neural differentiation, migration, and the development of synaptic connections in the setting of neural precursor cell transplantation. The ability to isolate and to maintain human neural stem cells in culture offers exciting possibilities for repair of neurodegenerative and other diseases of the nervous system. The rational maturation of cellular therapy using neural stem cells and other new cell sources as viable therapeutics for CNS disease will require the contributions of cell biologists and careful observations from clinical scientists.

REFERENCES

1. Björklund A, Stenevi U. Reconstruction of the nigrostriatal pathway by intracerebral nigral transplants. *Brain Res* 1979;177:555–560.
2. Perlow M, Freed W, Hoffer B, et al. Brain grafts reduce motor abnormalities produced by destruction of nigrostriatal dopamine system. *Neurosurgery* 1979;204:643–647.
3. Lindvall O, Rehncrona S, Gustuvii B, et al. Embryonic dopamine-rich mesencephalic grafts in Parkinson's disease. *Lancet* 1988;2:1483–1484.
4. Madrazo I, Leon V, Torres C, et al. Transplantation of embryonic substantia nigra and adrenal medulla to the caudate nucleus in two patients with Parkinson's disease. *N Engl J Med* 1988;318:51.
5. Lindvall O. Update on embryonic transplantation: the Swedish experience. *Mov Disord* 1998;13:83–87.
6. Freed C, Breeze R, Rosenberg N, et al. Survival of implanted embryonic dopamine cells and neurologic improvement 12 to 46 months after transplantation for Parkinson's disease. *N Engl J Med* 1992;237:1549–1555.
7. Hauser RA, Freeman TB, Snow BJ, et al. Long-term evaluation of bilateral embryonic nigral transplantation in Parkinson disease. *Arch Neurol* 1999;56:179–187.
8. Defer G, Geny C, Ricolfi F, et al. Long-term outcome of unilaterally transplanted parkinsonian patients. I. Clinical approach. *Brain* 1996;119:41–50.
9. Lindvall O, Sawle G, Widner H, et al. Evidence for long-term survival and function of dopaminergic grafts in progressive Parkinson's disease. *Ann Neurol* 1994;35:172–180.
10. Wenning G, Odin P, Morrish P, et al. Short- and long-term survival and function of unilateral intrastriatal dopaminergic grafts in Parkinson's disease. *Ann Neurol* 1997;42:95–107.
11. Freeman T, Olanow C, Hauser R, et al. Bilateral embryonic nigral transplantation into the postcommissural putamen in Parkinson's disease. *Ann Neurol* 1995;38:379–388.
12. Kordower J, Freeman T, Snow B, et al. Neuropathological evidence of graft survival and striatal reinnervation after the transplantation of embryonic mesencephalic tissue in a patient with Parkinson's disease. *N Engl J Med* 1995;332:1118–1124.
13. Piccini P, Brooks DJ, Björklund A, et al. Dopamine release from nigral transplants visualized *in vivo* in a Parkinson's patient. *Nat Neurosci* 1999;2:1137–1140.
14. Kordower J, Freeman TB, Chen EY, et al. Fetal grafts survive and mediate clinical benefit in a patient with Parkinson's disease. *Mov Disord* 1998:13:383–393.
15. Fisher LJ, Young SJ, Tepper JM, et al. Electrophysiological characteristics of cells within mesencephalic suspension grafts. *Neuroscience* 1991;40:109–122.
16. Doucet G, Murata Y, Brundin P, et al. Host afferents into intrastriatal transplants of fetal ventral mesencephalon. *Exp Neurol* 1989;106:1–19.
17. Mamelak AN, Eggerding FA, Oh DS, et al. Fatal cyst formation after fetal mesencephalic allograft transplant for Parkinson's disease. *J Neurosurg* 1998;89:592–598.
18. Folkerth RD, Durso R. Survival and proliferation of non-neural tissues, with obstruction of cerebral ventricles, in a parkinsonian patient treated with fetal allografts. *Neurology* 1996;46:1219–1225.
19. Freeman TB, Vawter DE, Leaverton PE, et al. Use of placebo controlled surgery in controlled clinical trials of a cellular-based therapy for Parkinson's disease. *N Engl J Med* 1999;341:988–992.
20. Freed CR, Greene PE, Breeze RE, et al. Transplantation of embryonic dopamine neurons for severe Parkinson's disease. *N Engl J Med* 2001;344:710–719.
21. Watts RL, Raiser CD, Stover NP, et al. Stereotactic intrastriatal implantation of retinal pigmented epithelial cells attached to microcarriers in advanced Parkinson's disease patients: a pilot study. *Neurology* 2001;8(Suppl 3):A283.
22. Kordower J, Styren S, Calrke M, et al. Fetal grafting for Parkinson's disease: expression of immune markers in patients with functional fetal nigral implants. *Cell Transplant* 1997;6:213–219.
23. Goetz CG, Stebbin GT III, Klawans HL, et al. United Parkinson Foundation neurotransplantation registry on adrenal medullary transplants: presurgical, and 1-year and 2-year follow up. *Neurology* 1991;41:1719–1722.
24. Advisory Group on the Ethics of Transplantation. *Animal tissues into humans.* Norwich, UK: Stationary Office, 1997:1–258.
25. Dunning J, White D, Wallwork J. The rationale for xenotransplantation as a solution to the donor organ shortage. *Pathol Biol* 1994;42:231–235.
26. Breimer M, Bjorck E, Svalander C, et al. Extracorporeal connection of pig kidneys to humans: clinical data and studies of platelet destruction. *Xenotransplantation* 1996;3:328–339.
27. Chari R, Collins B, Magee J, et al. Treatment of hepatic failure with *ex vivo* pig-liver perfusion followed by liver transplantation. *N Engl J Med* 1994;331:234–237.
28. Groth C, Korsgren O, Tibell A, et al. Transplantation of porcine embryonic pancreas to diabetic patients. *Lancet* 1994;344:1402–1404.

29. Rydberg L, Bjorck S, Hallberg E, et al. Extracorporeal ("ex vivo") connection of pig kidneys to human. II. The anti-pig antibody response. *Xenotransplantation* 1996;3:340–353.

30. Galpern WR, Burns LH, Deacon TW, et al. Xenotransplantation of porcine embryonic ventral mesencephalon in a rat model of Parkinson's disease: functional recovery and graft morphology. *Exp Neurol* 1996;140:1–13.

31. Isacson O, Deacon TW, Pakzaban P, et al. Transplanted xenogeneic neural cells in neurodegenerative disease models exhibit remarkable axonal target specificity and distinct growth patterns of glial and axonal fibres. *Nat Med* 1995;11:1189–1194.

32. Schumacher JM, Ellias SA, Palmer EP, et al. Transplantation of embryonic porcine mesencephalic tissue in patients with PD. *Neurology* 2000;14:1042–1050.

33. Fink JS, Schumacher JM, Ellias SA, et al. Porcine xenografts in Parkinson's disease and Huntington's disease patients: preliminary results. *Cell Transplant* 2000;9:273–278.

34. Deacon T, Schumacher J, Dinsmore J, et al. Histological evidence of embryonic pig neural cell survival after transplantation into a patient with Parkinson's disease. *Nat Med* 1997;3:350–353.

35. Kendall AL, Rayment FD, Torres E.M, et al. Functional integration of striatal allografts in a primate model of Huntington's disease. *Nat Med* 1998; 4:727–729.

36. Palfi S, Conde F, Riche D, et al. Fetal striatal allografts reverse cognitive deficits in a primate model of Huntington's disease. *Nat Med* 1998;4:963–966.

37. Quinn N, Brown R, Craufurd D, et al. Core Assessment Program for Intracerebral Transplantation in Huntington's Disease (CAPIT-HD). *Mov Disord* 1996;11:143–150.

38. Chapman L, Folks T, Salomon D, et al. Xenotransplantation and xenogenic infections. *N Engl J Med* 1995;333:1498–1501.

39. Akiyoshi D, Denaro M, Zhu H, et al. Identification of a full-length cDNA for an endogenous retrovirus of miniature swine. *J Virol* 1998;72:4503–4507.

40. LeTissier P, Stoye J, Yasuhiro Y, et al. Two sets of human-tropic pig retrovirus. *Nature* 1997;389:681–682.

41. Patience C, Takeuchi Y, Weiss R. Infection of human cells by an endogenous retrovirus of pigs. *Nat Med* 1997;3:282–286.

42. Wilson C, Wong S, Muller J, et al. Type C retrovirus released from porcine primary peripheral blood mononuclear cells infects human cells. *J Virol* 1998;72:3082–3087.

43. Heneine W, Tibell A, Switzer WM, et al. No evidence of infection with porcine endogenous retrovirus in recipients of porcine islet-cell xenografts. *Lancet* 1998;352:695–698.

44. Paradis K, Langford G, Long Z, et al. Search for cross-species transmission of porcine endogenous retrovirus in patients treated with living pig tissue. *Science* 1999;285:1236–1241.

45. Patience C, Patton G, Takeuchi Y, et al. No evidence of pig DNA or retroviral infection in patients with short-term extracorporeal connection to pig kidneys. *Lancet* 1998;352:699–701.

46. Auchincloss H Jr, Sachs DH. Xenogeneic transplantation. *Annu Rev Immunol* 1998;16:433–470.

47. Saporta S, Borlongan C, Moore J, et al. Microcarrier enhances survival of human and rat fetal ventral mesencephalon cells implanted in the rat striatum. *Cell Transplant* 1997;6:579–584.

48. Gage FH. Mammalian neural stem cells. *Science* 2000;287:1433–1438.

49. Van der Kooy D, Weiss S. Why stem cells? *Science* 2000;287:1439–1441.

50. Reynolds BA, Weiss S. Generation of neurons and astrocytes from isolated cells of the adult mammalian central nervous system. *Science* 1992;255:1707–1710.

51. Eriksson PS, Perfilieva E, Bjork-Eriksson T, et al. Neurogenesis in the adult human hippocampus. *Nat Med* 1998;4:1313–1317.

52. Kukekov VG, Laywell ED, Suslov O, et al. Multipotent stem/progenitor cells with similar properties arise from two different neurogenic regions of the adult human brain. *Exp Neurol* 1999; 156:333–344.

53. Johansson CB, Momma DL, Clarke DL, et al. Identification of a neural stem cell in the adult mammalian central nervous system. *Cell* 1999;96:25–34.

54. Chiasson BJ, Tropepe V, Morsheas CM, et al. Adult mammalian forebrain ependymal and subependymal cells demonstrate proliferative potential, but only subependymal cells have neural stem cell characteristics. *J Neurosci* 1999;19:4462–4471.

55. Doetsch F, Garcia-Verdugo JM, Alvarez-Buylla A. Regeneration of a germinal layer in the adult mammalian brain. *Proc Natl Acad Sci USA* 1999;96:11619–11624.

56. Gould E, Beylin A, Tanapat P, et al. Learning enhances adult neurogenesis in the hippocampal formation. *Nat Neurosci* 1999;2:260–265.

57. Van Praag H, Kempermann G, Gage FH. Running increases cell proliferation in the adult mouse dentate gyrus. *Nat Neurosci* 1999; 2:266–270.

58. Kempermann G, Kuhn HG, Gage FH. More hippocampal neurons in adult mice living in an enriched environment. *Nature* 1997;386:493–495.

59. Wagner JP, Black IB, DiCicco-Bloom E. Stimulation of neonatal and adult brain neurogenesis by subcutaneous injection of basic fibroblast growth factor. *J Neurosci* 1999;19:6006–6016.

60. Zigova T, Pencea V, Wiegand SJ, et al. Intraventricular administration of BDNF increase the number of newly generated neurons in the adult olfactory bulb. *Mol Cell Neurosci* 1998;11:234–245.

61. Fricker RA, Carpenter MK, Winkler C, et al. Site-specific migration and neuronal differentiation of human neural progenitor cells after transplantation in the adult rat brain. *J Neurosci* 1999;19:5990–6005.

62. Zhang SC, Ge B, Duncan ID. Adult brain retains the potential to generate oligodendroglial progenitors with extensive myelination capacity. *Proc Natl Acad Sci USA* 1999;96:4089–4094.

63. Yandava BD, Billiinghurst LL, Snyder EY. "Global" cell replacement is feasible via neural stem cell transplantation: evidence from the dysmyelinated shiverer mouse brain. *Proc Natl Acad Sci USA* 1999;96:7029–7034.

64. Struder L, Tabar V, McKay RDG. Transplantation of expanded mesencephalic precursors leads to recovery in parkinsonian rats. *Nat Neurosci* 1998;1:135–146.

65. Potter ED, Ling ZD, Carvey PM. Cytokine-induced conversion of mesencephalic-derived progenitor cells into dopamine neurons. *Cell Tissue Res* 1999;296:235–246.

66. Wagner J, Akerud P, Castro DS, et al. Induction of a midbrain dopaminergic phenotype in Nurr1-overexpressing neural stem cells by type 1 astrocytes. *Nat Biotech* 1999;17:653–659.

67. Suhonen JO, Peterson DA, Ray J, et al. Differentiation of adult hippocampus-derived progenitors into olfactory neurons *in vivo*. *Nature* 1996;383:624–627.

68. Gage FH, Coates PW, Palmer TD, et al. Survival and differentiation of adult neuronal progenitor cells transplanted to the adult brain. *Proc Natl Acad Sci USA* 1995;92:11879–11883.

69. Snyder EY, Yoon C, Flax JD, et al. Multipotent neural precursors can differentiate toward replacement of neurons undergoing targeted apoptotic degeneration in adult mouse neocortex. *Proc Natl Acad Sci USA* 1997;94:11663–11668.

70. Saporta A, Borlongan CV, Sanberg PR. Neural transplantation of human neuroteratocarcinoma (hNT) neurons into ischemic rats: a quantitative dose-response analysis of cell survival and behavioral recovery. *Neuroscience* 1999;91:519–525.

71. Kondziolka D, Wechsler LR, Goldstein S, et al. Neuronal transplantation for stroke: results of a phase 1 study. *Neurology* 2000;54:A1.

72. Zigova T, Wiling AE, Tedesco EM, et al. Lithiuim chloride induces the expression of tyrosine hydroxylase in hNT neurons. *Exp Neurol* 1999;157:251–258.

73. Brustle O, Jones KN, Learish RD, et al. Embryonic stem cell-derived glial precursors: a source of myelinating transplants. *Science* 1999;285:754–756.

74. Kopen GC, Prockop DJ, Phinney G. Marrow stromal cells migrate throughout forebrain and cerebellum after injection into neonatal mouse brain. *Proc Natl Acad Sci USA* 1999;96:10711–10716.

75. Espejo EF, Montoro RJ, Armengol AJ, et al. Cellular and functional recovery of Parkinsonian rats after intrastriatal transplantation of carotid body cell aggregates. *Neuron* 1998;20:197–206.

76. Fisher LJ, Jinnah HA, Kale LC, et al. Survival and function of intrastriatally grafted primary fibroblasts genetically modified to produce L-DOPA. *Neuron* 1991;371–380.

Surgery for Parkinson's Disease and Movement Disorders,
edited by J.K. Krauss, J. Jankovic, and R.G. Grossman.
Lippincott Williams & Wilkins, Philadelphia © 2001.

18

PRECLINICAL DEVELOPMENT OF TROPHIC FACTORS FOR TREATMENT OF PARKINSON'S DISEASE

PAUL A. LAPCHAK
DALIA M. ARAUJO

Neurotrophic factors are crucial to the development, guidance, and maintenance of distinct neuronal populations in the peripheral and central nervous system (CNS) (1–10). Neurotrophic factor–responsive neurons *in vivo* clearly have the ability to transport in retrograde fashion and accumulate neurotrophic factors, which are then transported to the cell body region in a specific receptor-mediated fashion (5,8,11–15). For example, [^{125}I]glial cell line–derived factor (GDNF) is transported from the dopaminergic target field in the striatum to the dopaminergic cell body in the substantia nigra (SN) (12,16,17). Whereas some neurons are responsive selectively to a specific neurotrophic factor, many others, like the SN dopaminergic neurons, are sensitive to more than one neurotrophic factor (1,5,7–10). Neurotrophic factors also can protect neurons from the degeneration that occurs subsequent to toxin exposure, injury, and neurodegenerative diseases, in which specific populations of CNS neurons are targeted for cell death, at least initially. In Parkinson's disease, for instance, the dopamine (DA) neurons of the SN undergo degeneration, the progression of which correlates with the neurologic abnormalities associated with the disease (18,19). In the rodent brain, the nigral DA neurons corresponding to those that deteriorate in Parkinson's disease are contained within the ventral mesencephalon. Neurons cultured from embryonic rat mesencephalon are responsive to several neurotrophic factors (1–10).

NEUROTROPHINS

Among the identified trophic factors for midbrain DA neurons are several members of the *neurotrophin* family of trophic factors (1–10). These neurotrophins stimulate high-affinity trk (A, B, C) receptors and a low-affinity p75 binding protein (2–10). Select neurotrophins appear to promote DA neuronal survival while at the same time depressing dopaminergic neurotransmission by reducing the synthesis of tyrosine hydroxylase (TH) (5,8,20). Brain-derived neurotrophic factor (BDNF), neurotrophin-3 (NT-3), and NT-4/5 all stimulate the survival and functional activity of these neurons *in vitro,* whereas nerve growth factor (NGF), the first neurotrophin identified (1,2,5,9,10,21), is ineffective (2,5,8,9,21–24). In addition, BDNF has been shown to protect DA neurons from 1-methyl-4-phenyl-1,2,3,6-tetrahydropyridine (MPTP) and 6-hydroxydopamine (6-OHDA) toxicity *in vitro* (25). However, *in vivo* animal studies have emphasized the role of neurotrophins in the adult nigrostriatal pathway. For example, *in vivo* studies have presented less promising results because of the limited diffusion of BDNF when it is administered by an intraventricular route, a result of binding to truncated trkB receptors (5,20). Moreover, different routes of delivery that circumvent the problems associated with BDNF binding to trkB along the ventricular wall have produced only transient responses (8). Similarly, the other neurotrophins have not yielded remarkable results in animal models of Parkinson's disease, even though they preferentially bind to different trk receptors within the CNS (8).

CILIARY NEUROTROPHIC FACTOR

Ciliary neurotrophic factor (CNTF), a member of the neuropoietic family of growth factors, is ubiquitously distributed throughout the CNS (26–29). The prediction that CNTF may be trophic for DA neurons of the nigrostriatal pathway was originally derived from indirect evidence demonstrating expression of CNTF in the SN (27–29). *In vitro* evidence indicates that CNTF can provide trophic support for various

P.A. Lapchak: Department of Neuroscience, Veterans Administration Hospital, La Jolla, California 92093.

D.M. Araujo: Department of Neuroscience, VASDHS, San Diego, California 92093.

neuronal populations, including midbrain DA neurons, but it requires cooperation from other factors (8). Results from *in vivo* studies, meanwhile, suggest that CNTF may protect nigrostriatal neurons after axotomy, but because the loss of nigral TH staining induced by axotomy was not affected by CNTF (30), it seems likely that CNTF exerts its trophic effects on non-DA neurons in the SN.

FIBROBLAST GROWTH FACTORS

Acidic and basic *fibroblast growth factor* (FGF) belong to a group of mitogenic growth factors that are potent effectors of glial cells, but they are also known to affect various neuronal populations in the CNS (31). However, the effects of FGF on neurons appear to be mediated indirectly, because suppression of astroglial growth also abolishes the neurotrophic activity (31). In the CNS, one of the areas of highest accumulation of basic FGF after intraventricular injection is the SN pars compacta (8,31), which is affected in Parkinson's disease (18,19,32), a finding suggesting that FGF may be an important DA trophic factor for DA neurons. However, many of the cells that transport FGFs in retrograde fashion, and nigrostriatal neurons are no exception, also transport other neurotrophins in retrograde fashion (8), a finding suggesting a redundancy of function. In a study that described the effects of basic FGF in MPTP-lesioned mice, the conclusion was that FGF protected neurons in young, but not aged, mice (33). Because Parkinson's disease affects predominantly the aged population, it can be argued that FGF may not be a clinically feasible prospect. Furthermore, as discussed for BDNF, the FGFs also suffer from limited penetration in the CNS because of their high avidity for binding to extracellular matrix components (34), thereby limiting their potential therapeutic usefulness.

TRANSFORMING GROWTH FACTOR-β

The *transforming growth factor-β* (TGF-β) superfamily of growth factors includes TGF-β1 to TGF-β3, as well as other potent trophic molecules (see later) (34–38). The TGF-β group signals through heteromeric serine/threonine kinase receptors (37), and their localization in the CNS has been studied extensively, with TGF-β3, especially, present in many neuronal populations, including the SN (35,36,38). In these neurons, TGF-β exhibits complex interactions and concomitant complicated effects with other trophic factors and cytokines (36,39). *In vitro* evidence showed that all members of the TGF-β group were equipotent in promoting the survival of midbrain DA neurons and in preventing *N*-methyl-4-phenylpyridinium (MPP$^+$)–induced toxicity (34,38,40). This effect was specific and did not involve glial-mediated effects, because glial proliferation and activation were not evident. In addition, it appears that TGF-β

requires other cooperative factors for its full neurotrophic potential to be realized (39). Although *in vivo* responses to TGF-β have not yet been reported, another member of the TGF-β superfamily, growth/differentiation factor 5 (GDF5), has been shown to prevent 6-OHDA–induced deficits in nigrostriatal DA markers (41,42).

GLIAL CELL LINE–DERIVED NEUROTROPHIC FACTOR

One of the most potent DA neurotrophic agents, *GDNF,* a remotely related member of the transforming growth factor beta (TGF-β) superfamily of peptide growth factors (43), was purified by means of an *in vitro* assay using embryonic mesencephalic cells (43,44). Subsequently, other GDNF-like members of this superfamily that exhibit varying degrees of trophic potency for DA neurons were isolated. *Neurturin* was the second member isolated and was shown to be present in several peripheral and central tissues (45–51). Like GDNF, neurturin supports the survival of midbrain DA neurons *in vitro* and in the adult rat after medial forebrain bundle axotomy (45,49,52). In addition, neurturin is a potent survival factor for motor, sympathetic, and enteric neurons *in vitro* (46–48,50). The more recently identified members of the GDNF family, artemin (53) and persephin (54,55), are also pleiotropic molecules that have been reported to exhibit varying degrees of trophic activity. Whereas artemin behaves essentially like GDNF, persephin does not appear to provide neurotrophic support for peripheral sympathetic, sensory, or enteric neurons (53–55). Naturally, because GDNF was the first of these family members to be identified, it has been the most thoroughly investigated to date. Because only limited accounts of the *in vivo* activity of neurturin and persephin have been reported thus far (54,55), this review focuses primarily on the pharmacology of GDNF and its potential application to the treatment of Parkinson's disease.

GLIAL CELL LINE–DERIVED NEUROTROPHIC FACTOR FAMILY LIGANDS AND RECEPTORS

High levels of GDNF mRNA expression were detected in the developing rat striatum, a major target of midbrain dopaminergic neurons (56), whereas lower levels were expressed in adults neurons (57–63). In the mouse CNS, GDNF mRNA appears to be expressed at similar levels in the striatum throughout the life span of the mouse (63). Similarly, expression of the other members of the GDNF family of ligands also appears to remain constant from development to adulthood in the mouse CNS (53–55). In addition to the nigrostriatal pathway, mRNA for GDNF and the other GDNF family members has been identified in a variety of brain structures, spinal cord, dorsal root ganglion, and many peripheral tissues (53–55,57,59–61,63–65). Moreover, the CNS distribution of GDNF mRNA suggests that nonneuronal cells such as basal forebrain astrocytes may be involved in the synthesis of GDNF (62). At present, it has not yet been reported whether other GDNF family ligands are also expressed in glial cells in the CNS.

All members of the GDNF family of ligands signal through a multicomponent receptor system composed of a specific glycosylphosphatidylinositol-linked (45,48,66–70) high-affinity binding cell-surface protein termed GFRα and a common constituent, the receptor tyrosine kinase ret (59,60,68,69,71–76). The latter was surprising because the related members of the TGF-β group signal through serine/threonine kinases (see earlier). Thus far, four different high-affinity GFRα (1 to 4) components have been characterized (59,67,68,70,71,77,78). On the basis of their preferential binding patterns, GFRα1 and GFRα2 have been designated the high-affinity receptors for GDNF and neurturin, respectively (59,68,71,78,79). However, the GFRα1/ret complex has been shown to be equally effective in mediating neurturin responses and *vice versa* (59,68,71,78,79). Unlike GFRα1 and GFRα2, GFRα3 is not expressed in the developing or adult CNS, but it is highly expressed in sensory and sympathetic ganglia (53,77). Artemin has been reported to be the preferential ligand for GFRα3 (53). However, its potent effects in the CNS, which lacks GFRα3 expression, suggest that alternative receptor interactions, at least in the CNS, also must be manifest. The latest high-affinity GFRα receptor to be characterized, the orphan receptor GFRα4, exhibits a similar nucleotide sequence and overlapping pattern of distribution to GFRα1 and GFRα2 (67). This finding suggests that, like the latter receptors, it may mediate the responses of more than one GDNF family member. Alternatively, it is possible that persephin (54,55), which does not appear to signal through either GFRα1 or GFRα2, or some other as yet unidentified member of the GDNF family may be the preferential ligand for GFRα4. The finding that ret can modulate binding to the high-affinity components of the GFRα/ret complex (80) has hampered the prediction of all GDNF family interactions obtained from binding studies alone. Nevertheless, these studies imply that the various members of the GDNF family may exert redundant trophic influences on CNS neurons.

EFFECTS OF GLIAL CELL LINE–DERIVED NEUROTROPHIC FACTOR FAMILY LIGANDS ON DOPAMINE NEURONS *IN VITRO*

Unlike the neurotrophin family of protein growth factors (see earlier), all members of the GDNF family of ligands isolated to date exhibit potent neurotrophic effects on ventral midbrain DA neurons in culture (22,24,43,53,54,81,82). The available data suggest that all four GDNF family ligands

identified so far may be equally potent and efficacious in promoting DA neuron survival (16,24,43,44,53,54,62,82–86). However, these results should be interpreted with some caution because exhaustive dose-response comparisons have not been reported. GDNF and neurturin interact with GFRα1 and GFRα2, respectively, to exert trophic effects on DA neurons (46,59,66,68–70,78,80,87). Because persephin does not signal through either GFRα1 or GFRα2 (54,67), its effects on midbrain DA neurons *in vitro* must be mediated through another receptor, possibly GFRα4 (see earlier). Conversely, artemin, the preferred ligand for GFRα3, appears to interact with either GFRα1 or GFRα2 to affect DA neurons (53).

The original claim (43) that GDNF is specific for midbrain DA neurons has been contested. In fact, in the CNS, GDNF has been shown to regulate a variety of neuronal cell types *in vitro* and *in vivo,* including noradrenergic (88), serotonergic (89), cholinergic (13,90,91), and γ-aminobutyric acid (GABA)-ergic (92,93) neurons. This lack of specificity makes GDNF a less than optimal candidate for preclinical and clinical development specifically for the treatment of DA-related diseases. The studies described earlier illustrate the survival-promoting effects of GDNF family ligands on DA neurons, but not whether these molecules also are neuroprotective against neurotoxic insults *in vitro*. In an elegant example of neuroprotection, GDNF was shown to enhance the survival of DA neurons, to prevent further cell death, and to stimulate the regrowth of dopaminergic fibers exposed previously to the neurotoxin MPP+ (94). This study represented an important step toward the development of GDNF as a potential candidate for Parkinson's disease therapy, because MPTP, the precursor to MPP+, is known to result in a Parkinson's-like syndrome in humans and is used frequently in nonhuman primate models of the disease (17,95–100).

EFFECTS OF GLIAL CELL LINE–DERIVED NEUROTROPHIC FACTOR FAMILY LIGANDS ON DOPAMINE NEURONS *IN VIVO*

Effects in Animal Models of Parkinson's Disease

In mice, the dopaminergic cell dysfunction, atrophy, and nerve terminal destruction consequent to exposure to MPTP were attenuated by intrastriatal administration of GDNF (16,101). A protective effect of GDNF given as a single injection before toxin exposure was reflected in increased levels of DA and the DA metabolites homovanillic acid (HVA) and dihydroxyphenylacetic acid (DOPAC) in the striatum and SN. Furthermore, GDNF restored DA, HVA, and DOPAC levels in the SN, even when it was given 1 week after MPTP (16). Similarly, GDNF has been shown to protect DA neurons against other neurotoxins. For instance, methamphetamine-induced lesions (102) of the nigrostriatal pathway in the rat were prevented by a pretreatment with GDNF.

Injecting GDNF intraventricularly in the rat has been demonstrated to be a suitable route of administration for effects on the striatonigral pathway to be manifest (12,17,90,95,103–105). Specifically, [^{125}I]GDNF injected into the lateral ventricle of the rat or monkey brain accumulates in SN cells (12,17). Moreover, after intraventricular injections, there is accumulation of [^{125}I]GDNF within the hypothalamus, medial septum, and cerebellum (12,17). Prior intraventricular treatment with GDNF protects against SN cell loss induced by 6-OHDA, one of the most commonly used DA neurotoxins in rodent models of Parkinson's disease (106–110). Moreover, recovery of toxin-induced dopaminergic hypofunction was observed with delayed administration of GDNF (85,90,95,97,103,105,111,112). The decrements in striatal DA levels and nigral TH activity induced by 6-OHDA lesions were reversed by long-term GDNF treatment (90,105,113). The effects of GDNF on neurochemical parameters of the nigrostriatal pathway were reflected by behavioral improvement (90,105,113). Apomorphine-induced rotations, which provide an index of the extent of the lesion produced by 6-OHDA, were reduced significantly by intraventricular administration of GDNF. More remarkably, with intranigral injection of GDNF, only a single dose resulted in marked, persistent reductions in rotations, up to 10 weeks after the injection (90,105,113). Because the effects induced by intraventricular injection were transitory and required subsequent bolus injections (13,14), the latter finding implies that a sustained effect by GDNF can be achieved in the nigrostriatal pathway, provided the agent is administered in the vicinity of DA cell bodies in the SN.

Gene therapy has been attempted using adenoviral vector–expressing GDNF in the rat CNS (114–119). *In vitro* studies have demonstrated that adenoviral GDNF prevents DA neuron death (119). *In vivo,* when injected into the nigrostriatal pathway, adenoviral GDNF exhibited essentially the same protective effects as natural GDNF (114–118). Thus, neurochemical parameters and behavioral correlates were elevated by virally delivered GDNF to a similar extent as intraventricular administration (104,114,118,120,121). Not only was there a protective effect after pretreatment with adenoviral-expressing GDNF (115), investigators also reported considerable prevention of further degeneration and partial reversal of neurochemcial and behavioral deficits when viral GDNF was injected weeks after the initial 6-OHDA insult (118). Furthermore, a single injection of adenovirus was capable of sustaining this neuroprotection for up to 3 weeks (118), a finding indicating that viral delivery may represent a feasible means by which to introduce GDNF into the CNS.

The prominent effects of GDNF on nigrostriatal dopaminergic neurons, despite extensive lesions of the pathway, were perplexing, given the finding that only few TH-positive nigral cells remain (15,120,122). This peculiarity

was addressed by an inventive study that used fluorogold retrograde labeling of the nigrostriatal pathway combined with TH immunocytochemistry to elucidate the mechanisms underlying the neuroprotective effects of GDNF (110). The results from this study showed that an initial loss of the dopaminergic phenotype throughout the SN preceded toxin-induced cell death. Moreover, GDNF induction of the DA phenotype in these "quiescent" cells directly correlated with the behavioral parameters affected (110). Thus, the loss of dopaminergic phenotype may represent the target for GDNF actions within the SN, and, further, a GDNF-responsive cell population may be present after an extensive lesion, even though the dopaminergic phenotype cannot be visualized using classic techniques. Clearly, the possibility that a similar phenomenon exists in patients with Parkinson's disease (18,98) would provide a possible therapeutic target for GDNF.

Whereas the other GDNF members have not been studied extensively, preliminary reports suggest that neurturin may be indistinguishable from GDNF in protecting nigral DA neurons in the rat from 6-OHDA damage (49). Thus, neurturin has been shown to augment striatal DA utilization and amphetamine-induced locomotor activity in rats with 6-OHDA lesions (49) and TH immunoreactivity after medial forebrain bundle axotomy (52). Persephin also appears to prevent the degeneration of nigral DA neurons after 6-OHDA lesions (54), but it has not yet been reported whether this translates into improved behavioral correlates. The ability of these GDNF family ligands, particularly GDNF, to promote the recovery of damaged DA neurons even after extensive degeneration has occurred suggests that they may be useful therapeutic agents to halt the progression of nigrostriatal degeneration in Parkinson's disease.

In the MPTP-lesioned hemiparkinsonian monkey, a model that is regarded widely as the most predictive preclinical model of Parkinson's disease (99), intranigral and intraventricular GDNF treatment significantly decreased the composite parkinsonian rating score after a single bolus injection (17,95,97,98). As was shown for the rodent brain, intraventricular injection of GDNF was deemed to be a suitable route of administration in the monkey brain. Again, this finding was supported by distribution studies, which showed that a bolus dose of [^{125}I]GDNF introduced into the lateral ventricle quickly distributes throughout the primate brain in a bilateral pattern (17). As early as 24 hours after the injection, [^{125}I]GDNF could be detected just ventral to the SN, a finding indicating that GDNF rapidly distributes in brain and can reach dopaminergic neuronal cell bodies of the nigrostriatal pathway rapidly. GDNF or vehicle was given as a single intracranial injection into the SN or the lateral ventricle, only after a stable level of motor dysfunction had been established (17).

Behavioral parameters associated with motor functions were assessed using a primate parkinsonian scale patterned after the human Unified Parkinson's Disease Rating Scale and were scored in the following categories: rigidity, bradykinesia, posture, balance, tremor, and food acquisition test (123). Improvement, attributable to ameliorations in rigidity, bradykinesia, posture balance, and fine regulation of motor control such as food acquisition, was apparent by 1 week after the injection, and as with the rodent model (see earlier), it persisted for a few weeks (17). Not surprisingly, the only category not affected by GDNF was tremor, a symptom that in patients with Parkinson's disease often responds better to anticholinergic than to dopaminergic agents (124). Immunocytochemical analysis revealed that the GDNF effects observed in MPTP-lesioned monkeys were likely the result of enhanced SN DA levels, because there was a significant elevation of TH-positive neurons within all regions of the SN, including the ventral tegmental area (VTA), where there is extensive loss of dopaminergic neurons and fibers (32). This finding was confirmed by neurochemical analyses, which measured increased DA levels in the SN and globus pallidus in response to GDNF (95,97,98,125). Additionally, in the caudate and putamen, the ratio of the DA metabolite, HVA, to DA was increased markedly compared with MPTP-lesioned controls (97).

Effects in Nonparkinsonian Animals

The pharmacology of GDNF in the various animal models of Parkinson's disease discussed earlier provides convincing evidence of the role of this agent in the regeneration and repair of the damaged nigrostriatal pathway. However, a complete understanding of the role of GDNF in the CNS necessitates a thorough examination of its effects in the intact animal, especially if potential unwanted side effects are to be identified. Morphologic changes in the nigrostriatal pathway were evident after GDNF administration (15,81). Intranigral injections resulted in robust increases in TH staining in the striatum and cell size in the SN ipsilateral to the injection site (15,81). Moreover, TH-positive processes, analogous to the growth cones of the developing nigrostriatal pathway (13–15,120), were considerably denser and more numerous. These results indicate that GDNF has the ability to invoke a state reminiscent of early development in the intact striatum.

Prominent effects on body weight were noted in response to either intraventricular or intranigral GDNF injections (12,120,125–127). In unlesioned GDNF-treated rats, weight gain was significantly curtailed compared with vehicle-injected rats (12,120). Because [^{125}I]GDNF has been shown to accumulate in the hypothalamus, investigators suggested that effects of GDNF on this brain structure may be responsible for the alterations in weight gain (104,105,120), a hypothesis confirmed by neurochemical analyses. The decreased weight gain correlated with increased hypothalamic DA function, which has been shown to correspond to decreased food intake (128). Thus, GDNF-induced effects on hypothalamic DA transmission and the consequent weight

loss may reflect an unwanted side effect of GDNF. In addition, increased locomotor activity, possibly resulting from overall enhanced DA activity in the CNS, was also noted (104,105,120). In addition to the hypothalamus, increased DA levels were detected in the SN, striatum, VTA, and frontal cortex of unlesioned rats (104,105,120). GDNF is also a neurotrophic factor for a variety of other neuronal types including septohippocampal cholinergic neurons (15,91), hypothalamic serotoninergic neurons (13–15,89,122), noradrenergic locus caeruleus neurons (88), and striatal GABAergic neuronal populations (92,93).

In unlesioned monkeys, as with rats (see earlier), intranigral administration of GDNF produced a persistent reduction in body weight (125–127). In addition, behavioral abnormalities manifested in response to GDNF included increased daytime and nocturnal activity, both of which could be attributed to elevated dopaminergic transmission (125). This finding was confirmed by neurochemical measures: the signal amplitude for potassium-evoked DA release was increased in the caudate and putamen 4 weeks after the intranigral injection of GDNF (95,125). The likely reason was an elevation of either presynaptic DA storage or DA synaptic efficiency, rather than increased DA synthesis, because striatal concentrations of DA and the DA metabolites DOPAC and HVA were unaffected by GDNF (95,125). In contrast, GDNF administration significantly augmented DA, DOPAC, and HVA levels in the SN and VTA. Furthermore, the GDNF-induced effects on DA levels in the SN may have been a consequence of increased TH activity, because immunocytochemical examination clearly revealed a proliferation of TH-positive staining, as well as enlarged DA neuronal perikarya and extensive neurite outgrowth in the SN after intranigral GDNF injections (125). Thus, the differential effects of GDNF in the striatum compared with the SN and VTA indicate that the mechanisms of GDNF action may differ depending on the particular region of the nigrostriatal pathway studied.

Effects in Combination with L-DOPA Therapy

Patients with Parkinson's disease are usually treated with L-DOPA, the precursor to DA synthesis. After prolonged therapy, these patients frequently develop complications such as dyskinesias and other toxic side effects, possibly resulting from unregulated levels of DA in the caudate and putamen. These side effects severely limit the tolerance of this medication as the disease progresses (129). In primates, side effects induced by L-DOPA include choreoathetoid movements (abnormal limb movements), buccolingual dyskinesia (protrusion of the tongue), akathisia (repeated shifting from one limb to the other), dystonia (dystonic posture), stereotypy (repeated behaviors), and vomiting (130).

In stable MPTP-lesioned hemiparkinsonian rhesus monkeys, presynaptic dopaminergic terminals in the striatum were significantly depleted, leading to decreased buffering and turnover (including storage and reuptake) of DA that can be synthesized from administered L-DOPA. After intraventricular administration of GDNF, these monkeys experienced a marked reduction in L-DOPA–induced side effects, such as dyskinesia and dystonia (127). Moreover, behavioral correlates, manifested by improved deficit, were clearly evident in the L-DOPA–treated animals that were given GDNF compared with the group that was given L-DOPA alone (127). Essentially, GDNF resulted in a shift in the L-DOPA dose-response curve, allowing a fivefold lower dose of L-DOPA to be administered and yet produce a similar benefit (127). Overall, it appears that GDNF makes the residual nigrostriatal dopaminergic neurons more responsive to L-DOPA, and the sequelae include improved behavioral performance such as decreased rigidity and bradykinesia, as well as improved fine motor control.

FUTURE PROSPECTS FOR GLIAL CELL LINE–DERIVED NEUROTROPHIC FACTOR THERAPY IN PARKINSON'S DISEASE

In the early stages of Parkinson's disease, patients respond remarkably well to symptomatic treatment with DA replacement therapy, usually given orally as a combination of L-DOPA and carbidopa, an inhibitor of peripheral metabolism of L-DOPA (i.e., Sinemet) (19,129). However, as the disease progresses, there is worsening of clinical symptoms and signs, at which point DA agonists with relative specificity, such as bromocriptine and pergolide, can be useful therapeutic agents. However, none of these drugs can prevent the degeneration of nigral dopaminergic neurons, which inexorably progresses and results in a consequent decline in the patient's clinical status. Whereas patients in the early stages of Parkinson's disease have sufficient active dopaminergic neurons and terminals to synthesize DA from the precursor L-DOPA, this is not the case in the late stages of the disease, when few functional DA neurons remain. In addition, continued L-DOPA treatment produces unwanted side effects such as abnormal movements (dyskinesia) resulting from excess DA (129,131). Thus, novel therapies that would address issues such as L-DOPA side effects and the lack of effect on the progressive degeneration of nigral DA neurons would be advantageous.

Because virtually every study to date has emphasized that GDNF is a potent trophic factor for nigrostriatal DA neurons, it was a logical candidate for the therapy of Parkinson's disease. As an added bonus, GDNF was shown to enhance the ability of DA neurons to use exogenous L-DOPA in the synthesis of DA and to prevent side effects induced by L-DOPA therapy, at least in MPTP-lesioned monkeys (127). Thus, the beneficial effects of GDNF may include the slowing of the neurodegeneration that occurs during the course

of Parkinson's disease, in addition to a possible restoration of dopaminergic function in the nigrostriatal pathway and subsequent improvement in motor functions. However exciting these findings, they should be interpreted with caution, because a thorough investigation of any potential side effects that may be manifest with GDNF treatment has not been reported. In particular, effects of GDNF on hypothalamic function (15,104,120,122), accompanied by significant weight loss, may prove to be serious enough to preclude the clinical use of this agent. GDNF injection sites also are characterized by an increased proliferation of glia (47,132). More troubling perhaps is the ubiquitous distribution (60,61,66,68,74,75,78,80) of GDNF receptors, GFRα1, GFRα2, and ret, particularly in peripheral organs, where GDNF may interact to cause unwanted side effects. In addition, evidence has implicated ret phosphorylation by GDNF in the stimulation of the mitogen-activated protein kinase signal transduction pathway (76) and, possibly, tumorigenesis. In conclusion, future studies of potential candidates for therapy of Parkinson's disease within the GDNF family of ligands may wish to focus on identifying potential members that will not interact with GFRα1 or GFRα2.

Nutt and colleagues have presented preliminary data of an experimental study on the intraventricular administration of GDNF in the treatment of Parkinson's disease. No improvements were seen in on or off UPDRS motor scores in 50 patients receiving placebo or 25–4000 micrograms intraventricular GDNF for 8 months. Nevertheless, there was clear evidence of biological effects including anorexia, weight loss, and sensory symptoms in most treated patients. There was no increase in tyrosine hydroxylase-positive fibers in the striatum in one patient who had died of unrelated causes (133).

REFERENCES

1. Araujo D, Lapchak P, Hefti F. Experimental systems to study neurotrophic factor effects on rat brain neurons. In: Bradley W, Crowell R, eds. *The yearbook of neurology and neurosurgery.* St. Louis: Mosby–Year Book, 1993:21–25.
2. Hefti F, Denton T, Knusel B, et al. Neurotrophic factors: what are they and what are they doing? In: Loughlin S, Fallon J, eds. *Neurotrophic factors.* New York: Academic, 1994:25–49.
3. Heumann R. Neurotrophin signalling. *Curr Opin Neurobiol* 1994;4:668–679.
4. Kupsch A, Oertel W, Earl C, et al. Neuronal transplantation and neurotrophic factors in the treatment of Parkinson's disease: update February 1995. *J Neural Transm* 1995;46:193–207.
5. Lapchak P, Araujo D, Hefti F. Neurotrophins in the CNS. *Rev Neurosci* 1992;3:1–12.
6. Lapchak P, Araujo D, Dugich-Djordjevic M, et al. Neurotrophins in the CNS: effects on hippocampal cholinergic function following deafferentation, regulation by pharmacological agents and lesions. In: Moody T, ed. *Growth factors, peptides and receptors.* New York: Plenum, 1993:241–254.

7. Lewin GR, Barde YA. Physiology of the neurotrophins. *Annu Rev Neurosci* 1996;19:289–317.

8. Mesulam E, Kroin J, Sendera T, et al. Distribution and retrograde transport of trophic factors in the central nervous system: functional implications for the treatment of neurodegenerative diseases. *Prog Neurobiol* 1999;57:451–484.

9. Snider W, Johnson E. Neurotrophic molecules. *Ann Neurol* 1989;26:489–506.

10. Thoenen H. The changing scene of neurotrophic factors. *Trends Neurosci* 1991;14:165-170.

11. Tomac A, Widenfalk J, Lin L, et al. Retrograde axonal transport of GDNF in the adult nigrostriatal system suggests a trophic role in the adult. *Proc Natl Acad Sci USA* 1995;92:8274–8278.

12. Lapchak PA, Jiao S, Collins F, et al. Glial cell line–derived neurotrophic factor: distribution and pharmacology in the rat following a bolus intraventricular injection. *Brain Res* 1997;747:92–102.

13. Lapchak PA. Therapeutic potentials for glial cell line–derived neurotrophic factor (GDNF) based upon pharmacological activities in the CNS. *Rev Neurosci* 1996;7:165–176.

14. Lapchak PA, Miller PJ, Jiao S, et al. Biology of glial cell line–derived neurotrophic factor (GDNF): implications for the use of GDNF to treat Parkinson's disease. *Neurodegeneration* 1996;5:197–205.

15. Lapchak PA, Jiao S, Miller PJ, et al. Pharmacological characterization of glial cell line–derived neurotrophic factor (GDNF): implications for GDNF as a therapeutic molecule for treating neurodegenerative diseases. *Cell Tissue Res* 1996;286:179–189.

16. Tomac A, Lindqvist E, Lin LF, et al. Protection and repair of the nigrostriatal dopaminergic system by GDNF *in vivo*. *Nature* 1995;373:335–339.

17. Lapchak PA, Araujo DM, Hilt DC, et al. Topographical distribution of [^{125}I]-glial cell line–derived neurotrophic factor in unlesioned and MPTP-lesioned rhesus monkey brain following a bolus intraventricular injection. *Brain Res* 1998;789:9–22.

18. Antonini A, Vontobel P, Psylla M, et al. Complementary positron emission tomographic studies of the striatal dopaminergic system in Parkinson's disease. *Arch Neurol* 1995;52:1183–1190.

19. Young AB, Penney JB Jr. Biochemical and functional organization of the basal ganglia. In: Jankovic J, Tolosa E, eds. *Parkinson's disease and movement disorders,* 3rd ed. Baltimore: Williams & Wilkins, 1998:1–13.

20. Lapchak PA, Beck KD, Araujo DM, et al. Chronic intranigral administration of brain-derived neurotrophic factor produces striatal dopaminergic hypofunction in unlesioned adult rats and fails to attenuate the decline of striatal dopaminergic function following medial forebrain bundle transection. *Neuroscience* 1993;53:639–650.

21. Hynes M, Poulsen K, Armanini M, et al. Neurotrophin-4/5 is a survival factor for embryonic midbrain dopaminergic neurons in enriched cultures. *J Neurosci Res* 1994;37:144–154.

22. Feng L, Wang CY, Jiang H, et al. Differential effects of GDNF and BDNF on cultured ventral mesencephalic neurons. *Brain Res Mol Brain Res* 1999;66:62–70.

23. Kaddis FG, Zawada WM, Schaack J, et al. Conditioned medium from aged monkey fibroblasts stably expressing GDNF and BDNF improves survival of embryonic dopamine neurons *in vitro*. *Cell Tissue Res* 1996;286:241–247.

24. Sautter J, Meyer M, Spenger C, et al. Effects of combined BDNF and GDNF treatment on cultured dopaminergic midbrain neurons. *Neuroreport* 1998;9:1093–1096.

25. Spina MB, Hyman C, Squinto S, et al. Brain-derived neurotrophic factor protects dopaminergic cells from 6-hydroxydopamine toxicity. *Ann NY Acad Sci* 1992;648:348–350.

26. Henderson J, Seniud N, Roder J. Localization of CNTF immunoreactivity to neurons and astroglia in the CNS. *Mol Brain Res* 1994;22:151–165.

27. MacLennan AJ, Vinson EN, Marks L, et al. Immunohistochemical localization of ciliary neurotrophic factor receptor alpha expression in the rat nervous system. *J Neurosci* 1996;16:621–630.

28. Davis S, Aldrich TH, Valenzuela DM, et al. The receptor for ciliary neurotrophic factor. *Science* 1991;253:59–63.

29. Ip NY, Maisonpierre P, Alderson R, et al. The neurotrophins and CNTF: specificity of action towards PNS and CNS neurons. *J Physiol Paris* 1991;85:123–130.

30. Hagg T, Varon S. Ciliary neurotrophic factor prevents degeneration of adult rat substantia nigra dopaminergic neurons *in vivo*. *Proc Natl Acad Sci USA* 1990;90:6315–6319.

31. Burgess WH, Maciag T. The heparin-binding (fibroblast) growth factor family of proteins. *Annu Rev Biochem* 1989;58:575–606.

32. Torack RM, Morris JC. Tyrosine hydroxylase-like (TH) immunoreactivity in Parkinson's disease and Alzheimer's disease. *J Neural Transm* 1992;4:165–171.

33. Date I, Notter MF, Felten SY, et al. MPTP-treated young mice but not aging mice show partial recovery of the nigrostriatal dopaminergic system by stereotaxic injection of acidic fibroblast growth factor (aFGF). *Brain Res* 1990;526:156–160.

34. Unsicker K, Suter-Crazzalora C, Krieglstein K. Growth factor function in the development and maintenance of midbrain dopaminergic neurons: concepts, facts and prospects for TGF-B. In: *Growth factors as drugs for neurological and sensory disorders.* Chichester, UK: Wiley, 1996.

35. Krieglstein K, Rufer M, Suter-Crazzolara C, et al. Neural functions of the transforming growth factors beta. *Int J Dev Neurosci* 1995;13:301–315.

36. Krieglstein K, Reuss B, Maysinger D, et al. Short communication: transforming growth factor-beta mediates the neurotrophic effect of fibroblast growth factor-2 on midbrain dopaminergic neurons. European *J Neurosci* 1998;10:2746–50.

37. Massague J, Attisano L, Wrana J. The TGF-B family and its composite receptors. Trends in Cell Biology 1994;4:172–178.

38. Unsicker K, Flanders KC, Cissel DS, et al. Transforming growth factor beta isoforms in the adult rat central and peripheral nervous system. *Neuroscience* 1991;44:613–625.

39. Krieglstein K, Henheik P, Farkas L, et al. Glial cell line–derived neurotrophic factor requires transforming growth factor-beta for exerting its full neurotrophic potential on peripheral and CNS neurons. *J Neurosci* 1998;18:9822–9834.

40. Unsicker K. GDNF: a cytokine at the interface of TGF-betas and neurotrophins. *Cell Tissue Res* 1996;286:175–178.

41. Sullivan AM, Pohl J, Blunt SB. Growth/differentiation factor 5 and glial cell line–derived neurotrophic factor enhance survival and function of dopaminergic grafts in a rat model of Parkinson's disease. *Eur J Neurosci* 1998;10:3681–3688.

42. Sullivan AM, Opacka-Juffry J, Pohl J, et al. Neuroprotective effects of growth/differentiation factor 5 depend on the site of administration. *Brain Res* 1999;818:176–179.

43. Lin LF, Doherty DH, Lile JD, et al. GDNF: a glial cell line–derived neurotrophic factor for midbrain dopaminergic neurons. *Science* 1993;260:1130–1132.

44. Lin LF, Zhang TJ, Colin F, et al. Purification and initial characterization of rat B49 glial cell line–derived neurotrophic factor. *J Neurochem* 1994;63:758–768.

45. Buj-Bello A, Adu J, Piñón LG, et al. Neurturin responsiveness requires a GPI-linked receptor and the Ret receptor tyrosine kinase. *Nature* 1997;387:721–724.

46. Creedon DJ, Tansey MG, Baloh RH, et al. Neurturin shares receptors and signal transduction pathways with glial cell line–derived neurotrophic factor in sympathetic neurons. *Proc Natl Acad Sci USA* 1997;94:7018–7023.

47. Heuckeroth RO, Lampe PA, Johnson EM, et al. Neurturin and GDNF promote proliferation and survival of enteric neuron and glial progenitors *in vitro*. *Dev Biol* 1998;200:116–129.

48. Heuckeroth RO, Enomoto H, Grider JR, et al. Gene targeting reveals a critical role for neurturin in the development and maintenance of enteric, sensory, and parasympathetic neurons. *Neuron* 1999;22:253–263.

49. Horger BA, Nishimura MC, Armanini MP, et al. Neurturin exerts potent actions on survival and function of midbrain dopaminergic neurons. *J Neurosci* 1998;18:4929–4937.

50. Kotzbauer PT, Lampe PA, Heuckeroth RO, et al. Neurturin, a relative of glial-cell-line–derived neurotrophic factor. *Nature* 1996;384:467–470.

51. Widenfalk J, Nosrat C, Tomac A, et al. Neurturin and glial cell line–derived neurotrophic factor receptor-beta (GDNFR-beta), novel proteins related to GDNF and GDNFR-alpha with specific cellular patterns of expression suggesting roles in the developing and adult nervous system and in peripheral organs. *J Neurosci* 1997;17:8506–8519.

52. Tseng JL, Bruhn SL, Zurn AD, et al. Neurturin protects dopaminergic neurons following medial forebrain bundle axotomy. *Neuroreport* 1998;9:1817–1822.

53. Baloh RH, Tansey MG, Lampe PA, et al. Artemin, a novel member of the GDNF ligand family, supports peripheral and central neurons and signals through the GFRalpha3-RET receptor complex. *Neuron* 1998;21:1291–1302.

54. Milbrandt J, de Sauvage FJ, Fahrner TJ, et al. Persephin, a novel neurotrophic factor related to GDNF and neurturin. *Neuron* 1998;20:245–253.

55. Jaszai J, Farkas L, Galter D, et al. GDNF-related factor persephin is widely distributed throughout the nervous system. *J Neurosci Res* 1998;53:494–501.

56. Heimer L, Zahm D, Alheid G. Basal ganglia. In: Paxinos G, ed. *The rat nervous system.* San Diego: Academic, 1995:579–628.

57. Nosrat CA, Tomac A, Lindqvist E, et al. Cellular expression of GDNF mRNA suggests multiple functions inside and outside the nervous system. *Cell Tissue Res* 1996;286:191–207.

58. Buj-Bello A, Buchman VL, Horton A, et al. GDNF is an age-specific survival factor for sensory and autonomic neurons. *Neuron* 1995;15:821–828.

59. Kokaia Z, Airaksinen MS, Nanobashvili A, et al. GDNF family ligands and receptors are differentially regulated after brain insults in the rat. *Eur J Neurosci* 1999;11:1202–1216.

60. Nosrat CA, Tomac A, Hoffer BJ, et al. Cellular and developmental patterns of expression of Ret and glial cell line–derived neurotrophic factor receptor alpha mRNAs. *Exp Brain Res* 1997;115:410–422.

61. Trupp M, Belluardo N, Funakoshi H, et al. Complementary and overlapping expression of glial cell line–derived neurotrophic factor (GDNF), c-ret proto-oncogene, and GDNF receptor-alpha indicates multiple mechanisms of trophic actions in the adult rat CNS. *J Neurosci* 1997;17:3554–3567.

62. Schaar DG, Sieber BA, Dreyfus CF, et al. Regional and cell-specific expression of GDNF in rat brain. *Exp Neurol* 1993;124:368–371.

63. Blum M, Weickert CS. GDNF mRNA expression in normal postnatal development, aging, and in Weaver mutant mice. *Neurobiol Aging* 1995;16:925–929.

64. Strömberg I, Björklund L, Johansson M, et al. Glial cell line–derived neurotrophic factor is expressed in the developing but not adult striatum and stimulates developing dopamine neurons *in vivo*. *Exp Neurol* 1993;124:401–412.

65. Schmidt-Kastner R, Tomac A, Hoffer B, et al. Glial cell line–derived neurotrophic factor (GDNF) mRNA upregulation in striatum and cortical areas after pilocarpine-induced status epilepticus in rats. *Mol Brain Res* 1994;26:325–330.

66. Baloh RH, Tansey MG, Golden JP, et al. TrnR2, a novel receptor that mediates neurturin and GDNF signaling through Ret. *Neuron* 1997;18:793–802.

67. Enokido Y, de Sauvage F, Hongo JA, et al. GFR alpha-4 and the tyrosine kinase Ret form a functional receptor complex for persephin. *Curr Biol* 1998;8:1019–1022.

68. Golden JP, Baloh RH, Kotzbauer PT, et al. Expression of neurturin, GDNF, and their receptors in the adult mouse CNS. *J Comp Neurol* 1998;398:139–150.

69. Klein RD, Sherman D, Ho WH, et al. A GPI-linked protein that interacts with Ret to form a candidate neurturin receptor [published erratum appears in *Nature* 1998;392:210]. *Nature* 1997;387:717–721.

70. Trupp M, Raynoschek C, Belluardo N, et al. Multiple GPI-anchored receptors control GDNF-dependent and independent activation of the c-Ret receptor tyrosine kinase. *Mol Cell Neurosci* 1998;11:47–63.

71. Yu T, Scully S, Yu Y, et al. Expression of GDNF family receptor components during development: implications in the mechanisms of interaction. *J Neurosci* 1998;18:4684–4696.

72. Durbec P, Marcos-Gutierrez CV, Kilkenny C, et al. GDNF signalling through the Ret receptor tyrosine kinase. *Nature* 1996;381:789–793.

73. Jing S, Wen D, Yu Y, et al. GDNF-induced activation of the ret protein tyrosine kinase is mediated by GDNFR-alpha, a novel receptor for GDNF. *Cell* 1996;85:1113–1124.

74. Trupp M, Arenas E, Fainzilber M, et al. Functional receptor for GDNF encoded by the c-ret proto-oncogene. *Nature* 1996;381:785–788.

75. Walker DG, Beach TG, Xu R, et al. Expression of the proto-oncogene Ret, a component of the GDNF receptor complex, persists in human substantia nigra neurons in Parkinson's disease. *Brain Res* 1998;792:207–217.

76. Worby CA, Vega QC, Zhao Y, et al. Glial cell line–derived neurotrophic factor signals through the RET receptor and activates mitogen-activated protein kinase. *J Biol Chem* 1996;271:23619–23622.

77. Baloh RH, Gorodinsky A, Golden JP, et al. GFRalpha3 is an orphan member of the GDNF/neurturin/persephin receptor family. *Proc Natl Acad Sci USA* 1998;95:5801–5806.

78. Jing S, Yu Y, Fang M, et al. GFRalpha-2 and GFRalpha-3 are two new receptors for ligands of the GDNF family. *J Biol Chem* 1997;272:33111–33117.

79. Hishiki T, Nimura Y, Isogai E, et al. Glial cell line–derived neurotrophic factor/neurturin-induced differentiation and its enhancement by retinoic acid in primary human neuroblastomas expressing c-Ret, GFR alpha-1, and GFR alpha-2. *Cancer Res* 1998;58:2158–2165.

80. Sanicola M, Hession C, Worley D, et al. Glial cell line–derived neurotrophic factor-dependent RET activation can be mediated by two different cell-surface accessory proteins. *Proc Natl Acad Sci USA* 1997;94:6238–6243.

81. Hudson J, Granholm AC, Gerhardt GA, et al. Glial cell line–derived neurotrophic factor augments midbrain dopaminergic circuits *in vivo*. *Brain Res Bull* 1995;36:425–432.

82. Clarkson ED, Zawada WM, Freed CR. GDNF reduces apoptosis in dopaminergic neurons *in vitro*. *Neuroreport* 1995;7:145–149.

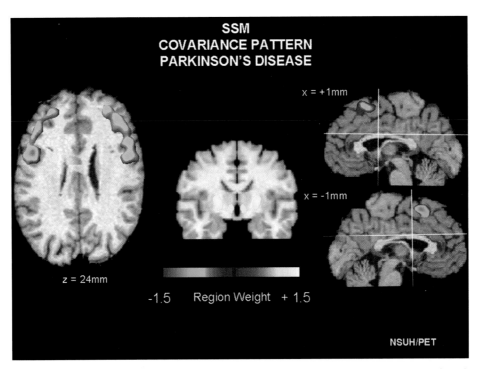

COLOR FIGURE 7.1. Display of the regional metabolic covariance pattern associated with Parkinson's disease (PD) identified using the Scaled Subprofile Model (SSM). Region weights for this PD-related pattern (PDRP) have been overlaid on standard Talairach transformed magnetic resonance imaging (MRI) sections. The pattern is characterized by relative lentiform and thalamic hypermetabolism *(yellow)* covarying negatively with bilateral metabolic reductions *(blue)* in motor and premotor regions and in the supplementary motor area (SMA).

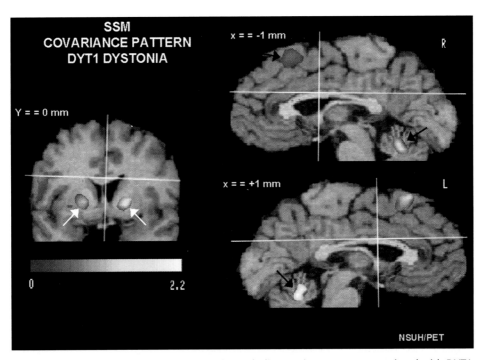

COLOR FIGURE 7.2. Display of the regional metabolic covariance pattern associated with DYT1 dystonia identified using the Scaled Subprofile Model (SSM). Region weights have been mapped on standardized Talairach magnetic resonance imaging sections. This pattern was characterized by relatively increased metabolism in the lentiform nucleus, supplementary motor area (SMA), and cerebellar hemispheres.

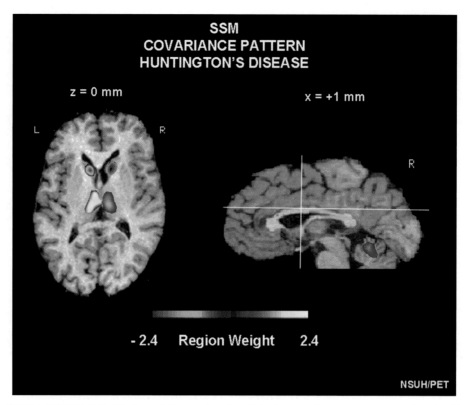

COLOR FIGURE 7.3. Display of the regional metabolic covariance pattern associated with Huntington's disease identified using the Scaled Subprofile Model (SSM). Region weights have been mapped on standardized Talairach magnetic resonance imaging sections. This pattern was characterized by caudate hypometabolism covarying with relative metabolic increases in the thalamus and cerebellum.

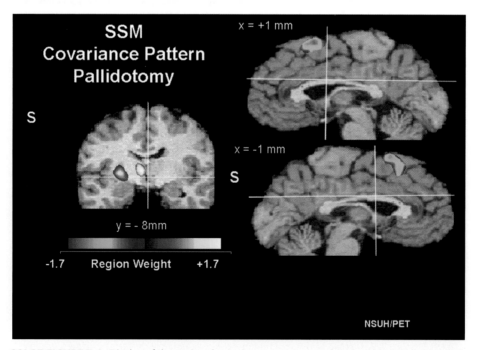

COLOR FIGURE 7.4. Display of the regional covariance pattern associated with surgical changes in glucose metabolism after pallidotomy identified using the Scaled Subprofile Model (SSM). Region weights have been overlaid on standardized Talairach transformed magnetic resonance imaging sections. This pattern was characterized by operative declines in lentiform metabolism covarying with bilateral metabolic increases in the supplementary motor area (SMA).

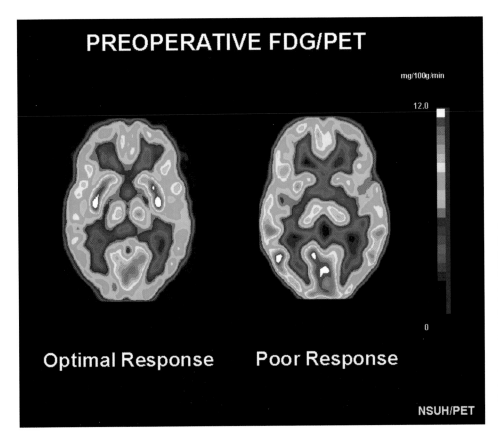

PREOPERATIVE FDG/PET

mg/100g/min

12.0

0

Optimal Response   **Poor Response**

NSUH/PET

COLOR FIGURE 7.5. Preoperative [18F] fluorodeoxyglucose (FDG) positron emission tomography images from two patients with idiopathic Parkinson's disease who underwent right unilateral pallidotomy. **Left:** A patient with preoperative lentiform glucose hypermetabolism had an optimal surgical outcome. **Right:** A patient with a lower rate of metabolism in the lentiform nucleus had no therapeutic response to surgery. Both pallidotomy lesions were comparable in size and location. (The *color stripe* represents regional rates of glucose metabolism in mg/min/100g.)

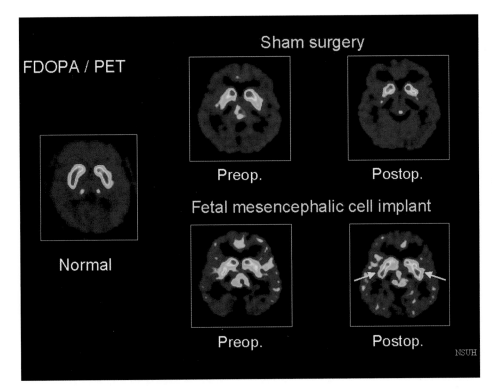

FDOPA / PET

Sham surgery

Preop.   Postop.

Fetal mesencephalic cell implant

Normal

Preop.   Postop.

NSUH

COLOR FIGURE 7.6. [15F] fluorodopa (FDOPA) positron emission tomography (PET) images from a normal volunteer **(left)** and from two patients studied in the course of a blinded sham-controlled study of fetal nigral dopamine cell implantation for advanced Parkinson's disease **(right)**. The **upper tier** represents baseline and 15 month follow-up FDOPA/PET scans from a patients with Parkinson's disease who was randomized to sham surgery. The **lower tier** represents baseline and 15-month postoperative scans from another patient who was randomized to bilateral implantation in the putamen. At baseline, both patients demonstrated bilateral increases in putamen FDOPA uptake compatible with engraftment *(arrows)*.

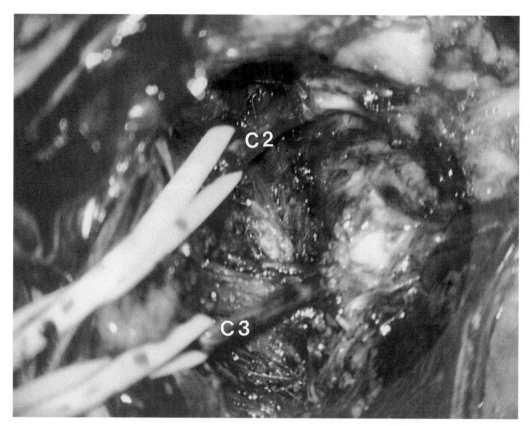

COLOR FIGURE 31.3. Posterior branch of C-2 and C-3 on the left.

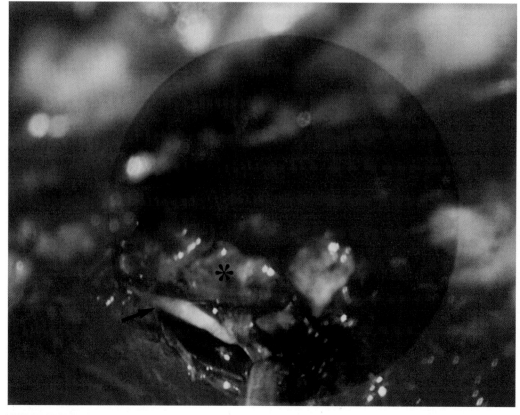

COLOR FIGURE 31.5. Intraoperative view of C-1 *(arrow)* on the left side, beneath the vertebral artery (*).

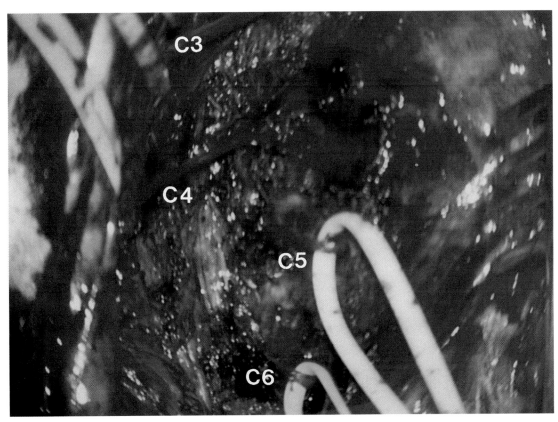

COLOR FIGURE 31.6. Posterior branches of C3-6 on the left side.

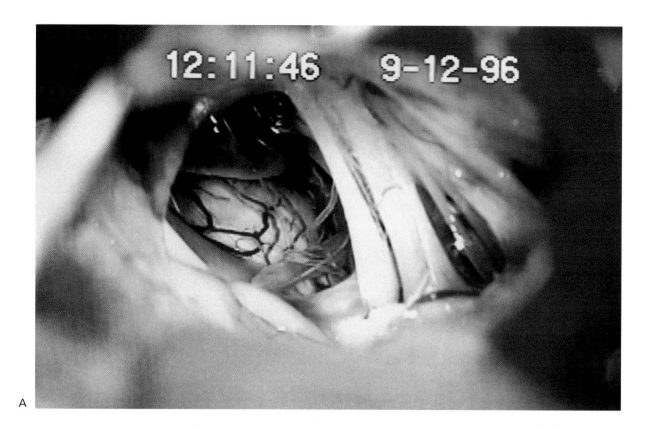

A

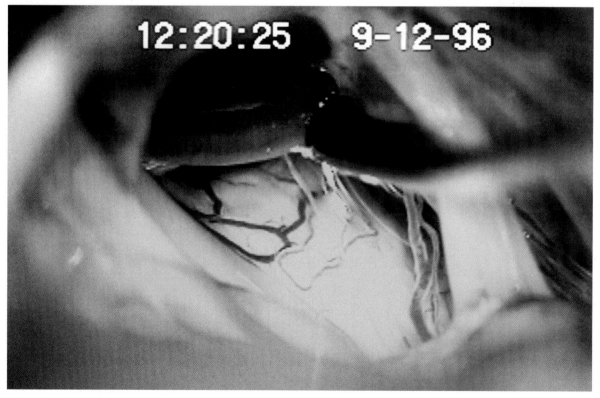

B

COLOR FIGURE 34.4. A: This is an operative photograph from a patient with typical right-sided hemifacial spasm. Note the arterial loop compressing the nerve as it emerges from the pons on its caudal and lateral aspect. **B:** The vessel can be mobilized away from the root entry zone with gentle manipulation. A piece of Teflon felt is then placed under the artery to hold it away from the facial nerve. Care must be taken not to damage any perforating vessels in this region.

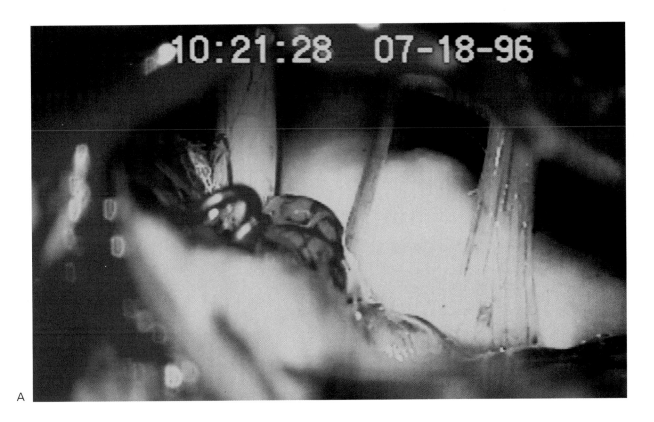

A

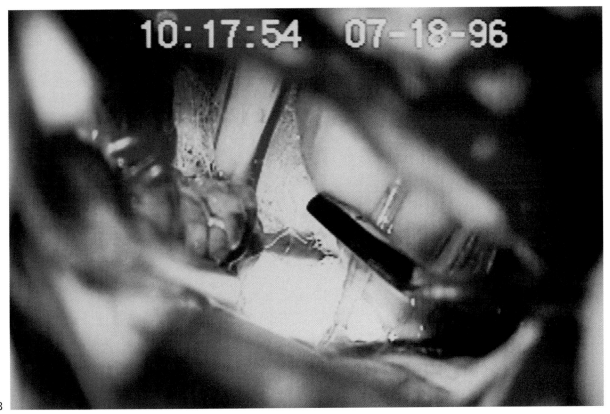

B

COLOR FIGURE 34.5. A: This photograph, also from a patient with typical hemifacial spasm, demonstrates compression of the nerve by an ectatic vertebral artery. **B:** Decompression in this case is accomplished by gradual mobilization of the vessel beginning caudal to the lower cranial nerves and moving progressively rostrally. Felt is used to lift the artery gradually and carefully off the facial root entry zone.

83. Clarkson ED, Zawada WM, Freed CR. GDNF improves survival and reduces apoptosis in human embryonic dopaminergic neurons *in vitro. Cell Tissue Res* 1997;289:207–10.

84. Engele J, Franke B. Effects of glial cell line–derived neurotrophic factor (GDNF) on dopaminergic neurons require concurrent activation of cAMP-dependent signaling pathways. *Cell Tissue Res* 1996;286:235–240.

85. Sauer H, Rosenblad C, Björklund A. Glial cell line–derived neurotrophic factor but not transforming growth factor beta 3 prevents delayed degeneration of nigral dopaminergic neurons following striatal 6-hydroxydopamine lesion. *Proc Natl Acad Sci USA* 1995;92:8935–8939.

86. Zurn AD, Baetge EE, Hammang JP, et al. Glial cell line–derived neurotrophic factor (GDNF), a new neurotrophic factor for motoneurones. *Neuroreport* 1994;6:113–118.

87. Jomary C, Thomas M, Grist J, et al. Expression patterns of neurturin and its receptor components in developing and degenerative mouse retina. *Invest Ophthalmol Vis Sci* 1999;40:568–574.

88. Arenas E, Trupp M, Akerud P, et al. GDNF prevents degeneration and promotes the phenotype of brain noradrenergic neurons *in vivo. Neuron* 1995;15:1465–1473.

89. Galter D, Unsicker K. Regulation of the transmitter phenotype of rostral and caudal groups of cultured serotonergic raphe neurons. *Neuroscience* 1999;88:549–559.

90. Lapchak PA, Miller PJ, Jiao S. Glial cell line–derived neurotrophic factor induces the dopaminergic and cholinergic phenotype and increases locomotor activity in aged Fischer 344 rats. *Neuroscience* 1997;77:745–752.

91. Araujo DM, Hilt DC, Miller PJ, et al. Ret receptor tyrosine kinase immunoreactivity is altered in glial cell line–derived neurotrophic factor-responsive neurons following lesions of the nigrostriatal and septohippocampal pathways. *Neuroscience* 1997;80:9–16.

92. Araujo DM, Hilt DC. Glial cell line–derived neurotrophic factor attenuates the excitotoxin-induced behavioral and neurochemical deficits in a rodent model of Huntington's disease. *Neuroscience* 1997;81:1099–1110.

93. Araujo DM, Hilt DC. Glial cell line–derived neurotrophic factor attenuates the locomotor hypofunction and striatonigral neurochemical deficits induced by chronic systemic administration of the mitochondrial toxin 3-nitropropionic acid. *Neuroscience* 1998;82:117–127.

94. Hou JG, Mytilineou C. Secretion of GDNF by glial cells does not account for the neurotrophic effect of bFGF on dopamine neurons *in vitro. Brain Res* 1996;724:145–148.

95. Gerhardt GA, Cass WA, Huettl P, et al. GDNF improves dopamine function in the substantia nigra but not the putamen of unilateral MPTP-lesioned rhesus monkeys. *Brain Res* 1999;817:163–171.

96. Ballard PA, Tetrud JW, Langston JW. Permanent human parkinsonism due to 1-methyl-4-phenyl-1,2,3,6-tetrahydropyridine (MPTP): seven cases. *Neurology* 1985;35:949–956.

97. Gash DM, Zhang Z, Ovadia A, et al. Functional recovery in parkinsonian monkeys treated with GDNF. *Nature* 1996;380:252–255.

98. German DC, Manaye KF, Sonsalla PK, et al. Midbrain dopaminergic cell loss in Parkinson's disease and MPTP-induced parkinsonism: sparing of calbindin-D28k-containing cells. *Ann NY Acad Sci* 1992;648:42–62.

99. Langston JW, Forno LS, Rebert CS, et al. Selective nigral toxicity after systemic administration of 1-methyl-4-phenyl-1,2,5,6-tetrahydropyrine (MPTP) in the squirrel monkey. *Brain Res* 1984;292:390–394.

100. Tetrud JW, Langston JW, Garbe PL, et al. Mild parkinsonism in persons exposed to 1-methyl-4-phenyl-1,2,3,6-tetrahydropyridine (MPTP). *Neurology* 1989;39:1483–1487.

101. Date I, Aoi M, Tomita S, et al. GDNF administration induces recovery of the nigrostriatal dopaminergic system both in young and aged parkinsonian mice. *Neuroreport* 1998;9:2365–2369.

102. Cass WA. GDNF selectively protects dopamine neurons over serotonin neurons against the neurotoxic effects of methamphetamine. *J Neurosci* 1996;16:8132–139.

103. Gash DM, Zhang Z, Gerhardt G. Neuroprotective and neurorestorative properties of GDNF. *Ann Neurol* 1998;44:S121–S125.

104. Lapchak P, Araujo D. Glial cell line–derived neurotrophic factor: drug development. *Drug News Perspect* 1997;10:347–353.

105. Lapchak PA, Miller PJ, Collins F, et al. Glial cell line–derived neurotrophic factor attenuates behavioural deficits and regulates nigrostriatal dopaminergic and peptidergic markers in 6-hydroxydopamine-lesioned adult rats: comparison of intraventricular and intranigral delivery. *Neuroscience* 1997;78:61–72.

106. Cass WA, Manning MW. GDNF protection against 6-OHDA-induced reductions in potassium-evoked overflow of striatal dopamine. *J Neurosci* 1999;19:1416–1423.

107. Opacka-Juffry J, Ashworth S, Hume SP, et al. GDNF protects against 6-OHDA nigrostriatal lesion: *in vivo* study with microdialysis and PET. *Neuroreport* 1995;7:348–352.

108. Kearns CM, Cass WA, Smoot K, et al. GDNF protection against 6-OHDA: time dependence and requirement for protein synthesis. *J Neurosci* 1997;17:7111–7118.

109. Kearns CM, Gash DM. GDNF protects nigral dopamine neurons against 6-hydroxydopamine *in vivo. Brain Res* 1995;672:104–111.

110. Bowenkamp KE, David D, Lapchak PA, et al. 6-hydroxydopamine induces the loss of the dopaminergic phenotype in substantia nigra neurons of the rat: a possible mechanism for restoration of the nigrostriatal circuit mediated by glial cell line–derived neurotrophic factor. *Exp Brain Res* 1996;111:1–7.

111. Winkler C, Sauer H, Lee CS, et al. Short-term GDNF treatment provides long-term rescue of lesioned nigral dopaminergic neurons in a rat model of Parkinson's disease. *J Neurosci* 1996;16:7206–7215.

112. Björklund A, Rosenblad C, Winkler C, et al. Studies on neuroprotective and regenerative effects of GDNF in a partial lesion model of Parkinson's disease. *Neurobiol Dis* 1997;4:186–200.

113. Hoffer BJ, Hoffman A, Bowenkamp K, et al. Glial cell line–derived neurotrophic factor reverses toxin-induced injury to midbrain dopaminergic neurons *in vivo. Neurosci Lett* 1994;182:107–111.

114. Choi-Lundberg DL, Lin Q, Chang YN, et al. Dopaminergic neurons protected from degeneration by GDNF gene therapy. *Science* 1997;275:838–841.

115. Bilang-Bleuel A, Revah F, Colin P, et al. Intrastriatal injection of an adenoviral vector expressing glial-cell-line–derived neurotrophic factor prevents dopaminergic neuron degeneration and behavioral impairment in a rat model of Parkinson disease. *Proc Natl Acad Sci USA* 1997;94:8818–8823.

116. Barkats M, Nakao N, Grasbon-Frodl EM, et al. Intrastriatal grafts of embryonic mesencephalic rat neurons genetically modified using an adenovirus encoding human Cu/Zn superoxide dismutase. *Neuroscience* 1997;78:703–713.

117. Horellou P, Bilang-Bleuel A, Mallet J. *In vivo* adenovirus-mediated gene transfer for Parkinson's disease. *Neurobiol Dis* 1997;4:280–287.

118. Lapchak PA, Araujo DM, Hilt DC, et al. Adenoviral vector-mediated GDNF gene therapy in a rodent lesion model of late stage Parkinson's disease. *Brain Res* 1997;777:153–160.

119. Fan D, Ogawa M, Ikeguchi K, et al. Prevention of dopaminergic neuron death by adeno-associated virus vector-mediated GDNF

gene transfer in rat mesencephalic cells *in vitro. Neurosci Lett* 1998;248:61–64.

120. Lapchak PA. A preclinical development strategy designed to optimize the use of glial cell line–derived neurotrophic factor in the treatment of Parkinson's disease. *Mov Disord* 1998;13 [Suppl 1]:49–54.

121. Lapchak PA, Gash DM, Jiao S, et al. Glial cell line–derived neurotrophic factor: a novel therapeutic approach to treat motor dysfunction in Parkinson's disease. *Exp Neurol* 1997;144:29–34.

122. Lapchak PA, Gash DM, Collins F, et al. Pharmacological activities of glial cell line–derived neurotrophic factor (GDNF): preclinical development and application to the treatment of Parkinson's disease. *Exp Neurol* 1997;145:309–321.

123. Smith R, Zhang Z, Kurlan R, et al. Developing a stable model of Parkinsonism in the rhesus monkey. *Neuroscience* 1993;52: 7–16.

124. Paré D, Curro'Dossi R, Steriade M. Neuronal basis of the parkinsonian resting tremor: a hypothesis and its implications for treatment. *Neuroscience* 1990;35:217–226.

125. Gash DM, Zhang Z, Cass WA, et al. Morphological and functional effects of intranigrally administered GDNF in normal rhesus monkeys. *J Comp Neurol* 1995;363:345–358.

126. Zhang Z, Miyoshi Y, Lapchak PA, et al. Dose response to intraventricular glial cell line–derived neurotrophic factor ad-ministration in parkinsonian monkeys. *J Pharmacol Exp Ther* 1997;282:1396–1401.

127. Miyoshi Y, Zhang Z, Ovadia A, et al. Glial cell line–derived neurotrophic factor-levodopa interactions and reduction of side effects in parkinsonian monkeys. *Ann Neurol* 1997;42:208–214.

128. Gillard E, Dang D, Stanley B. Evidence that neuropeptide Y and dopamine in the perifornical hypothalamus interact antagonistically in the control of food intake. *Brain Res* 1993;628:128–136.

129. Marsden CD, Parkes JD. "On-off" effects in patients with Parkinson's disease on chronic levodopa therapy. *Lancet* 1976;1:292–296.

130. Kurlan R, Kim M, Gash D. Oral levodopa dose-response study in MPTP-lesioned hemiparkinsonian monkeys: assessment with a new rating scale for monkey parkinsonism. *Mov Disord* 1991; 6:111–118.

131. Maloteaux JM, Vanisberg MA, Laterre C, et al. [^{3}H]GBR 12935 binding to dopamine uptake sites: subcellular localization and reduction in Parkinson's disease and progressive supranuclear palsy. *Eur J Pharmacol* 1988;156:331–340.

132. Franke B, Figiel M, Engele J. CNS glia are targets for GDNF and neurturin. *Histochem Cell Biol* 1998;110:595–601.

133. Nutt JG, Bronstoin JM, Carter JH, et al. Intraventricular administration of GDNF in the treatment of Parkinson's disease. *Neurology* 2001;56[Suppl 3]:546–601.

Surgery for Parkinson's Disease and Movement Disorders,
edited by J.K. Krauss, J. Jankovic, and R.G. Grossman.
Lippincott Williams & Wilkins, Philadelphia © 2001.

19

POTENTIALS OF GENE AND CELL THERAPY FOR TREATMENT OF PARKINSON'S DISEASE

UN JUNG KANG
OLE ISACSON

The development of molecular biologic techniques has resulted in the discovery of genetic mutations that are responsible for various neurodegenerative disorders including Parkinson's disease (PD) (1–3). Molecular biologic technologies have also led to the development of genetic engineering methods as potential therapeutic modalities for various disorders (4–6). These advances should lead to a better understanding of the pathogenesis of and new treatments for many disorders that have not been amenable to traditional therapies. The idea of gene therapy was proposed decades ago, but a successful clinical application has not yet been fully implemented (4). As with most scientific developments, the initial implementation of ideas reveals unanticipated problems, and further improvements and modifications follow. This chapter discusses the basic concepts and methodology of gene therapy including limitations of the current techniques and recent promising advances. The potential of gene therapy for PD is then illustrated through specific examples in animal models of PD.

BASIC CONCEPTS OF GENE THERAPY

To put it in simple terms, *gene therapy* delivers DNA materials into the host instead of the final desired product. It uses internal machinery to transcribe the DNA information into RNA, then to translate RNA to protein, which, in turn, may be a therapeutic molecule or may synthesize a desired product. Delivery of DNA can provide a more efficient, sustained, and localized supply of the product than delivery of the product itself. An abnormal gene in genetic disorders could have a defective function that could be complemented by inserted normal genetic information. When the genetic abnormality leads to new toxic function, a strategy to intervene and to neutralize the toxic function is necessary. In other cases, gene therapy does not directly address the consequences of genetic mutations, but rather it provides a biologic minipump that delivers therapeutic pharmacologic compounds directly into specific sites of the body (7).

GENE THERAPY METHODS FOR THE NERVOUS SYSTEM

Two general approaches have been employed for delivering therapeutic genes into target tissues. With *ex vivo* gene therapy, cells are genetically modified *in vitro,* and then they are transplanted into the host. With *in vivo* gene therapy, the therapeutic gene is introduced directly into the host somatic cells *in situ,* by using viral vectors (Fig. 19.1).

Ex Vivo Modality of Gene Transfer

For *ex vivo* gene transfer, the cells to be transduced with the genes should be easily obtainable, readily cultured, able to express the transgenes, and able to withstand the selection processes used to enrich for transduced cells. The cells should be nononcogenic and immunologically compatible with the recipient, and they should survive well in the brain. The cells then are genetically modified to secrete neuroactive substances such as neurotransmitters and neurotrophic factors, which serve as a biologic pump at a localized site in the brain. Primary skin fibroblasts taken from adult animals satisfy most of the criteria outlined earlier (7). Fibroblasts can be easily obtained from patients: their own skin biopsy specimen is modified into customized immunocompatible donor cells. The astrocyte is also an attractive cell type for grafting in the central nervous system (CNS) because of its intrinsic supportive role in that system. These cells are

U.J. Kang: Departments of Neurology and Neurobiology, Pharmacology, and Physiology, University of Chicago, Chicago, Illinois 60637.

O. Isacson: Neuroregeneration Laboratory, Harvard Medical School/McLean Hospital, Boston, Massachusetts 02115.

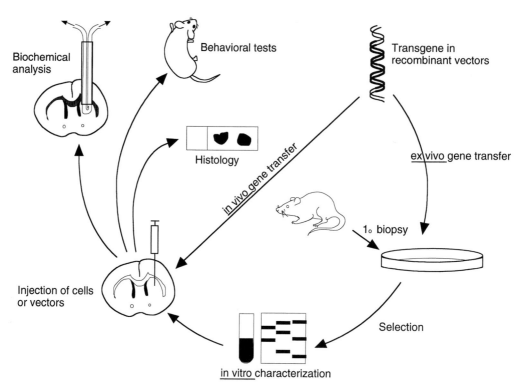

FIGURE 19.1. Experimental schemes for transferring genes into the central nervous system. Two general methods of gene transfer, *in vivo* and *ex vivo*, are schematically depicted. For details, please see the text.

not as easy to transduce with retroviruses as are fibroblasts, however (8).

The advantages of *ex vivo* gene transfer include the ability to control and to monitor the gene transfer process before the cells are placed back into the subjects. The biochemical effect of the transgene can be characterized, and potential tumorigenesis can be assessed. Toxicity of the virus can be screened. In addition, grafted cells may provide useful functions beyond those provided by the transgene, such as serving as a substrate for axonal growth or restoring synaptic contacts with the host neurons. For certain applications, however, direct *in vivo* gene therapy may be more suitable, as discussed in the next section.

A more desirable cell for CNS somatic gene therapy would be one of CNS origin with neuronal features such as a storage mechanism, secretory machineries, and regulatory signal transduction pathways for the final product. The most commonly used CNS cells are primary neurons from fetal tissues. However, because of the logistical and ethical dilemma of using fetal tissues, alternatives have been vigorously sought. Primary neurons can be genetically modified to boost their survival or their phenotypes to maximize their utility. They have also been conditionally immortalized using nontransforming oncogenes to generate neuronal cell lines with low risk of tumor formation (9,10). More recently, neuronal stem cells have been discovered and deserve special attention as

potential powerful gene therapy vehicles (11), as discussed in the next section.

Neuronal Stem Cells

Neuronal stem cells are multipotent, capable of self-renewal, and present in neurogenic areas of both embryonic and adult brains. These cells are also referred to as progenitor cells when they are more committed to mature phenotypes than stem cells, or as CNS precursor cells to more loosely refer to either type (12). Neuronal stem cells were initially isolated from fetal and adult rodent brains, from regions that undergo neurogenesis beyond the developmental ages such as subventricular zone and hippocampal dentate gyrus (13,14). These neuronal stem cells can be propagated in culture in the presence of epidermal growth factor (EGF) or basic fibroblast growth factor (bFGF, FGF-2) (14,15). The presence of dividing cells in adult human hippocampus suggests the existence of neuronal stem cells in adult human brains as well (16). Human CNS stem cells were isolated from the developing human forebrain initially by transducing a population of dividing cells with retroviruses expressing an oncogene, v-*myc* (17), and then more recently, by growth in a combination of EGF, FGF-2, and leukemia inhibitory growth factor (18). The properties of neuronal stem cells are similar to those of the bone marrow stem cells (12).

In fact, there are hints of the existence of common neuro-hematopoietic stem cells—hematopoietic cells can emerge after transplantation of neuronal stem cells (19), and bone marrow–derived cells can differentiate into glial cells in the brain (20).

Neuronal stem cells can differentiate into glial or neuronal phenotypes in culture and also in both neurogenic and nonneurogenic sites of adult rat brain after transplantation (15,21). Human progenitor cells that are transplanted into neurogenic regions of rodent brain such as the subventricular zone and hippocampus migrate specifically along the routes normally taken by the endogenous neuronal precursors in rodent brain (18). They seem to respond to local cues to differentiate into site-specific neuronal phenotypes. When they are transplanted within nonneurogenic areas such as the striatum, they migrate in an apparently nondirected manner and differentiate into both neuronal and glial phenotypes.

Understanding proper differentiation signals for the desired neuronal phenotypes would ultimately provide a means of generating unlimited supply of transplant donor cells. For example, Nurr1 is a critical transcriptional factor in the development of dopaminergic neurons (22,23). It induces expression of the first and rate-limiting step of dopamine synthesis, tyrosine hydroxylase (TH) in neuronal precursor cells (24). Therefore, Nurr1 was introduced into neuronal stem cells in an attempt to generate dopaminergic neurons (24–26). Nurr1 alone, however, was insufficient to induce full-fledged dopaminergic phenotypic expression. This finding indicates that other differentiation signals are necessary for transcription of additional molecules involved in dopamine synthesis and processing. Although the understanding of such transcriptional signals is limited at this point, partially differentiated neuronal stem cells could be further modified by additional genes to achieve desired phenotypes, as outlined later in this chapter.

In Vivo or Direct Gene Transfer

Host CNS cells may be better equipped to produce the desired products from the genetic information than foreign donor cells because they may possess the machinery necessary for the posttranslational modification of the gene products, the appropriate cofactors, and the ability to secrete the neurotransmitters or other neuroactive compounds. Viral solutions may also be less intrusive than grafts to normal brain physiology because grafts of genetically engineered cells could disrupt the normal architecture. Moreover, grafting genetically modified cells is more suitable for delivery of secretable products that act on cell-surface receptors such as neurotransmitters and neurotrophic factors, but not for delivery of intracellular proteins such as protein kinases, receptors, and transporters. Conversely, the consequence of delivering therapeutic molecules (e.g., dopamine) directly into host cells (e.g., striatal neurons) that do not normally express

such molecules is not as predictable as delivering them extracellularly by grafts serving as a biologic minipump. Expression of the gene product could lead to untoward alteration of the host cell function. The major disadvantages of *in vivo* gene transfer also include the safety of using viruses directly. The use of neurotrophic viruses such as herpesvirus, adenovirus, adenoassociated virus (AAV), and lentivirus has been shown to be effective in gene transfer into neurons.

Vector Constructs

Although many viruses have been explored as vector systems, the following virus vectors have been most extensively applied to CNS gene transfer. Each has its own advantages and disadvantages, and there does not seem to be a clear universal vector system of choice at this point. A simplified general scheme of virus vectors is described in Fig. 19.2.

Neurotrophic Virus Vectors for In Vivo Gene Therapy

Herpes simplex type 1 virus (HSV-1) vectors infect a wide range of host cells including postmitotic neurons, and they can establish latency indefinitely within the neuron. Two general approaches include (a) use of recombinant HSV with various deletions that render the virus replication-defective (27,28) and (b) use of an amplicon based on plasmid vectors containing the transgene plus minimal HSV genes such as origin of DNA replication and packaging site. Because of the large size of HSV, development of safe vectors will require extensive understanding of the genome to be able to reduce neurovirulence and cytotoxicity (29,30). Conversely, the large size of the HSV viral genome (152 kb pairs) also allows insertion of a large foreign DNA, which may prove very useful for certain types of *in vivo* CNS gene therapy.

Adenovirus represents an attractive candidate for direct gene transfer into the CNS because of its high-titer virus stocks, efficient infection of postmitotic cells, and the relatively benign nature of the viral infection (31). Adenovirus is a double-stranded, linear DNA virus that, in its wild-type form, causes a variety of mild, flulike ailments. The potential for adenovirus vectors to achieve efficient gene transfer to neurons, microglial cells, and astrocytes *in vivo* has been noted (32,33). Host immune reactions to the viral protein remain the major risk of the adenovirus vector and are also partly responsible for the limited duration of transgene expression (34). Better long-term expression has been noted in neonatal or immunocompromised animals (35). Recent constructs of adenovirus vectors that delete all viral genes show high levels of stable expression with minimal toxicity and allow inserts of up to 37 kb (36).

AAV is a nonpathogenic DNA virus, which requires helper viruses such as adenovirus and herpesvirus for productive infection. AAV vectors have minimal viral sequences

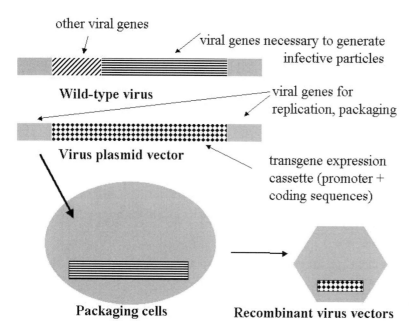

other viral genes

viral genes necessary to generate infective particles

Wild-type virus

viral genes for replication, packaging

Virus plasmid vector

transgene expression cassette (promoter + coding sequences)

Packaging cells

Recombinant virus vectors

FIGURE 19.2. An idealized scheme for general virus vectors. Wild-type viruses are engineered to produce virus plasmid vector, which has minimal viral genes necessary for packaging the vector into the virus particles. Other viral genes are deleted to reduce the deleterious effect and to make room for insertion of therapeutic genes. Viral components necessary to generate infective particles are introduced into the packaging cells separate from the virus plasmid vector. Packaging cells then produce infective virus particles containing the therapeutic transgene, but minimal or no virus genes.

of their own and therefore have minimal deleterious consequences. Because of the small genome, AAV can accommodate only about 5-kb inserts. AAV integrates into a specific site in the chromosome 19q13.3 (37), and long-term expression of various neural genes has been noted in the CNS with minimal host reactions (38–41). Despite its limited capacity for transgenes, AAV is the safest vector capable of long-term *in vivo* expression at this point.

Retrovirus Vectors for Ex Vivo Therapy

Disabled *murine leukemia retroviruses* have been most widely used for gene therapy, especially for most *ex vivo* applications. Retroviruses infect a broad range of cells with high efficiency. Many generations of modified vectors have been developed to lower the chance of a recombination event that can lead to wild-type virus generation (42). The integration of provirus into the chromosome is stable and precise, but the location is apparently random, and therefore it could produce an insertional mutation by disrupting a normal gene. Homologous recombination of the retroviral vectors with the retroviral genome in the packaging cells could generate the wild-type virus, which could lead to the formation of tumors (43). However, current generation of packaging cells has minimal overlap of sequences with helper viruses, and the helper virus genes are separated into two separate plasmids to minimize the possibility of recombination further (44). Disadvantages of retroviral vectors include relatively low viral titers, usually less than 10^6 infectious units per milliliter. The size of the gene that can be inserted is limited to 8 to 10 kb. Retroviruses also require dividing cells with active replication and DNA synthesis for the provirus integration to occur (45). Therefore, retroviruses are not useful for *in vivo* gene trans-

fer into nondividing cells, but they remain the mainstay of *ex vivo* therapies.

Hybrid Vectors

Hybrid vectors combine advantageous properties of different virus vectors (46). A good example of hybrid vectors is lentiviral vector, which combines the ability of the *human immunodeficiency virus* (HIV-1) to insert a provirus copy into the genome of nondividing cells with wide host range and high infectivity of stomatitis virus G surface glycoprotein. Unlike other retroviruses, lentiviruses can infect nondividing cells by using nuclear import machinery to gain entry into the nucleus in quiescent cells and then integrating viral DNA into the host chromosome. Stable transgene expression in neurons was noted *in vivo* for up to 3 months without appreciable pathologic changes and host immune response (47). Because HIV prevents cells from undergoing mitosis, development of packaging cell lines that can facilitate vector generation has been hampered. Further safety of the vectors must be ensured before clinical use of these HIV-based vectors can be contemplated. Another example of hybrid viruses is the HSV/AAV vector. The AAV rep gene and inverted terminal repeats of AAV are incorporated into HSV amplicon vectors to enable amplification and specific integration of desired gene into chromosome (48). These new-generation hybrid vectors may provide ideal tools that circumvent the safety issues and achieve long-term expression of the transgenes.

Further Development of Gene Therapy Vectors

Before these gene therapy methods can be applied to human neurodegenerative disorders, several issues need to be resolved. Safety issues of gene therapy vectors are discussed earlier, and much progress has been made in this regard. Another safety issue concerns the transgene itself. Expression of the transgenes and secretion of the transgene products into the serum can lead to immune responses to the transgene products. However, it is not clear whether the immune system can recognize the transgene products that are expressed intracellularly but are not secreted. Another problem of gene therapy has been the inability to obtain long-term stable transgene expression *in vivo* (49). Long-term expression is easily achieved in cultures throughout many passages of donor cells. Once the cells are implanted in animals, however, transgene expression diminishes rapidly (49). Although this remains an unresolved problem, several possibilities appear promising. Vectors that lead to integration of the transgenes into the chromosomes are more likely to be stable than vectors that stay episomal. In addition, integration sites used by the vectors play a significant role in the transcriptional activity of the transgene. Retroviruses integrate into the chromosome during active division, but the integration site may become dormant in the quiescent state that grafted cells assume *in vivo*. Taking advantage of the ability of lentivirus to enter into the nucleus of nondividing neurons, and to integrate into sites that are active during quiescence, investigators have been able to achieve long-term expression of transgenes in neurons of the CNS (47). AAV also integrates into the genome of host neurons and has shown promise in its ability to sustain long-term gene expression *in vivo* (38–40).

Promoter types may also significantly influence long-term expression. Most gene therapy vectors contain viral promoters to express the transgenes, but their transcriptional activity may be suppressed in the somatic cells. Promoters of endogenous cellular genes such as constitutive housekeeping gene promoters (50), or cell type–specific promoters (51), have had some initial success. However, most tissue-specific promoters have a low basal activity. A more recent approach has shown enhanced transcriptional activity from synthetic promoters engineered from a combination of operator elements (52). The effect of the promoter may depend on the cell type and the vectors used (53,54).

Although the current focus is on achievement of high and stable expression of transgenes, excessive levels of products could result in adverse side effects. Optimal levels are critical for physiologic function of many substances, and the ability to regulate the transgene expression is important. Promoters that can be regulated externally or have a built-in feedback mechanism will be an important advance for the future. One such system was developed to express the transgene by promoters whose activities can be either turned on or off by administration of tetracycline both *in vitro* (10) and *in vivo* (55). Other combinations of nontoxic substances and heterologous transcription factors that bind to regulable promoters have been developed (56,57).

STRATEGIES OF GENE THERAPY FOR PARKINSON'S DISEASE

Dopamine Replacement by Delivering Neurotransmitter Synthesizing Genes

The pathogenesis of PD is well understood, and the efficacy of replacing the neurotransmitter dopamine is well established. However, long-term treatment with the precursor, L-3,4-dihydroxyphenylalanine (L-DOPA) produces dyskinesia and fluctuations in most patients. These problems can be either prevented or reduced by continuous delivery of dopamine into striatum (58). Various dopamine-producing cells including dopaminergic fetal neurons can also provide continuous and site-specific dopamine delivery (59). However, given the limitations in obtaining proper fetal tissues in sufficient amounts, alternative sources of donor cells such as xenografts and genetically engineered cells have been proposed. To provide L-DOPA in the brain by gene therapy, initial studies have focused on introducing the TH gene, which is the first and rate-limiting step of dopamine synthesis, by using established cell lines such as rat fibroblast 208F cells (60), NIH3T3 cells, and endocrine cell lines, AtT-20 and RIN cells (61). Subsequently, to overcome the problems with the tumor cell lines, primary cells such as fibroblast cells (62), or astrocytes (8) have been shown to produce long-term graft survival without tumor formation or immunologic rejection. More recently, neuronal precursor cells have been genetically modified to express dopaminergic phenotype, but their efficacy in *in vivo* models is not clear yet. In addition, direct *in vivo* TH gene transfer into the brain cells using viral vectors has also been attempted (63,64). Most of these studies have shown partial reversal of apomorphine-induced rotation, which is used as a rodent behavioral model of PD.

Further refinement of the L-DOPA delivery has been achieved by using the gene guanosine triphosphate cyclohydrolase I (GCH1), which is the first and rate-limiting step in the biosynthesis of tetrahydrobiopterin, an essential cofactor for TH. Experimental gene therapy studies have shown that double transduction with TH and GCH1, by either *ex vivo* (65) or *in vivo* (40) gene transfer, is necessary for sufficient L-DOPA and dopamine production in rat models of PD (Fig. 19.3A). Microdialysis studies have shown direct biochemical evidence for the efficacy. These studies have also pointed out the limitations of the rotational behavioral model, which have contributed to misleading conclusions of previous studies about the efficacy of using TH gene alone. The importance of GCH1 has been underlined by the finding that mutations in GCH1 in patients with L-DOPA–responsive dystonia (DRD) lead to loss of its function to generate cofactor, tetrahydrobiopterin (BH$_4$) (66). The absence of cofactor results in the lack of L-DOPA and dopamine production and, consequently, parkinsonism and dystonia. The symptoms of DRD patients can be almost completely ameliorated by L-DOPA therapy without development of the long-term complications that are commonly observed in

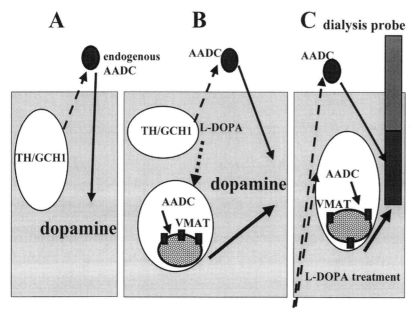

FIGURE 19.3. Dopamine replacement strategy for Parkinson's disease by gene transfer. **(A):** Cells expressing tyrosine hydroxylase (TH) and guanosine triphosphate cyclohydrolase 1 (GCH1) are grafted into the striatum. The L-DOPA produced by these cells *(dotted line)* is converted by endogenous aromatic L-amino acid decarboxylase (AADC) to dopamine *(solid line).* **(B):** Cells expressing AADC and vesicular monoamine transporter (VMAT) could be cografted with L-DOPA–producing cells to provide additional source of decarboxylation and storage of dopamine. **(C):** An alternative strategy combines the use of AADC/VMAT cells with exogenous administration of L-DOPA. These cells increase the efficacy of L-DOPA by providing additional decarboxylation and increased storage and sustained release of dopamine.

PD. Such an ideal response to L-DOPA in DRD abrogates any need for gene therapy, but it provides us with an insight into the importance of events that occur downstream from production of L-DOPA in the therapy of PD.

The second step in dopamine synthesis is decarboxylation of L-DOPA to dopamine by aromatic L-amino acid decarboxylase (AADC). Although there seems to be some decarboxylation of L-DOPA to dopamine even with severe dopaminergic neuronal loss in animal models and patients with PD (67,68), the exact source and sites of AADC *in vivo* are not clear (69). When additional AADC was provided within the genetically modified grafts producing L-DOPA, the final levels of L-DOPA and dopamine decreased, presumably because of the feedback inhibition of dopamine on TH (70). Therefore, keeping the cytoplasmic dopamine levels low by sequestering it into the vesicles at high concentrations seems to be a critical strategy of dopamine delivery (71). The combination of L-DOPA–producing cells with cells that can decarboxylate L-DOPA to dopamine and their storage in vesicles may be more optimal, but this has not yet been tested directly (Fig. 19.3B).

In the strategies of providing a source of L-DOPA or dopamine as described earlier, the precise control of the exact amount of L-DOPA or dopamine given by gene therapy will be critical and may be difficult to achieve. Excessive dopamine will be detrimental to patients. One could attempt to control the precise levels by using the regulable promoters described earlier. We proposed another approach of combining the precursor L-DOPA administration with genetic machinery to process L-DOPA more efficiently (72). Providing additional AADC in the denervated striatum of rat models of PD resulted in higher levels of dopamine produced from L-DOPA (41). However, increasing the level of dopamine is not as critical as prolonging the duration of ele-

vation and buffering the fluctuating levels of dopamine after the administration of L-DOPA. Combined use of AADC for decarboxylation of L-DOPA and vesicular monoamine transporter for efficient storage of dopamine within cells sustained high levels of dopamine from L-DOPA administration compared with using only AADC (71) (Fig. 19.3C). This finding underlines the importance of storage and gradual release of dopamine in the pathogenesis and treatment of fluctuating responses in PD.

Although site-specific and sustained delivery of dopamine would provide a major advance in PD therapy, it is not clear whether this approach will be sufficient to restore the entire symptom complex of PD including some of the L-DOPA-associated complications such as dyskinesia. The role of nondopaminergic systems in PD needs to be explored further. In addition, restoration of neuronal connectivity and complex functions such as feedback interaction of dopaminergic neurons with striatal neurons may be important. However, it is not clear whether such proper interactions could be restored even with fetal dopaminergic neurons or dopaminergic neuronal cell lines generated by *ex vivo* gene therapy.

Repair and Protection Strategy by Neurotrophic Factor Delivery

The peptidergic growth factors have wide-ranging effects on the survival of neuronal populations as well as on regulation of neurotransmitter release and modulation of neural activities in the adult CNS. Although the precise mechanism of the neuronal degeneration of PD is not known, *neurotrophic factors or growth factors* may prevent or may slow the cell death cascade regardless of the initial triggering event. Several growth factors that have shown to possess trophic activity in the dopaminergic system include brain-derived neurotrophic factor (BDNF), neurotrophin-3 (NT-3), NT-4/5, bFGF, transforming growth factor-β, and glial cell line–derived factor (GDNF) (73–78). All these factors have been shown to enhance dopamine neuronal cell viability *in vitro,* although this in some cases appears to be mediated by indirect effects on other cell types (77,79). *In vivo* effects have been mostly noted by neurotrophin and GDNF family members. *In vivo* delivery of BDNF enhances striatal dopamine turnover and decreases nigral dopamine turnover, and it also causes contralateral rotations and locomotor activity in amphetamine-treated rats (80, 81). Direct infusion of BDNF above the substantia nigra (SN) increases the firing rate and even the number of electrically active dopamine neurons in this pivotal brain region (82). The presence and expression of BDNF and its receptor, TrkB, in the adult SN indicates that BDNF may regulate dopamine function under normal physiologic conditions (74,83,84). As in the developing CNS, striatal BDNF is transported in retrograde fashion to dopamine neurons in adult brain (85). Infusion of NT-4/5 into the ventral mesencephalon also causes increased striatal dopamine turnover and release and locomotor activation after amphetamine stimulation (86). The NT-3 molecule also enhances amphetamine-induced contralateral turning and decreases SN dopamine turnover (81). One of the most potent factors for SN dopamine is GDNF. In normal animals, GDNF increases both spontaneous and amphetamine-induced motor behavior. These motor effects occur in parallel with increased dopamine levels and turnover in the SN and enhanced dopamine turnover and consequent reduction in striatal dopamine levels (87). Infusion of GDNF into the striatum results in retrograde transport to the SN dopamine neurons (88).

These results support the concept that even in the adult brain, developmentally dependent growth factors may be able to augment dopamine neuronal function. The problem with pharmacologic delivery of the peptidergic growth factors is access to the brain. The nonoral delivery methods of these substances frequently require methods that circumvent the blood-brain barrier, for instance by neurosurgical intraparenchymal or intraventricular infusions. These methods are site-specific but invasive and often unpredictable. Moreover, effective delivery is limited by diffusion properties of the factor within the brain (89). Intraventricular administration of the TrkB ligand BDNF is ineffective because of binding by truncated TrkB receptors that are present in the ependymal lining of the ventricles.

As an alternative to direct infusion, methods for cell-mediated delivery of therapeutic proteins have been developed including *ex vivo* as well as *in vivo* gene transfer. Implants of BDNF-producing fibroblast cells protected against neurotoxins such as 6-hydroxydopamine (6-OHDA) (90) and 1-methyl-4-phenylpyridinium (91). In addition, sprouting of dopaminergic fiber has been demonstrated in BDNF-transduced fibroblasts implanted into the midbrain (92).

GDNF has been delivered into rat SN neurons by adenovirus or AAV vectors, and it has protected these neurons from progressive degeneration induced by 6-OHDA lesion of the dopaminergic terminals in the striatum (33,93). A more practical approach of injecting the viruses into the striatum resulted in cellular and behavioral protection from striatal 6-OHDA lesions (94,95).

Other Potential Targets of Gene Therapy for Parkinson's Disease: Intervention of Pathogenesis

Understanding the origin and pathogenesis of PD may allow us to intervene directly at the level of pathogenesis and may forestall the clinical manifestations or stop progression of the disease. Although the origin of PD is still not known in most cases, recent discoveries of mutations in α-synuclein in families with autosomal dominant inheritance of PD (1,2) and *parkin* in families with autosomal recessive juvenile parkinsonism (3) may provide us new clues. Knowledge of the precise steps by which these mutations lead to dopaminergic neuronal death could allow us to apply these findings to sporadic forms of PD as well.

Although the precise strategy awaits further understanding of the mechanism of toxicity by genetic mutations, general therapeutic approaches for a known genetic defect can be outlined. For autosomal recessive genetic disorders, which commonly confer a "loss of function," augmentation of the missing genetic information may restore the abnormalities. Conversely, a dominant disorder may involve a "gain of function" induced by the mutant protein. For these disorders, it is not possible simply to replace the defective gene with a normal one. Techniques for specifically targeting the abnormal sequence and replacing it with a normal sequence exist and are applied in generation of transgenic animals with "knockout, knock-in" strategy (96). However, these techniques are not easily applicable to humans. The intervention of gene expression at the level of messenger RNA could be attempted. It may be possible to integrate viral or nonviral vectors carrying catalytic antisense RNAs or ribozymes that bind to, and irreversibly cleave, abnormal mRNAs (97). Antisense RNA has been used to hamper transcription, processing, transport, or translation of mRNAs in a variety of cell types.

Intervention further downstream of the abnormal protein expression will be possible once the normal physiology of the mutant protein is known. Pharmacologic blockade of the effects of the mutated protein may be envisaged by introducing genes that will produce inhibitory substances. In addition, even when the exact function of the mutant protein is unknown, understanding the general process of dopaminergic cell death could lead to other approaches in preventing disease progression. For example, the genes preventing apoptosis could be expressed in dopaminergic neurons to save them from their demise (98). Given the possible role of oxidative stress in dopaminergic neuronal degeneration in

PD, overexpression of a free radical scavenging enzyme, such as superoxide dismutase (SOD), may protect dopaminergic neurons from degeneration. Experimental models show that SOD overexpression protects dopaminergic neurons from neurotoxicity (99). In addition, SOD enhances the survival of the grafted neurons (100).

CONCLUSIONS

In summary, gene therapy has the potential to provide efficient delivery of various genes and products into a localized site. Along with new genetic discoveries and advances in understanding of the pathogenesis of PD, this approach may provide the most efficient means of therapeutic intervention at appropriate levels. In addition, gene therapy experiments contribute to further understanding of the biology of the diseases. Gene therapy is an evolving concept that could correlate the new molecular understanding of the diseases with current modalities of PD therapy.

REFERENCES

1. Polymeropoulos MH, Lavedan C, Leroy E, et al. Mutation in the α-synuclein gene identified in families with Parkinson's disease. *Science* 1997;276:2045–2047.
2. Leroy E, Boyer R, Auburger G, et al. The ubiquitin pathway in Parkinson's disease [Letter]. *Nature* 1998;395:451–452.
3. Kitada T, Asakawa S, Hattori N, et al. Mutations in the parkin gene cause autosomal recessive juvenile parkinsonism. *Nature* 1998;392:605–608.
4. Friedmann T. The road toward human gene therapy: a 25-year perspective. *Ann Med* 1997;29:575–577.
5. Hermens WTJM, Verhaagen J. Viral vectors, tools for gene transfer in the nervous system. *Prog Neurobiol* 1998;55:399–432.
6. Kang UJ. Potential of gene therapy for Parkinson's disease: neurobiologic issues. *Mov Disord* 1998;13[Suppl 1]:59–72.
7. Gage FH. Intracerebral grafting of genetically modified cells acting as biological pumps. *Trends Pharmacol Sci* 1990;11:437–439.
8. Lundberg C, Horellou P, Mallet J, et al. Generation of DOPA-producing astrocytes by retroviral transduction of the human tyrosine hydroxylase gene: *in vitro* characterization and *in vivo* effects in the rat Parkinson model. *Exp Neurol* 1996;139:39–53.
9. Renfranz PJ, Cunningham MG, McKay DG. Region-specific differentiation of the hippocampal stem cell line HiB5 upon implantation into the developing mammalian brain. *Cell* 1991; 66:713–729.
10. Hoshimaru M, Ray J, Sah DWY, et al. Differentiation of the immortalized adult neuronal progenitor cell line HC2S2 into neurons by regulatable suppression of the v-myc oncogene. *Proc Natl Acad Sci USA* 1996;93:1518–1523.
11. Svendsen CN, Smith AG. New prospects for human stem-cell therapy in the nervous system. *Trends Neurosci* 1999;22:357–364.
12. Scheffler B, Horn M, Blumcke I, et al. Marrow-mindedness: a perspective on neuropoiesis. *Trends Neurosci* 1999;22:348–357.
13. Reynolds BA, Weiss S. Generation of neurons and astrocytes from isolated cells of the adult mammalian central nervous system. *Science* 1992;255:1707–1710.
14. Tropepe V, Sibilia M, Ciruna BG, et al. Distinct neural stem cells proliferate in response to EGF and FGF in the developing mouse telencephalon. *Dev Biol* 1999;208:166–188.
15. Gage FH, Coates PW, Palmer TD, et al. Survival and differentiation of adult neuronal progenitor cells transplanted to the adult brain. *Proc Natl Acad Sci USA* 1995;92:11879–11883.
16. Eriksson PS, Perfilieva E, Bjork-Eriksson T, et al. Neurogenesis in the adult human hippocampus. *Nat Med* 1998;4:1313–1317.
17. Flax JD, Aurora S, Yang C, et al. Engraftable human neural stem cells respond to developmental cues, replace neurons, and express foreign genes. *Nat Biotechnol* 1998;16:1033–1039.
18. Fricker RA, Carpenter MK, Winkler C, et al. Site-specific migration and neuronal differentiation of human neural progenitor cells after transplantation in the adult rat brain. *J Neurosci* 1999;19:5990–6005.
19. Bjornson CR, Rietze RL, Reynolds BA, et al. Turning brain into blood: a hematopoietic fate adopted by adult neural stem cells *in vivo*. *Science* 1999;283:534–537.
20. Eglitis MA, Mezey E. Hematopoietic cells differentiate into both microglia and macroglia in the brains of adult mice. *Proc Natl Acad Sci USA* 1997;94:4080–4085.
21. Winkler C, Fricker RA, Gates MA, et al. Incorporation and glial differentiation of mouse EGF-responsive neural progenitor cells after transplantation into the embryonic rat brain. *Mol Cell Neurosci* 1998;11:99–116.
22. Zetterstrom RH, Solomin L, Jansson L, et al. Dopamine neuron agenesis in Nurr1-deficient mice. *Science* 1997;276:248–250.
23. Saucedo-Cardenas O, Quintana-Hau JD, Le WD, et al. Nurr1 is essential for the induction of the dopaminergic phenotype and the survival of ventral mesencephalic late dopaminergic precursor neurons. *Proc Natl Acad Sci USA* 1998;95:4013–4018.
24. Wagner J, Akerud P, Castro DS, et al. Induction of a midbrain dopaminergic phenotype in Nurr1-overexpressing neural stem cells by type 1 astrocytes. *Nat Biotechnol* 1999;17:653–659.
25. Sakurada K, Ohshima-Sakurada M, Palmer TD, et al. Nurr1, an orphan nuclear receptor, is a transcriptional activator of endogenous tyrosine hydroxylase in neural progenitor cells derived from the adult brain. *Development* 1999;126:4017–4026.
26. Daadi MM, Weiss S. Generation of tyrosine hydroxylase-producing neurons from precursors of the embryonic and adult forebrain. *J Neurosci* 1999;19:4484–4497.
27. Dobson AT, Margolis TP, Sedarati F, et al. A latent, nonpathogenic HSV-1–derived vector stably expresses β-galactosidase in mouse neurons. *Neuron* 1990;5:353–360.
28. Johnson PA, Yoshida K, Gage FH, et al. Effects of gene transfer into cultured CNS neurons with a replication-defective herpes simplex virus type 1 vector. *Mol Brain Res* 1992;12:95–102.
29. Johnson PA, Miyanohara A, Levine F, et al. Cytotoxicity of a replication-defective mutant of herpes simplex virus type 1. *J Virol* 1992;66:2952–2965.
30. Kennedy PG. Potential use of herpes simplex virus (HSV) vectors for gene therapy of neurological disorders. *Brain* 1997;120:1245–1259.
31. Neve RL. Adenovirus vectors enter the brain. *Trends Neurosci* 1993;16:251–253.
32. Davidson BL, Allen ED, Kozarsky KF, et al. A model system for *in vivo* gene transfer into the central nervous system using an adenoviral vector. *Nat Genet* 1993;3:219–223.
33. Choi-Lundberg DL, Lin Q, Chang YN, et al. Dopaminergic neurons protected from degeneration by GDNF gene therapy. *Science* 1997;275:838–841.
34. Byrnes AP, MacLaren RE, Charlton HM. Immunological instability of persistent adenovirus vectors in the brain: peripheral exposure to vector leads to renewed inflammation, reduced gene expression, and demyelination. *J Neurosci* 1996;16:3045–3055.

35. Tripathy SK, Goldwasser E, Lu MM, et al. Stable delivery of physiologic levels of recombinant erythropoietin to the systemic circulation by intramuscular injection of replication-defective adenovirus. *Proc Natl Acad Sci USA* 1994;91:11557–11561.

36. Burcin MM, Schiedner G, Kochanek S, et al. Adenovirus-mediated regulable target gene expression *in vivo*. *Proc Natl Acad Sci USA* 1999;96:355–360.

37. Samulski RJ, Zhu X, Xiao X, et al. Targeted integration of adeno-associated virus (AAV) into human chromosome 19 [published erratum appears in *EMBO J* 1992;11:1228]. *EMBO J* 1991;10:3941–3950.

38. McCown TJ, Xiao X, Li J, et al. Differential and persistent expression patterns of CNS gene transfer by an adeno-associated virus (AAV) vector. *Brain Res* 1996;713:99–107.

39. Samulski RJ, During MJ, Kaplitt MG, et al. Adeno-associated virus vectors yield long-term expression and delivery of potentially therapeutic genes into non-dividing neuronal cells. *J Neurovirol* 1997;3[Suppl 1]:S72–S72.

40. Mandel RJ, Rendahl SK, Spratt SK, et al. Characterization of intrastriatal recombinant adeno-associated virus–mediated gene transfer of human tyrosine hydroxylase and human GTP-cyclohydrolase 1 in a rat model of Parkinson's disease. *J Neurosci* 1998;18:4271–4284.

41. Leff SE, Spratt SK, Snyder RO, et al. Long-term restoration of striatal L-aromatic amino acid decarboxylase activity using recombinant adeno-associated viral vector gene transfer in a rodent model of Parkinson's disease. *Neuroscience* 1999;92:185–196.

42. Miller AD, Miller DG, Garcia JV, et al. Use of retroviral vectors for gene transfer and expression. *Methods Enzymol* 1993;217:581–599.

43. Kolberg R. Gene-transfer virus contaminant linked to monkeys' cancer. *J NIH Res* 1992;4:43–44.

44. Miller AD, Rosman GJ. Improved retroviral vectors for gene transfer and expression. *Biotechniques* 1989;7:980–989.

45. Miller DG, Adam MA, Miller AD. Gene transfer by retrovirus vectors occurs only in cells that are actively replicating at the time of infection. *Mol Cell Biol* 1990;10:4239–4242.

46. Jacoby DR, Fraefel C, Breakefield XO. Hybrid vectors: a new generation of virus-based vectors designed to control the cellular fate of delivered genes [Editorial]. *Gene Ther* 1997;4:1281–1283.

47. Naldini L, Blomer U, Gallay P, et al. *In vivo* gene delivery and stable transduction of nondividing cells by a lentiviral vector. *Science* 1996;272:263–267.

48. Johnston KM, Jacoby D, Pechan PA, et al. HSV/AAV hybrid amplicon vectors extend transgene expression in human glioma cells. *Hum Gene Ther* 1997;8:359–370.

49. Palmer TD, Rosman GJ, Osborne WRA, et al. Genetically modified skin fibroblasts persist long after transplantation but gradually inactivate introduced genes. *Proc Natl Acad Sci USA* 1991;88:1330–1334.

50. Scharfmann R, Axelrod JH, Verma IM. Long-term *in vivo* expression of retrovirus-mediated gene transfer in mouse fibroblast implants. *Proc Natl Acad Sci USA* 1991;88:4626–4630.

51. Dai Y, Roman M, Naviaux RK, et al. Gene therapy via primary myoblasts: long-term expression of factor IX protein following transplantation *in vivo*. *Proc Natl Acad Sci USA* 1992;89:10892–10895.

52. Li X, Eastman EM, Schwartz RJ, et al. Synthetic muscle promoters: activities exceeding naturally occurring regulatory sequences. *Nat Biotechnol* 1999;17:241–245.

53. Roemer K, Johnson PA, Friedmann T. Activity of the simian virus 40 early promoter-enhancer in herpes simplex virus type 1 vectors is dependent on its position, the infected cell type, and the presence of Vmw175. *J Virol* 1991;65:6900–6912.

54. Blomer U, Naldini L, Verma IM, et al. Applications of gene therapy to the CNS. *Hum Mol Genet* 1996;5:1397–1404.

55. Dhawan J, Rando TA, Elson SL, et al. Tetracycline-regulated gene expression following direct gene transfer into mouse skeletal muscle. *Somat Cell Mol Genet* 1995;21:233–240.

56. Suhr ST, Gil EB, Senut MC, et al. High level transactivation by a modified Bombyx ecdysone receptor in. *Proc Natl Acad Sci USA* 1998;95:7999–8004.

57. Ye X, Rivera VM, Zoltick P, et al. Regulated delivery of therapeutic proteins after *in vivo* somatic cell gene transfer. *Science* 1999;283:88–91.

58. Mouradian MM, Heuser IJ, Baronti F, et al. Modification of central dopaminergic mechanisms by continuous levodopa therapy for advanced Parkinson's disease. *Ann Neurol* 1990;27:18–23.

59. Olanow CW, Kordower JH, Freeman TB. Fetal nigral transplantation as a therapy for Parkinson's disease. *Trends Neurosci* 1996;19:102–109.

60. Wolff JA, Fisher LJ, Jinnah HA, et al. Grafting fibroblasts genetically modified to produce L-dopa in a rat model of Parkinson disease. *Proc Natl Acad Sci USA* 1989;86:9011–9014.

61. Horellou P, Brundin P, Kalen P, et al. *In vivo* release of DOPA and dopamine from genetically engineered cells grafted to the denervated rat striatum. *Neuron* 1990;5:393–402.

62. Fisher LJ, Jinnah HA, Kale LC, et al. Survival and function of intrastriatally grafted primary fibroblasts genetically modified to produce L-DOPA. *Neuron* 1991;6:371–380.

63. During MJ, Naegele JR, O'Malley KL, et al. Long-term behavioral recovery in parkinsonian rats by an HSV vector expressing tyrosine hydroxylase. *Science* 1994;266:1399–1403.

64. Kaplitt MG, Leone P, Samulski RJ, et al. Long-term gene expression and phenotypic correction using adeno-associated virus vectors in the mammalian brain. *Nat Genet* 1994;8:148–54.

65. Bencsics C, Wachtel SR, Milstien S, et al. Double transduction with GTP cyclohydrolase I and tyrosine hydroxylase is necessary for spontaneous synthesis of L-DOPA by primary fibroblasts. *J Neurosci* 1996;16:4449–4456.

66. Ichinose H, Ohye T, Takahashi E, et al. Hereditary progressive dystonia with marked diurnal fluctuation caused by mutations in the GTP cyclohydrolase 1 gene. *Nat Genet* 1994;8:236–242.

67. Abercrombie ED, Bonatz AE, Zigmond MJ. Effects of L-DOPA on extracellular dopamine in striatum of normal and 6-hydroxydopamine-treated rats. *Brain Res* 1990;525:36–44.

68. Zhu MY, Juorio AV. Aromatic L-amino acid decarboxylase: biological characterization and functional role. *Gen Pharmacol* 1995;26:681–696.

69. Melamed E, Hefti F, Pettibone DJ, et al. Aromatic L-amino acid decarboxylase in rat corpus striatum: implications for action of L-DOPA in parkinsonism. *Neurology* 1981;31:651–655.

70. Wachtel SR, Bencsics C, Kang UJ. The role of aromatic L-amino acid decarboxylase for dopamine replacement by genetically modified fibroblasts in a rat model of Parkinson's disease. *J Neurochem* 1997;69:2055–2063.

71. Lee WY, Chang JW, Nemeth NL, et al. Vesicular monoamine transporter-2 and aromatic L-amino acid decarboxylase enhance dopamine delivery after L-3,4-dihydroxyphenylalanine administration in Parkinsonian rats. *J Neurosci* 1999;19:3266–3274.

72. Kang UJ, Fisher LJ, Joh TH, et al. Regulation of dopamine production by genetically modified primary fibroblasts. *J Neurosci* 1993;13:5203–5211.

73. Hyman C, Hofer M, Barde YA, et al. BDNF is a neurotrophic factor for dopaminergic neurons of the substantia nigra. *Nature* 1991;350:230–232.

74. Hyman C, Juhasz M, Jackson C, et al. Overlapping and distinct actions of the neurotrophins BDNF, NT-3, and NT-4/5 on

cultured dopaminergic and GABAergic neurons of the ventral mesencephalon. *J Neurosci* 1994;14:335–347.

75. Hynes MA, Poulsen K, Armanini M, et al. Neurotrophin-4/5 is a survival factor for embryonic midbrain dopaminergic neurons in enriched cultures. *J Neurosci Res* 1994;37:144–154.

76. Lin LFH, Doherty DH, Lile JD, et al. GDNF: a glial cell line–derived neurotrophic factor for midbrain dopaminergic neurons. *Science* 1993;260:1130–1132.

77. Knusel B, Michel PP, Schwaber JS, et al. Selective and nonselective stimulation of central cholinergic and dopaminergic development *in vitro* by nerve growth factor, basic fibroblast growth factor, epidermal growth factor, insulin and the insulin-like growth factors I and II. *J Neurosci* 1990;10:558–570.

78. Poulsen KT, Armanini MP, Klein RD, et al. TGFb2 and TGFb3 are potent survival factors for midbrain dopaminergic neurons. *Neuron* 1994;13:1245–1252.

79. Engele J, Bohn MC. The neurotrophic effects of fibroblast growth factors on dopaminergic neurons *in vitro* are mediated by mesencephalic glia. *J Neurosci* 1991;11:3070–3078.

80. Altar CA, Boylan CB, Jackson C, et al. Brain-derived neurotrophic factor augments rotational behavior and nigrostriatal dopamine turnover *in vivo*. *Proc Natl Acad Sci USA* 1992;89:11347–11351.

81. Martin-Iverson MT, Todd KG, Altar CA. Brain-derived neurotrophic factor and neurotrophin-3 activate striatal dopamine and serotonin metabolism and related behaviors: Interactions with amphetamine. *J Neurosci* 1994;14:1262–1270.

82. Shen RY, Altar CA, Chiodo LA. Brain-derived neurotrophic factor increases the electrical activity of pars compacta dopamine neurons *in vivo*. *Proc Natl Acad Sci USA* 1994;91:8920–8924.

83. Gall CM, Gold SJ, Isackson PJ, et al. Brain-derived neurotrophic factor and neurotrophin-3 messenger RNAs are expressed in ventral midbrain regions containing dopaminergic neurons. *Mol Cell Neurosci* 1992;3:56–63.

84. Seroogy KB, Lundgren KH, Tran TM, et al. Dopaminergic neurons in rat ventral midbrain express brain-derived neurotrophic factor and neurotrophin-3 mRNAs. *J Comp Neurol* 1994;342:321–334.

85. Mufson EJ, Kroin JS, Sobreviela T, et al. Intrastriatal infusions of brain-derived neurotrophic factor: retrograde transport and colocalization with dopamine containing substantia nigra neurons in rat. *Exp Neurol* 1994;129:15–26.

86. Altar CA, Boylan CB, Fritsche M, et al. The neurotrophins NT-4/5 and BDNF augment serotonin, dopamine, and GABAergic systems during behaviorally effective infusions to the substantia nigra. *Exp Neurol* 1994;130:31–40.

87. Hudson J, Granholm AC, Gerhardt GA, et al. Glial cell line–derived neurotrophic factor augments midbrain dopaminergic circuits *in vivo*. *Brain Res Bull* 1995;36:425–432.

88. Tomac A, Widenfalk J, Lin LFH, et al. Retrograde axonal transport of glial cell line–derived neurotrophic factor in the adult nigrostriatal system suggests a trophic role in the adult. *Proc Natl Acad Sci USA* 1995;92:8274–8278.

89. Morse JK, Wiegand SJ, Anderson K, et al. Brain-derived neurotrophic factor (BDNF) prevents the degeneration of medial septal cholinergic neurons following fimbria transection. *J Neurosci* 1993;13:4146–4156.

90. Levivier M, Przedborski S, Bencsics C, et al. Intrastriatal implantation of fibroblasts genetically engineered to produce brain-derived neurotrophic factor prevents degeneration of dopaminergic neurons in a rat model of Parkinson's disease. *J Neurosci* 1995;15:7810–7820.

91. Frim DM, Uhler TA, Galpern WR, et al. Implanted fibroblasts genetically engineered to produce brain-derived neurotrophic factor prevent 1-methyl-4-phenylpyridinium toxicity to dopaminergic neurons in the rat. *Proc Natl Acad Sci USA* 1994;91:5104–5108.

92. Lucidi-Phillipi CA, Gage FH, Shults CW, et al. BDNF-transduced fibroblasts: production of BDNF and effects of grafting to the adult rat brain. *J Comp Neurol* 1995;354:361–376.

93. Mandel RJ, Spratt SK, Snyder RO, et al. Midbrain injection of recombinant adeno-associated virus encoding rat glial cell line–derived neurotrophic factor protects nigral neurons in a progressive 6-hydroxydopamine-induced degeneration model of Parkinson's disease in rats. *Proc Natl Acad Sci USA* 1997;94:14083–14088.

94. Bilang-Bleuel A, Revah F, Colin P, et al. Intrastriatal injection of an adenoviral vector expressing glial cell-line–derived neurotrophic factor prevents dopaminergic neuron degeneration and behavioral impairment in a rat model of Parkinson disease. *Proc Natl Acad Sci USA* 1997;94:8818–8823.

95. Choi-Lundberg DL, Lin Q, Schallert T, et al. Behavioral and cellular protection of rat dopaminergic neurons by an adenoviral vector encoding glial cell line–derived neurotrophic factor. *Exp Neurol* 1998;154:261–275.

96. Westphal CH, Leder P. Transposon-generated "knock-out" and "knock-in" gene-targeting constructs for use in mice. *Curr Biol* 1997;7:530–533.

97. Blaese RM. Gene therapy for cancer. *Sci Am* 1997;XX:107–115.

98. Linnik MD, Zahos P, Geschwind MD, et al. Expression of bcl-2 from a defective herpes simplex virus-1 vector limits neuronal death in focal cerebral ischemia. *Stroke* 1995;26:1670–1674.

99. Przedborski S, Kostic V, Jackson-Lewis V, et al. Transgenic mice with increased Cu/Zn-superoxide dismutase activity are resistant to N-methyl-4-phenyl-1,2,3,6-tetrahydropyridine-induced neurotoxicity. *J Neurosci* 1992;12:1658–1667.

100. Nakao N, Frodl EM, Widner H, et al. Overexpressing Cu/Zn superoxide dismutase enhances survival of transplanted neurons in a rat model of Parkinson's disease. *Nat Med* 1995;1:226–231.

Surgery for Parkinson's Disease and Movement Disorders,
edited by J.K. Krauss, J. Jankovic, and R.G. Grossman.
Lippincott Williams & Wilkins, Philadelphia © 2001.

20

POLYMER-ENCAPSULATED CELLS AS A TOOL FOR DRUG DELIVERY AND NEURAL TRANSPLANTATION IN PARKINSON'S DISEASE

J.C. BENSADOUN
H.R. WIDMER
A.D. ZURN
PATRICK AEBISCHER

Parkinson's disease (PD) is a neurodegenerative disorder characterized by motor disturbances resulting from dopamine deficiency within the striatum after degeneration of dopaminergic neurons of the substantia nigra (SN). Although symptomatic treatment with L-DOPA to restore dopamine levels in the basal ganglia has initial beneficial effects, it leads to severe side effects after a few years (1). Efforts are therefore being pursued to develop alternative strategies such as local delivery of dopamine or neuroprotective molecules such as neurotrophic factors. However, direct injection of dopamine or recombinant proteins into the brain is limited by (a) the poor stability of the molecules, (b) the need for a continuous release, and (c) the infectious complications and surgical trauma associated with repetitive administration. Moreover, although embryonic neural graft transplantation to replace the degenerated dopaminergic neurons has demonstrated promising results, immunologic, ethical, and tissue availability problems limit broad application of these techniques (2). Thus, development of an efficient drug delivery system in the central nervous system represents a challenging problem for the treatment of PD. To optimize the delivery of therapeutic molecules in specific areas of the brain as well as to obviate immunologic rejection, a cell encapsulation technique allowing the local and continuous release of molecules was developed (3). Primary cells or cell lines are sequestered in a hollow fiber made of a permselective polymer membrane that allows the inward diffusion of nutrients and the outward diffusion of biotherapeutic molecules. The molecular weight

cutoff of the encapsulating membrane is set to prevent the inward diffusion of immunoglobulins and lytic factors of the complement, as well as the cell-to-cell contact between the transplanted cells and the host immunocompetent cells. The major advantage of this system relies on the possibility of using cell lines of either allogeneic or xenogeneic donor origin without immunosuppression. This chapter describes this cell encapsulation technique and reviews the *in vivo* studies that have demonstrated its efficacy for the delivery of dopamine and neurotrophic factors in animal models of PD. Furthermore, its potential clinical use for the treatment of PD is also discussed.

CELL ENCAPSULATION

Cell encapsulation is generally divided in two classes: microencapsulation and macroencapsulation. *Microencapsulation* allows one to confine small clusters of cells within a thin, spheric, semipermeable polyelectrolyte-based membrane. Bead diameter varies from 300 to 1,500 μm. Implantation of polyelectrolyte-based microcapsules containing dopamine-secreting cells such as PC12 or of bovine chromaffin cells has been shown to reduce behavioral deficits in animal models of PD (4,5). This technique presents several advantages: (a) ideal shape for neurochemical diffusion, (b) soft fabrication process for the cells, (c) and ease of the procedure. These polyelectrolyte-based microcapsules are, however, mechanically and chemically fragile, and they are difficult to retrieve once implanted. Thermoplastic-based microcapsules show improved mechanical behavior (6). Use of organic solvent in their fabrication process is, however, often associated with cell cytotoxicity. In general, the unretrievability of the microcapsules constitutes

J.C. Bensadoun, A.D. Zurn, and P. Aebischer: Division of Surgical Research and Gene Therapy Center, Centre Hospitalier Universitaire Vaudois, 1011 Lausanne, Switzerland.
H.R. Widmer: Department of Neurosurgery, University Hospital, 3010 Bern, Switzerland.

the major limitation of microencapsulation for clinical applications.

Macroencapsulation represents another cell immunoisolation system involving preformed hollow, cylindric, permselective polymer membranes that can be loaded with cells. Polymer membranes must have specific characteristics such as acceptable biocompatibility, durability, and appropriate mechanical properties to allow optimal cell survival as well as induce a minimal host tissue reaction. To date, two synthetic polymers have been commonly used for macroencapsulation: (a) polyacrylonitrile-polyvinyl chloride and (b) polyether sulfone. These thermoplastic polymers offer the advantage of being chemically stable. Moreover, compared with microcapsules, macrocapsules can be retrieved and replaced, provided tethering systems are adequate.

The polymer membrane represents a physical barrier preventing any cell-to-cell contact with host immunocompetent cells. The presence of pores allows the inward diffusion of oxygen, glucose, and other nutrients as well as the outward secretion of therapeutic compounds. Ideally, the pore size is selected to limit the diffusion of immunoglobulins and lytic

factors of the complement inside the capsule. In this context, membranes with a molecular weight cutoff between 50 and 280 kDa have been commonly used.

The shape of the device is also an important parameter. To support cell viability, the maximal distance between encapsulated cells and metabolic supply should not exceed 500 μm. Optimal results have been obtained with fiber diameters between 600 and 900 μm and a membrane thickness of 50 to 100 μm. The length of the capsule depends on (a) the number of cells needed, (b) the implantation site, and (c) the type of hosts. Hence, it varies from a minimum of 0.5 cm in rats to 5 cm in humans (7,8).

To support optimal cell survival and differentiation, an extracellular matrix can be introduced inside the hollow fiber (Fig. 20.1). Depending on the cell type, collagen, hydrogels such as alginate or agarose, or polyvinyl alcohol are commonly used. Polyvinyl alcohol has to be placed inside the fiber before cell encapsulation, whereas collagen, alginate, and agarose are mixed with the cells before loading. Finally, loading is performed by slowly injecting the cell suspension into the fiber and sealing the ends with a photopolymerizable

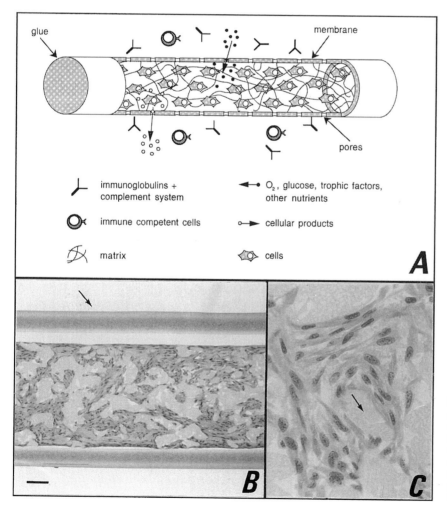

FIGURE 20.1. Cell encapsulation system. **A:** Schematic representation of a polymer capsule. **B:** Micrograph showing a longitudinal section of a polymeric capsule loaded with C$_2$C$_{12}$ cells and maintained for 4 weeks *in vitro* (scale bar: 100 μm). *Arrow:* polymer membrane. **C:** Higher magnification ($\times$10) of **B.** Note the homogenous distribution of the cells in the supporting matrix *(arrow)*.

acrylic glue. A schematic representation and photomicrographs of the capsule are shown in Fig. 20.1.

POLYMER-ENCAPSULATED DOPAMINE-SECRETING CELLS FOR NEUROTRANSMITTER REPLACEMENT THERAPY

One of the strategies to improve parkinsonian symptoms is to provide dopamine to the depleted striatum. Although often associated with beneficial effects, systemic administration of L-DOPA leads to side effects within 5 to 10 years. Direct infusion of dopamine into the striatum partially prevents these side effects, but the rapid oxidation of dopamine compromises its long-term application. Transplantation of polymer-encapsulated dopamine-secreting cells represents an attractive alternative to direct infusion. PC12 cells, a catecholaminergic cell line derived from rat pheochromocytoma, synthesize, store, and release catecholamines, in particular dopamine (9). *In vitro* studies have revealed that polymer-encapsulated PC12 cells survive, synthesize, and release dopamine for up to 6 months (10). Similarly, encapsulated PC12 cells survive at least 6 months when they are implanted either in rat (11,12) or monkey striatum (13), with no lymphocytic infiltration and a minimal astrocytic reaction. Unencapsulated PC12 cells did not survive implantation in these species, a finding demonstrating that polymer capsules provide effective immunoisolation for xenogeneic cells in the central nervous system.

The efficacy of polymer-encapsulated dopaminesecreting cells in reversing behavioral symptoms was subsequently evaluated in a rodent model of PD (12,14). Polyacrylonitrile-polyvinyl chloride capsules containing PC12 cells were implanted unilaterally into the striatum of 6-hydroxydopamine (6-OHDA)–lesioned rats (12). A significant reduction in apomorphine-induced rotation was observed for up to 24 weeks in the presence of PC12 cell–containing capsules, but not with empty polymer devices. Released dopamine was detectable up to a distance of 200 to 250 μm from the implant (12). In another study, intrastriatal, but not intraventricular, implantation of PC12 cells reduced apomorphine-induced rotation in rats (14). Thus, appropriate localization of the capsule is required to induce behavioral recovery in these animals. Polymer-encapsulated dopamine-secreting cells have also been tested in a nonhuman primate model of PD (13,15). Adult cynomolgus monkeys (*Macaca fascicularis*) lesioned with a unilateral intracarotid injection of 1-methyl-4-phenyl-1,2,3,6-tetrahydropyridine (MPTP) underwent implantation in the putamen (three capsules) and in the anterior portion of the caudate nucleus (one capsule) with hollow-fiber capsules loaded with PC12 cells. Behavioral tests showed that upper limb movement and the ability to perform a food-picking task were significantly improved in the animals that had received encapsulated PC12 cells. The

lack of tyrosine hydroxylase (TH)-positive fibers sprouting in the implanted sites suggested that the functional recovery was directly caused by the dopamine release from the encapsulated PC12 cells.

Taken together, these data indicate that encapsulated dopamine-releasing cells survive and provide behavioral recovery in various animal models of PD in the absence of any side effects. In the perspective of clinical applications, this approach is limited by (a) the choice of the implantation site and (b) the low stability of dopamine. Although striatum appears to be the most appropriate site for implantation of encapsulated dopamine-releasing cells, surgical complications potentially associated with repetitive replacements of the device in the parenchyma hamper the usefulness of this approach for humans. To date, ventricular placement represents the safest site available for capsule implantation into the brain. However, intraventricular implantation of encapsulated PC12 cells does not improve parkinsonian symptoms as compared with the intraparenchymal procedure (14). The likely reason is a dilution effect within the cerebrospinal fluid or poor diffusibility of the dopamine within the brain parenchyma. Strategies to increase the amount of dopamine released by the capsule may allow better availability of the molecule throughout the whole striatal tissue, essential to attenuate parkinsonian symptoms. Conversely, this rise in circulating dopamine may induce severe side effects associated with diffusion into other brain structures. In summary, experiments with encapsulated dopamine-releasing cells have demonstrated the feasibility and efficacy of the encapsulation technique for the local release of molecules into the brain. The invasiveness of this solely symptomatic approach, however, prevents its use for clinical application.

POLYMER ENCAPSULATION OF GENETICALLY ENGINEERED CELL LINES FOR NEUROPROTECTIVE STUDIES

Although effective in minimizing parkinsonian symptoms, dopamine replacement therapy does not impede the progressive degeneration of the nigral dopaminergic neurons. With the discovery of trophic factors acting on midbrain dopaminergic neurons, neuroprotective approaches have been developed to slow down or to prevent this degenerative process. *Glial cell line–derived neurotrophic factor* (GDNF) is one of the most potent survival factors for dopaminergic neurons *in vitro*. *In vivo,* GDNF protects dopaminergic neurons against induced cell death in several animal models of PD (16–20). Because GDNF does not act only on dopaminergic neurons (21–25), delivery of large boluses of GDNF diffusing in various brain structures may potentially lead to side effects. In this context, transplantation of encapsulated cells genetically engineered to release GDNF was used to provide a localized and continuous release of small quantity of the neurotrophic factor in a restricted area of the brain.

Genetically Engineered Cell Lines

Baby hamster kidney (BHK) cells have been transfected with an expression vector containing the cDNA for human GDNF or neurturin, a close relative of GDNF (26). More recently, we used a mouse myoblast cell line (C_2C_{12}) for transfection because of its capacity to differentiate into myotubes *in vitro,* thereby avoiding the long-term accumulation of cell debris in the capsule typically observed with the use of a continuously dividing cell line (27). In both cell lines, a suicide gene, the herpes simplex virus thymidine kinase (HSV-tk) gene, was inserted into the expression vector to ensure additional safety of the system. In the unlikely event of capsule breakage and ineffectiveness of the host immune system, cells can be eliminated by systemic administration of ganciclovir.

Polymer-Encapsulated GDNF-Secreting Cells in a Rat Model of Parkinson's Disease

We have investigated the neuroprotective effect of GDNF released by encapsulated BHK cells in a rat model of PD (8). Medial forebrain bundle (MFB) axotomy leads to the rapid degeneration of nigral dopaminergic neurons and, as a consequence, to a massive loss of striatal dopamine. We implanted either a single 5-mm capsule containing BHK cells releasing approximately 5 ng of GDNF per day or BHK control cells unilaterally lateral to the MFB and rostral to the SN. One week after capsule implantation, MFB axotomy was performed on the same side. Seven days later, the animals were tested for amphetamine-induced rotational behavior. Rotations were significantly reduced in the presence of BHK-GDNF capsules, but not with control BHK capsules (8). Immunohistochemical analysis of the SN revealed that animals implanted with BHK-GDNF capsules had 64.9±7.2% TH-immunoreactive cells on the lesioned side as compared with the nonlesioned side, whereas control animals had only 27.2±3.5% positive cells (Fig. 20.2). These data indicate that polymer-encapsulated GDNF-secreting cells can protect nigral dopaminergic neurons from MFB axotomy-induced cell death and can reverse drug-induced rotational behavior by a mechanism that is not mediated by striatal dopamine. By using the same lesion model, neuroprotective effects were also obtained with neurturin released by encapsulated BHK cells (28).

POLYMER-ENCAPSULATED CELLS FOR NEURAL GRAFT MAINTENANCE

Transplantation of autologous *adrenal medullary chromaffin cells* that secrete catecholamines or fetal ventral mesencephalic grafts containing dopaminergic neurons was previ-

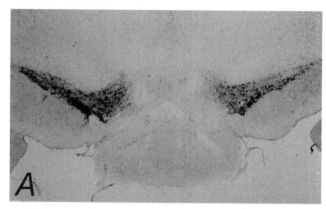

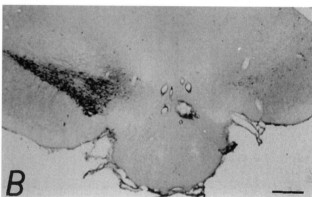

FIGURE 20.2. Effect of glial cell line–derived neurotrophic factor (GDNF) released by encapsulated baby hamster kidney (BHK) cells on the number of nigral neurons (revealed by tyrosine hydroxylase staining) after a unilateral (right) medial forebrain bundle axotomy in the rat. Note the important protection against cell loss in the BHK-GDNF group **(A)** as compared with the parent BHK-implanted animals **(B)** (scale bar: 100 μm).

ously shown to exert beneficial effects in animal models of PD and in patients with parkinsonism (29–33). However, grafts of chromaffin cells survive poorly and tend to lose their capacity to secrete dopamine over time. Similarly, only 5% to 20% of the implanted embryonic mesencephalic neurons survive transplantation into the striatum of various host species including humans (2,32,34). Different compounds such as free radical scavengers, antioxidants, antiapoptotic molecules, and neurotrophic factors were previously assessed to improve graft survival and function, as well as to reduce the amount of tissue needed (35–38). In this context, encapsulated genetically engineered cells continuously releasing low amounts of neurotrophic factors were tested in cografting experiments to support graft survival and function in animal models of PD (39,40).

Because nerve growth factor (NGF) was shown to increase chromaffin cell survival (41), polymer-encapsulated human NGF-secreting BHK (BHK-hNGF) cells were used in cografting experiments in a rat model of PD (39). The experiment involved unilateral implantation of either a single capsule containing BHK cells releasing approximately 10 ng of NGF per day or BHK control cells into the striatum of

6-OHDA–lesioned rats. Concurrently, adrenal medullary tissue from 6-week-old Sprague-Dawley rats was grafted at a 1.5-mm distance from the polymer capsule. Apomorphine-induced rotational behavior, morphologic analysis of the retrieved capsules, and chromaffin cell survival were assessed at 1, 6, and 12 months after transplantation. Results showed that drug-induced turns were significantly decreased in animals cografted with the BHK-hNGF cells, but not with control BHK cells. Consistent with these behavioral results, the mean number of surviving chromaffin cells was 26- to 32-fold higher in animals cografted with the BHK-hNGF capsule as compared with controls. The retrieved capsules secreted 2 to 3 ng of NGF per day, that is, approximately one-third of the initial amount at time of implantation. These data suggest that cografting of NGF-secreting polymer capsules with adrenal chromaffin cells provides graft survival and function as compared with chromaffin grafts alone. However, this approach is made difficult in elderly patients with PD, in whom the disease process has been shown to affect tissue integrity. The generally poor outcome of clinical results reported for transplantation of chromaffin cells constitutes sufficient rationale not to proceed with this strategy clinically.

Similarly, polymer-encapsulated GDNF-secreting BHK cells were used in an attempt to improve survival and function of fetal mesencephalic grafts in a rat model of PD (40). Investigators implanted either a single 5-mm capsule containing BHK cells releasing approximately 50 ng of GDNF per day or BHK control cells into the striatum of 6-OHDA–lesioned rats. One week later, rat fetal ventral mesencephalic tissue grown as free-floating roller tube cultures (42) was transplanted into the striatum, 1.5 mm anterior to the capsule. Amphetamine-induced rotation was assessed at 3 and 6 weeks after grafting. The animals were sacrificed at the end of the last behavioral test. Drug-induced rotations were significantly decreased at 3 and 6 weeks in animals cografted with GDNF-releasing capsules, whereas mesencephalic grafts combined with BHK control cells did not significantly reverse rotation. GDNF led to a 2.6-fold increase in the number of TH-positive cells per graft as well as a 1.5-fold increase in the TH-positive fiber network around the graft as compared with the control group. In addition, TH-positive fibers had a tendency to grow toward the source of GDNF (Fig. 20.3). These data indicate that the continuous delivery of GDNF by encapsulated cells is an efficient system to support long-term survival and function of dopaminergic grafts in the rat brain. In a clinical perspective, this technique could be very useful to decrease the amount of fetal tissue needed for patients with PD. Presumably, through its action on cell survival, GDNF released by the capsulated cells should help the graft to integrate and form synapses within the host tissue during the critical phase after cotransplantation. In this context, the perspective of a clinical trial based on striatal cotransplantation of GDNF-releasing capsule and embryonic mesencephalic tissue remains fully conceivable.

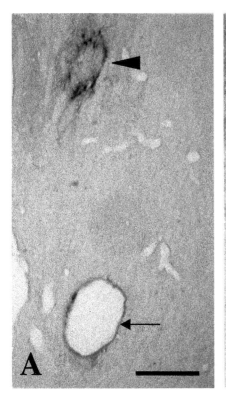
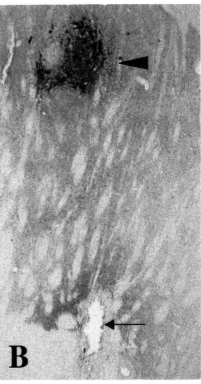

FIGURE 20.3. Microphotographs of horizontal sections through rat striatum stained with antibodies against tyrosine hydroxylase (TH) showing ventral mesencephalic grafts *(arrowheads)* and the site of capsule implantation *(arrows)* in the BHK (baby hamster kidney) control **(A)** and BHK-GDNF (glial cell line–derived neurotrophic factor) **(B)** group. Notice the larger size of the grafts, the larger number of TH-immunoreactive neurons, and the pronounced sprouting of nerve fibers from the grafts toward the GDNF-producing capsule in **B** as compared with **A** (scale bar: 500 μm).

TOWARD A CLINICAL TRIAL USING POLYMER-ENCAPSULATED GENETICALLY ENGINEERED CELLS RELEASING GDNF IN PATIENTS WITH PARKINSON'S DISEASE

Study in Late-Stage Parkinsonian Baboons

To validate encapsulated GDNF-secreting cells as a functional treatment for patients with parkinsonism, this delivery method was evaluated in a monkey model of PD. Because of surgical complications associated with striatal localization, intraventricular implantation was assessed in this study. Chronic MPTP treatment in monkeys leads to behavioral features closely mimicking parkinsonian symptoms (43). Baboons chronically lesioned with MPTP for 12 to 18 months underwent bilateral implantation into the lateral ventricles of one 2-cm capsule containing BHK cells releasing approximately 200 ng of GDNF per day (44). Hypokinetic and bradykinetic behaviors were tested at 1, 2, 3, and 4 months after capsule implantation using a video-movement tracking and analyzing system. Animals were sacrificed at the end of the last behavioral test. GDNF treatment almost completely reversed MPTP-induced hypokinesia in these animals. However, GDNF treatment had only a small effect on the bradykinetic behavior. Histologic analyses revealed that GDNF induced sprouting of the remaining TH-positive neurites in the SN and in the putamen. The capsules were well tolerated, and no side effects such as weight loss were observed during the 4-month implantation period. These data suggest that long-term intracerebroventricular delivery of small amounts of GDNF using polymer-encapsulated cells can provide behavioral benefits in chronically lesioned monkeys, an animal model with deficits closely resembling parkinsonian symptoms. The slow continuous release of small quantities of GDNF is not associated with the marked side effects observed with large intracerebroventricular bolus injection of GDNF. Conversely, the poor diffusion of GDNF from the ventricles probably keeps this molecule from reaching distant structures of the striatum, a finding explaining the partial behavioral improvement observed in the monkey study. The "ideal" therapeutic dose of intracerebroventricular GDNF conferring maximal behavioral recovery, while avoiding any side effect, has yet to be determined.

Phase I/II Clinical Trial in Patients with Parkinson's Disease

Based on the promising results obtained in rat and monkey models of PD with GDNF, a phase I/II clinical trial is being initiated in patients with PD at the University Hospital in Lausanne (Switzerland). The goal of this trial is to evaluate the safety and tolerability of intracerebroventricular delivery of GDNF using the polymer encapsulation technology. For this purpose, a master cell bank of C_2C_{12} cells releasing 200 ng GDNF/10^6 cells per day has been prepared. Microbiologic tests to exclude bacterial and fungal contaminants,

mycoplasma, and viruses, as well as tumorigenicity studies in rats and sheep, are currently being performed. Authorization for the trial has to be obtained from the Ethical Committee of the Faculty of Medicine and the Federal Commission for Biologic Safety. Based on the results of these tests, patients will undergo bilateral implantation into the ventricles of one 2-cm capsule containing C_2C_{12} cells releasing 100 to 200 ng GDNF per day. The patients will be followed-up over a period of 12 months. For clinical evaluation, the methodology suggested by the Core Assessment Program for Intracerebral Transplantation in PD (CAPIT-PD) will be used (45). Positron emission tomography studies will also be performed to evaluate the effects of GDNF on striatal dopamine levels during the course of the treatment.

CONCLUSION

In vitro and *in vivo* experiments using cell encapsulation have demonstrated the efficacy of this technique for local and continuous release of small quantities of molecules for long periods while avoiding immunologic rejection. Studies with polymer-encapsulated dopamine-secreting cells for neurotransmitter replacement therapy have illustrated the ability of such technique to reduce behavioral deficits in animal models of PD. Besides symptomatic approaches, neuroprotective therapy using neurotrophic factors such as GDNF represents an important advance to slow down or prevent the degenerative process of the disease, but it requires an appropriate delivery system. Polymer encapsulation of genetically engineered cell lines has demonstrated promising cellular and functional results in various animal models of PD, including primates. In this context, the local and continuous release of small quantities of GDNF using cell encapsulation technique may potentially be of benefit in patients with PD, especially in the context of neural transplantation approaches.

REFERENCES

1. Luquin MR, Scipioni O, Vaamonde J, et al. Levodopa-induced dyskinesias in Parkinson's disease: clinical and pharmacological classification. *Mov Disord* 1992;7:117–124.
2. Borlongan CV, Stahl CE, Cameron DF, et al. CNS immunological modulation of neural graft rejection and survival. *Neurol Res* 1996;18:297–304.
3. Aebischer P, Winn SR, Galletti PM. Transplantation of neural tissue in polymer capsules. *Brain Res* 1988;448:364–368.
4. Winn SR, Tresco PA, Zielinski B, et al. Behavioral recovery following intrastriatal implantation of microencapsulated PC12 cells. *Exp Neurol* 1991;113:322–329.
5. Aebischer P, Tresco PA, Sagen J, et al. Transplantation of microencapsulated bovine chromaffin cells reduces lesion-induced rotational asymmetry in rats. *Brain Res* 1991;560:43–49.
6. Roberts T, De Boni U, Sefton MV. Dopamine secretion by PC12 cells microencapsulated in a hydroxyethyl methacrylate-methyl methacrylate copolymer. *Biomaterials* 1996;17:267–275.

7. Aebischer P, Schluep M, Déglon N, et al. Intrathecal delivery of CNTF using encapsulated genetically modified xenogeneic cells in amyotrophic lateral sclerosis patients. *Nat Med* 1996;2:696–699.

8. Tseng JL, Baetge EE, Zurn AD, et al. GDNF reduces drug-induced rotational behavior after medial forebrain bundle transection by a mechanism not involving striatal dopamine. *J Neurosci* 1997;17:325–333.

9. Greene LA, Rein G. Release, storage and uptake of catecholamines by a clonal cell line of nerve growth factor (NGF) responsive pheochromocytoma cells. *Brain Res* 1977;129:247–263.

10. Jaeger CB, Greene LA, Tresco PA, et al. Polymer encapsulated dopaminergic cell lines as "alternative neural grafts." *Prog Brain Res* 1990;82:41–46.

11. Jaeger CB, Aebischer P, Tresco PA, et al. Growth of tumour cell lines in polymer capsules: ultrastructure of encapsulated PC12 cells. *J Neurocytol* 1992;21:469–480.

12. Tresco PA, Winn SR, Tan S, et al. Polymer-encapsulated PC12 cells: long-term survival and associated reduction in lesion-induced rotational behavior. *Cell Transplant* 1992;1:255–264.

13. Kordower JH, Liu YT, Winn S, et al. Encapsulated PC12 cell transplants into hemiparkinsonian monkeys: a behavioral, neuroanatomical, and neurochemical analysis. *Cell Transplant* 1995;4:155–171.

14. Emerich DF, Winn SR, Lindner MD. Continued presence of intrastriatal but not intraventricular polymer-encapsulated PC12 cells is required for alleviation of behavioral deficits in parkinsonian rodents. *Cell Transplant* 1996;5:589–596.

15. Aebischer P, Goddard M, Signore AP, et al. Functional recovery in hemiparkinsonian primates transplanted with polymer-encapsulated PC12 cells. *Exp Neurol* 1994;126:151–158.

16. Lin LF, Doherty DH, Lile JD, et al. GDNF: a glial cell line–derived neurotrophic factor for midbrain dopaminergic neurons. *Science* 1993;260:1130–1132.

17. Beck KD, Valverde J, Alexi T, et al. Mesencephalic dopaminergic neurons protected by GDNF from axotomy-induced degeneration in the adult brain. *Nature* 1995;373:339–341.

18. Sauer H, Rosenblad C, Björklund A. Glial cell line–derived neurotrophic factor but not transforming growth factor beta 3 prevents delayed degeneration of nigral dopaminergic neurons following striatal 6-hydroxydopamine lesion. *Proc Natl Acad Sci USA* 1995;92:8935–8939.

19. Tomac A, Lindqvist E, Lin LF, et al. Protection and repair of the nigrostriatal dopaminergic system by GDNF *in vivo*. *Nature* 1995;373:335–339.

20. Gash DM, Zhang Z, Ovadia A, et al. Functional recovery in parkinsonian monkeys treated with GDNF. *Nature* 1996;380:252–255.

21. Henderson CE, Phillips HS, Pollock RA, et al. GDNF: a potent survival factor for motoneurons present in peripheral nerve and muscle. *Science* 1994;266:1062–1064.

22. Zurn AD, Baetge EE, Hammang JP, et al. Glial cell line–derived neurotrophic factor (GDNF), a new neurotrophic factor for motoneurones. *Neuroreport* 1994;6:113–118.

23. Arenas E, Trupp M, Akerud P, et al. GDNF prevents degeneration and promotes the phenotype of brain noradrenergic neurons *in vivo*. *Neuron* 1995;15:1465–1473.

24. Farkas LM, Suter-Crazzolara C, Unsicker K. GDNF induces the calretinin phenotype in cultures of embryonic striatal neurons. *J Neurosci Res* 1997;50:361–372.

25. Meyer M, Zimmer J, Seiler RW, et al. GDNF increases the density of cells containing calbindin but not of cells containing calretinin in cultured rat and human fetal nigral tissue. *Cell Transplant* 1999;8:25–36.

26. Kotzbauer PT, Lampe PA, Heuckeroth RO, et al. Neurturin, a relative of glial-cell-line–derived neurotrophic factor. *Nature* 1996;384:467–470.

27. Déglon N, Heyd B, Tan SA, et al. Central nervous system delivery of recombinant ciliary neurotrophic factor by polymer encapsulated differentiated C2C12 myoblasts. *Hum Gene Ther* 1996;7:2135–2146.

28. Tseng JL, Bruhn SL, Zurn AD, et al. Neurturin protects dopaminergic neurons following medial forebrain bundle axotomy. *Neuroreport* 1998;9:1817–1822.

29. Fiandaca MS, Kordower JH, Hansen JT, et al. Adrenal medullary autografts into the basal ganglia of *Cebus* monkeys: injury-induced regeneration. *Exp Neurol* 1988;102:76–91.

30. Backlund EO, Granberg PO, Hamberger B, et al. Transplantation of adrenal medullary tissue to striatum in parkinsonism: first clinical trials. *J Neurosurg* 1985;62:169–173.

31. Olanow CW, Freeman TB, Kordower JH. Neural transplantation as a therapy for Parkinson's disease. *Adv Neurol* 1997;74:249–269.

32. Lindvall O. Update on fetal transplantation: the Swedish experience. *Mov Disord* 1998;13[Suppl 1]:83–87.

33. Hauser RA, Freeman TB, Snow BJ, et al. Long-term evaluation of bilateral fetal nigral transplantation in Parkinson disease. *Arch Neurol* 1999;56:179–187.

34. Kordower JH, Freeman TB, Snow BJ, et al. Neuropathological evidence of graft survival and striatal reinnervation after the transplantation of fetal mesencephalic tissue in a patient with Parkinson's disease. *N Engl J Med* 1995;332:1118–1124.

35. Nakao N, Frodl EM, Duan WM, et al. Lazaroids improve the survival of grafted rat embryonic dopamine neurons. *Proc Natl Acad Sci USA* 1994;91:12408–12412.

36. Barkats M, Nakao N, Grasbon-Frodl EM, et al. Intrastriatal grafts of embryonic mesencephalic rat neurons genetically modified using an adenovirus encoding human Cu/Zn superoxide dismutase. *Neuroscience* 1997;78:703–713.

37. Schierle GS, Hansson O, Leist M, et al. Caspase inhibition reduces apoptosis and increases survival of nigral transplants. *Nat Med* 1999;5:97–100.

38. Rosenblad C, Martinez-Serrano A, Björklund A. Glial cell line–derived neurotrophic factor increases survival, growth and function of intrastriatal fetal nigral dopaminergic grafts. *Neuroscience* 1996;75:979–985.

39. Date I, Shingo T, Ohmoto T, et al. Long-term enhanced chromaffin cell survival and behavioral recovery in hemiparkinsonian rats with co-grafted polymer-encapsulated human NGF-secreting cells. *Exp Neurol* 1997;147:10–17.

40. Sautter J, Tseng JL, Braguglia D, et al. Implants of polymer-encapsulated genetically modified cells releasing glial cell line–derived neurotrophic factor improve survival, growth, and function of fetal dopaminergic grafts. *Exp Neurol* 1998;149:230–236.

41. Unsicker K, Skaper SD, Varon S. Developmental changes in the responses of rat chromaffin cells to neuronotrophic and neurite-promoting factors. *Dev Biol* 1985;111:425–433.

42. Meyer M, Widmer HR, Wagner B, et al. Comparison of mesencephalic free-floating tissue culture grafts and cell suspension grafts in the 6-hydroxydopamine-lesioned rat. *Exp Brain Res* 1998;119:345–355.

43. Varastet M, Riche D, Maziere M, et al. Chronic MPTP treatment reproduces in baboons the differential vulnerability of mesencephalic dopaminergic neurons observed in Parkinson's disease. *Neuroscience* 1994;63:47–56.

44. Palfi S, Joseph JM, Condé F, et al. Transplantation of polymer encapsulated GDNF-secreting xenogeneic cells leads to prolonged functional recovery in late-stage parkinsonian baboons (submitted).

45. Langston JW, Widner H, Goetz CG, et al. Core assessment program for intracerebral transplantations (CAPIT). *Mov Disord* 1992;7:2–13.

Surgery for Parkinson's Disease and Movement Disorders,
edited by J.K. Krauss, J. Jankovic, and R.G. Grossman.
Lippincott Williams & Wilkins, Philadelphia © 2001.

21

APOMORPHINE INFUSIONS FOR TREATMENT OF ADVANCED PARKINSON'S DISEASE

A.J. LEES

Apomorphine is a nonnarcotic dopamine receptor agonist that was first synthesized in 1869 and was originally used in veterinary medicine to treat behavioral vices in farm animals. Although it was suggested as a potential therapy for Parkinson's disease in 1884, its early use in clinical medicine was as an emetic, sedative, anticonvulsant, and treatment for narcotic and alcohol dependence (1). Aporphine alkaloids are present in the tubers and petals of water lilies (species *Nymphaea*), and it has been suggested that the mystical and magical properties ascribed to these plants by the Maya and Ancient Egyptians may relate to the effects of apomorphine on the central nervous system. Schwab and colleagues showed that subcutaneous injections of apomorphine produced a marked but short-lived improvement in Parkinson's disease (2), but because of nausea, postural hypotension, sedation, and ephemeral therapeutic effects, the drug did not catch on in clinical practice. In 1967, the structural similarity to dopamine was noted, and ever since then apomorphine has found wide application in preclinical neuropharmacology as the prototype dopamine agonist.

After the successful introduction of high-dose dopa as an effective therapy for Parkinson's disease, Cotzias and colleagues reinvestigated apomorphine as a dopamine analog with properties potentially complementary to those of dopa (3). These investigators confirmed the drug's potent effects on all the motor disabilities, especially tremor, and made the interesting suggestion that it may possess antidyskinetic properties . The subsequent success of L-dopa and the advent of the first orally active dopamine receptor agonists in the early 1970s, however, led to further neglect of apomorphine's potential as an antiparkinsonian drug. In 1979, investigators showed that pretreatment with the newly developed peripheral dopamine receptor antagonist domperidone effectively prevented apomorphine-induced nausea and orthostatic hy-

potension, although it had no effect on yawning (4). Apomorphine reliably reverses refractory L-dopa–induced "off"-period disabilities, a finding indicating that striatal dopamine receptors remain responsive to stimulation at these times and that the peripheral and central handling of L-dopa must be important in the pathogenesis of the "on-off" phenomenon (5). When apomorphine, a dopamine agonist, is administered before pallidotomy, it has been found to suppress the abnormal hyperactivity of the internal segment of the globus pallidus and the subthalamic nucleus and to enhance the activity of the external segment of the globus pallidus based on intraoperative cellular recordings (6). However, marked or complete suppression of activity of the internal segment of the globus pallidus is associated with the emergence of dyskinesias. This finding suggests that dopaminergic drugs and pallidotomy improve parkinsonian symptoms through a similar mechanism.

APOMORPHINE IN THE MANAGEMENT OF L-DOPA–PROVOKED MOTOR FLUCTUATIONS

The availability of domperidone and the development of new drug delivery systems encouraged us to reinvestigate apomorphine in the management of patients with brittle, oscillating disease that cannot be controlled with optimum oral drug regimens. These patients are asked to keep detailed diaries of their motor performance over a representative week at home and to indicate the times and duration of their dyskinetic bursts and "off" periods. They are then admitted to the hospital for further assessment including an apomorphine challenge test to determine the amplitude and quality of their dopaminergic motor response and the pattern and severity of associated dyskinesias. Although domperidone, 20 mg three times daily, as pretreatment for 48 hours is routinely recommended, most patients who are responding to long-term L-dopa therapy do not experience serious adverse reactions

A.J. Lees: Reta Lila Weston Institute of Neurological Studies, Windeyer Institute of Medical Science, University College London, London W1P 6DB, United Kingdom.

to apomorphine. The dose of subcutaneous apomorphine to which the patient clearly responds is also a helpful guide to the initial maintenance hourly apomorphine infusion rate. If the amplitude of motor response to apomorphine is small or if severe-onset and end-of-dose biphasic dyskinesias occur, then a good response to long-term apomorphine infusion is unlikely. Dementia, severe neurobehavioral problems, and marked postural instability are other important limitations. Some patients are also reluctant to embark on a program of treatment that they fear may limit their freedom of movement or "make them feel like invalids"; a few patients are also needle phobic. The success of apomorphine therapy depends on detailed explanation of what can be achieved, support and educational backup, and an optimistic commitment to the therapeutic approach by patient and physician.

Techniques of Subcutaneous Apomorphine Infusion

Numerous different minipump systems are available for apomorphine administration (Graseby MS26 and MS16A, Diesetronic, Deltec, Cane). The small delivery needle is inserted subcutaneously in the flanks of the abdominal wall, and the site is changed at least once a day. Oral medication is initially left unchanged, and the apomorphine is started usually at a rate of 1 to 3 mg per hour. The rate is then altered to obtain the best reduction in daily "off" time, and oral medication is slowly reduced, starting with oral dopamine agonists and other adjuvant therapy and then finally diminishing the dose of L-dopa at an average rate of 50 mg per day at weekly intervals. The reduction of oral medication has to be done slowly, flexibly, and patiently, often over a 6-month period if success is to be achieved. Some patients find it impossible to discontinue all their L-dopa, and others find the need to use a booster device on the pump to give them extra pulses of dopaminergic stimulation during "off" phases. Most patients find a 12- to 18-hour infusion period most satisfactory (they remove the pump before retiring to bed), but some rotate the needle site and use a lower dose rate overnight to overcome nocturnal immobility, cramps, and restless legs. Most of the patients who use the waking day regimen supplement their therapy with a nocturnal dose of L-dopa, and many also use another early morning dose of L-dopa to start the day while they wait for the apomorphine pump to take effect. Patients and their families are usually able to manage the preparation of the apomorphine, the setting of the pump, and the insertion of the needle themselves, but some patients require help from visiting nurses. A week's admission to the hospital to assess the patient's response to the drug and to resolve difficulties with adherence to the protocols is ideal, but intelligent, motivated patients may not require a hospital stay. After hospital discharge, the ideal schedule consists of an appointment in the outpatient clinic a week later and again in a month.

Problems of Apomorphine Infusion

When the pump treatment was started in 1986, it was initially used to reduce the burden of "off"-period disability in L-dopa–treated patients with severely fluctuating disease who could not be improved by L-dopa dosage modification or the introduction of orally active dopamine agonists. Patients with severe interdose chorea were considered to be relatively poor candidates for the pump, and no attempts to reduce the daytime L-dopa dosage markedly were made, even though studies had shown that the degree of motor benefit seen with apomorphine was comparable to that seen with L-dopa (7). In fact, in our 5-year review, the mean dose of L-dopa increased from 986 mg preapomorphine to 1141 mg at review (8). This strategy, in part, stemmed from our desire to keep the apomorphine dose as low as possible, to reduce the risk of itchy red nodules of panniculitis at the injection sites. These nodules represent the most common complication of therapy, and in addition to their unsightliness, they may scab over, bruise, or break down, and they sometimes ulcerate or become infected. Occasionally, surgical débridement with closure of ulcers has been required. Scrupulous aseptic insertion of the needle, dilution of the apomorphine solution to 5 mg/mL, and the use of abdominal wall ultrasound therapy with application of silicone gel patches have all helped to minimize this problem. Although drug dosage is probably important in the pathogenesis of nodules, there appear to be some additional factors, possibly including local allergies associated with eosinophilia (9). Whereas some patients develop red itchy nodules as soon as the apomorphine is infused, other patients have pristine, virtually unblemished skin after more than 5 years of continuous drug delivery. Another rare complication that has been encountered is marked edema of the legs and abdominal wall with generalized erythema.

Clinical Results

With the strategy of "add-on" apomorphine therapy, it was possible to reduce the amount of "off"-period disability markedly. This advance enabled many people who had become dependent on others for everyday survival to return to independent lives. Some reported that it had turned the clock back 3 or 4 years, and some of the more dramatic results were reminiscent of the awakenings achieved with L-dopa in severely handicapped patients with parkinsonism after the introduction of this agent. Patients who had been "off" for up to 70% of the waking day despite large doses of L-dopa, during which time they would find it difficult to walk, speak, or think clearly, reported that with apomorphine, they were "on" for all but 2 or 3 hours, with marked reductions in other problems such as "off"-period bowel and bladder dysfunction, depression, drooling, and painful dystonia. An overall reduction in peak dose chorea was also noted. Neuropsychiatric morbidity presented a further

TABLE 21.1. APOMORPHINE INFUSION RESULTS

Author and Group (yr)	No. of Patients	Mean Duration of Disease (yr)	Mean Apomorphine Daily Dose (mg)	Mean % L-Dopa Dose Reduction	Mean % Reduction in "Off" Time	Mean Duration of Apomorphine (mo)
Hughes et al. (1993)	22	19	93	15	60	37
Pollak et al. (1990), Grenoble	9	15	100	53	67	10
Pietz et al. (1998), Lund	25	16	112	50	50	44
Wenning et al. (1999), Innsbruck	16	11	162	60	55	57
Chaudhuri et al. (1999), King's, London (unpublished)	34	10	70	18	42	30
Kanovsky et al. (1999), Brno	12	14	30	23	41	9
Vanderheyden et al. (1999), Montigny-le-	11	13	48	30	40	12

challenge. Nevertheless, the drug was generally well tolerated, and the only serious—very rare—adverse event reported was autoimmune hemolytic anemia, which has also been reported with L-dopa (10). The results of our own early studies in reducing "off"-period disability and the results of other colleagues in Europe are shown in Table 21.1 (8,11–16). These studies showed that even in patients who were considered unmanageable by medical means, a further 50% reduction in "off"-period time could be achieved, often with a concomitant reduction in L-dopa dosage. Furthermore, our published 5-year review showed that 79% of patients had maintained their response over the follow-up period. In 1996, we carried out a 10-year review of all patients treated with apomorphine at University College London Hospitals based on detailed review of the clinical dossiers and interviews with patients and caregivers. At the time of this review, 68 patients were using apomorphine pumps, although many of these patients had initially used intermittent apomorphine injections before switching to the pump (only 20 had started apomorphine by continuous infusion). A further 26 patients had discontinued apomorphine, most commonly because of neuropsychiatric complications, severe dyskinesias, more sudden and severe "off" periods, serious frequent falls, or a wish to return to oral medication. Sedation and weight gain were other common adverse events, but these did not usually lead to discontinuation of apomorphine.

Most of the patients treated with the pump had been taking levodopa therapy for more than 10 years and were receiving between 30 and 300 mg of apomorphine a day (mean, 90 mg). Of the total number of 161 patients treated with apomorphine either by intermittent injection or pump over the 10-year period, 26 had died: bronchopneumonia was reported as the cause of death in 9, and sudden deaths from either pulmonary embolism or myocardial infarction occurred in 6. At the end of this review, it was concluded that it could be possible to treat bradykinesia, tremor, and rigidity successfully with dopaminergic therapy in many patients indefinitely. However, postural instability with falls, increasing cognitive impairment, personality change, and dyskinesias were regarded as ongoing therapeutic challenges.

CONTINUOUS SUBCUTANEOUS APOMORPHINE AS A TREATMENT FOR L-DOPA–INDUCED DYSKINESIAS

Although often remarkably well tolerated by patients, L-dopa–induced dyskinesias compromise motor function, interfere with walking, posture, and balance, and lead to embarrassment for both patients and their families. Occasionally, they can lead to traumatic musculoskeletal injuries or can predispose patients to cervical root or spinal cord damage.

Pathophysiology of L-Dopa–Induced Dyskinesias

The mechanisms that underlie L-dopa–induced dyskinesias are still unclear, but even short periods of drug exposure may prime dyskinesias in severely disabled patients. Once dyskinesias are primed, the message for their production seems to be stored through some form of molecular encoding, which is then difficult to reverse. Alterations in the chemical striatal output circuitry have been proposed as important pathogenic mechanisms, and stereotactic lesioning or deep brain stimulation in the thalamus or globus pallidus is the most effective remedy when the abnormal movements are incapacitating. Long-term, intermittent L-dopa therapy can lead to alterations in the balance of neuronal activity in the striatal output pathways to the globus pallidus. The direct striopallidal pathway, which is mainly regulated by D_1 dopamine receptors, contains the inhibitory neurotransmitter γ-aminobutyric acid (GABA), but it also colocalizes two neuropeptides, substance P and dynorphin. In contrast, the indirect pathway from the striatum to the globus pallidus external segment is predominantly regulated by D_2 receptors and colocalizes GABA and enkephalin (17). Alterations in activity of these output pathways have now been demonstrated using *in situ* hybridization techniques to measure mRNA neuropeptide expression. In the 1-methyl-4-phenyl-1,2,3,6-tetrahydropyridine (MPTP)-treated primate, a pronounced decrease in mRNA for preprotachykinin in the direct pathway and an increase in preproenkephalin in the indirect pathway are found. After L-dopa administration, the preprotachykinin decrease disappears, but there is no effect on the increased enkephalin expression (18). These findings have also been confirmed in L-dopa–treated patients with Parkinson's disease, in whom an additional diminution in GABA expression in the indirect pathway also occurs (19,20). Using positron emission tomography, Piccini and colleagues showed reduced putamen and thalamic opioid binding in dyskinetic, but not nondyskinetic, patients (21). These findings raise the possibility that continuing increased expression of enkephalin in the indirect striopallidal pathway after reversal of the substance P/dynorphin abnormality in the direct pathway may be an important trigger for the emergence of dyskinesias and suggests that drugs that could reduce enkephalin overexpression could be of potential interest as selective antidyskinetic agents. The capacity of pulsed intermittent long-term L-dopa administration to increase preprotachykinin expression back to normal, but not alter the excess preproenkephalin expression in animal models of Parkinson's disease, is not a property shared by all dopaminergic agonists, and some of the dopamine agonists have different effects (22). This finding is also of interest in view of the clinical observation that dopamine receptor agonists given to patients with *de novo* Parkinson's disease have an extremely low proclivity to introduce interdose dyskinesias (23). Furthermore, in the 6-hydroxydopamine rodent model, continuous steady-state levodopa administration restores neuropeptide levels much more closely to normal than does intermittent L-dopa administration (24). It is not known what effect long-term continuous apomorphine administration has on striatal neuropeptide expression, but it seems reasonable to assume that when administered as monotherapy, this approach may lead to a more tonic physiologic stimulation of the dopamine receptors than oral L-dopa therapy.

Clinical Results

These observations encouraged us to explore the additional role of continuous subcutaneous apomorphine monotherapy in antidyskinetic therapy. Since 1995, we have been attempting to increase the dyskinesia threshold in patients with fluctuating disease with distressing and disabling interdose chorea by slowly but relentlessly reducing all oral antiparkinsonian medication to nothing. Adjunctive drugs

such as oral agonists, selegiline, and anticholinergic drugs are first gradually withdrawn, and then L-dopa is tapered at a rate of about 50 mg daily per week, with concomitant increase in the apomorphine infusion rate. Not all patients can achieve complete withdrawal, and much encouragement and explanation of what is hoped to be achieved are needed to achieve success. Reductions in dyskinesias, with weight gain occurring in all patients over several months, are sustained for several years, provided the patient does not develop erratic absorption of apomorphine because of marked nodule formation, and oral L-dopa and subcutaneous apomorphine injections can be avoided (25). The results can be as striking as those achieved by pallidotomy without the associated morbidity. These results, confirmed by several groups, indicate that this approach should be offered as an alternative to functional neurosurgery to all patients with severe refractory "on-off" oscillations and L-dopa–induced dyskinesias. Apart from the development of abdominal wall panniculitis, the main long-term problem with this strategy is the emergence of neurobehavioral problems including hypersexuality and mania, paranoia, and excessive daytime somnolence (8).

ALTERNATIVE ROUTES OF APOMORPHINE ADMINISTRATION

Stocchi and colleagues used an implantable venous catheter into the superior vena cava (Portacath system) that was implanted using local anesthesia in eight patients who had benefited greatly from subcutaneous apomorphine but in whom the drug had become less effective after the development of abdominal wall nodules. Switching to the intravenous route restored an excellent and predictable response in all patients, with a marked decrease in "off" time. The catheter was changed routinely on an annual basis. Other benefits of the intravenous route were the efficacy and rapid onset of the booster device (26). We confirmed these findings in six patients with a mean age of 56 years and mean duration of Parkinson's disease of 14.5 years who had received subcutaneous apomorphine for 4.1 years. A mean reduction of "off" time of 58% occurred, with an average 57% reduction of adjunctive oral antiparkinsonian medication and a 3% reduction in apomorphine dose. In contrast to the study of Stocchi et al., however, there was a high incidence of complications, including postoperative wound infection, aggregation of apomorphine on the catheter tip, venous thrombosis, and translocation of the catheter tip. Four patients required relocation of the catheter. These serious complications mean that this approach should be used only with great caution, and further research is needed to determine whether the complications can be minimized by more frequent flushing of the catheter, echocardiographic screening of the catheter tip, and trials of less acidic—more dilute—apomorphine solutions (27). Patients' consistent observations of greater and more reliable motor response by the intravenous route, however, suggest that this approach to apomorphine use should be explored further. It may also be possible to use the intravenous route for 6 months, to allow the abdominal wall to recover, and then revert to the subcutaneous route. Programmable pump implantation inside the abdominal peritoneum is feasible in monkeys, with an outflow catheter inserted directly into a cerebral ventricle. Preliminary results indicate that apomorphine administered intracerebrally can reverse MPTP-induced akinesia. However, long-term toxicity remains a major potential problem with this route of administration, particularly because the therapeutic dose of apomorphine can be reduced only approximately twofold compared with the parenteral route (28); transdermal administration using iontophoresis at different current densities has also been explored. Although therapeutic effects can be seen without skin toxicity, it seems unlikely that high enough doses can be reliably delivered by this route (29).

CONCLUDING REMARKS

Long-term experience with continuous subcutaneous infusions of apomorphine has shown that this approach is a safe and effective treatment for severe L-dopa–induced fluctuations and peak-dose dyskinesias. In contrast to the currently available orally administered dopamine agonists, apomorphine is as potent as L-dopa even in the late stages of disease. As a result, with persistence and reassurance, it is often possible to withdraw L-dopa completely during the apomorphine infusion period, with marked reduction in refractory "off" periods and a gradual resetting of the dyskinesia threshold to higher than that needed for motor improvement. Trials have not yet taken place to see whether early therapy with apomorphine infusions could prevent the development of these complications. The level of disability can be pushed back by 2 to 5 years, and in some instances this can make the difference between a virtually independent existence at home and long-term residential care in a nursing home. The treatment is expensive, and it requires for its success continuous committed support from a medical team and nurse specialist, but the results can be as good as the best results seen with deep cerebral stimulation or lesioning of the globus pallidus or subthalamic nucleus. Although the pump is not acceptable to all patients, it should be available in specialized centers as a further therapeutic option to consider in the management of patients with late-stage L-dopa–treated Parkinson's disease.

REFERENCES

1. Neumeyer JL, Lal S, Baldessarini RJ. Historical highlights of the chemistry, pharmacology and early clinical uses of apomorphine. In: Gessa GL, Corsini GU, eds. *Basic pharmacology,* vol 1: *Apomorphine and other dopaminomimetics.* New York: Raven, 1981: 1–17.
2. Schwab RS, Amador LV, Lettvin YJ. Apomorphine in Parkinson's disease. *J Pharm Pharmacol* 1967;19:627–629.
3. Cotzias GC, Papavasiliou PD, Tolosa ES, et al. Treatment of Parkinson's disease with aporphines. *N Engl J Med* 1976;294:567–572.
4. Corsini GU, Del Zompo M, Gessa GL, et al. Therapeutic efficacy of apomorphine combined with an extracerebral inhibitor of dopamine receptors in Parkinson's disease. *Lancet* 1979;1:954–956.
5. Hardie RJ, Lees AJ, Stern GM. On-off fluctuations in Parkinson's disease: a clinical and neuropharmacological study. *Brain* 1984;107:487–506.
6. Lozano AM, Lang AE, Levy R, et al. Neuronal recordings in Parkinson's disease patients with dyskinesias induced by apomorphine. *Ann Neurol* 2000;47[Suppl 1]:S141–S146.
7. Stibe CM, Lees AJ, Stern GM. Subcutaneous infusion of apomorphine and lisuride in the treatment of Parkinson's disease. *Lancet* 1987;1:871.
8. Hughes AJ, Bishop S, Turjanski L, et al. Subcutaneous apomorphine in Parkinson's disease: response to chronic administration for up to five years. *Mov Disord* 1993;8:165–170.
9. Kempster PA, Frankel JP, Bovindon M, et al. Comparison of motor response to apomorphine and levodopa in Parkinson's disease. *J Neurol Neurosurg Psychiatry* 1990;53:1004–1007.
10. Frankel JP, Lees AJ, Kempster PA, et al. Subcutaneous apomorphine in the treatment of Parkinson's disease. *J Neurol Neurosurg Psychiatry* 1990;53:96–101.
11. Pollak P, Champay AS, Gaio JM, et al. Administration souscutanée dans les fluctuations motrices de la maladie de Parkinson. *Rev Neurol (Paris)* 1990;146:116–123.
12. Pietz K, Hagell P, Odin P. Subcutaneous apomorphine in late stage Parkinson's disease: a long term follow up. *J Neurol Neurosurg Psychiatry* 1998;65:709–716.
13. Wenning GK, Bosch S, Liginger E, et al. Effects of long-term, continuous subcutaneous apomorphine infusions on motor complications in advanced Parkinson's disease. *Adv Neurol* 1999;80:545–548.
14. Reuter I, Ellis CN, Ray Chaudhuri K. Nocturnal subcutaneous apomorphine infusion in Parkinson's disease and restless legs syndrome. *Acta Neurol Scand* 1999;100:163–167.
15. Kanovsky P, Kubova D, Hertova H, et al. Suppression of L-dopa–induced dyskinesias by subcutaneous infusions of apomorphine. In: *International Congress on Parkinson's Disease.* Vancouver, 1999 (abst).
16. Vanderheyden JE, Vesale B. Usefulness of apomorphine subcutaneous continuous infusion in severely disabling Parkinson's disease: short-term, long-term benefits and side-effects observed in 50 cases. In: *International Congress on Parkinson's Disease.* Vancouver, 1999 (abst).
17. Albin RL, Young AB, Penney JB. The functional anatomy of the basal ganglia disorders. *Trends Neurosci* 1989;12:36–374.
18. Herrero M, Augood SJ, Hirsch EC, et al. Effect of L-dopa on pre-proenkephalin and pre-protachykinin gene expression in the MPTP-treated monkey striatum. *Neuroscience* 1995;68:1189–1119.
19. Nisbet AP, Foster OJ, Kingsbury A, et al. Pre-proenkephalin and pre-protachykinin mRNA expression in normal human basal ganglia and in Parkinson's disease. *Neuroscience* 1995;6:361–376.
20. Nisbet AP, Eve DJ, Kingsbury A, et al. Glutamate decarboxylase-67 messenger RNA expression in normal human basal ganglia and in Parkinson's disease. *Neuroscience* 1996;75:389–406.

21. Piccini P, Weeks RA, Brooks DJ. Alterations in opioid receptor binding in Parkinson's disease patients with levodopa-induced dyskinesias. *Ann Neurol* 1997;42:720–726.

22. Jenner P. The rationale for the use of dopamine agonists in Parkinson's disease. *Neurology* 1995;4[Suppl 3]:S12.

23. Lees AJ, Stern GM. Sustained bromocriptine therapy in previously untreated patients with Parkinson's disease. *J Neurol Neurosurg Psychiatry* 1981;44:1020–1023.

24. Engber TM, Suzel Z, Juncos JL, et al. Continuous and intermittent levodopa differentially affect rotation induced by D_1 and D_2 dopamine agonists. *Eur J Pharmacol* 1989;168:291–298.

25. Colzi A, Turner K, Lees AJ. Continuous subcutaneous waking day apomorphine in the long-term treatment of levodopa induced interdose dyskinesias in Parkinson's disease. *J Neurol Neurosurg Psychiatry* 1998;64:573–576.

26. Stocchi F, Farina C, Nordera GP, et al. Implantable venous access systems for apomorphine infusion in complicated Parkinson's disease. *Mov Disord* 1999;14:358.

27. Manson AJ, Hanagasi H, Turner K, et al. Intravenous apomorphine therapy in Parkinson's disease. Clinical and Pharmacotinotic observations. *Brain* 2001;124:331–340.

28. Pollak P, Benabid AL, Limousin P, et al. External and implanted pumps for apomorphine infusion in Parkinsonism. *Acta Neurochir Suppl (Wien)* 1993;58:48–52.

29. van der Geest R, van Laar T, Gubens-Stibbe JM, et al. Iontophoretic delivery of apomorphine. II: an *in vivo* study in patients with Parkinson's disease. *Pharm Res* 1997;14:1804–1810.

Surgery for Parkinson's Disease and Movement Disorders,
edited by J.K. Krauss, J. Jankovic, and R.G. Grossman.
Lippincott Williams & Wilkins, Philadelphia © 2001.

22

STEREOTACTIC RADIOSURGERY IN THE TREATMENT OF PARKINSON'S DISEASE

GERHARD M. FRIEHS
BEVERLY C. WALTERS
VASILIOS ZERRIS

When Lars Leksell started developing the *gamma knife* in the 1950s, he was the first to realize the potential benefits of radiosurgery for functional disorders. As early as 1951, he used an orthovoltage x-ray tube to treat trigeminal neuralgia (1). In 1968, the gamma knife was introduced in its present form, and from that time forward, functional disorders of different types were treated on a routine basis. These disorders include obsessive compulsive disorder (2,3), trigeminal neuralgia (4), intractable pain (2,5–7), and movement disorders (6–22). Poor localization techniques dependent on pneumoencephalography initially led to disappointing results (17). This finding, coupled with the emergence of oral L-dopa therapy, caused general interest in neurosurgical treatment of Parkinson's disease (PD) to decrease dramatically. However, several more recent factors have contributed to the resurrection of neurosurgical and, specifically, radiosurgical treatment of PD, including severe side effects of long-term pharmacologic treatment of the disorder, such as bothersome dyskinesias. Other factors influencing the resurgence of interest in neurosurgical and radiosurgical treatment of PD include development of different targets for the treatment of different symptoms of PD and refinement in target localization techniques with the advent of computed tomography (CT) and magnetic resonance imaging (MRI). By the end of 1998, 814 cases of gamma knife treatment for PD had been reported worldwide to the gamma knife manufacturer from about 30 treatment centers (Elekta, personal communication).

GAMMA KNIFE TECHNIQUE

The gamma knife is a radiosurgical instrument that uses 201 cobalt-60 emitters as radiation sources that are arranged in a hemispheric array. The emitted radiation intersects at a fixed focus point (Fig. 22.1). To reach any given coordinate, the patient's head has to be moved about the focus. Therefore, a stereotactic frame has to be securely affixed to the patient's head, with markers provided for computation. It is desirable to approximate the frame angle to the plane of the anterior and posterior commissures (the AC-PC plane). For that purpose, the anterior margin of the frame is angled superiorly with respect to the posterior frame margin. An imaginary line between the lateral canthus and the external auditory canal is a good external landmark for this angulation so the imaging studies performed will be aligned parallel to the AC-PC plane without having to change the gantry angle of the imaging machine (Fig. 22.2A). For functional radiosurgery, MRI is preferable to CT for target localization because some of the target structures and many surrounding critical structures can be better visualized directly. It is of utmost importance to ensure that the distortion generated by any given MRI machine in combination with a stereotactic frame is within negligible limits. Ideally, as in most gamma knife centers, this quality assurance process is performed on a daily basis. This involves taking MRI images of a phantom in at least two planes and shimming of the MRI magnet if there is inaccuracy that is unacceptable. Typically, the highest geometric accuracy is found on axial images in which the distortion is in the 1-mm range. Coronal images have a slightly higher tendency for distortion, especially in the X-Z direction. Sagittal images are not recommended as a basis for treatment planning because they carry the highest risk of image distortion. Although different MRI sequences can be helpful, inversion recovery sequences in the axial and coronal planes with a slice thickness of 2 mm or less without interslice gaps are most useful in delineating the target area with its surrounding structures.

In a case report in which an 8-mm collimator was used for a radiosurgical thalamotomy (17), an unpredictably large

G.M. Friehs, B.C. Walters, and V. Zerris: Department of Clinical Neurosciences (Neurosurgery), Brown University School of Medicine, Providence, Rhode Island 02906.

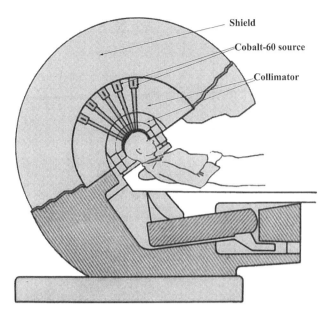

FIGURE 22.1. Schematic cross section through a gamma knife. The patient is in a supine position on the couch with the head fixed in a stereotactic frame *(not shown)* docked onto the inner (secondary) collimator helmet. The outer (primary) collimator contains the 201 radiation sources, which are arranged in a hemispheric array. The cobalt-60 sources are shielded externally by a thick steel cover.

lesion volume was created. A retrospective multicenter study on lesion sizes after functional radiosurgery demonstrated that more than one shot with the 4-mm collimator is potentially dangerous and advised against using this technique (23). Animal experiments have demonstrated that radiation

of less than 100 Gy does not produce necrosis in white or gray matter and therefore does not result in a visible lesion (24). Experience in human patients strongly indicates that a dose of less than 160 Gy with a 4-mm collimator is the safest way to perform functional radiosurgery and is very likely to result in a predictable lesion volume (23). Therefore, the current recommendation is to use single 4-mm collimator shots for radiosurgical treatment of PD. A maximum dose of 140 to 160 Gy is prescribed, and care is taken not to expose the surrounding critical structures to high levels of radiation. In pallidal radiosurgery, the 10% isodose line representing 14 to 16 Gy should barely touch the optic tract (Fig. 22.3A and B); the more radioresistant internal capsule can be touched by the 20% isodose line with 28 to 32 Gy (Fig. 22.2B and C). If necessary, the isodose configuration must be adapted by introducing certain plugging patterns in an attempt to drive the isodose lines away from critical structures (Fig. 22.3C and D). In a gamma knife unit with new cobalt-60 sources, treatment time for a typical thalamotomy or pallidotomy is approximately 1 hour. Aging of the cobalt sources naturally increases treatment time; it is doubled after 5 years of operation, which is the approximate half-life of cobalt-60. Treatment itself produces absolutely no pain. There are no immediate side effects; there is also no immediate primary therapeutic effect because the development of a radionecrotic lesion requires at least 4 to 6 weeks. After treatment and removal of the stereotactic frame, patients are typically kept in the hospital overnight. No evidence indicates that any medication in the immediate perioperative period such as dexamethasone is necessary or helpful.

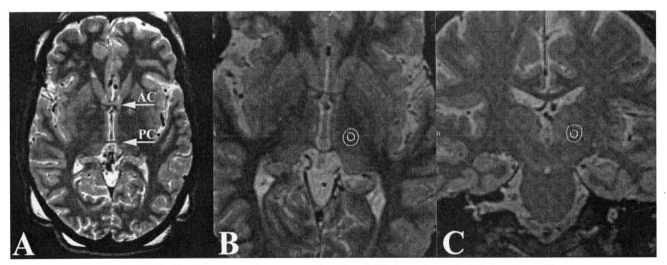

FIGURE 22.2. Planning magnetic resonance imaging (MRI) for radiosurgical thalamotomy. The axial MRI sections shown (**A** and **B**) are in the plane of the anterior commissure (AC) and posterior commissure (PC). The left ventrolateral thalamus is targeted (**B** and **C**) 2 mm superior to the AC-PC plane. The isodose distribution of the 80% (**B** and **C**; *inner circle*) and 20% (**B** and **C**; *outer circle*) isodose lines from a single 4-mm collimator shot are depicted. The internal capsule is barely touched by the 20% isodose line.

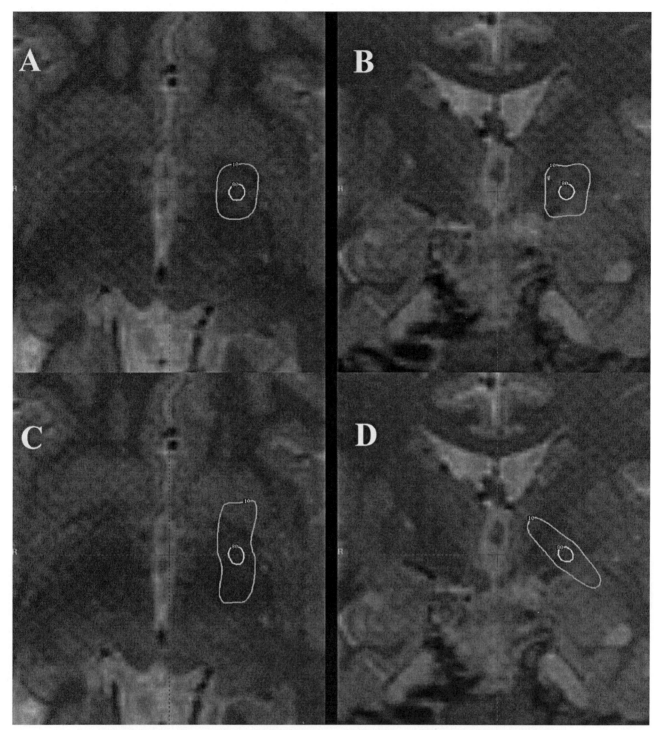

FIGURE 22.3. Planning magnetic resonance imaging (MRI) for radiosurgical pallidotomy. The 80% *(inner circle)* and 10% isodose line *(outer circle)* are outlined. The original plan with a single 4-mm collimator shot showed the 10% isodose line covering most of the optic tract (**A:** Axial MRI, inversion recovery [IR] sequence; **B:** coronal MRI, IR sequence). After introducing a plugging pattern to protect the optic apparatus, the isodose configuration was projected in a more favorable location with the 10% isodose line barely touching the optic tract. The appearance of the 80% isodose line is slightly more oval but unchanged in location. (**C:** Axial MRI, IR sequence, with plugging pattern; **D:** axial MRI, IR sequence, with plugging pattern).

TARGET STRUCTURES

The two targets commonly used for radiosurgery for PD are identical to the target areas employed for open functional stereotactic ablation or stimulation: the ventrolateral thalamus (VL) and the internal segment of the globus pallidum (GPi).

Thalamus

The posterior part of the VL, which is often identified as a separate subnucleus ventralis intermedius (VIM) according to older nomenclature, is found to be the best target for alleviation of tremor of the contralateral extremities (Figs. 22.2 and 22.4). Because the VIM area is not directly visible on MRI or CT images, it has to be determined through stereotactic calculations. Our target coordinates for VIM are approximately as follows:

- 4 to 8 mm anterior to the posterior commissure
- 12 to 16 mm lateral from the midline, which is 2 to 3 mm medial to the posterior limb of the internal capsule
- 0 to 2 mm above the AC-PC plane

Other areas in the main motor thalamic nucleus VL that have also been targeted are just anterior to the VIM. These areas correspond to the ventralis oralis posterior and ventralis oralis anterior nuclei.

Globus Pallidus Internal Segment

The GPi is located in a triangle described by the internal capsule medially, the optic tract inferiorly, and the external segment of the GP laterally (Fig. 22.5). The GPi itself and the surrounding structures are all visualized on coronal MRI images. Another method of defining the target area is to follow the guidelines given for open stereotactic pallidotomies. Briefly, the approximate coordinates are as follows:

- 3 mm anterior to the mid–AC-PC plane
- 18 to 21 mm lateral of the midline
- 3 to 6 mm inferior to the AC-PC plane

A radiosurgical lesion in the GPi after gamma knife pallidotomy is shown in Fig. 22.6.

Caudate Nucleus

In addition to these commonly used targets, a target in the caudate nucleus has also been used in patients with PD (11,12) (Fig. 22.7). The placement of a 4-mm collimator lesion at the base of the caudate nucleus head was reported to improve symptoms of PD. Although the goal of radiosurgical thalamotomy or pallidotomy is the destruction of tissue and interruption of pathways, the caudatotomy is believed to be a procedure that relies on tissue regeneration that follows a radiosurgical destructive lesion. The exact coordinates for the lesion were not reported, but placement of bilateral lesions into the most basal aspect of the head of the caudate nucleus has been recommended.

CLINICAL ASPECTS

Specific Indications

Indications for radiosurgical thalamotomy are the same as for open stereotactic ablative or stimulation procedures. Patients with tremor refractory to medication are good candidates for radiosurgical thalamotomy in the contralateral thalamic VIM. Moreover, lesions placed in the VIM region have been reported to alleviate contralateral rigidity (16), in addition to improving tremor. For parkinsonian rigidity, tremor, and bradykinesia, the GPi is the preferred target in radiosurgery. To date, no report has been published on radiosurgical lesioning of the subthalamic nucleus, which is reported to be the most promising target for neurostimulation therapy. The reports on radiosurgical caudate nucleus lesioning identified patients with non–tremor-dominant parkinsonism as good candidates for that treatment. The most significant improvements were seen in increased movement speed, in the ability to walk, and in improved independence in activities of daily living (12). As a general rule, radiosurgery can be performed irrespective of the general health of the patient, even in intubated patients. However, the technical limitations of radiosurgery preclude the use of the gamma knife in some patients. The Leksell stereotactic frame cannot accommodate extremely large head sizes. The cutoff limit is the equivalent of a hat size 61-62, which, in reality, is only very rarely encountered. Certain preexisting spinal deformities such as pronounced thoracic kyphosis or extreme cervical spinal immobility can make it difficult or even impossible to position the patient with the stereotactic frame in the MRI unit. In these circumstances, a noncontrast CT scan with very thin slices 1 mm thick can be obtained to identify the AC-PC plane. Determination of the target structure is then performed by relying on calculation of stereotactic coordinates based on stereotactic atlases alone.

Bilateral Surgery

Because functional radiosurgery is a tissue-destroying procedure, the same limitations identified for open stereotaxy apply to bilateral surgery. If bilateral radiosurgical thalamotomies, which have been described (11), are contemplated, the risk of side effects can be expected to increase significantly. This is especially true for the occurrence of dysarthria or hypophonia, both of which are known to be much more likely with bilateral thalamic lesions than with unilateral lesions. Staging of radiosurgical thalamotomies is recommended, with an interval of about 6 months between procedures (11). Bilateral pallidotomies have also been performed successfully with radiosurgery. The limiting factor here remains radiation exposure to the optic apparatus (20).

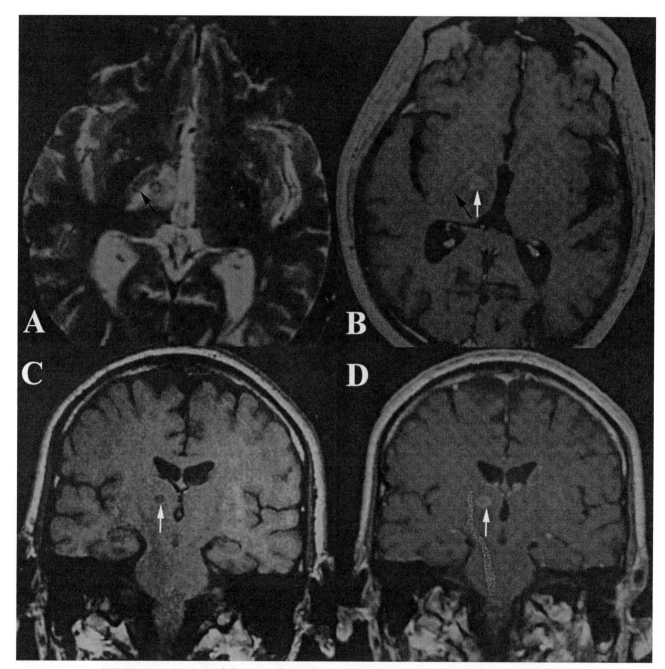

FIGURE 22.4. One-year follow up after radiosurgical gamma knife thalamotomy on the right side. **A:** Axial T2-weighted magnetic resonance imaging (MRI) showing the hypointense lesion with surrounding hyperintense signal involving most of the ventrolateral and anterior medial thalamus. Note the proximity of the lesion to the internal capsule *(black arrow)*. **B:** Axial T1-weighted MRI with contrast enhancement. Again, the lesion is noted *(white arrow)* in close proximity to, but without extension into, the internal capsule *(black arrow)*. **C:** Coronal T1-weighted MRI without contrast enhancement. The lesion *(white arrow)* appears as a hypointensity. **D:** Coronal T1-weighted MRI with contrast enhancement. The course of the corticospinal tract is outlined *(shaded area)* with the lesion just medial to it *(white arrow)*. Note the difference in lesion size compared with the noncontrast MRI **(C)**.

In the case of caudate lesioning, the procedures have always been performed bilaterally in a nonstaged design, without reports of morbidity.

Currently, there are two strong indications for stereotactic radiosurgery for PD, as follows:

1. Contraindication to open surgical procedures because of bleeding disorders, anticoagulation therapy, or very poor general health
2. The patient's explicit wish to have a noninvasive procedure performed

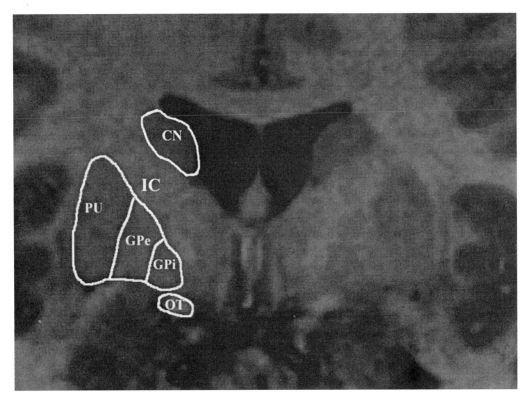

FIGURE 22.5. Higher-magnification inversion recovery (IR) magnetic resonance imaging sequence, coronal section, at the level of the mamillary bodies. The structures within the corpus striatum are directly visible. The optic tract is in direct contact with the medial globus pallidum (GPi). CN, caudate nucleus; GPe, globus pallidum external segment; GPi, globus pallidum internal segment; IC, internal capsule; OT, optic tract; PU, putamen.

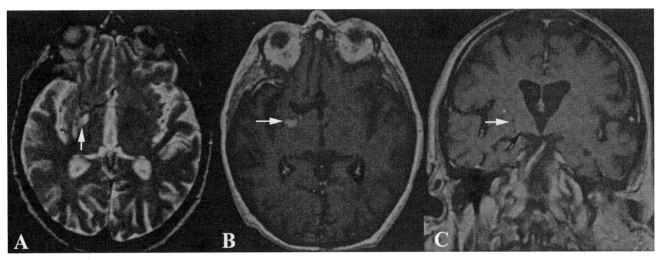

FIGURE 22.6. Follow-up after radiosurgical gamma knife pallidotomy on the right side. **A:** Axial T2-weighted magnetic resonance imaging (MRI), 1 year after radiosurgery, showing the lesion isointense to cerebrospinal fluid *(white arrow)*. There is visible hyperintense signal change around the lesion. **B:** Axial T1-weighted MRI with contrast enhancement, 1 year after treatment. The contrast-enhancing lesion is clearly identified *(white arrow)*. **C:** Coronal T1-weighted MRI with contrast enhancement, 2 years after gamma knife radiosurgery. The lesion *(white arrow)*, which is still slightly contrast enhancing, is close to the optic tract *(black arrow)*.

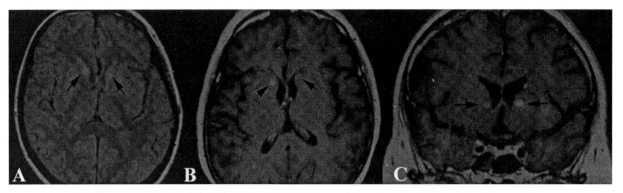

FIGURE 22.7. Magnetic resonance imaging (MRI) scans 6 months after bilateral caudate nucleus lesions. The axial proton density MRI **(A)** indicates some signal hyperintensity around the heads of the caudate nuclei. The lesions are brightly contrast enhancing, round areas located at the base of the caudate nucleus head. (**B**: Axial T1-weighted MRI with contrast enhancement; **C**: coronal T1-weighted MRI with contrast enhancement; the lesions are indicated by the *black arrows*).

In addition, nonscientific factors such as local availability of gamma knife units and patient or physician bias play a role in matching the appropriate patient to the ideal treatment modality. Unfortunately, insurance approval or denial for radiosurgery has influenced patient selection even further. There is a tremendous regional variation in the United States in insurance authorization for gamma knife treatment for PD; even federal insurance agencies have no uniform regulation or acceptance of the procedure.

Advantages and Disadvantages of Gamma Knife Radiosurgery

When radiosurgery is compared with open stereotactic ablative surgery (thalamotomy, pallidotomy) or neurostimulation (thalamic stimulation, pallidal stimulation, and subthalamic nucleus stimulation), the main difference observed is the less invasive nature of radiosurgery (Table 22.1). Although it is a lesion-generating procedure, it does not require

surgical penetration of the skull or brain tissues, and therefore there is no associated risk of infection or hemorrhage.

Side Effects of the Procedure

Complications or side effects from radiosurgical treatment are rare. There is a theoretic risk of developing radiation necrosis that could result in a lesion much larger than expected. This occurrence has been reported in the literature (8-mm collimator shot) (17). In this publication, the authors reported unexpectedly large treatment volumes after functional radiosurgery with an 8-mm collimator formerly used for functional procedures. With the currently used 4-mm collimators, this risk is more theoretic than real. Other specific risks of radiosurgical thalamotomy or pallidotomy are the same as for their open stereotactic equivalents and include damage to the optic tract resulting in visual field cuts and damage to the internal capsule with consequent hemiparesis or dysarthria. There have been no published

TABLE 22.1 ADVANTAGES AND DISADVANTAGES OF GAMMA KNIFE RADIOSURGERY IN COMPARISON WITH STEREOTACTIC RADIOFREQUENCY LESIONING AND DEEP BRAIN STIMULATION

	Radiosurgey	Stereotactic Radiofrequency Lesioning	Deep Brain Stimulation
Surgery type	Noninvasive	Invasive	Invasive
Modulation of effect	Irreversible; cannot be modified once lesion has been placed	Irreversible; cannot be modified once lesion has been placed	Fully reversible; can be modified through stimulator program
Onset of effect	Delayed by ~6 wk	Immediate	Immediate
Target areas	Thalamus; globus pallidum	Thalamus; globus pallidum; subthalamic nucleus	Thalamus; globus pallidum; subthalamic nucleus
Lesion visibility on magnetic resonance imaging	Visible contrast enhancement for years	Visible contrast enhancement for months	No lesion; electrode visible
Limitations	Basically none	Bleeding disorder; patient willing to undergo invasive procedure	Bleeding disorder; patient willing to undergo invasive procedure

reports or personal communications of mortality as a result of radiosurgical treatment of PD.

REVIEW OF OUTCOME

Problems in Assessment of Clinical Studies

In reviewing relevant literature to assess the ability of radiosurgical treatment of PD to achieve the desired outcomes, it is important to examine the published reports critically for study validity. Outcome studies, which are not randomized controlled trials, are generally longitudinal follow-up studies of patients treated with the intervention of interest. In other words, these are studies of patient prognosis with treatment. As such, the rules of evidence in effect for such studies apply. What this means is that the studies should conform to certain study design criteria that are meant to reduce or eliminate systematic or random error. Random error is usually avoided by the use of and adherence to a randomized study design, but because no such studies have been done with radiosurgical treatment of PD, prognosis with treatment studies are all that are available for determining outcome. Systematic error, or bias, is the influence of certain factors in a certain direction all the time. An example of systematic error would be the use of radiosurgery in only patients with the most refractory parkinsonism, after all else has failed. In this circumstance, the outcomes could be systematically shown to be poorer than those with treatments available to all patients regardless of previous treatment failures. Another bias could be introduced by patients who had long-standing PD with associated debilitation, both social and physical.

To diminish the effect of bias, certain criteria have been established by which articles of the highest quality are judged (25). These criteria are as follows.

- Patients should be studied from a uniform time in their disease, such as from the first diagnosis, point of refractoriness, time of development of intolerable side effects to pharmacologic treatments, and so forth, to form an "inception cohort."
- The severity of illness should be categorized, and objective outcome measures should be applied.
- Outcome assessment should be done in a blinded fashion or should be so completely objective that blinding is not necessary.
- Referral patterns should be defined; that is, is the reporting center one that receives the worst or the best patients, clinically speaking, or all patients suitable for the treatment?
- Follow-up of patients should be complete and for a reasonable period of time.
- Adjustment should be made (usually with multivariate analysis) for factors in the patient that could influence the outcome but that are extraneous to the PD, such

as cerebrovascular disease, other neurodegenerative disorders, cardiac disease, or malignant disease.

Literature Review

Using these criteria, a review of the literature on gamma knife radiosurgery for treatment of PD was conducted. The search terms used were "parkinsonism and radiosurgery" and "parkinsonism and gamma knife." Additional articles were found by examining the reference lists in the articles identified in this primary search. Each of these articles was evaluated, and those not pertaining to the question of interest, that is, outcomes of radiosurgery for PD, were discarded. All articles reporting experience with five or more patients were included. This left a total of nine articles for critical appraisal of study quality and for deriving an understanding of the expected outcomes of treatment with radiosurgery for PD. The critical evaluation of the methodologic quality of these studies applying the established rules of evidence listed earlier is shown in Table 22.2.

Generally, the patients treated with radiosurgery were those who chose this route over a more invasive approach or those who could not be treated with open surgical procedures because of the presence of factors contraindicating invasive treatment, as described earlier. They were patients who had demonstrated refractoriness to medical management, who had intolerable side effects to medication, who could not be treated with radiofrequency lesioning because of, for example, advanced age or anticoagulant use, who elected to undergo gamma knife radiosurgery. Outcome measures reported included radiographic findings such as lesion size (23) and postoperative intracerebral hemorrhage (22), clinical improvement using the Unified Parkinson Disease Rating Scale (26) or Hoehn and Yahr stage ratings (27), neurologic deficit such as homonymous hemianopia or behavioral changes including confusion, disorientation, somnolence, and combativeness (22), and mild symptoms such as headache (11). Sometimes, clinical improvement was described in the form of testimonials; for example, "Her energy level has improved and speech is stronger. She is very happy about the operation" (19). Others included descriptors such as "improvement" or "tremor-free" without using recognized objective measures of outcomes.

Those articles that met most of the criteria applied indicated that, overall, gamma knife radiosurgery is effective and safe. With respect to relief of the symptoms under treatment, 88% to 90% of patients with tremor, 85% of patients with dyskinesias, and 65% of patients with bradykinesias or rigidity improved, using objective, blinded, or independent outcome measurements (20). Complications were rare; a single patient was reported with homonymous hemianopia, and no patients exhibited cognitive worsening (20). Another patient experienced delayed-onset dysarthria, which remained permanent (9).

TABLE 22.2 CRITICAL EVALUATION OF THE PERTINENT LITERATURE ON PROGNOSIS WITH GAMMA KNIFE RADIOSURGERY FOR TREATMENT OF PARKINSON'S DISEASE

Author (yr)	No. Patients with Parkinsonism	Inception Cohort	Referral Pattern Described	Complete Follow-up Achieved	Objective Outcome Criteria	Outcome of Assessment Blinded	Extraneous Variables Adjusted for
Rand et al. (1993)	15	Unknown	No	Unknown	No: testimonial descriptive terminology	No	No
Friehs et al. (1995)	12	Unknown	No	Yes	Yes: UPDRS, videos	No	No
Ohye et al. (1996)	6	Unknown	No	Unknown	No: testimonial, descriptive terminology	No	No
Pan et al. (1996)	8	Usual indications for gamma knife	No	6/8 (75%)	No: testimonial, descriptive terminology	No	No
Young et al. (1996)	20	Unknown	No	Unknown	No: descriptive terminology	No	No
Young (1996)	5	Unknown	No	Unknown	No: descriptive terminology	No	No
Friehs et al. (1997)	10	Unknown	No	Unknown	Yes: UPDRS, Hoehn and Yahr, videos, independent assessment	No	No
Duma et al. (1998)	34	Usual indications for gamma knife	No	Unknown	Yes: UPDRS	Unknown: "independent neurologist" evaluation	No
Young et al. (1998)	44	Unknown	No	Unknown	Yes: UPDRS, Hoehn and Yahr	Yes	No
Young et al. (1998)	29	Usual indications for gamma knife	No	Yes	Yes: UPDRS, Hoehn and Yahr	Yes	No
Duma et al. (1999)	56	Usual indications for gamma knife; excluded from radiofrequncy	No	Unknown	Yes: UPDRS	Unknown: "independent neurologist" evaluation	No

UPDRS, Unified Parkinson's Disease Rating Scale.

CONCLUSIONS AND RECOMMENDATIONS

Gamma knife radiosurgery for PD is a valid alternative to open stereotactic ablation or deep brain stimulation therapy. Based on the literature reviewed, gamma knife treatment is far from experimental. In the United States, studies such as randomized controlled trials are hardly feasible when there are reimbursement restrictions such as those described earlier. Resolution of this problem would facilitate the development of multicenter studies of large numbers of patients and would thereby elucidate the relative roles of each currently available treatment for PD. Such high-quality experimental research should be the goal of the twenty-first century.

REFERENCES

1. Leksell L. The stereotactic method and radiosurgery of the brain. *Acta Chir Scand* 1951;102:316–319.
2. Leksell L. Cerebral radiosurgery. I. Gamma thalamotomy in two cases of intractable pain. *Acta Chir Scand* 1968;134:585–595.
3. Kihlstrom L, Guo WY, Lindquist C, et al. Radiobiology of radiosurgery for refractory anxiety disorders. *Neurosurgery* 1995;36:294–302.
4. Kondziolka D, Lundsford LD, Flickinger JC, et al. Stereotactic radiosurgery for trigeminal neuralgia: a multi-institutional study using the gamma unit. *J Neurosurg* 1996;84:940–945.
5. Steiner L, Forster D, Leksell L, et al. Gamma thalamotomy in intractable pain. *Acta Neurochir (Wien)* 1980;52:173–184.
6. Young RF. Functional neurosurgery with the Leksell gamma knife. *Stereotact Funct Neurosurg* 1996;66:19–23.
7. Young RF. Functional disease of the brain: treatment by gamma knife radiosurgery. In: DeSalles AAF LR, ed. *Minimally invasive therapy of the brain.* New York: Thieme, 1997:225–234.
8. Duma CM, Jacques DB, Kopyov OV, et al. Gamma knife radiosurgery for thalamotomy in parkinsonian tremor: a five-year experience. *J Neurosurg* 1998;88:1044–1049.
9. Duma CM, Jacques D, Kopyov OV. The treatment of movement disorders using gamma knife stereotactic radiosurgery. *Neurosurg Clin North Am* 1999;10:379–389.
10. Friedman JH, Epstein M, Sanes JN, et al. Gamma knife pallidotomy in advanced Parkinson's disease. *Ann Neurol* 1996;39:535–538.
11. Friehs GM, Ojakangas CL, Pachatz P, et al. Thalamotomy and caudatotomy with the gamma knife as a treatment for parkinsonism with a comment on lesion sizes. *Stereotact Funct Neurosurg* 1995;64:209–221.
12. Friehs GM, Ojakangas CL, Schrottner O, et al. Radiosurgical lesioning of the caudate nucleus as a treatment for parkinsonism: a preliminary report. *Neurol Res* 1997;19:97–103.
13. Pendl G, Schrottner O, Friehs GM, et al. Radiosurgery with the first Austrian cobalt-60 gamma unit: a one year experience. *Acta Neurochir (Wien)* 1994;127:170–179.
14. Hirato M, Ohye C, Shibazaki T, et al. Gamma knife thalamotomy for the treatment of functional disorders. *Stereotact Funct Neurosurg* 1995;64:164–171.
15. Ohye C, Shibazaki T, Hirato M, et al. Gamma thalamotomy for parkinsonian and other kinds of tremor. *Stereotact Funct Neurosurg* 1996;66:333–342.
16. Li P, Dai JZ, Wang BJ, et al. Stereotactic gamma thalamotomy for the treatment of parkinsonism. *Stereotact Funct Neurosurg* 1996;66:329–332.
17. Lindquist C, Steiner L, Hindmarsh T. Gamma knife thalamotomy for tremor: report of two cases. In: Steiner L, ed. *Radiosurgery: baseline and trends.* New York: Raven, 1992:237–243.
18. Otsuki T, Jokura H, Takahashi K, et al. Stereotactic gamma-thalamotomy with a computerized brain atlas: technical case report. *Neurosurgery* 1994;35:764–767.
19. Rand RW, Jacques DB, Melbye RW, et al. Gamma knife thalamotomy and pallidotomy in patients with movement disorders: preliminary results. *Stereotact Funct Neurosurg* 1993;61:65–92.
20. Young RF, Shumway-Cook A, Vermeulen SS, et al. Gamma knife radiosurgery as a lesioning technique in movement disorder surgery. *J Neurosurg* 1998;89:183–193.
21. Young RF, Vermeulen SS, Grimm P, et al. Electrophysiological target localization is not required for the treatment of functional disorders. *Stereotact Funct Neurosurg* 1996;66:309–319.
22. Young RF, Vermeulen SS, Posewitz A, et al. Pallidotomy with the gamma knife: a positive experience. *Stereotact Funct Neurosurg* 1998;70:218–228.
23. Friehs GM, Noren G, Ohye C, et al. Lesion size following gamma knife treatment for functional disorders. *Stereotact Funct Neurosurg* 1996;66:320–328.
24. Kondziolka D, Lundsford LD, Claassen D, et al. Radiobiology of radiosurgery. I. The normal rat brain model. *Neurosurgery* 1992;31:271–279.
25. Sackett DL, Hellstrand E, Tugwell PX. *Clinical epidemiology: a basic science for clinical medicine.* Toronto: Little, Brown, 1985.
26. Fahn S, Elton RL, members of the UPDRS Development Committee. Unified Parkinson's Disease Rating Scale. In: Fahn S, Marsden C, Goldstein M, eds. *Recent developments in Parkinson's disease,* 2nd ed. New York: Macmillan, 1987:153–163.
27. Hoehn MM, Yahr MD. Evaluation of the long term results of surgical therapy. In: Gillingham FJ, Donaldson IML, eds. *Third symposium on Parkinson's disease.* Edinburgh: E & S Livingstone, 1969:274–280.

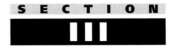

TREMOR DISORDERS

Surgery for Parkinson's Disease and Movement Disorders,
edited by J.K. Krauss, J. Jankovic, and R.G. Grossman.
Lippincott Williams & Wilkins, Philadelphia © 2001.

23

THALAMOTOMY FOR TREATMENT OF ESSENTIAL TREMOR

KEVIN A. WALTER
JUNG-IL LEE
FREDERICK A. LENZ

Essential tremor is a relatively common movement disorder, affecting 415 per 100,000 persons older than the age of 40 years (1). It is marked by a low-frequency tremor (4 to 8 Hz) that is precipitated by volitional movement, but it often disappears on repose (2). The tremor preferentially affects the upper extremities, with the head and lower extremities affected to lesser extents. Although the origin of the phenomenon is not well understood, a familial form of the disease does exist (1,2). It is transmitted in an autosomal dominant pattern with high penetrance in such cases.

Investigations into the neurophysiologic mechanisms underlying essential tremor have taken several pathways. Animal studies with β-carboline drugs such as harmaline produce a tremor similar to essential tremor (3,4). Harmaline-induced tremor has been shown to originate in the inferior olive and to be expressed through the cerebellobulbospinal pathways. Studies with positron emission tomography have shown that the cerebellum, contralateral red nucleus, thalamus, and sensorimotor cortex show overactivity in essential tremor (5). Additionally, surgical lesions performed in the ventralis intermedius (VIM) nucleus of the thalamus have controlled tremor in these patients, a finding implicating the role of thalamocortical connections in essential tremor (6–8).

Thalamic single neuron activity recorded during thalamotomy has been compared with forearm electromyographic (EMG) activity (Fig. 23.1) (9). These studies indicate that thalamic cells have tremor frequency firing patterns that are linearly related to forearm EMG signals during essential tremor. Three models could account for this correlation: thalamic activity drives EMG activity, thalamic activity is driven by sensory input generated by tremor movement, or an oscillator outside the thalamus drives both thalamic

and EMG activity. Because surgical lesions in the thalamus abolish tremor (6–8), it would seem most likely that some population of thalamic cells is responsible for driving the tremor (9).

INDICATIONS

Stereotactic thalamotomy has been employed for patients with disabling tremors in whom medical treatment has failed or who are unable to tolerate medical therapy (6–8). Approximately two-thirds of patients have satisfactory control of their condition with first-line therapy consisting of β-blockers and anxiolytics; approximately one-third of patients are candidates for surgical therapy (1).

The average functional status of patients with essential tremor undergoing stereotactic thalamotomy in our institution is outlined in Table 23.1 (6). The functional measure was obtained by grading speech, hygiene, eating, drinking, dressing, writing, and work separately from 1 to 4 where 1 was normal activity and 4 represented maximal assistance. A score of 28 represented complete dependence. Writing, drawing, and straight-line tests were administered and graded, by a blinded assessor, from 0 to 4 where 4 indicated inability to complete the task. The three scores were added together to obtain the composite writing score out of 12. Postural tremor amplitude and action tremor amplitude were rated by the surgeon where 0 was no tremor and 4 was more than 2 cm of tremor amplitude. Examples of preoperative and postoperative drawing samples are given in Fig. 23.2. Overall, the average patient was moderately disabled by tremor before coming to surgical treatment.

TARGET POINTS

To target the thalamic neurons involved in tremor, initial coordinates are taken from radiographic studies. The anterior

K.A. Walter and F.A. Lenz: Department of Neurosurgery, Johns Hopkins Hospital, Baltimore, Maryland 21287-7713.

J-I Lee: Department of Neurosurgery, Samsung Medical Center, Sungkyunkwan University School of Medicine, Seoul 135-710 Korea.

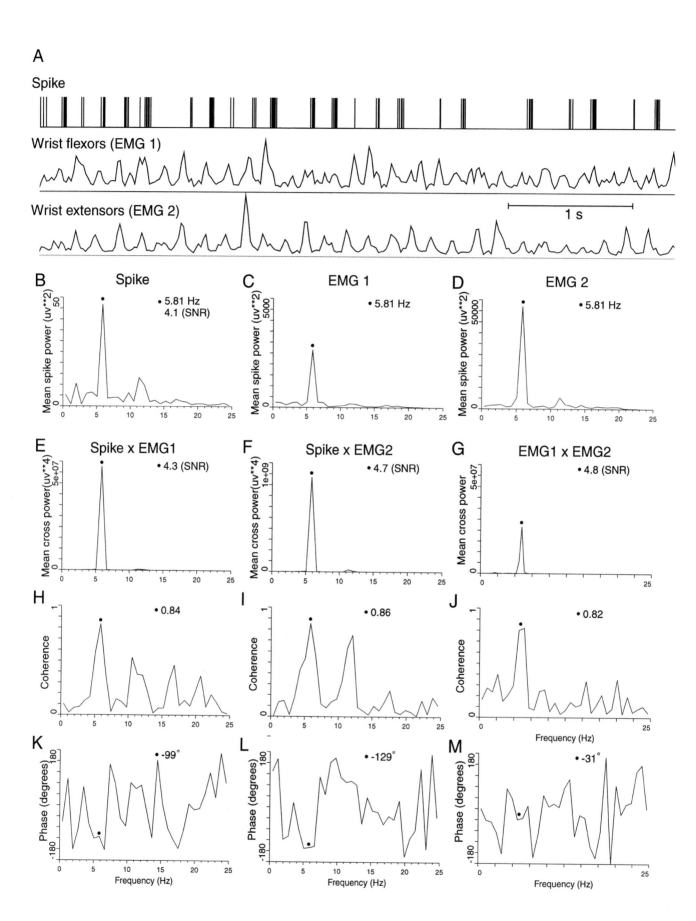

TABLE 23.1. TOTAL FUNCTIONAL, BLINDED HANDWRITING/DRAWING, AND AMPLITUDE (ACTION AND POSTURE) SCORES FOR 21 PATIENTS WITH ESSENTIAL TREMOR BEFORE AND AFTER UNILATERAL THALAMOTOMY[a]

Average Score Mean (SD)	Functional	Blinded Handwriting/ Drawing	Postural Tremor Amplitude	Action Tremor Amplitude
Preoperative	13.4 (1.8)	6.3 (0.7)	3.0 (0.3)	3.5 (0.2)
Postoperative: 3 mo	4.7 (1.5)	2.8 (0.4)	0.7 (0.4)	0.6 (0.4)
Postoperative: 1 yr	4.5 (1.3)	2.9 (0.3)	0.9 (0.4)	0.6 (0.4)
Significance				
Preoperative versus 3 mo	$p < .001$	$p < .001$	$p < .05$	$p < .05$
Preoperative versus 3 mo	$p < .001$	$p < .001$	$p < .05$	$p < .05$

[a]For scoring, see text.
From Zirh AT, Reich SG, Dougherty PM, et al. Stereotactic thalamotomy in the treatment of essential tremor of the upper extremity: reassessment including a blinded measure of outcome. *J Neurol Neurosurg Psychiatry* 1999;66:772–775, with permission.

commissure–posterior commissure (AC-PC) line is delineated by either computed tomography or magnetic resonance imaging while the patient's head is held in a stereotactic frame. One study suggested that the optimal target for thalamotomy in parkinsonian tremor is the site where cells with tremor activity are located (10). In a group of patients with parkinsonism, this site was located 2 mm anterior to the principal sensory nucleus and 3 mm above the AC-PC line (10).

Other approaches have been applied to define the optimal site for thalamotomy as well. Lesions have been placed anterior to the site at which evoked potentials can be recorded in response to cutaneous stimulation of the fingers (11). Lesions have been made in the region where electrical stimulation produces effects on tremor and anterior to the region where electrical stimulation evokes sensations (12). Finally, lesions have been made in the region where cells respond to somatosensory stimulation of muscle, joint, and tendon and where electrical stimulation produces effects on tremor (13).

Our approach has been to define the position of the ventral caudal nucleus (6,10,14,15), identified as the region where most cells exhibit small, well-circumscribed receptive fields to manual somatosensory stimulation. The region anterior to this location is then explored to locate sites where tremor-related neuronal discharges can be recorded (16). Lesions are made among these tremor related cells using radiofrequency coagulation (10). Our technique produces

individual lesions with a radius of 2.0 and 5.0 mm with a volume of 60 mL. Lesions of these volumes have been shown to achieve good tremor control in patients with relatively low-amplitude tremors such as parkinsonian or essential tremor, whereas larger lesions were said to be required in patients with tremors resulting from cerebrovascular or posttraumatic causes. Figure 23.3 shows a lesion 1 day after surgical treatment (17) in a patient who underwent left VIM stereotactic thalamotomy for essential tremor at our institution.

CLINICAL RESULTS

The results of several large clinical series of stereotactic thalamotomy for essential tremor have been published (Table 23.2). Although these studies have been conducted using different intraoperative protocols, each has demonstrated that most patients undergoing the procedure experience a significant reduction in tremor. Furthermore, this tremor control is maintained for extended periods (10 years or more).

Nagaseki et al. reported the outcome for 43 patients undergoing stereotactic lesioning of the VIM thalamic nucleus between August 1975 and April 1982 (18). Of these patients, 16 had essential tremor, whereas the remainder had Parkinson's disease. In patients with essential tremor, the authors

←

FIGURE 23.1. Simultaneous recording of thalamic single neuron activity and peripheral electromyography (EMG) during tremor in a patient with essential tremor. **A:** Digitized spike train **(upper trace)** and demodulated EMG channels **(lower two traces)**. **B:** Smoothed spike autopower spectrum of the spike train illustrated in **A. C:** and **D:** Smoothed autopower spectra for the two demodulated EMG channels. The *dot* indicates the frequency at which the maximum spectral component occurs in the EMG autopower spectrum, that is, tremor frequency (5.81 Hz). **E–F:** Cross-power spectra; **H–J:** coherence spectra; and **K–M:** phase spectra between spike×EMG1, spike×EMG2, and EMG1×EMG2, respectively. The numbers to the *right* of the spectra indicate the frequency with highest autopower **(B–D)** and the value at tremor frequency of cross-power SNR **(E–G)**, coherence **(H–J)**, and phase **(K–M)**. (From Hua S, Lenz FA, Zirh TA, et al. Thalamic activity correlated with essential tremor. *J Neurol Neurosurg Psychiatry* 1998;64:273–276, with permission.)

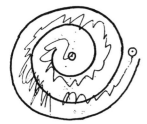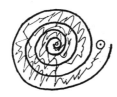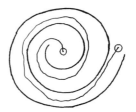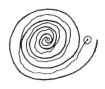

FIGURE 23.2. Sample drawing tasks performed preoperatively **(A)** and 1 year postoperatively **(B)** in a right-handed patient undergoing left ventralis intermedius stereotactic thalamotomy for essential tremor.

reported complete abolition of tremor in 11 patients and significant reduction of tremor in the remaining five patients. One patient subsequently underwent a contralateral procedure, and one patient had a recurrence and had a second procedure on the same side. Fifteen of 16 patients returned to work, and 11 patients were able to discontinue their pharmacologic therapy. The mean follow-up period for this series was 6.25 years.

Although these authors did not segregate their complications between patients with essential tremor and those with Parkinson's disease, it is likely that the complication rate for the two indications was similar (18). Among the 43 patients treated, three long-term residual deficits were encountered. Two patients experienced persistent dysarthria, and one pa-

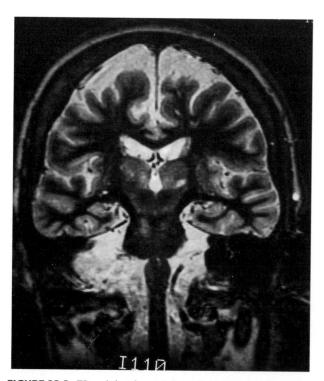

FIGURE 23.3. T2-weighted coronal magnetic resonance imaging scan at the level of the thalamus. The scan was obtained on postoperative day 1 in a patient undergoing stereotactic thalamotomy for essential tremor. The lesion is demonstrated by the hyperintense *(white)* signal in the ventrolateral thalamus.

tient experienced perioral numbness. Five patients who had contralateral weakness and five who experienced cerebellar signs saw their symptoms resolve in the immediate postoperative period.

Mohadjer et al. reported on 105 patients with essential tremor operated on between 1964 and 1984 at the University of Freiburg, Germany (19). The anatomic target was the zona incerta either alone or in combination with other target points. These surgeons reported a 93.7% improvement in tremor control in the immediate postoperative period. A follow-up questionnaire was sent to all 105 patients, with a mean follow-up period of 8.6 years. Of the 65 patients who responded, 68.7% believed that they were still enjoying a significant benefit from the surgery; however, nine patients experienced persistent side effects. Five patients had contralateral weakness, one had dysarthria, and three showed signs of cerebellar dysfunction.

In a series of 60 patients undergoing stereotactic thalamotomy for tremor, Jankovic et al. reported on six patients with essential tremor (7). These investigators targeted the VIM-thalamus in all six patients. Outcome was determined based on a global scale measuring improvement in tremor, and functional status ranged from 0 (no effect) to 4 (marked improvement in movement disorder and function). The mean outcome for essential tremor patients was 3.3, corresponding to a moderate improvement in tremor and functional status with a mean follow-up of 59.2 months. Overall, 83% (five of six) of patients experienced improvements in their tremor. Complications of the procedure in these 60 patients included persistent contralateral weakness (nine patients); dysarthria (six patients); increased ipsilateral tremor (one patient); blepharospasm (one patient); and death due to pulmonary embolism (one patient).

Eight patients were treated for essential tremor at the Mayo Clinic in Rochester, Minnesota from 1984 to 1991 (8). Preoperative and postoperative assessments were made for each patient with regard to disability in handwriting, speaking, feeding, hygiene, dressing, and working. Maximum disability represented a score of 28, and minimum disability was scored as 0. The mean follow-up was 17.3 months postoperatively. All eight patients experienced improvement postoperatively. The mean disability score was reduced from 21.1 preoperatively to 3.9 postoperatively. Furthermore, voice tremor

TABLE 23.2 CLINICAL SERIES OF STEREOTACTIC THALAMOTOMY FOR ESSENTIAL TREMOR

Author (yr)	No. Patients	% Marked Improvement	Follow-up (yr)	Complications
Nagaseki et al. (1986)	16	100%	6.5	2/43[a] dysarthria 1/43[a] perioral numbness 5/43[a] transient hemiparesis
Mohadjer et al. (1990)	105	68.7%	8.6	1 dysarthria 5 hemiparesis 3 ataxia
Jankovic et al. (1995)	6	83%	4.9	9/60[a] hemiparesis 6/60[a] dysarthria 1/60[a] blepharospasm 1/60[a] death
Goldman and Kelly (1992)	8	100%	1.5	2 dysarthria 1 cognitive verbal deficit
Zirh et al. (1999)	21	100%	1	1 perioral numbness 2 dysarthria 1 ataxia

[a]The number of complications refers to the total number of patients in these reports including patients with Parkinson's disease.

was abolished or was significantly improved in 71.4% of patients. Two patients had persistent dysarthria, and one had a verbal cognitive deficit after the operation.

We employed a similar disability scale to report the outcome of 21 patients treated at the Johns Hopkins Hospital in Baltimore between 1990 and 1993 (6). We achieved a reduction in mean functional disability score from 13.4 preoperatively to 4.5 postoperatively, with a follow-up of 1 year in all patients. Patients experienced significant improvements in all the categories tested (tremor amplitude, blinded assessment of handwriting/drawing, functional disability). In these 21 patients, complications of the operation were persistent perioral numbness (one patient); mild dysequilibrium (one patient); and cerebellar dysarthria (two patients).

ALTERNATIVES

The primary alternative to stereotactic VIM thalamotomy for essential tremor is implantation of *deep brain stimulating electrodes* (DBS) into the VIM. Although thalamotomy produces good tremor control for this condition, it was postulated that using stimulation rather than thermal coagulation would reduce the frequency of the long-term side effects of these procedures. Unlike the radiofrequency lesion of thalamotomy, which is permanent, DBS can be adapted to tailor the stimulation patterns to match the patient's symptoms and clinical concerns (20,21). By reducing, modifying, or stopping stimulation, unpleasant or disabling side effects can be reduced or eliminated. This is particularly advantageous for bilateral procedures in which the incidence of dysarthria approaches 30% to 60% of patients postoperatively (6–8).

Tasker et al. retrospectively reviewed their case series of DBS implants and thalamotomies for both Parkinson's disease and essential tremor (22). Because of the small number of patients with essential tremor in each series, the results were evaluated pooled with the patients with parkinsonism. These investigators reported complete abolition of tremor in 42% of both groups and near abolition of tremor in 79% of patients who had DBS and 69% of patients who underwent thalamotomy. Tremor recurrence was 5% in the DBS-treated patients and 15% in the thalamotomy-treated group. Ataxia, dysarthria, and gait disturbance occurred in 42% of the thalamotomy-treated patients and 26% of the DBS-treated patients; 15% of patients required a repeat thalamotomy, but none required a second DBS procedure. Based on these results, the authors concluded that DBS and thalamotomy produce equivalent degrees of tremor control, but DBS produces these results with less morbidity. However, several authors have reported a lower complication rate for thalamotomy than the 42% mentioned by Tasker, and this study was neither prospective nor randomized.

Additionally, implantation of a stimulating electrode includes the long-term maintenance of the stimulator. The burden of this maintenance can be estimated from large single-institution studies of DBS (141 patients followed-up over 20 years) (23) and spinal cord stimulation for the treatment of pain (249 patients followed-up over 14 years) (24). The accumulated complications in these studies included infection, erosion, foreign body reaction, lead fracture, and stimulator failure. The total morbidity rate in the two studies was 17% and 36%. In their most recent review (117 patients followed-up over 8 years), Benabid et al. noted complications of this type in 7% of cases (20). This lower

Functional Scores

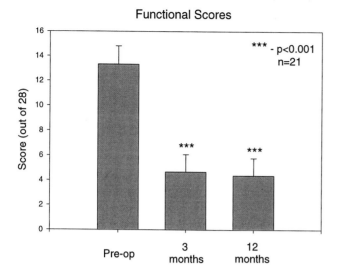

Blinded Writing and Drawing Scores

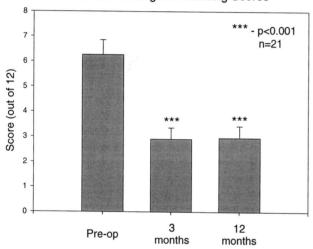

FIGURE 23.4. Preoperative and postoperative functional scores in patients undergoing stereotactic thalamotomy for essential tremor. **A:** Global function scores graded 0 to 28 for handwriting, postural tremor amplitude, and action tremor amplitude. **B:** Subset of handwriting and drawing scores comprising part of the overall global function score given in **A.** Stereotactic thalamotomy significantly improved both global functioning and handwriting/drawing ability (n = 21; p < . 001).

figure may result from technical improvement, or it may reflect the shorter follow-up in that study. Finally, there are the cost and inconvenience of readjusting the stimulator at intervals and of changing the battery at 3- to 5-year intervals. For all these reasons, the cost and inconvenience of VIM DBS are higher than those of thalamotomy. However, it is clearly the preferred procedure when bilateral procedures are required because of the high morbidity rate of bilateral thalamotomy.

CONCLUSION

Stereotactic VIM thalamotomy produces good long-term tremor control among patients with essential tremor in whom medical therapy has failed. Its primary advantage over DBS is the lack of costly implanted hardware that must be maintained and is subject to infection, wound breakdown, or irritation. However, it may carry a slightly higher risk of permanent neurologic deficit as has been shown in the study of Schuurman and Colleagues (25). In the interim, however, it appears that DBS is advantageous for at least one side of a bilateral procedure to reduce the risk of speech disturbance.

ACKNOWLEDGMENTS

This work is supported by grants to FAL from the Eli Lilly Corporation and the National Institutes of Health (NS28598, P01 NS32386-Proj. 1, NS 40059, R0 1NS38493).

REFERENCES

1. Koller WC, Busenbark KL. Essential tremor. In: Watts RL, Koller WC, eds. *Movement disorders.* New York: McGraw-Hill, 1997:365–386.
2. Elble RJ, Koller W. *Tremor.* Baltimore: Johns Hopkins University Press, 1990.
3. Lamarre Y. Central mechanisms of experimental tremor and their clinical relevance. In: Findley LJ, Capildeo R, eds. *Handbook of tremor disorders.* New York: Marcel Dekker, 1995:103–118.
4. Elble RG. The pathophysiology of tremor. In: Watts RL, Koller WC, eds. *Movement disorders.* New York: McGraw Hill, 1997:405–417.
5. Jenkins IH, Bain PB, Colebatch JG, et al. A positron emission tomography study of essential tremor: evidence of overactivity of cerebellar connections. *Ann Neurol* 1993;34:82–90.
6. Zirh AT, Reich SG, Dougherty PM, et al. Stereotactic thalamotomy in the treatment of essential tremor of the upper extremity: re-assessment including a blinded measure of outcome. *J Neurol Neurosurg Psychiatry* 1999;66:772–775.
7. Jankovic J, Cardoso F, Grossman RG, et al. Outcome after stereotactic thalamotomy for parkinsonian, essential and other types of tremor. *Neurosurgery* 1995;37:680–687.
8. Goldman MS, Kelly PJ. Symptomatic and functional outcome of stereotactic ventralis lateralis thalamotomy for intention tremor. *J Neurosurg* 1992;77:223–229.
9. Hua S, Lenz FA, Zirh TA, et al. Thalamic activity correlated with essential tremor. *J Neurol Neurosurg Psychiatry* 1998;64:273–276.
10. Lenz FA, Normand SL, Kwan HC, et al. Statistical prediction of the optimal lesion site for thalamotomy in parkinsonian tremor. *Mov Disord* 1995;10:318–328.
11. Kelly PJ, Derome P, Guiot G. Thalamic spatial variability and the surgical results of lesions placed with neurophysiologic control. *Surg Neurol* 1976;9:307–315.
12. Tasker RR, Organ LW, Hawrylyshyn P. *The thalamus and midbrain*

in man: a physiologic atlas using electrical stimulation. Springfield, IL: Charles C Thomas, 1982.

13. Ohye C, Fukamachi A, Miyazaki M, et al. Physiologically controlled selective thalamototomy for the treatment of abnormal movement by Leksell's open method. *Acta Neurochir* 1977;37:93–104.

14. Lenz FA, Tasker RR, Kwan HC, et al. Single unit analysis of the human ventral thalamic nuclear group: correlation of thalamic "tremor cells" with the 3–6 Hz component of parkinsonian tremor. *J Neurosci* 1988;8:754–764.

15. Lenz FA, Dostrovsky JO, Kwan HC, et al. Methods for microstimulation and recording of single neurons and evoked potentials in the human central nervous system. *J Neurosurg* 1988;68:630–634.

16. Lenz FA, Kwan HC, Martin RL, et al. Single neuron analysis of the human ventral thalamic nuclear group: tremor-related activity in functionally identified cells. *Brain* 1994;117:531–543.

17. Tomlinson FH, Jack CR Jr, Kelly PJ. Sequential magnetic resonance imaging following stereotactic radiofrequency ventralis lateralis thalamotomy. *J Neurosurg* 1991;74:579–584.

18. Nagaseki Y, Shibazaki T, Hirai T, et al. Long-term follow-up results of selective VIM-thalamotomy. *J Neurosurg* 1986;65:296–302.

19. Mohadjer M, Goerke H, Milios E, et al. Long term results of stereotaxy in the treatment of essential tremor. *Stereotact Funct Neurosurg* 1990;54–55:125–129.

20. Benabid AL, Pollak P, Gao D. Chronic electric stimulation of the ventralis intermediate nucleus of the thalamus as treatment of movement disorders. *J Neurosurg* 1996;84:203–214.

21. Koller W, Pahwa R, Busenbark K, et al. High frequency unilateral thalamic stimulation in the treatment of essential and parkinsonian tremor. *Ann Neurol* 1997;42:292–299.

22. Tasker RR, Munz M, Junn FSCK, et al. Deep brain stimulation and thalamotomy for tremor compared. *Acta Neurochir Suppl (Wien)* 1997;68:49–53.

23. Schvarcz JR. Chronic self-stimulation of the medial posterior inferior thalamus for the alleviation of deafferentation pain. *Acta Neurochir Suppl (Wien)* 1980;30:295–301.

24. North RB, Kidd DH, Zahurak M, et al. Spinal cord stimulation for chronic intractable pain: experience over two decades. *J Neurosurg* 1993;32:384–395.

25. Schuurman PR, Bosd DA, Bossuyt PM, et al. A comparison of continuous thalamic stimulation and thalamotary for suppression of severe tumor. *N Engl J Med* 2000;342:461–468.

Surgery for Parkinson's Disease and Movement Disorders,
edited by J.K. Krauss, J. Jankovic, and R.G. Grossman.
Lippincott Williams & Wilkins, Philadelphia © 2001.

24

THALAMIC STIMULATION FOR TREATMENT OF ESSENTIAL TREMOR

RAJESH PAHWA
WILLIAM C. KOLLER

During thalamotomy, electrical stimulation has been used for years to determine the optimal target for tumor control. It has long been known that electrical stimulation can inhibit tremor. The effect is immediately reversible when the stimulation is discontinued and is obtained only at high frequencies (100 Hz and higher). Because of the concerns of side effects and complications associated with bilateral ablative surgery, Benabid and his associates initially proposed the use of chronic deep brain stimulation (DBS) for patients who had thalamotomy on one side and who requested the procedure on the contralateral side (1). Since then, many investigators have reported the safety and efficacy of chronic thalamic stimulation (2–6).

THALAMIC STIMULATION FOR TREMOR CONTROL

The Activa tremor control therapy (Medtronics, Minneapolis) uses a DBS lead, the extension that connects the DBS lead to an implantable pulse generator (IPG), and the Itrel II IPG (7). Stimulation is usually initiated 1 day postoperatively and is programmed by using an external programming device. Adjustable parameters include pulse width, amplitude, stimulation frequency, and the choice of active contacts. The patient can turn the stimulator on or off using a handheld magnet.

Clinical Results of Thalamic Deep Brain Stimulation in Essential Tremor

A summary of the studies that have reported the efficacy of DBS in ET is shown in Table 24.1. In 1993, Benabid and his colleagues reported major benefit in 68% of their 13 patients

with essential tremor (ET) who underwent DBS of the thalamus (8). By 1996, these investigators had operated on 20 patients with ET: 13 patients underwent bilateral thalamic stimulation and two patients had contralateral thalamotomy (3). Although the results continued to be satisfactory, tremor control deteriorated in 18.5% of the cases, mainly for the action component of the tremor. These surgeons reported complications of the entire cohort of 117 patients who also had diagnoses other than ET. Three patients had microhematomas that caused reversible neurologic deficits. Another three patients had asymptomatic hematomas. Three patients had skin infections, two patients had granulomas along the connector extension tract, and one patient had a transient fluid collection in the subclavicular pocket of the stimulator. The side effects of stimulation were mild and reversible. Paresthesia, foot dystonia, dysarthria, and disequilibrium were reported effects of stimulation.

Blond et al. reported four ET patients with unilateral DBS (9). Two of the patients had major tremor suppression, one patient had moderate improvement, and one patient had mild improvement. There were no complications, and side effects included hand tonic posture (one patient) and persistent paresthesia (one patient) in a total of 14 cases (all types of tremor).

Koller et al. reported the results of a multicenter study of unilateral thalamic stimulation in ET and tremor associated with Parkinson's disease (PD) (5). At 3 months, 90% of the 29 patients with ET reported marked to moderate improvement. Results of formal assessments of writing, drawing spirals, drawing straight lines, pouring liquids, and bringing liquids to the mouth were significantly improved. Complications and adverse effects were reported for the entire group of patients with ET and PD. Six patients with ET and PD who underwent surgical treatment did not have the device implanted for the following reasons: lack of tremor suppression during surgery (two patients), intracranial hemorrhage during surgery (one patient), persistent microthalamotomy effect (one patient), subdural hematoma during bur-hole

R. Pahwa and W.C. Koller: Department of Neurology, University of Kansas Medical Center, Kansas City, Kansas 66160.

TABLE 24.1. THALAMIC STIMULATION FOR ESSENTIAL TREMOR

Author (yr)	Summary of Results
Blond et al. (1992)	4/4 improved
Benabid et al. (1996)	20/20 improved
Koller et al. (1997)	27/29 improved, significant improvement in ADL and tremor scores, 56% in hand functions
Ondo et al. (1998)	12/14 data analyzed, 82% improvement in arm tremor, 83% improvement in leg tremor, 55% improvement in head tremor, 59% improvement in writing and pouring
Limousin et al. (1999)	37 patients (some bilateral), 80% improvement in ADL scores, 53% in tremor scores, 44% in hand functions

ADL, activities of daily living.

trephination (one patient), and withdrawal of consent on the operating table (one patient). Other complications included lead dislodgment of the lead during surgery (one patient) requiring reimplantation, ischemic changes on the electrocardiogram (one patient), and generalized seizures (one patient). Adverse effects of stimulation were mild and included paresthesia, headache, disequilibrium, paresis, gait disorder, dystonia, dysarthria, and localized pain. Skin infection (two patients), IPG malfunction (one patient), and skin erosion from the extension wire (one patient) were other complications associated with the device that occurred during the first year.

Ondo et al. reported 14 patients with ET who had undergone unilateral thalamic DBS 3 months earlier (6). There was an 83% reduction in the contralateral arm tremor. All measures of tremor including writing samples, pouring tests, subjective functional surveys, and disability scores improved significantly. There was a 55% improvement in head tremor. Adverse effects to stimulation were mild and responded to parameter adjustment. There were no significant surgical complications. Two patients underwent reimplantation because of wire breakage.

Limousin et al. performed a multicenter trial of thalamic stimulation in ET and PD in Europe (10). Thirty-seven patients with ET were included. At 12 months, there was a 79% reduction in the upper limb tremor and a 64% improvement in the lower limb tremor. Drawing, writing, pouring, and other activities of daily living were also significantly improved. Head tremor was significantly improved at 3-month follow-up, and bilateral stimulation was more effective. Voice tremor was not significantly reduced postoperatively. Complications were reported both for patients with ET and for those with PD (n = 110). Four patients had major adverse effects unrelated to surgical treatment or stimulation. Three patients died of causes unrelated to surgery or

stimulation, and one patient had a stroke 3 months postoperatively. Two patients had subdural hematomas that resolved without intervention, and one patient had a subdural and thalamic hematoma that also resolved without sequelae. Infection (two patients), subcutaneous hematomas (two patients), electrode replacement (five patients), and transient attention and cognitive deficit (one patient) were other complications that were reported. Adverse effects to stimulation, including dysarthria, disequilibrium, and dystonia, were mild and reversible with change in stimulation parameters.

We reported results of staged bilateral thalamic stimulation in nine patients with ET (11). There was a 35% improvement in total tremor scores after the first surgical procedure and an additional 34% improvement 1 year after the second operation. When the postural and kinetic hand tremor scores were summarized for the target limb, there was a 68% improvement after the first surgical procedure and a 75% improvement on the opposite side after the second operation. Five patients had head tremor preoperatively. After the first operation, only two patients had head tremor, and after the second surgical procedure, only one patient had head tremor. Five patients had surgical complications including asymptomatic intracranial hematoma (one patient), hematoma over the implanted pulse generator (one patient), postoperative seizures (one patient), lead displacement (one patient), and pulse generator malfunction requiring replacement (one patient). Adverse effects related to the stimulation included paresthesia (nine patients), dysarthria (four patients) disequilibrium (three patients), headaches (two patients), dyspraxia (one patient), and word finding difficulty (one patient).

Carpenter et al. studied the effects of thalamic stimulation on voice tremor in patients with ET who had surgical treatment for hand tremor (12). Seven patients had voice tremor. Five of these patients received unilateral implants, and two patients received bilateral implants. Four of the seven patients reported improvement in voice tremor. Voice gains were typically restricted to patients with severe symptoms and did not parallel improvement in hand tremor.

We evaluated the effect of unilateral DBS of the thalamus in 38 patients with essential head tremor. Preoperative head tremor scores were compared with scores at 3, 6, and 12 months after implant with stimulation "on" and "off." There was a significant improvement in head tremor at all postimplant evaluations compared with baseline measurements. The improvement was 52% at 3 months, 35% at 6 months, and 50% at 12 months.

Mechanism of Action of Thalamic Stimulation

The precise mechanism of action of thalamic stimulation is unknown. Stimulation may cause a depolarization block and may thereby inactivate the region where stimulation is applied (13). Tremor suppression could also be the result of inhibiting or jamming rhythmic neuronal activity. This could occur either by desynchronization (9) or by blocking transmission of neuronal activity (14). This could also occur by an unknown mechanism on cerebellar and brainstem circuits through antidromic or orthodromic activation of cells or fibers (14,15).

Tolerance to Thalamic Stimulation

Tolerance to thalamic stimulation can be seen in some patients. Tolerance implies an increase in stimulation intensity with good control of tremor, although worsening over a period of days or weeks and requiring frequent readjustments. The appearance of tolerance may be dose related and usually occurs in patients who require high intensities initially to control the tremors (16). In some patients, the lead may not be in the ideal position. Turning the device off at night may prolong the appearance of tolerance, and occasionally stimulation holidays may help for short periods. Repositioning of the lead (if it is not in the ideal location) or thalamotomy may be considered in patients who show tolerance to chronic stimulation.

Advantages and Disadvantages of Thalamic Stimulation

Thalamic stimulation has advantages compared with ablative procedures including reversibility, adaptability, the ability to change stimulus parameters to increase efficacy or to reduce side effects, and the ability to perform bilateral procedures with less risk of permanent morbidity. The disadvantages of stimulation include the cost of the system, implantation of a foreign body that increases the risk of infections, the need to replace battery in the future, the time, effort, and training required to optimize stimulus parameters, breakage or malfunction of the hardware, and possible problems related to external magnetic fields (5).

Thalamic Stimulation or Thalamotomy?

Although thalamic stimulation is considered a newer surgical approach to treat tremor compared with thalamotomy, clinical studies are lacking to help us decide whether one procedure is superior to another. In the retrospective study by Tasker et al., complications were more common in the thalamotomy group (42%) as compared with the thalamic stimulation group (26%) (17). We compared 17 patients who had undergone thalamotomy for ET and matched them with 17 patients who had undergone thalamic stimulation (18). Although there were no significant differences among any efficacy outcome variables, the complications were higher for the thalamotomy group. Although these studies have certain drawbacks, at the present time it appears that thalamotomy

may have a higher complication rate as compared with thalamic DBS. This was also confirmed by the recent randomized prospective study by Schuurman and Colleagues (19).

CONCLUSIONS

Patients with ET who have disabling medication-resistant tremor are reasonable candidates for thalamic stimulation. Contraindications include marked cognitive problems, an unstable medical diagnosis that would increase the surgical risk significantly, and the presence of a pacemaker.

REFERENCES

1. Benabid AL, Pollak P, Louveau A, et al. Combined (thalamotomy and stimulation) stereotactic surgery of the VIM thalamic nucleus for bilateral Parkinson disease. *Appl Neurophysiol* 1987;50:344–346.
2. Alesch F, Pinter MM, Helscher RJ, et al. Stimulation of the ventral intermediate thalamic nucleus in tremor dominated Parkinson's disease and essential tremor. *Acta Neurochir (Wien)* 1995;136:75–81.
3. Benabid AL, Pollak P, Gao D, et al. Chronic electrical stimulation of the ventralis intermedius nucleus of the thalamus as a treatment of movement disorders. *J Neurosurg* 1996;84:203–214.
4. Hubble JP, Busenbark KL, Wilkinson S, et al. Deep brain stimulation for essential tremor. *Neurology* 1996;46:1150–1153.
5. Koller W, Pahwa R, Busenbark K, et al. High-frequency unilateral thalamic stimulation in the treatment of essential and parkinsonian tremor. *Ann Neurol* 1997;42:292–299.
6. Ondo W, Jankovic J, Schwartz K, et al. Unilateral thalamic deep brain stimulation for refractory essential tremor and Parkinson's disease tremor. *Neurology* 1998;51:1063–1069.
7. Medtronics. *Activa tremor control therapy reference guide.* Minneapolis: Medtronics, 1997.
8. Benabid AL, Pollak P, Seigneuret E, et al. Chronic VIM thalamic stimulation in Parkinson's disease, essential tremor and extrapyramidal dyskinesias. *Acta Neurochir Suppl (Wien)* 1993;58:39–44.
9. Blond S, Caparros-Lefebvre D, Parker F, et al. Control of tremor and involuntary movement disorders by chronic stereotactic stimulation of the ventral intermediate thalamic nucleus. *J Neurosurg* 1992;77:62–68.
10. Limousin P, Speelman JD, Gielen F, et al. Multicentre European study of thalamic stimulation in parkinsonian and essential tremor. *J Neurol Neurosurg Psychiatry* 1999;66:289–296.
11. Pahwa R, Lyons KE, Wilkinson SB, et al. Bilateral thalamic stimulation for essential tremor. *Neurology* 1998;50[Suppl 4]:A19.
12. Carpenter MA, Pahwa R, Miyawaki KL, et al. Reduction in voice tremor under thalamic stimulation. *Neurology* 1998;50:796–798.
13. Vitek JL. Stereotaxic surgery and deep brain stimulation for Parkinson's disease and movement disorders. In: Watts RL, Koller WC, eds. *Movement disorders: neurologic principles and practice.* New York: McGraw-Hill, 1997:237–255.
14. Deiber MP, Pollak P, Passingham R, et al. Thalamic stimulation and suppression of parkinsonian tremor: evidence of a cerebellar deactivation using positron emission tomography. *Brain* 1993;116:267–279.

15. Ohye C, Shibazaki T, Hirai T, et al. Possible descending pathways mediating spontaneous tremor in monkeys. *Adv Neurol* 1984;40:181–188.
16. Benabid AL, Pollak P, Hoffmann D, et al. Chronic high-frequency thalamic stimulation in parkinson's disease. In: Koller WC, Paulson G, eds. *Therapy of Parkinson's disease.* New York: Marcel-Dekker, 1995:381–401.
17. Tasker RR, Munz M, Junn FS, et al. Deep brain stimulation and thalamotomy for tremor compared. *Acta Neurochir Suppl (Wien)* 1997;68:49–53.
18. Pahwa R, Lyons KE, Troster AI, et al. Comparison of thalamotomy to deep brain stimulation (dbs) of the thalamus in essential tremor (ET). *Neurology* 1999;52[Suppl 2]:A457(abst).
19. Schuurman PR, Bosd DA, Bossuyt PM, et al. A comparison of continuous thalamic stimulation and thalamotomy for suppression of severe tumor. *N Engl J Med* 2000;342:461–468.

Surgery for Parkinson's Disease and Movement Disorders,
edited by J.K. Krauss, J. Jankovic, and R.G. Grossman.
Lippincott Williams & Wilkins, Philadelphia © 2001.

25

SURGICAL TREATMENT OF TREMOR
SECONDARY TO MULTIPLE SCLEROSIS

JEAN-PAUL NGUYEN
A. FÈVE
C. LEGUERINEL
B. POLLIN
P. CESARO
Y. KERAVEL

The development of tremor during the course of *multiple sclerosis* is a relatively frequent event. The functional repercussions of this tremor are generally severe, because it is almost always an action tremor (1). Medical treatment is usually ineffective (2), and for this reason, stereotactic surgery is often considered when the tremor induces functional disability. Up until recently, the main stereotactic procedure was thalamotomy (3–8). Although this technique achieves excellent results on tremor, it has largely been superseded by chronic thalamic stimulation (9–12). In this chapter, we discuss the respective advantages and disadvantages of the two techniques.

INCIDENCE AND PREVALENCE

Cerebellar and brainstem lesions are demonstrated in more than 80% of patients with multiple sclerosis (13), a finding suggesting that many patients may develop tremor. It is therefore surprising that some authors report tremor in fewer than 3% of cases (14). This discordance could be related to the finding that the main functional assessment scales for multiple sclerosis do not take tremor into account (15). Furthermore, the incidence and prevalence of tremor during the course of multiple sclerosis are difficult to establish because the type and severity of the tremor are not always clearly specified in the literature. In the most detailed study (5),

moderate tremor was present in 32% of cases, and severe tremor was present in 6% of cases.

CLINICAL CLASSIFICATION

Action tremor is the most typical form of tremor encountered in multiple sclerosis. It essentially involves the upper extremities, but it can also affect the lower extremities and the head and neck. Action tremor is a complex tremor (1), combining a postural component and an intention component. *Severe postural tremor* (severe postural cerebellar tremor, rubral tremor, superior cerebellar peduncle tremor, peduncular tremor, cerebellar outflow tremor) is characterized by large-amplitude and relatively slow (2.5 to 4 Hz) oscillations, mainly affecting the proximal part of the upper extremities. Tremor affects rotation and abduction-adduction movements at the shoulder and flexion-extension movements at the elbow. Tremor is observed when the forearms are flexed with the arms in abduction.

When postural tremor is less severe (mild postural cerebellar tremor, postural tremor), it essentially involves the distal part of the upper extremities, especially the wrist and fingers (flexion-extension movements). The tremor is usually rapid (2.5 to 10 Hz) and essentially occurs when the patient keeps the upper extremities extended. *Intention tremor* (cerebellar intention tremor, kinetic cerebellar tremor, ataxic tremor, hyperkinetic tremor) is a tremor that appears as the finger approaches its target and is well demonstrated by the finger-nose maneuver.

Action tremor is typically related to lesions of the cerebellar peduncles (16,17). It can also be caused by lesions of the lateral cerebellar nuclei or vermis (18). Theoretically, any lesion situated on the efferent pathways of the cerebellum (especially cerebellothalamic tracts) can induce action tremor.

J-P. Nguyen, A. Fève, C. Leguerinel, and Y. Keravel: Service de Neurochirurgie, Hôpital Henri Mondor, Créteil 94000, France.
B. Pollin: Laboratoire de Physiologie de la Manducation, Université Denis Diderot, Paris, France.
J-P Nguyen and P. Cesaro: INSERM U421, Facultéde Médecine, Créteil 94000, France.
P. Cesaro: Service de Neurologie, Hôpital Henri Mondor, Créteil 94000, France.

It is often very difficult to determine the lesion responsible for tremor in multiple sclerosis because of the presence of multiple plaques.

These multiple lesions also mean that isolated tremor is rare and is frequently associated with a cerebellar syndrome characterized, in particular, by dysmetria, which may be difficult to differentiate from intention tremor (19,20). The presence of hypotonia and the Stewart-Holmes maneuver can help to demonstrate and assess the severity of the cerebellar syndrome. Tremor is also frequently associated with a motor deficit, especially affecting the lower extremities. In the case of paraplegia, the motor deficit masks the tremor.

Other abnormal movements may be observed during the course of multiple sclerosis. Tranchant et al. (21), in particular, reported 14 cases, including nine cases of dystonia, three cases of parkinsonian syndrome, and two cases of myoclonus and also reviewed 135 cases published in the literature. The most frequent abnormal movements are paroxysmal dystonia. A few rare cases of paroxysmal tremor have been reported (22).

Assessment

Clinical assessment is essential in patients who are potential candidates for surgery. Because of the risk related to any surgical procedure, it is essential to assess the severity of the tremor and its repercussions on everyday activities, as well as the relative severity of associated disorders. Surgical treatment is primarily indicated when tremor is the predominant symptom, with a large amplitude and major functional repercussions.

The intensity of the tremor can be clinically assessed by accelerometry, electromyography, and analysis of video recordings. Webster's score can be used to quantify the amplitude of the tremor (23). This assessment must be performed during several maneuvers because of the complexity of the action tremor: maintenance of the arms extended, arms flexed, and finger-nose maneuver. The repercussions of the tremor on everyday activities can be assessed by Brown's scale (24), based on 25 activities, some of which involve the use of the upper extremities. This scale is well adapted to cases of unilateral tremor, because the benefit of treatment can be clearly demonstrated. In the case of unilateral treatment in a patient with bilateral tremor, this scale only poorly reflects postoperative clinical improvement. Bain's visual analog scale (25), which is well correlated with everyday activity assessment scales, appears to be better adapted to patients with bilateral action tremor. We also use the following five-point functional self-assessment scale (global disability scale): 0, normal activities; 1, moderate handicap; 2, marked handicap; 3, major handicap; 4, no activity possible.

In very severe forms, the slightest movement often induces major oscillations of the entire body, responsible for marked fatigue. This fatigue is added to that directly related to the disease and to the patient's generally debilitated state.

Reduction of fatigue is one of the objectives of surgery in these patients (26).

SURGICAL TREATMENT

The results of medical treatment are often very disappointing (2). Surgical treatment is therefore considered because of the functional repercussions of the tremor. Selection criteria and indications are globally the same for thalamotomy and for chronic thalamic stimulation.

Objectives of Surgery and Selection Criteria

The objectives of surgery differ in patients with relatively limited disease and in patients with very advanced disease. In the first group, tremor may be isolated, it is frequently unilateral, and the patient has little or no other permanent neurologic signs. The tremor is often a postural tremor, with no major intention component, and it resembles essential tremor. The objective of treatment is to obtain marked functional improvement, allowing the patient to eat unassisted and to write legibly (10,11). At this stage, the disease usually has an episodic course, and the patient should not undergo operation after a recent acute episode. When tremor is strictly unilateral, thalamotomy can be theoretically proposed, but chronic thalamic stimulation is generally preferred.

In the second group, tremor is usually bilateral and is accompanied by axial tremor. Patients usually present with other permanent deficits. They very often have disorders of balance and paraparesis that make walking almost impossible. The tremor usually is of very large amplitude, comprising distal and proximal postural components and an intention component. Tremor generally masks the other symptoms affecting the upper extremities: motor deficit and cerebellar syndrome. The presence of a severe cerebellar syndrome constitutes a relative contraindication to surgery. At this stage of the disease, magnetic resonance imaging usually shows multiple subcortical and brainstem plaques. Thalamic plaques are relatively rare. A large lesion in the thalamic region, considered as a target for stereotactic treatment, is generally a contraindication for thalamotomy and chronic stimulation.

Resolution of the tremor at this stage of the disease generally does not allow complete functional improvement. However, the patient will, one hopes, be able to grasp and easily use an object. If a cerebellar syndrome persists, it is unlikely that the patient will be able to write legibly. Patients with untreated contralateral tremor will also be unlikely to be able to eat unassisted easily. In every case, disappearance of the large oscillations, especially affecting the proximal part of the limb, will reduce physical fatigue related to tremor and will provide greater comfort during active or passive mobilization (26). The possibility to grasp and use certain objects may restore a certain degree of autonomy to the patient (10,11).

Indications

It is usually recommended that surgeons not operate too early in these cases, because some tremors resolve spontaneously. It seems reasonable to wait for at least 1 year. In addition, surgical treatment should not be performed until at least 6 months after the patient's last acute episode.

In relatively limited forms of tremor, surgery is generally indicated when patients have difficulties in writing and eating. In advanced forms, surgery may be indicated when the patient is unable to grasp an object and experiences marked oscillations (amplitude greater than 30 cm) during the slightest attempt to mobilize the upper extremity.

Stereotactic Targets and Technical Considerations

The ventral part of the thalamus represents the usual stereotactic target to treat tremor (27). The target is situated in the ventrooralis posterior nucleus or nucleus ventralis intermedius (VIM), depending on the surgeon. Because cerebellar afferents preferentially terminate in the VIM (28), this nucleus is adopted by most surgeons to treat action tremors (29,30).

Studies by Guiot et al. (31), followed by those by Ohye et al. (32), demonstrated the existence of a somatotopic arrangement in the VIM, especially in the mediolateral direction. According to Ohye et al. (30,32), the best target to treat tremor of the upper extremity is situated laterally, near the lateral edge of the thalamus. In a previous study (29), we showed that high-frequency stimulation of the inferior part of VIM (close to the anterior commissure–posterior commissure or AC-PC line) controlled distal tremors, whereas stimulation of the superior or middle part of VIM was more effective on

proximal tremors. The use of a four-contact electrode (3387 Medtronic, Minneapolis) allowing simultaneous or separate stimulation of these various zones of the VIM is therefore essential for the treatment of action tremors.

The somatotopic arrangement of the VIM is probably not the only element that must be taken into account in the choice of the target. In a recent study (10), the postural component and intention component of the action tremor appeared to be controlled by stimulation of various zones of the VIM. The postural component is generally easy to control. Several targets can be effective in the same patient, and they tend to be situated in the lateral part of the VIM (*gray circles,* Fig. 25.1), as well as in the inferior and superior parts of the nucleus. On a lateral view, they are distributed along the long axis of the VIM (Fig. 25.2). The zone allowing control of the intention component of the tremor is more difficult to identify and is very limited (*white triangles,* Fig. 25.1). The postural and intention components can sometimes be controlled by acting on a single target. Intraoperative stimulation using a classic bipolar semimicroelectrode induces marked improvement of the tremor and thus confirms the position of the target. The intensity of stimulation is generally less than 1 mA with a pulse width of 1 millisecond and a frequency of 100 Hz. When distinct targets need to be stimulated to improve all components of the tremor, we use a semimicroelectrode (PK08-06 AS Dixi Medical, Besançon, France) with several contacts that can be activated simultaneously (Fig. 25.3).

It is also sometimes necessary simultaneously to stimulate several contacts postoperatively. In a series of 37 patients (10), including 29 patients with marked long-term improvement, stimulation used only one contact in 13 cases, two adjacent contacts in 13 cases, and three adjacent contacts in three cases.

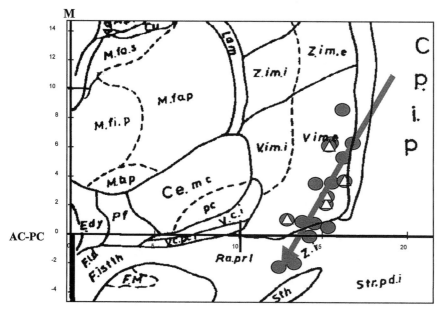

FIGURE 25.1. Effective contact positions on proximal postural tremor *(gray circles)* and intentional tremor *(white triangles),* in six patients. Frontal view of the ventralis intermedius nucleus (VIM) (Schaltenbrandt's atlas). The mean tract *(arrow)* is oblique medially, forming an angle of 25 degrees with the midline and intersecting the anterior commissure–posterior commissure (AC-PC) plane 13.5 mm lateral to the midline (M).

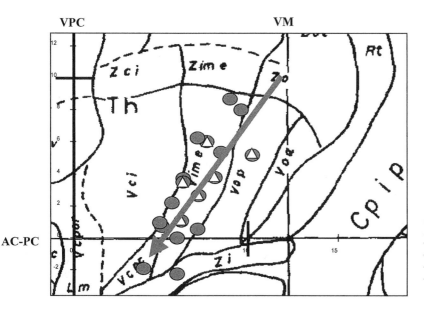

FIGURE 25.2. Same positions and abbreviations as in Fig. 25.1. Lateral view of the VIM. The mean tract *(arrow)* forms an angle of 55 degrees with the AC-PC line and intersects this line 5 mm anteriorly to the CP. The VPC line is perpendicular to the PC; the VM line is perpendicular to the midpoint of the AC-PC line.

We use a double oblique tract to follow the outline of the long axis of the VIM. On lateral views of the VIM, the mean tract forms an angle of 55 degrees with the AC-PC line and intersects this line 5 mm anteriorly to the PC (Fig. 25.2). On anteroposterior views, the tract is oblique medially, forming an angle of 25 degrees with the midline and intersecting the plane of the AC-PC line 13.5 mm lateral to the midline (Fig. 25.1).

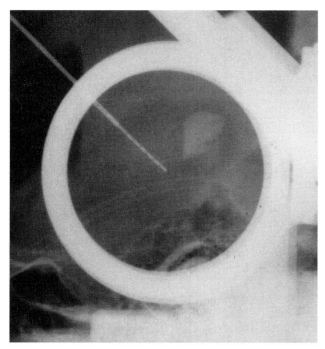

FIGURE 25.3. Semimicroelectrode with several contacts used for intraoperative stimulation. Several contacts can be stimulated simultaneously.

Review of the Literature

Thalamotomy

For a long time, thalamotomy represented the only surgical treatment option for tremor (3–8). The results of thalamotomies performed to treat parkinsonian tremors showed that the improvement was often remarkable and the operation was well tolerated. However, action tremor observed in the context of multiple sclerosis was rapidly shown to be more difficult to control, and the operation was often associated with complications. Hirai and Jones demonstrated that thalamotomy was effective on action tremor when the volume of the lesion was greater than in other tremors, a finding that explains treatment failure or tremor recurrence when small lesions are created and the complications observed when a larger lesion is created (33).

In most series, the initial result was relatively satisfactory in 65% to 96% of patients, but, probably for the reasons indicated earlier, the tremor recurred fairly frequently, in about 20% of patients (34). Haddow et al. reviewed the main publications reporting the results of thalamotomy performed for this indication (5). They analyzed 14 articles published between 1960 and 1992. The results, based on 243 patients, indicate satisfactory short-term improvement of the tremor in more than 75% of cases and a long-term benefit in 50% to 70% of patients. The reason for this discrepancy in the assessment of results could be that the functional handicap and its repercussions on everyday activities were not precisely evaluated in any of these series. More recently, Critchley and Richardson reported the results in a series of 24 patients and took into account the functional status of the upper extremities and patient satisfaction (35). The functional status was improved in 62% of cases in the long term (mean follow-up, 2.2 years), and 61% of patients declared to be satisfied with the operation.

The morbidity related to thalamotomy performed for this indication is high. Transient complications are observed in 27% to 78% of patients, and permanent complications are observed in 18% to 57% of cases (27). The most frequent complications are motor deficits, dysarthria, and gait disorders. In only one case, the operation was considered responsible for triggering an acute exacerbation of the disease. In many cases, these complications affect patients with advanced disease who have a history of major neurologic deficits. The operation may be sufficient to decompensate patients and to accelerate an already progressively unfavorable clinical course. In the series reported by Hooper and Whittle (36), four of the ten patients studied died of their disease during the year after the operation.

Whittle and Haddow reported the results of a series of nine surgical patients, with no major complications, but with very disappointing results on tremor (only 22% of patients were improved) (8). Another series reported a complication rate of 45% (35), which corresponds to the mean rate reported in the major published trials.

Thalamic Stimulation

As early as 1980, Brice and McLellan showed that chronic stimulation of the thalamic and subthalamic region could improve the action tremor of multiple sclerosis on a long-term basis (9). The results on tremor were subsequently confirmed by Andy (37), and then Benabid et al. (38). In 1996, Benabid et al. reported the results of a series of 117 patients treated by chronic high-frequency stimulation of the VIM (39). Only four patients in this series presented a tremor related to multiple sclerosis. Two of these patients were improved. During the same period, Siegfried and Lippitz reported the results of a series of 60 patients, including ten patients with multiple sclerosis (40). Tremor was perfectly controlled in seven patients, with no complications.

We reported a first series of 13 patients with severe tremor related to multiple sclerosis and treated by chronic stimulation of the VIM (11). The severity of the disease was assessed by the Expanded Disability Status Scale (EDSS) (15), and functional impairment of the upper extremities was evaluated by a score based on that proposed by Speelman and Van Manen (7). Tremor was significantly improved in the long term (mean follow-up, 13 months) in 69.2% of patients, with no significant modification of EDSS scores and no permanent complications. In the four less severely affected patients (EDSS less than 6), the functional improvement enabled them to eat unassisted.

More recently, we analyzed a series of 37 patients submitted to detailed clinical assessment (10). In addition to EDSS, this assessment (prospective in 20 patients) comprised Webster's score, Brown's functional scale, Bain's visual analog scale, and a self-assessment scale: 78.3% of patients were improved at long-term follow-up (mean, 21 months). This improvement was statistically significant on three of the four scales. Brown's functional scale was not significantly improved, undoubtedly because this scale comprises many bimanual tasks, which remain difficult to perform even when tremor has been controlled on one side. Five patients underwent operation on both sides, and contralateral operations were performed an average of 1 year after the first operation. Tremor gradually returned in three patients (recurrence rate, 8.1%).

One patient experienced permanent, but incomplete deterioration of a motor deficit of the lower extremity contralateral to site of the operation. Gait deteriorated transiently in two patients, and there was one case of infection.

Advantages and Disadvantages of the Various Techniques

Thalamotomy is a more straightforward procedure. It is almost as effective as thalamic stimulation, but it presents a higher risk of postoperative unwanted effects. Complications of bilateral thalamotomy are even more frequent and more serious. Chronic stimulation of the VIM is associated with a lower operative risk. The stimulation parameters can be adapted to the patient's clinical state, and this is a major advantage in the context of an evolving disease. The cost of stimulators is one of the disadvantages of this technique. However, battery life span is relatively long, because the stimulator can almost always be stopped at night, given that, in contrast to certain cases of resting tremor, there is no "rebound" tremor after stopping the stimulator.

CONCLUSIONS

Thalamotomy and thalamic stimulation provide long-term improvement in 60% to 80% of patients with action tremor related to multiple sclerosis. The complication rate is much lower with thalamic stimulation (10.8%) than with thalamotomy (about 45%). These results indicate that it is preferable to propose thalamic stimulation as first-line treatment. In patients with relatively limited disease, the objective of surgery is to obtain functional improvement allowing them to eat unassisted. In patients with more advanced disease, the objective is to allow them to grasp an object easily and to minimize fatigue related to the tremor.

REFERENCES

1. Sabra AF, Hallett M. Action tremor with alternating activity in antagonist muscles. *Neurology* 1984;34:151–156.
2. Lou JS, Goldfarb L, McShane L, et al. Use of Buspirone for treatment of cerebellar ataxia: an open-label study. *Arch Neurol* 1995;52:982–988.
3. Barnett GH, Kinkel RP, Bashin C, et al. Stereotactic thalamotomy for intractable tremor in multiple sclerosis. *Neurology* 1992;42[Suppl 3]:327.

4. Broager B, Fog T. Thalamotomy for the relief of intention tremor in multiple sclerosis. *Acta Neurol Scand* 1962;38:153–156.

5. Haddow LJ, Mumford C, Whittle IR. Stereotactic treatment of tremor due to multiple sclerosis. *Neurosurg Q* 1997;7:23–24.

6. Shazadi S, Tasker RR, Lozano A. Thalamotomy for essential and cerebellar tremor. *Stereotact Funct Neurosurg* 1996;65:11–17.

7. Speelman JD, Van Manen J. Stereotactic thalamotomy for the relief of intention tremor in multiple sclerosis. *J Neurol Neurosurg Psychiatry* 1984;47:596–599.

8. Whittle IR, Haddow LJ. CT guided thalamotomy for movement disorders in multiple sclerosis: problems and paradoxes. *Acta Neurochir (Wien)* 1995;64:13–16.

9. Brice J, McLellan L. Suppression of intention tremor by contingent deep-brain stimulation. *Lancet* 1980;7:1221–1224.

10. Caparros-Lefebvre D, Blond S, Nguyen JP, et al. Chronic deep brain stimulation for movement disorders. In: Cohadon F, eds. *Advances and technical standards in neurosurgery,* vol 25. Vienna: Springer, 1999:61–138.

11. Geny C, Nguyen JP, Pollin B, et al. Improvement of severe postural cerebellar tremor in multiple sclerosis by chronic thalamic stimulation. *Mov Disord* 1996;11:489–494.

12. Whittle IR, Hooper J, Pentland B. Thalamic deep-brain stimulation for movement disorders due to multiple sclerosis. *Lancet* 1998;351:109–110.

13. Bauer HJ. Problems of symptomatic therapy in multiple sclerosis. *Neurology* 1978;28:8–20.

14. Kelly R. Clinical aspects of multiple sclerosis. In: *Handbook of clinical neurology: demyelinating diseases,* vol 3. New York: Elsevier Science, 1988:49–78.

15. Kurtzke JF. Rating neurological impairment in multiple sclerosis: an expanded disability status scale (EDSS). *Neurology* 1983;33:1444–1452.

16. Geny C, Nguyen JP, Cesaro P, et al. Thalamic stimulation for severe action tremor after lesion of the superior cerebellar peduncle. *J Neurol Neurosurg Psychiatry* 1995;59:641–642.

17. Remy P, DeRecondo A, Defer G, et al. Peduncular "rubral" tremor and dopaminergic denervation: a PET study. *Neurology* 1995;45:472–477.

18. Anouti A, Koller WC. Tremor disorders: diagnosis and management. *West J Med* 1995;162:510–513.

19. Manto M, Jacquy J, Hildebrand J, et al. Recovery of hypermetria after a cerebellar stroke occurs as a multistage process. *Ann Neurol* 1995;38:437–445.

20. Rondot P, Jedynak CP, Ferrey G. Pathological tremors: nosological correlates. *Prog Clin Neurophysiol* 1978;5:95–113.

21. Tranchant C, Bhatia P, Marsden CD. Movement disorders in multiple sclerosis. *Mov Disord* 1995;4:418–423.

22. Nardocci N, Zorzi G, Savoldelli M, et al. Paroxysmal dystonia and paroxysmal tremor in a young patient with multiple sclerosis. *Ital J Neurol Sci* 1995;16:315–319.

23. Webster DD. Critical analysis of the disability in Parkinson's disease. *Mod Treatment* 1968;5:257–282.

24. Brown RJ, MacCarthy B, Jahanshahi M, et al. Accuracy of self reported disability in patients with parkinsonism. *Arch Neurol* 1989;46:955–959.

25. Bain PG, Findley LJ, Atchison P, et al. Assessing tremor severity. *J Neurol Neurosurg Psychiatry* 1993;56:868–873.

26. Nguyen JP, Fève A, Pollin B, et al. Severe action tremor in multiple sclerosis: assessment and follow-up of 25 patients treated by chronic thalamic stimulation. *Mov Disord* 1996;11:94(abst).

27. Speelman JD, Schuurman PR, DeBie RMA, et al. Thalamic surgery and tremor. *Mov Disord* 1998;13:103–106.

28. Hirai T, Miyazaki M, Nakajima H, et al. The correlation between tremor characteristics and predicted volume of effective lesion in stereotactic Vim-thalamotomy. *Brain* 1983;106:1001–1018.

29. Nguyen JP, Degos JD. Thalamic stimulation and proximal tremor: a specific target in the nucleus ventrointermedius thalami. *Arch Neurol* 1993;50:498–500.

30. Ohye C, Fukamachi A, Miyazaki M, et al. Physiologically controlled selective thalamotomy for the treatment of abnormal movement by Leksell's open system. *Acta Neurochir (Wien)* 1977;37:93–104.

31. Guiot G, Derome P, Arfel G, et al. Electrophysiological recordings in stereotactic thalamotomy for parkinsonism. *Prog Neurol Surg* 1973;5:189–221.

32. Ohye C, Shibazaki T, Hirai T, et al. Further physiological observations on the ventralis intermedius neurons in the human thalamus. *J Neurophysiol* 1989;61:488–500.

33. Hirai T, Jones EG. A new parcellation of the human thalamus on the basis of histochemical staining. *Brain Res Rev* 1989;14:1–34.

34. Alusi SH, Glickman S, Aziz TZ, et al. Tremor in multiple sclerosis. *J Neurol Neurosurg Psychiatry* 1999;66:131–134.

35. Critchley GR, Richardson PL. Vim thalamotomy for the relief of the intention tremor of multiple sclerosis. *Br J Neurosurg* 1998;12:559–562.

36. Hooper J, Whittle IR. Long-term outcome after thalamotomy for movement disorders in multiple sclerosis. *Lancet* 1998;352:1984.

37. Andy OJ. Thalamic stimulation for control of movement disorders. *Appl Neurophysiol* 1983;46:107–111.

38. Benabid AL, Pollak P, Gervason C, et al. Long-term suppression of tremor by chronic stimulation of the ventral intermediate thalamic nucleus. *Lancet* 1991;337:403–406.

39. Benabid AL, Pollak P, Gao D, et al. Chronic electrical stimulation of the ventralis intermedius nucleus of the thalamus as a treatment of movement disorders. *J Neurosurg* 1996;84:203–214.

40. Siegfried J, Lippitz B. Chronic electrical stimulation of the VL-VPL complex and of the pallidum in the treatment of movement disorders: personal experience since 1982. *Stereotact Funct Neurosurg* 1994;62:71–75.

Surgery for Parkinson's Disease and Movement Disorders,
edited by J.K. Krauss, J. Jankovic, and R.G. Grossman.
Lippincott Williams & Wilkins, Philadelphia © 2001.

26

SURGICAL TREATMENT OF POSTTRAUMATIC TREMOR

JOACHIM K. KRAUSS
FRITZ A. NOBBE
FRITZ MUNDINGER

Head trauma may cause a variety of movement disorders (1,2). Posttraumatic movement disorders are more frequently associated with severe craniocerebral trauma (3–5). The frequency of *posttraumatic tremor* has varied considerably among different studies on the long-term follow-up after head injury (6). Tremors were reported in 66% of the responders in a questionnaire-based survey screening severely head-injured children for the presence of "significant tremor" (7). Taking into account that tremors may not have been present in those not responding to the survey, the frequency of tremor in this pediatric population still was thought to be as high as 45%. Tremors were the most frequent movement disorders in survivors of severe head injury at a mean follow-up of 3.9 years after trauma (3). Tremors with higher frequencies resembling enhanced physiologic or essential tremor were more often transient and, in general, did not contribute to additional disability. Transient tremors occurred in 10% of the 225 patients who were available for long-term follow-up. Persistent tremors were found in 9.1% of patients, of whom 3.2% had low-frequency postural or kinetic tremors.

Postural and kinetic tremors of the upper extremities may interfere with any goal-directed motor function. Typically, the tremor is present during the whole range of moving the upper extremity but increases in amplitude toward reaching the goal. The frequency of these coarse tremors usually ranges between 2.5 and 4 Hz, with varying amplitudes. The rhythmic oscillatory movements are sometimes interrupted by irregular jerking movements that may show a "myoclonic" appearance or may even resemble "hemiballistic" movements (8,9). Some patients also have tremor at rest, in particular when the limb is unsupported. Although this may appear as "cerebellar tremor at rest" in some instances, other patients

have a combined tremor with genuine resting tremor. Such slow posttraumatic tremors have been categorized as "midbrain," "rubral," or "Holmes" tremors or "myorhythmias" (10–12). In a series of 35 patients with severe posttraumatic tremor, the kinetic component of the tremor was the most evident feature (13). Tremor at rest was observed in 21 patients but appeared to imply some degree of postural maintenance in the majority of cases. Bilateral tremor was evident in ten patients. Commonly, posttraumatic tremor affects predominantly or exclusively the upper extremity. In about half the patients, there is also accompanying tremor of the head or of the upper trunk that occasionally can manifest as titubation. Functional stereotactic surgery targeting the thalamus can effectively abate the disabling tremor, and persistent improvement of the tremor has been achieved in most patients. This is a problematic group of patients, however, because there has been a striking incidence of postoperative side effects. Several issues related to the high occurrence of side effects deserve special consideration.

CLINICAL PROFILE OF PATIENTS WITH POSTTRAUMATIC TREMORS

The planning of surgical treatment of posttraumatic tremors has to take into account several features that are unique to this group of patients. Patients with posttraumatic tremors differ from other patients who undergo movement disorders surgery with regard to age, the widespread cerebral damage from severe head injury, the high frequency of other neurologic and psychologic symptoms, and the associated disability. The posttraumatic "midbrain syndrome" was first outlined by Kremer and colleagues in 1947 (11).

The most frequent cause of persistent posttraumatic tremor has been severe closed head injury in autopedestrian accident with a history of deceleration trauma. In a series of 35 patients with persistent tremors, the mean age at trauma was 11 years, with a range from 3 to 29 years (13). The

J.K. Krauss: Department of Neurosurgery, University Hospital, Klinikum Mannheim, 68167 Mannheim, Germany.
F.A. Nobbe: Department of Neurology, RWTH Aachen, 52057 Aachen, Germany.
F. Mundinger: Department of Functional and Stereotactic Neurosurgery, St. Josefs-Krankenhaus, 79114 Freiburg, Germany.

male-to-female ratio, with male sex being two to three times more predominant than female, reflects the higher occurrence of severe head injury in boys and men. Most patients are comatose for weeks and often exhibit transient apallic syndromes or akinetic mutism during recovery. The delay between the trauma and the manifestation of the tremor is variable, ranging between 4 weeks and 1 year. Initial hemiparesis may have a masking effect, and the tremor will often become manifest only when the paresis resolves.

The history of deceleration trauma and associated clinical findings indicate that most patients with posttraumatic tremor suffer diffuse axonal injury. This is also supported by neuroradiologic findings. In a series of 19 patients with posttraumatic kinetic tremor, there was evidence of diffuse axonal injury in 18 patients according to late-phase magnetic resonance imaging (MRI) studies revealing corpus callosal atrophy, ventriculomegaly, and subcortical and brainstem lesions (12). The appearance of tremor is usually related to lesions of the dentatothalamic pathways. The dentate nucleus ipsilateral to the tremor was involved in 4% of patients, the dentatothalamic pathway within the ipsilateral superior cerebellar peduncle or in its predecussational mesencephalic course was involved in 56%, and the intramesencephalic postdecussational dentatothalamic pathway contralateral to the tremor was affected in 28% (12) (Fig. 26.1). Patients with an accompanying parkinsonian-like rest tremor may also have lesions involving the substantia nigra (Fig. 26.2). Occasionally, thalamic lesions are found (14). There is no convincing evidence that lesioning of the red nucleus is involved in posttraumatic tremor. The crescendo appearance

with goal-directed movements may be the result of amplification of the tremor in reverberating circuits caused by impaired thalamic relay. Marked decrease in $[^{18}F]$-dopa uptake in the contralateral striatum without significant changes in the D_2-specific binding was found in patients with posttraumatic "midbrain" tremor who improved with levodopa therapy (15).

Commonly, patients with severe posttraumatic tremors present with a variety of other symptoms. With few exceptions, appendicular tremors are associated with at least some degree of ataxia of the affected limb. Psychologic and cognitive alterations were found in 91% of patients with persistent tremor at a mean of 7 years after head injury, dysarthria in 86%, oculomotor nerve deficits in 69%, truncal ataxia in 91%, and residual hemiparesis or tetraparesis in 91% (13). Other movement disorders such as hemidystonia, focal dystonias, or galloping tongue were present in 46% of patients.

INDICATIONS FOR SURGICAL TREATMENT

The prognosis of posttraumatic tremor is difficult to predict early after its onset. It may lessen or resolve spontaneously within 1 year after its manifestation. The natural history of posttraumatic tremor in the majority of patients, however, appears to be characterized by persistence of the violent shaking movements. Medical treatment of posttraumatic tremor is notoriously difficult. Few patients have been reported to respond favorably to medical treatment. Drugs reported to

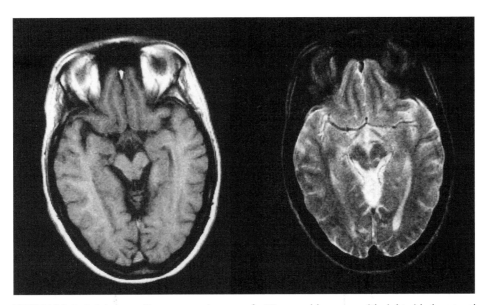

FIGURE 26.1. Axial magnetic resonance images of a 30-year-old woman with right-sided postural and kinetic tremor 12 years after she sustained a severe head injury. Spin-echo (SE) 450/17 **(A)** and SE 2500/90 **(B)** images show a lesion affecting the left postdecussational dentatothalamic pathway but not affecting the substantia nigra. (From Krauss JK, Wakhloo AK, Nobbe F, et al. MR pathological correlations of severe posttraumatic tremor. *Neurol Res* 1995;17:409–416, with permission.)

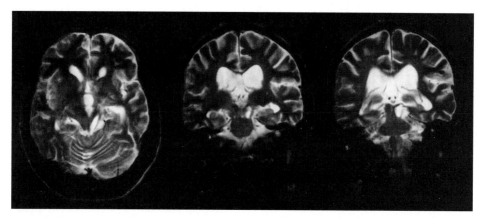

FIGURE 26.2. RARE 3710/32 magnetic resonance images of a 37-year-old man with right-sided tremor at rest, postural, and kinetic tremor 33 years after a severe head injury. Axial **(A)** and coronal **(B, C)** coronal images reveal a lesion both of the contralateral postdecussational dentatothalamic pathway and of the substantia nigra. (From Krauss JK, Wakhloo AK, Nobbe F, et al. MR pathological correlations of severe posttraumatic tremor. *Neurol Res* 1995;17:409–416, with permission.)

improve posttraumatic tremor include glutethimide, isoniazid, L-tryptophan, propranolol, benzodiazepines, carbamazepine, levodopa/carbidopa, and anticholinergics (6,15–18). Systematic studies, however, are lacking. Botulinum toxin injections may be helpful to relieve the tremor temporarily, but the high doses administered to both proximal and distal arm muscles limit the usefulness of this treatment (19).

Because functional stereotactic surgery, in particular radiofrequency lesioning, is associated with a significant risk of postoperative side effects in these vulnerable patients, the possible gains as well as the adverse effects of surgery should be discussed in detail with patients and their caretakers. The indication to undergo surgical treatment should consider both the social embarrassment that is associated with the shaking movements and the secondary functional disability. Patients must clearly understand the possibility of worsening of preexistent gait ataxia and of dysarthria with the use of lesioning techniques. It is best to decide on a case-by-case basis what treatment option is the best suited for the individual patient. For example, worsening of dysarthria may be unacceptable in one patient, whereas it would not contribute to additional disability in another patient who has no ability for useful communication as a result of severe dysarthria preoperatively.

Moreover, the age of the patient should be considered. It is useful to wait until children with severe posttraumatic tremor reach adolescence so they can understand the rationales of the surgical procedure and cooperate during the operation to facilitate confirmation of the optimal target. Once the decision to operate has been made, the procedure should not be deferred too long, because the tremor may be so disabling that it precludes professional development. The indication for bilateral surgery should be conservative. If deemed necessary, deep brain stimulation (DBS) techniques may be considered. In patients with bilateral tremor, handedness determines the side to undergo operation.

FUNCTIONAL NEUROSURGERY FOR POSTTRAUMATIC TREMOR

Before the advent of functional stereotactic surgery, few attemps were made to treat posttraumatic tremor surgically. Bucy performed ablations of the contralateral motor cortex to abate posttraumatic tremor as early as in 1937 (20). Functional stereotactic surgery was introduced only relatively late in the treatment of posttraumatic tremor. We summarize the available data on lesioning and DBS in Tables 26.1 and 26.2.

Clinical Studies on Ablative Surgery

Cooper was the first to report on thalamotomy for treatment of posttraumatic tremor in 1960 (21). He claimed complete relief of tremor without side effects after chemothalamectomy in two patients. Since then, targets in the ventrolateral thalamus or the subthalamic region have been used almost exclusively. In 1969, Nashold and Slaughter reported on mild improvement of ipsilateral posttraumatic intention tremor in a patient after high-frequency lesioning dentatectomy (22). Several case reports and smaller series were published from 1963 to 1980 (23–27). Whereas the number of functional stereotactic procedures for treatment of Parkinson's disease and for other movement disorders declined in the 1970s and 1980s, there was a relative increase in the number of patients operated on for posttraumatic tremor (28–41). The evaluation of many of these publications is mainly limited by the absence of data on long-term follow-up. In several reports, it remains unclear whether the improvement of tremor was also accompanied by improvement of daily living activities. This is of particular interest with regard to both the relatively high frequency of persistent side effects and the high prevalence of neurologic deficits in posttraumatic tremor. Studies providing more detail on outcome were published only in the 1980s and 1990s (9,13,28,36,39).

TABLE 26.1. FUNCTIONAL STEREOTACTIC SURGERY FOR POSTTRAUMATIC TREMOR: LESIONING PROCEDURES

Author (yr)	Target	Cases	Immediate Improvement	Long-Term Follow-up	Last Follow-up, Mean Yr (Range)	Symptomatic Improvement (%)	Functional Improvement (%)	Persistent Side Effects (%)
Cooper (1960)	VL	2	2	1	1.3	1/1	1/1	NA
Spiegel et al. (1963)	STR	1	1	1	NA	0/1	NA	NA
Fox and Kurtzke (1966)	VL	1	1	1	0.5	1/1	1/1	0/1
Samra et al. (1970)	VL	5	5	NA	NA	5/5 (100)	NA	NA
Van Manen (1974)[a]	VL	2	2	2	7	1/2	NA	1/2
Eiras and Garcia (1980)	GP, VOP	1	1	1	2.5	1/1	1/1	0/1
Andrew et al. (1982)	VL	8	8	NA	NA	8/8 (100)	8/8 (100)	5/8 (63)
Kandel (1982)[a]	VL, STR, GP	10	NA	NA	NA	NA	NA	NA
Niizuma et al. (1982)[a]	VIM, Sub-VIM	3	3	NA	NA	NA	NA	NA
Ohye et al. (1982)	VIM	8	8	NA	NA	NA	NA	1/8 (13)
Hirai et al. (1983)	VL	5	4	NA	NA	NA	NA	0/5
Bullard and Nashold (1984)	VL	7	7	7	1.5 (0.2 to 3)	7/7 (100)	6/7 (86)	3/7 (43)
Bullard and Nashold (1988)[b]	VL	10	10	8	1.3 (0.2 to 3)	8/8 (100)	7/8 (90)	4/8 (50)
Iwadate et al. (1989)	VL	3	2	NA	NA	2/3 (66)	NA	NA
Richardson (1989)	VL	1	1	NA	NA	1/1	NA	NA
Goldman and Kelly (1992)	VL	4	4	4	3 (1.4 to 4.5)	3/4 (75)	3/4 (75)	0/4 (0)
Marks (1993)	VIM	7	6	NA	NA	6/7 (86)	NA	1/7 (14)
Taira et al. (1993)	VOP, VIM	3	1	3	0.5	1/3 (33)	NA	2/3 (66)
Krauss et al. (1994)	VL, Zi	35	35	32	10.5 (0.5 to 24)	28/32 (88)	26/29 (90)	12/32 (38)
Jankovic et al. (1995)	VIM	6	6	6	4	6/6 (100)	3/6 (50)	3/6 (50)
Shahzadi et al. (1995)[a]	VIM	11	11	NA	NA	NA	NA	6/11 (55)
Louis et al. (1996)	VL	2	2	2	0.3 and 4	2/2	NA	NA
Total		128	113/118 (96%)	68 (53%)		81/92 (88%)	56/65 (86%)	38/103 (37%)

GP, globus pallidus; NA, not available; STR, subthalamic region; VIM, (nucleus) ventralis intermedius (thalami); VL, ventrolateral thalamus; VOP, (nucleus) ventrooralis posterior (thalami); Zi, zona incerta.
[a]Series with tremors of different origins, usually cerebellar-type tremors; specific data for posttraumatic tremor not always available.
[b]The series of Bullard and Nashold from 1988 includes the patients in the series from 1984.

TABLE 26.2. FUNCTIONAL STEREOTACTIC SURGERY FOR POSTTRAUMATIC TREMOR: DEEP BRAIN STIMULATION

Author (yr)	Target	Cases	Immediate Improvement	Long-Term Follow-up	Last Follow-up (yr)	Symptomatic Improvement	Functional Improvement	Persistent Side Effects
Andy (1983)	CM-PF, Zi	1	1	NA	NA	1/1	1/1	0/1
Broggi et al. (1993)	VIM	1	1	1	0.8	1/1	1/1	0/1
Nguyen and Degos (1993)	VIM	1	1	1	1	1/1	1/1	0/1
Benabid et al. (1996)[a]	VIM	X/7	NA	NA	NA	"Inconsistently, less significantly, or not improved"	"Significant improvement observed in the quality of daily living"	NA
Standhart et al. (1998)	VIM	1	0	NA	NA	0/1	NA	NA
Nobbe (2000)[b]	VOP	1	1	1	0.5	1/1	1/1	0/1
Krauss (2000)[b]	VOP/VIM	1	1	1	1.5	1/1	1/1	0/1
Vesper et al. (2000)	VOP/VIM	4	4	4	0.5	4/4	4/4	NA

CM-PF, centrum medianum–(nucleus) parafascicularis (thalami); NA, not available; VIM, (nucleus) ventralis intermedius; VOP, (nucleus) ventrooralis posterior (thalami); Zi, zona incerta.
[a]Series with tremors of different origins, usually cerebellar-type tremors; specific data for posttraumatic tremor not always available.
[b]Unpublished data.

Our literature review detected a total of 128 patients who were reported to have undergone ablative stereotactic surgery for posttraumatic tremor since 1960 (Table 26.1). Evaluation of the reported data often is difficult because many patients were grouped in series undergoing thalamotomy for tremors of different origin. Overall, immediate intraoperative or postoperative improvement of tremor was obtained in almost all instances. Amelioration of the tremor on follow-up examinations was reported in 81 of 92 instances (88%). However, few studies have assessed true long-term follow-up, and in many cases, the duration of follow-up was unclear or was limited to 0.5 to 3 years postoperatively. Functional improvement, in general, paralleled the reduction of the kinetic tremors and was described in 56 of 65 patients in whom it was assessed (86%). Both transient and persistent side effects were reported frequently. Transient side effects included worsening of preoperative dysarthria and dysphagia, gait disturbance, and contralateral motor deficits. In the multipatient studies on posttraumatic tremor, the frequency of transient side effects varied from 50% to 90%. Worsening of dysarthria was observed in 70% of patients in the early postoperative period in the series of Bullard and Nashold (9). Decreased velopharyngeal functioning, a decrease in the oronasal pressure differential, and decreased range of motion of the tongue were characteristic findings. Although many patients have a subsequent improvement of adverse effects in the first few weeks or months after the operation, postoperative morbidity tends to persist in a considerable proportion of patients. Overall, persistent side effects have been reported to occur in 37% of patients, with a range between 0% and 66% in different studies.

Symptomatic and Functional Outcome in a Series of 35 Patients

We reported elsewhere on the symptomatic and functional long-term outcome in a series of 35 patients who underwent thalamic and subthalamic region radiofrequency lesioning for severe posttraumatic appendicular tremors (13). The tremors were most evident on activity in all but one of these patients. The amplitude of the kinetic tremor was greater than 5 cm in 33 patients (94%) and greater than 12 cm in 19 patients (54%). All these patients were severely incapacitated in daily living activities by the tremors. The 35 patients underwent a total of 42 stereotactic operations for the tremors. Twenty-two patients underwent left-sided procedures only (63%), and 11 patients had surgical treatment on the right side only (31%), whereas two patients were operated on bilaterally by a staged procedure (6%). The contralateral zona incerta was the stereotactic target in 12 instances and was targeted in combination with the base of the ventrolateral (oroventral) thalamus in 25 instances. Five patients were reoperated on the same side on recurrence of the tremor. Immediate intraoperative abolition or reduction of the tremor was achieved in 98% of the procedures. Side effects, however, were observed in as many as 25 pa-

tients (71%) in the early postoperative period. Worsening of preoperative dysarthria was seen in ten patients (29%), and increased dysphagia occurred in two patients (6%). Nine patients (26%) had a transient increase in hemiparesis on the surgical side. Truncal ataxia worsened in five patients (14%), and increased lack of initiative was noted in eight patients (23%). Postoperative long-term follow-up was obtained in 32 patients (mean follow-up period, 10.5 years). Persistent improvement of tremor was noted in 88%. The tremor was absent or markedly reduced in 65%. In only two patients, control of the tremor was considered minor. Tremor at rest was completely abolished in all but five patients, but the most striking improvement was the reduction in postural and kinetic tremor. Tremor ipsilateral to the lesion site improved in five patients, as did head tremor and body rocking in 14 patients. As in previous studies, the frequency of persistent side effects was relatively high (38%). These side effects consisted mainly in the aggravation of preoperative symptoms with increased dysarthria in 11 patients (34%) and increased truncal ataxia in three patients (9%). All patients with persistent morbidity had had immediate postoperative side effects. There was a trend for patients with left-sided surgical treatment to present more frequently with increased dysarthria than patients who had right-sided procedures. Surprisingly, four other patients benefited from marked amelioration of their dysarthria after placement of the lesions. Two patients developed postoperative hemiballism, which was associated with an infection in one case. Seven patients with preoperative dystonic postures had an increase in dystonia on long-term evaluation, and seven other patients developed dystonic postures or hemidystonia during follow-up. It is unclear whether this effect was related to the surgical procedure or whether it was related primarily to the trauma, because the interval between trauma and the stereotactic operation was relatively shorter in those patients who developed clinically relevant dystonia in the long term. It has been well documented that dystonia may become manifest with a delay of several years after a static cerebral lesion has occurred (42,43). Functional disability, which was assessed and quantified with a modified form of an established rating scale for patients with tremor (44), was reduced from a mean value of 57% of maximal disability preoperatively to 37% in the long term ($p < .001$). Improvement was more striking in patients who had severe incapacitating tremor and who had comparatively fewer other neurologic or mental symptoms preoperatively.

Technical Considerations

As described in thalamotomy for other tremors (45), a wide variability regarding the optimal lesioning site within the thalamus was evident among different surgeons. Lesions most often were placed in the ventrolateral thalamus, but they were also placed in Forel's field, the sub VIM region, the subthalamic area, and the zona incerta (Table 26.1). Targets also varied within the ventrolateral nucleus, and some authors preferred the ventralis intermedius. The limited number of cases and follow-up data on posttraumatic tremor precluded any considerations on which structure may be "best" for stereotactic surgery with respect to reduction of tremor and side effects.

Investigators have stated that in patients with low-frequency high-amplitude kinetic tremors, larger lesions are required as compared with other types of tremor to achieve long-term control (31,32). However, larger lesions may also result in more frequent and severe side effects, in particular in patients with posttraumatic tremor who have additional neurologic deficits. Under such circumstances, combined stereotactic lesions in the zona incerta and the basal ventrolateral thalamus may offer some advantages to create smaller lesions. The zona incerta as a stereotactic target was introduced by Mundinger in the early 1960s to keep lesions smaller (46,47). In our series of functional stereotactic surgery for treatment of posttraumatic tremor, all patients underwent lesioning of the zona incerta, which was combined with placement of a lesion in the base of the ventrolateral thalamus in 23 patients (13). There was a trend for better long-term improvement in patients with combined lesions as compared with those with lesions in the zona incerta alone. MRI studies were obtained in 18 patients who had undergone successful lesioning of the ventral thalamus or the zona incerta at a mean of 11 years postoperatively (range 3 to 20 years). In all patients but one, a lesion could be identified (Fig. 26.3). The mean lesion size was 18 mm³ (range, 10 to 60 mm³), which indeed was comparatively smaller than reported in other studies.

Deep Brain Stimulation for Treatment of Posttraumatic Tremor

Thalamic DBS has been used in only a limited number of patients with posttraumatic tremors (48–53). Andy, in 1983, apparently was the first to describe successful thalamic DBS, in a 39-year-old patient who had developed a "flapping tremor" of the left arm after a severe head injury (48). The patient achieved complete relief of the tremor on chronic DBS and had no untoward side effects. Nguyen and Degos reported on a 15-year-old patient who was severely incapacitated by a right-sided kinetic posttraumatic tremor (51). With chronic DBS over 12 months, the patient achieved both symptomatic and functional improvement and regained the ability to write. Broggi et al. described a 19-year-old man who had unilateral posttraumatic postural and kinetic tremor associated with bradykinesia (49). Chronic thalamic DBS markedly improved the tremor but not the bradykinesia. Benabid and colleagues found thalamic DBS for posttraumatic tremor less effective as compared with its effect on parkinsonian tremor or essential tremor (52). They noted that various tremors and dyskinetic movement disorders, including those in seven patients with posttraumatic or posthemorrhagic midbrain tremors, were "inconsistently, less significantly or not improved." Nevertheless, these investigators reported that even though the improvement of the tremor in their patients was not apprehended by standard clinical rating scales for tremor, "there was significant improvement observed in the quality of daily living." In only one instance, thalamic DBS was found completely ineffective for treatment of posttraumatic tremor (50). In contrast to thalamic lesioning, none of the patients with posttraumatic tremor who underwent thalamic DBS reported to suffer from adverse effects postoperatively.

The possible advantages of thalamic DBS in this group of patients as compared with lesioning may be best illustrated by the following case report. A 31-year-old woman presented with a disabling posttraumatic tremor of her left arm. She had sustained a severe head injury at age 9 years that had rendered her comatose for about 7 weeks. The tremor was first noted several months postoperatively during recovery. On hospital admission, mental and psychologic alterations were

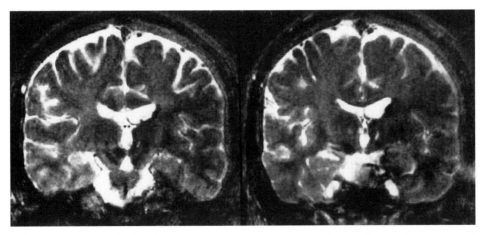

FIGURE 26.3. Coronal spin-echo (SE) 5600/30 magnetic resonance images 3 years after functional stereotactic surgery in the left basal ventrolateral thalamus and zona incerta showing a small lesion that effectively abated this patient's contralateral kinetic posttraumatic tremor. (From Krauss JK, Mohadjer M, Nobbe F, et al. The treatment of posttraumatic tremor by stereotactic surgery. *J Neurosurg* 1994;80:810–819, with permission.)

evident. She obtained a score of 26 out of 30 on the Mini-Mental Status Examination. She had marked dysarthria, and walking was impeded by gait ataxia and postural instability. The right arm adopted a dystonic posture, whereas there was a low-frequency tremor of the left arm on movement with a terminal amplitude of about 5 cm. The tremor was accompanied by ataxia and other cerebellar symptoms. MRI scans showed the aftermath of diffuse axonal injury. The patient underwent stereotactic placement of a quadripolar DBS electrode in the right thalamic ventrooralis posterior/ventralis intermedius nucleus that was connected subcutaneously to a subclavicular impulse generator. There were no adverse events intraoperatively or in the postoperative course. The impulse generator was programmed on the first postoperative day, and this resulted in almost complete abolition of the tremor with bipolar stimulation using a voltage of 1.6 v at a pulse width of 210 microseconds and a frequency of 130 Hz. In the following weeks, there was a partial recurrence of the tremor, which was well controlled, however, by increasing the voltage of stimulation to 3.5 v in several steps. During the subsequent programming sessions, the preliminary amplitude was determined with regard to both control of the tremor and its effect on the patient's dysarthria and gait ataxia. The voltage below the threshold that worsened the patient's preexistent deficits was chosen, respectively. With this regimen, sustained improvement of the tremor was achieved over a follow-up of 2.5 years without the occurrence of adverse effects.

CONCLUSIONS

Functional stereotactic surgery targeting the ventrolateral or ventrointermediate thalamus is a highly effective treatment option for disabling persistent posttraumatic tremor. The major limitation of thalamotomy is the relatively high occurrence of increased preoperative dysarthria and of gait ataxia even with unilateral procedures. The experience with DBS is limited. Nevertheless, DBS appears to be associated with fewer side effects than radiofrequency lesioning in posttraumatic tremor, and its effect can be titrated to balance between improvement of tremor and the induction of stimulation-induced increases in the patients' neurologic deficits. More knowledge of the long-term outcome in these patients is needed.

REFERENCES

1. Krauss JK, Jankovic J. Head injury and posttraumatic movement disorders. *Neurosurgery* 2001; in press.
2. Jankovic J. Post-traumatic movement disorders: central and peripheral mechanisms. *Neurology* 1994;44:2006–2014.
3. Krauss JK, Traenkle R, Kopp KH. Posttraumatic movement disorders in survivors of severe head injury. *Neurology* 1996;47:1488–1492.
4. Krauss JK, Traenkle R, Kopp KH. Movement disorders secondary to moderate and mild head injury. *Mov Disord* 1997;12:428–431.
5. Samie MR, Selhorst JB, Koller WC. Post-traumatic midbrain tremors. *Neurology* 1990;40:62–66.
6. Curran TG, Lang AE. Trauma and tremor. In: Findley LJ, Koller WC, eds. *Handbook of tremor disorders.* New York: Marcel Dekker, 1995;411–428.
7. Johnson SLJ, Hall DMB. Post-traumatic tremor in head injured children. *Arch Dis Child* 1992;67:227–228.
8. Obeso JA, Narbona J. Post-traumatic tremor and myoclonic jerking. *J Neurol Neurosurg Psychiatry* 1983;46:788.
9. Bullard DE, Nashold BS Jr. Stereotaxic thalamotomy for treatment of posttraumatic movement disorders. *J Neurosurg* 1984; 61:316–321.
10. Holmes G. On certain tremors in organic cerebral lesions. *Brain* 1904;27:327–375.
11. Kremer M, Russell WR, Smyth GE. A mid-brain syndrome following head injury. *J Neurol Neurosurg Psychiatry* 1947;10:49–60.
12. Krauss JK, Wakhloo AK, Nobbe F, et al. MR pathological correlations of severe posttraumatic tremor. *Neurol Res* 1995;17:409–416.
13. Krauss JK, Mohadjer M, Nobbe F, et al. The treatment of posttraumatic tremor by stereotactic surgery. *J Neurosurg* 1994;80:810–819.
14. Krauss JK, Traenkle R, Raabe A. Tremor and dystonia after penetrating diencephalic-mesencephalic trauma. *Park Rel Disord* 1997;3:117–119.
15. Remy P, de Recondo A, Defer G, et al. Peduncular 'rubral' tremor and dopaminergic denervation: a PET study. *Neurology* 1995;45:472–477.
16. Aisen ML, Adelstein BD, Romerco J, et al. Glutethimide treatment of disabling action tremor in patients with multiple sclerosis and traumatic brain injury. *Arch Neurol* 1991;48:513–515.
17. Ellison PH. Propranolol for severe post-head injury action tremor. *Neurology* 1978;28:197–199.
18. Sandyk R, Iacono RP, Fisher H. Posttraumatic cerebellar syndrome: response to L-tryptophan. *Int J Neuroscience* 1989;47:301–302.
19. Jankovic J, Schwartz K, Clemence W, et al. A randomized, double-blind, placebo-controlled study to evaluate botulinum toxin type A in essential hand tremor. *Mov Disord* 1996;11:250–256.
20. Bucy PC. Relation to abnormal involuntary movements. In: Bucy PC, ed. *The precentral motor cortex,* 2nd ed. Urbana, IL: University of Illinois Press, 1949:395–408.
21. Cooper IS. Neurosurgical alleviation of intention tremor of multiple sclerosis and cerebellar disease. *N Engl J Med* 1960;263:441–444.
22. Nashold BS, Slaughter DG. Effects of stimulating or destroying the deep cerebellar regions in man. *J Neurosurg* 1969;31:172–186.
23. Spiegel EA, Wycis HT, Szekely EG, et al. Campotomy in various extrapyramidal disorders. *J Neurosurg* 1963;20:871–884.
24. Fox JL, Kurtzke JF. Trauma-induced intention tremor relieved by stereotaxic thalamotomy. *Arch Neurol* 1966;15:247–251.
25. Samra K, Waltz JM, Riklan M, et al. Relief of intention tremor by thalamic surgery. *J Neurol Neurosurg Psychiatry* 1970;33:7–15.
26. Van Manen J. Stereotaxic operations in cases of hereditary and intention tremor. *Acta Neurochirur* 1974;21[Suppl]:49–55.
27. Eiras J, Cosamalon JG. Síndrome mioclónico posttraumático: efectividad de las lesiones talámicas sobre las mioclonías de acción. *Arch Neurobiol* 1980;43:17–28.
28. Andrew J, Fowler CJ, Harrison MJG. Tremor after head injury and its treatment by stereotaxic surgery. *J Neurol Neurosurg Psychiatry* 1982;45:815–819.
29. Kandel EI. Treatment of hemihyperkinesias by stereotactic operations on basal ganglia. *Appl Neurophysiol* 1982;45:225–229
30. Niizuma H, Kwak R, Ohyama H, et al. Stereotactic thalamotomy

for postapoplectic and posttraumatic involuntary movements. *Appl Neurophysiol* 1982;45:295–298.

31. Ohye C, Hirai T, Miyazaki M, et al. VIM thalamotomy for the treatment of various kinds of tremor. *Appl Neurophysiol* 1982;45:275–280.

32. Hirai T, Miyazaki, Nakajima H, et al. The correlation between tremor characteristics and the predicted volume of effective lesions in stereotaxic nucleus ventralis intermedius thalamotomy. *Brain* 1983;106:1001–1018.

33. Bullard DE, Nashold BS. Posttraumatic movement disorders. In: Lunsford LD, ed. *Modern stereotactic neurosurgery.* Boston: Martinus Nijhoff, 1988:341–352.

34. Iwadate Y, Saeki N, Namba H, et al. Post-traumatic intention tremor—clinical features and findings. *Neurosurg Rev* 1989; 12[Suppl 1]:500–507.

35. Richardson RR. Rehabilitative neurosurgery: posttraumatic syndromes. *Stereotact Funct Neurosurg* 1989;53:105–112.

36. Goldman MS, Kelly PJ. Symptomatic and functional outcome of stereotactic ventralis lateralis thalamotomy for intention tremor. *J Neurosurg* 1992;77:223–229.

37. Marks PV. Stereotactic surgery for post-traumatic cerebellar syndrome: an analysis of seven cases. *Stereotact Funct Neurosurg* 1993;60:157–167.

38. Taira T, Speelman JD, Bosch DA. Trajectory angle in stereotactic thalamotomy. *Stereotact Funct Neurosurg* 1993;61:24–31.

39. Jankovic J, Cardoso F, Grossman RG, et al. Outcome after stereotactic thalamotomy for parkinsonian, essential, and other types of tremor. *Neurosurgery* 1995;37:680–686.

40. Shahzadi D, Tasker RR, Lozano A. Thalamotomy for essential and cerebellar tremor. *Stereotact Funct Neurosurg* 1995;65:11–17.

41. Louis ED, Lynch T, Ford B, et al. Delayed-onset cerebellar syndrome. *Arch Neurol* 1996;53:450–454.

42. Krauss JK, Mohadjer M, Braus DF, et al. Dystonia following head trauma: a report of nine patients and review of the literature. *Mov Disord* 1992:7:263–272.

43. Pettigrew LC, Jankovic J. Hemidystonia: a report of 22 patients and a review of the literature. *J Neurol Neurosurg Psychiatry* 1985; 48:650–657.

44. Fahn S, Tolosa E, Marín C. Clinical rating scale for tremor. In: Jankovic J, Tolosa E, eds. *Parkinson's disease and movement disorders.* Baltimore: Urban & Schwarzenberg, 1988:225–234.

45. Laitinen LV. Brain targets in surgery for Parkinson's disease. *J Neurosurg* 1985;62:349–351.

46. Mundinger F. Stereotaxic interventions on the zona incerta area for treatment of extrapyramidal motor disturbances and their results. *Confin Neurol* 1965;26:222–230.

47. Mundinger F. 30 Jahre stereotaktische Hirnoperationen beim Parkinsonismus (Ergebnisse im Vergleich pallido-thalamo-subthalamischer Ausschaltungen und Indikationen). In: Gänshirt H, Berlit P, Haack G, eds. *Pathophysiologie, Klinik und Therapie des Parkinsonismus.* Basel: Editiones Roche, 1983:331–357.

48. Andy OJ. Thalamic stimulation for control of movement disorders. *Appl Neurophysiol* 1983;46:107–111.

49. Broggi G, Brock S, Franzini A, et al. A case of posttraumatic tremor treated by chronic stimulation of the thalamus. *Mov Disord* 1993;8:206–208.

50. Standhart H, Pinter MM, Volc D, et al. Chronic electrical stimulation of the nucleus ventralis intermedius of the thalamus for the treatment of tremor. *Mov Disord* 1998;13[Suppl 3]:141.

51. Nguyen JP, Degos JD. Thalamic stimulation and proximal tremor: a specific target in the nucleus ventrointermedius thalami. *Arch Neurol* 1993;50:498–500.

52. Benabid AL, Pollak P, Gao D et al. Chronic electrical stimulation of the ventral intermedius nucleus of the thalamus as a treatment of movement disorders. *J Neurosurg* 1996;84:203–214.

53. Vesper J, Funk T, Kean BC, et al. Thalamic deep brain stimulation: present state of the art. *Neurosurg Quart* 2000;10:252–260.

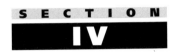

DYSTONIA

Surgery for Parkinson's Disease and Movement Disorders,
edited by J.K. Krauss, J. Jankovic, and R.G. Grossman.
Lippincott Williams & Wilkins, Philadelphia © 2001.

27

PALLIDOTOMY AND THALAMOTOMY FOR DYSTONIA

WILLIAM G. ONDO
MICHAEL DESALOMS
JOACHIM K. KRAUSS
JOSEPH JANKOVIC
ROBERT G. GROSSMAN

Dystonia is defined as patterned involuntary muscle contraction. Although the diagnosis is based solely on clinical examination, electromyographic cocontraction of agonist and antagonist muscles is characteristic. Dystonia can occur in any part of the body, and thus initially it was thought to represent several distinct diseases. The nomenclature is still largely based on anatomic distribution. Different classifications include generalized dystonia (entire body), hemidystonia (one side, usually from a structural lesion), segmental dystonia (multiple but contiguous body parts), or focal dystonia (one body part). The focal dystonias are named according to anatomic site. The most common include cervical dystonia (often called torticollis, which actually means pure rotation of the neck), blepharospasm (periocular), and writer's cramp (hand and arm during writing).

Dystonic muscle activity is usually precipitated, or at least exacerbated, by planned volitional muscle actions. Some focal dystonias that first occur only with very specific actions are termed *task-specific dystonias.* Any act requiring repetitive motions, such as writing, stenography, or playing musical instruments can evolve into a task-specific dystonia. Of these, writer's cramp is the most common.

As a general rule, focal dystonias begin in the fourth to sixth decade and remain focal. In contrast, dystonia that begins in childhood typically occurs in the limbs, and it often spreads to become generalized. It is not clear whether this variation results from different pathophysiologic processes or whether it is a true age-dependent phenomenon.

Several other distinct forms of dystonia are separately classified. *Tardive dystonia* (seen after exposure to dopamine-blocking drugs) often results in neck and trunk extension and can be severe (1). *Paroxysmal dyskinesias,* which can occur in a setting of action (kinesiogenic) or rest (nonkinesiogenic), are predominately dystonic and may represent seizure activity within the basal ganglia (2). *Dopa-responsive dystonia* (Segawa's dystonia) actually represents several different enzymatic perturbations that impede the production of endogenous dopamine (3,4). This condition responds dramatically to levodopa replacement.

Dystonia may be primary or secondary. Although many *genetic* (primary) forms of dystonia have been linked, only *DYT-1,* which codes for the protein torsion A, is available for testing (5,6). This specific condition is most commonly seen in eastern Europeans, especially Ashkenazi Jews. It usually presents in childhood with limb involvement before it spreads to become generalized. The other genetic generalized dystonias have heterogeneous characteristics and demographics (Table 27.1). Because most of these conditions have only partial penetrance, the absence of a clear family history does not irrefutably preclude their existence (7–11).

Various *neurologic conditions* such as static encephalopathies (dystonic cerebral palsy), Wilson's disease, and Hallervorden-Spatz disease can include dystonia as part of their phenotype (12,13). Any structural lesion within the basal ganglia, thalamus, or brainstem can also cause secondary dystonia, especially in younger people (14). Peripheral nerve injuries occasionally cause dystonia that tends to be painful and segmental (15).

PATHOPHYSIOLOGY OF DYSTONIA

The exact pathophysiologic mechanisms resulting in both primary and secondary dystonia are unknown. Increasing evidence, however, suggests that altered signaling through

W.G. Ondo and J. Jankovic: Department of Neurology, Baylor College of Medicine, Houston Texas 77030.

M. Desaloms and R.G. Grossman: Department of Neurosurgery, Presbyterian Hospital of Dallas, Dallas, Texas 75231.

J.K. Krauss: Department of Neurosurgery, University Hospital, Klinikum Mannheim, 68167 Mannheim, Germany.

TABLE 27.1. GENETIC DYSTONIAS

Dystonia	Pattern of Inheritance	Linkage Site	Ethnic Origins	Phenotype and Additional Features
DYT-1[a]	AD	9q34.1	Ashkenazi Jewish	C.O., generalized, limb onset
DYT-2	AR	—	Spanish	—
DYT-3[b]	X-linked	Xq13	Filipino	Young A.O., cranial, generalized, parkinsonism
DYT-4	AD	—	Australia	Hypophonia
DYT-5[c]	AD	14q22.1		C.O., diurnal, L-dopa responsive
DYT-6	AD	8p21–q22**	Mennonite, Amish	A.O., cranial, arm, dysarthria
DYT-7	AD	18p	German	A.O., cranial, cervical, arm tremor
DYT-8	AD	2q33–q25	—	C.O., paroxysmal choreoathetosis
DYT-9	AD	11p	—	C.O., paroxysmal ataxia
DYT-10	AD		—	C.O., paroxysmal kinesigenic
DYT-11	AD	11q23	—	C.O., myoclonus, alcohol responsive
DYT-12	AD	19q13	—	Rapid-onset dystonia-parkinsonism

AD, autosomal dominant; A.O., adult onset; AR, autosomal recessive, C.O., child onset.
[a]Oppenheim's dystonia: GAC deletion in torsinA protein (an adenosine triphosphate–binding protein).
[b]Lubag's disease: striatal gliosis.
[c]Segawa's dopa-resonsive dystonia: (guanosine triphosphate cyclohydrolase deficiency); other defects also identified.

the basal ganglia circuitry causes changes within the supplementary motor area (SMA) and sensorimotor cortex. The dopaminergic system is specifically implicated by positron emission tomography (PET) studies that show a moderate reduction in putamen $[^{18}F]$-dopa uptake in familial dystonia (16). Perlmutter et al. reported reduced putaminal binding of $[^{18}F]$-spiperone, a radioligand relatively specific for D_2 receptors, thus implicating the "indirect" basal ganglia pathway in the pathophysiology of dystonia (17). The "indirect" pathway may also play a key role in the production of levodopa-induced dyskinesias in patients with Parkinson's disease (PD) (18), and it is generally thought to inhibit unwanted movement (19).

According to current basal ganglia models, reduced dopaminergic input into both the "indirect" and "direct" pathway results in increased activity of the internal segment of the globus pallidus (GPi). In 1-methyl-4-phenyl-1,2,3,6-tetrahydropyridine models of PD, microelectrode recordings of the GPi have consistently demonstrated increased GPi activity in the "off" state. It is also generally assumed that patients with PD have increased GPi activity, although "normal" control data do not actually exist in human patients. GPi recordings in patients with dystonia have been more variable. Overall, the GPi firing rate is less than that seen in "off" patients with PD, and it is even less than that seen in normal nonhuman primates. Importantly, however, the firing pattern is irregular and clumped (20). Moreover, patients with dystonia show a higher number of GPi cells that respond to sensory stimulation (20,21). This increased response to sensory input is also seen in the ventralis intermedius (VIM) nucleus of the thalamus (20,22).

Our own data also show that GPi firing in dystonia is less than that seen in PD (31.8 ± 14.8 versus 84.7 ± 29.6 per minute; $p < .001$; Mann-Whitney Rank Sum test). The dystonia firing pattern does appear to be irregular and clumped. However, no clear correlation exists between absolute GPi firing rate and surgical outcome.

The GPi, which is the main basal ganglia outflow nucleus, functionally inhibits the ventrolateral/ventroanterior thalamus (VL/VA), which then stimulates the SMA. In PD, SMA activity is reduced, as predicted by this model, and it can be increased by both dopaminergic treatment and pallidotomy (23–27). In dystonia, however, the relationship between GPi output and cortical activity is less clear. Studies suggests that rostral SMA (rostral premotor and dorsolateral prefrontal cortex) activity is increased with limb movement in both primary and secondary dystonia (16,28). Primary dystonia demonstrates decreased primary motor cortex activity, whereas dystonia secondary to basal ganglia lesions results in increased activity of the primary motor cortex (16,28).

Kumar et al. recently compared $[^{15}O]H_2O$ PET images in a single patient with primary but not clearly genetic dystonia, before and after activation of bilateral GPi deep brain stimulation (DBS), which mimics the effects of lesioning (29). During joystick movements, activation of the GPi DBS reduced PET activity bilaterally in the primary motor, lateral premotor, SMA, anterior cingulate, and prefrontal areas and ipsilaterally in the lentiform nucleus. There were no differences while at rest.

Therefore, it appears that GPi lesioning improves pathologic irregular GPi firing patterns in a manner that reduces cortical overactivity. Specific differences in the pathophysiology of various dystonia types remain unclear.

HISTORY OF CENTRAL NERVOUS SYSTEM ABLATIVE SURGERY FOR DYSTONIA

Russell Meyers, during the 1940s, was arguably the first to perform lesioning of the basal ganglia to treat movement disorders (30). He targeted several different sites, including the ansa lenticularis and the GP. Shortly thereafter, Spiegel first used a stereotactic frame in conjunction with pneumoencephalography for human surgery (31). As stereotactic techniques improved over the next two decades, basal ganglia surgery was performed for a variety of movement disorders including dystonia. Cooper reported the largest early series using thalamotomy for dystonia, and for many years, this was clearly considered the surgical procedure of choice (32). More recently, pallidotomy regained popularity as a treatment for fluctuating PD because its dramatic effect is the reduction of levodopa-induced dyskinesia. Because dyskinesia are clinically, and possibly physiologically, similar to dystonia, pallidotomy has been reconsidered for the treatment of dystonia, for which it has demonstrated initial success.

PATIENT SELECTION FOR CENTRAL NERVOUS SYSTEM ABLATIVE SURGERY

Only a few patients with dystonia should be considered for central nervous system (CNS) ablative surgery. Whereas loose selection guidelines can be proposed for pallidotomy and thalamotomy, several principles apply to both procedures.

First, the dystonia must be severe enough to warrant surgical intervention. Typically, we consider only patients with generalized and hemidystonias, because these patients are the most severely affected, and these conditions are most refractory to therapy. Few good data are available regarding the treatment of focal dystonia with CNS ablation, and most focal dystonias can be treated satisfactorily with botulinum toxin (BTX) and medications.

Second, in all cases patients must have had unsatisfactory responses to more conventional and less invasive treatments. These include various pharmacologic agents including anticholinergics (trihexyphenidyl, benztropine), benzodiazepines (e.g., diazepam, clonazepam), baclofen, tizanidine, levodopa, and in some cases dantrolene. Other muscle relaxants including cyclobenzaprine, methocarbamol, carisoprodol, and metaxalone are also occasionally helpful. These medications are dose dependent, so in most cases the dose should be augmented until adverse events become prohibitive. Furthermore, polytherapy with agents employing different mechanisms of action is usually superior to monotherapy. Again, adverse events eventually limit the dosing.

BTX is currently the mainstay of treatment for most focal dystonias, with or without adjunctive pharmacotherapy. It is effective for discrete anatomic areas, especially in the face and neck. Involvement of larger anatomic areas, such as the legs, significantly increases the required dose of BTX and makes the use of this agent more problematic for several reasons. The cost of therapy increases greatly from approximately $100 per injection for the small doses used in hemifacial spasm to more than $2,500 per injection for the large amounts needed for generalized dystonia. Because these injections are administered three to four times per year, the cost of treated generalized dystonia can be prohibitive. Furthermore, the development of neutralizing antibodies against the toxin correlates with higher and more frequent dosing (33). Although additional strains of BTX are now available, it appears that resistance will remain a problem. Other less well studied treatment alternatives include phenol injections, physical therapy, and electrical stimulation. Peripheral denervation procedures are discussed in Chapters 30 and 31.

Third, CNS ablation may be limited by the usual contraindications and restrictions of surgery and anesthesia. In contrast to patients with PD, who usually undergo similar procedures while awake, the severe muscle contractions seen in patients with dystonia often necessitate general anesthesia.

PALLIDOTOMY FOR DYSTONIA

The surgical methods for *pallidotomy* in dystonia are identical to those used for PD (34–36). They are described in Chapters 5 and 6. Briefly, localization of the GPi is performed using a Leskell G head frame and 1-mm computed tomography axial scans. The initial target is 19 to 21 mm lateral to the midline, 4 to 5 mm inferior to the anterior commissure–posterior commissure (AC-PC) line, and 2 to 3 mm anterior to the midcommissural point. Single-unit extracellular recordings help to guide lesion placement when high-frequency discharges are identified. Photic stimulation is used to identify the optic pathways. The electrical recording techniques are described in more detail separately. Finally, two radiofrequency lesions are made 2 mm apart along the same trajectory for 60 seconds at 75°C.

To date, we have adequate follow-up data on 12 patients, aged 5 to 56 years, who underwent GPi lesioning for general dystonia or hemidystonia (Table 27.2). Of these patients, three were older than 21 years. The patients were taking a total of 30 medications for dystonia at the time of surgery, and 11 patients had received BTX injections within the previous year.

The pathogenesis of dystonia varied. Three patients had a clear genetic dystonia, and two of them tested positive for *DYT-1*. Three patients had idiopathic dystonia, but they did not have a clear genetic history of dystonia, and six cases were believed to be symptomatic (secondary) from hypoxia (three patients), focal hemorrhage (one patient), and peripheral nerve injury (one patient). In one patient, the pathogenesis was not clear because he had a mild perinatal hypoxic event that did not have a sequela until the appearance of rapidly progressive generalized dystonia when he was 5 years old. There was no family history, and no other cause could be found.

Patients were evaluated preoperatively and at 3 to 6 months postoperatively. Results of 1- and 2-year follow-up examinations were available in some of these patients. In addition to general neurologic evaluation, patients underwent unblinded dystonia assessments with the Burke-Marsden-Fahn Dystonia Scale (BMFDS) and the Unified Dystonia Rating Scale (37,38). The UDRS is a detailed rating of dystonia amplitude (0 to 4) and duration (0 to 4) in 14 different body areas. An activity of daily living scale based on the UDRS was also used and included questions (each scored from 0 to 5) regarding the patient's ability to write, eat, drink from a cup, and walk. The UDRS is currently being validated by the Dystonia Study Group.

TABLE 27.2. CHARACTERISTICS OF 12 PATIENTS UNDERGOING PALLIDOTOMY

Patient	Age at Surgery (yr)	Age at Onset (yr)	Initial Site of Dystonia	Current Site of Dystonia	Cause	Surgical Site
1	56	41	Left arm	Cervical > Generalized	Trauma	Left
2	51	10	Right arm	Generalized	Idiopathic	Bilateral (s)
3	18	13	Oral	Generalized	Trauma	Bilateral(s)
4	9	6	Right foot	Generalized (right > left)	Genetic	Bilateral (s)
5	16	10	Oral	Generalized	Probably hypoxic	Bilateral (c)
6	20	12	Right arm	R hemisphere	Trauma	Left
7	14	7	Right arm	Generalized	Genetic	Bilateral (c)
8	13	10	Right arm	Generalized	Genetic	Bilateral (c)
9	14	8	Generalized	Generalized	Hemorrhage	Bilateral (c)
10	6	4	Bilateral legs	Generalized	Idiopathic	Bilateral (2)
11	25	7	Right arm	Right hemisphere	Hypoxic[a]	Left
12	7	6	Right side	Generalized (right > left)	Idiopathic[b]	Bilateral (s)
Total	20.8 (11.6)	11.6 (7.1)				

(c), concurrent; (s), staged.
[a]Gunshot wound severing carotid artery.
[b]Cognitive developmental delay, hypertelorism.

Ten patients had bilateral procedures (staged in three patients and concurrent in seven). Both patients who had unilateral procedures had symptomatic hemidystonia. Overall, ten of 12 patients demonstrated significant improvement (Table 27.3). One male patient who experienced global hypoxia secondary to drowning did not improve at all after simultaneous bilateral pallidotomy. He demonstrated a mixed movement disorder consisting of generalized dystonia, chorea, and myoclonus. A second girl with an area of hemosiderin in the GPi and external segment of the GP had mild improvement in one arm after a bilateral procedure, but no other change.

All the patients with genetic and idiopathic dystonias (both *DYT-1* positive and *DYT-1* negative) demonstrated marked improvement, whereas improvement in the symptomatic dystonias tended to be less dramatic and less consistent. Nevertheless, some patients with symptomatic dystonias still had robust benefit.

It is difficult to compare the efficacy of unilateral operations with that of concurrent bilateral procedures because this decision was clinically based on the anatomic distribution of the dystonia. All patients with oromandibular and axial dystonia had bilateral procedures, and therefore it is difficult to know what, if any, improvement unilateral pallidotomy would have had on their midline dystonia. The patients who underwent staged bilateral procedures experienced predominantly contralateral improvement after the first procedure and further axial and bilateral improvement after the second procedure.

Improvement in different anatomic areas has been relatively consistent. The most dramatic benefit occurs in the hands and arms, which return to normal levels of function

TABLE 27.3. INDIVIDUAL OUTCOME MEASURES: 3-MONTH FOLLOW-UP

Patient	Preoperative BMF	Postoperative BMF	Preoperative UDRS	Postoperative UDRS	Preoperative ADL	Postoperative ADL	No. Preoperative Medications	No. Postoperative Medications
1	34	13	51	16	12	6	3	1
2	57	9	83	20	16	8	3	1
3	56	46	86	58	18	16	3	2
4	26	13	36	12	10	5	2	0
5	59	17	101	27	19	9	3	0
6	23	6	38	11	10	6	2	1
7	50	17	68	21	18	7	3	0
8	48	17	81	20	17	6	3	0
9	56	45	82	74	19	18	3	3
10	58	36	88	54	19	18	3	3
11	25	13	37	15	13	10	1	0
12	31	25	51	34	15	11	1	1
Mean	43.6	21.5	66.8	32.2	15.5	9.8	2.5	1.0
(SD)	13.2	10.0	20.2	15.7	2.9	3.5	0.7	0.8

ADL, Activity of Daily Living Scale; BMF, Burke Marsden Fahn Scale; UDRS, Unified Dystonia Rating Scale.

in many cases. Lower extremity function and gait also consistently improve. Midline structures, however, especially the jaw, do not respond as consistently, even with bilateral procedures.

The course of improvement is interesting and has led to considerable speculative debate. Pallidotomy performed for PD immediately improves motor tone and dyskinesia. Motor tone in patients with dystonia may improve almost immediately, but the actual dystonia does not begin to improve for 2 to 7 days. Improvement continues for up to 3 months. It is unknown whether this finding represents a relearning effect or some ongoing pathophysiologic change. The improvement has been generally maintained over time, but we have seen some mild recrudescence, especially in the midline structures (jaw and neck). All patients who initially responded are still much improved after a mean of 1.5 years of follow-up.

Complications related to surgery were limited to transient postoperative lethargy in one patient and mild unilateral weakness in another patient. Postoperative magnetic resonance imaging demonstrated lesions that were confined within the GPi in all cases except in the patient with transient weakness, in whom the lesion extended slightly into the internal capsule. There was no clear difference in adverse events between unilateral and bilateral procedures. The patient with postoperative lethargy had a bilateral procedure. No bulbar symptoms or cognitive compromise occurred in any case.

Therefore, from our experience, we consider the ideal candidate for pallidotomy to (a) have a primary genetic generalized dystonia, (b) have no surgical contraindications, (c) be refractory to other treatments, and (d) have considerable disability referable to the limbs rather than midline structures. However, patients who do not meet all these criteria may still have a dramatic benefit from pallidotomy.

Our results have been generally consistent with those seen in others centers that perform pallidotomy for dystonia (39–48). The delayed improvement has been consistently observed. Most series, however, are too small to assess factors that may otherwise predict response.

Iacono et al. first published an account of striking improvement after bilateral pallidotomies in a 17-year-old boy with primary generalized dystonia (42), and they subsequently reported mixed results in four additional cases (43). "Marked improved" was noted in two adults with craniocervical dystonia. One of these underwent bilateral pallidotomies, and the other, who had isolated cervical dystonia, underwent a left pallidotomy. A 48-year-old patient with primary spasmodic dysphonia and left lower extremity dystonia experienced moderate improvement in leg dystonia, but no change in dysphonia, after a right pallidotomy. A 24-year-old patient with secondary generalized dystonia, primarily appendicular in distribution, did not improve.

Vitek et al. reported marked improvement in contralateral dystonic symptoms, with significant reductions in the BMFDS of 72% to 80% after unilateral pallidotomy in three patients (20). Comparison of preoperative and postoperative surface electromyographic studies of overactive muscle groups revealed decreased coactivation of agonist-antagonist muscle groups during movement and a dramatic reduction in resting electromyographic activity after pallidotomy. One year postoperatively, there was better residual improvement in appendicular signs, and these investigators speculated that axial symptoms may be better treated with bilateral pallidotomies. Vitek also experienced more favorable results with pallidotomy in patients with primary dystonia who tested positive for the *DYT-1* gene (personal communication).

Lozano and associates reported remarkable improvement in an 8-year-old Ashkenazi boy with familial (*DYT-1*-negative) primary generalized dystonia after simultaneous bilateral pallidotomies (40). Improvement continued for 3 months postoperatively. Lin et al. also observed progressive postoperative improvement leading to an excellent functional outcome after staged bilateral pallidotomies in a 36-year-old woman with severe secondary generalized dystonia (46).

THALAMOTOMY

Patient Selection

In most instances, guidelines similar to those used for pallidotomy govern the selection process for potential candidates for *thalamotomy*. Patients must be severely incapacitated by their dystonic symptoms and must be refractory to medical management. There are numerous potential surgical risks, and bilateral procedures are often indicated, with their additional risk of dysarthria and other bulbar signs. The origin of dystonia, whether primary or secondary, must be clearly elucidated if possible because certain subgroups of patients dystonia may respond differently to thalamotomy and pallidotomy.

Surgical Technique

The surgical technique for thalamotomy in dystonia is similar to that in patients with PD in most centers (50–54). The target is usually in the VIM nucleus. At our center, the target is slightly more anterior and medial in the ventrolateral thalamus. The lesion therefore lies in the area designated the ventralis oralis (VOA/VOP) in the Hassler terminology.

General anesthesia is often required to ensure the patient's safety during the procedure. In addition, patients with dystonia are usually children and may not tolerate stereotactic procedures done using local anesthesia. Performing stereotactic procedures without patient feedback, however, makes target localization more difficult.

Briefly, the procedure begins with placement of the stereotactic frame to align the frame parallel to the patient's AC-PC line using a Leksell G head frame. A computed tomography scan is then performed with contiguous 1-mm axial slices through the basal ganglia and ventricular system. The images are then transferred to a workstation that reconstructs the data on sagittal and coronal views. The AC and PC are identified, and the AC-PC line is used as a reference for targeting. Patients with dystonia may have narrow third ventricles, and adjustments need to be made accordingly (51). The most common coordinate setting for the VOA/VOP nuclei is 12 mm lateral, 1 mm above, and 2 mm posterior to the midcommissural point. This situation places the lesion along the border between these two nuclei. A bur hole is made 2 cm anterior to the coronal suture and 3 cm lateral to the midline. In awake patients, stimulation induces increased dystonic movements in the contralateral extremities. A lesion is made with a 1.1×3.0 mm bare-tip electrode at $75°C$ for 60 seconds.

The surgical procedure usually provides a degree of relaxation of the dystonic symptoms immediately in awake patients, although the full effect is not apparent until weeks or months postoperatively. If an additional lesion is made, it is usually extended slightly anteriorly and medially. Although microelectrode recording has been very helpful in performing pallidotomies for dystonia, we do not use it for targeting the thalamus (50).

Outcomes

In our experience of 17 patients with dystonia who underwent VOA/VOP thalamotomy, 47% showed early moderate improvement that was sustained over time (50). Further improvement was noted in 12% of patients with time. Patients with secondary dystonia tended to fare better than those with primary dystonia, with a moderate to marked improvement in 50% versus 43%. In addition, as with pallidotomy for dystonia, improvement is often delayed and gradual. This finding, again, contrasts with thalamotomy used to treat tremor in PD. Comparison of our results with those of others (Table 27.4) is difficult because of the differences in the rating scales, the nuclei targeted, the lengths of follow-up, and the heterogeneous groups of patients studied. Regardless, the results appear similar to those of others, with a moderate improvement seen overall.

Cooper reported the first large series of thalamotomy for generalized dystonia. One hundred four patients underwent unilateral surgical procedures, and 122 patients underwent bilateral surgery (55,56). His usual target was in the VIM, ventral caudal, and centromedian nuclei. The lesions were typically large, and the procedure was often repeated if not effective. Overall, 69.7% of patients showed mild to moderate improvement in the short term. Cooper noted a consistent deterioration in improvement with time in many of his patients. Axial and appendicular symptoms responded equally well. The mortality rate in this series was 2%.

Kandel performed 272 procedures on 188 patients with primary dystonia. His lesions were typically located in the ventrolateral nucleus, although he sometimes added lesions into both the GPi and subthalamic nucleus (57). Overall, 54% of patients showed significant improvement, and 22% showed good improvement in dystonic symptoms. The reported mortality rate was 1.8%, and the morbidity rate was 10%.

Tasker et al. reported thalamotomy results in 49 patients, 20 with primary dystonia and 29 with secondary dystonia (52). These surgeons used physiologic guidance using microelectrode recording and stimulation to identify dystonic cells. The ideal location was essentially the VIM nucleus, which is used for patients with tremor. These surgeons noted that 68% of patients with secondary dystonia showed a greater than 25% improvement, whereas only 50% of patients with primary dystonia showed similar improvement. Most of the improvement was seen in appendicular symptoms, with the axial symptoms of gait, speech, and facial movement showing more modest results.

Gros and associates observed an immediate improvement in 51% of their patients, but after 6 years, only 33% remained improved (58). The various other series reported similarly modest results overall (59,60).

Complications

Surgical complications were seen in 35% of patients in our thalamotomy series. Confusion and contralateral hemiparesis were the most series problems, but dysarthria and pseudobulbar palsy were also encountered. One patient (6%)

TABLE 27.4. THALAMOTOMY FOR DYSTONIA: PUBLISHED OUTCOMES

Author (yr)	Diagnosis	No.	Improved (%)	Complications (%)
Laitinen (1965)	Cerebral palsy, dystonia	10	50	n/a
Cooper (1969, 1976)	Various dystonia	208	69.7	n/a
Gros et al. (1976)	Primary	25	33	16
Tasker et al. (1983)	Generalized	56	34	21
Kandel (1989)	Primary dystonia	188	76	10
Cardoso et al. (1995)	Various dystonia	17	47	35
Andrew et al. (1983)	Various dystonia	55	47	n/a
Krauss et al. (1992)	Traumatic	9	50	0

suffered persistent neurologic deficits after a second procedure to enlarge the lesion. Other series report complication rates of 16% to 47% (58–60). Additional complications that have been reported include dysphagia, gait disturbances, transient numbness, seizures, and death.

CONCLUSIONS

Overall, thalamotomy results in moderate to good improvement in ameliorating the symptoms of dystonia. Because of the relatively small numbers of patients undergoing thalamic lesioning, the varied methods used, and the inconsistent outcome assessments, no definitive recommendations about the surgical indications and ideal lesion placement can be made.

Recent experience with pallidotomy for dystonia, when compared with thalamotomy, suggests that patients may respond better to one or the other procedure, based on pathogenesis. Thalamotomy may be somewhat more efficacious in patients with secondary dystonia as opposed to primary dystonia. Conversely, patients with primary dystonia, especially related to *DYT-1*, probably respond more favorably to pallidotomy. These findings may suggest that pallidotomy is more appropriate for patients with primary dystonia and that thalamotomy is the possible procedure of choice in secondary dystonia.

FUTURE DIRECTIONS

Both pallidotomy and thalamotomy have a place in the treatment of dystonia, because they appear to best treat different types of the disease. Their concurrent use on the same side, or the use of pallidotomy on one side and thalamotomy on the other side, may improve efficacy and may reduce adverse events. In our own experience, we had one patient with secondary hemidystonia after acute ischemic injury (severed carotid artery) who had a thalamotomy, with modest improvement, followed years later by a same-side pallidotomy, and who did very well after the second procedure. We also have a patient who had a thalamotomy on one side and a pallidotomy on the other who did well and did not suffer any adverse events.

DBS, discussed in detail elsewhere, mimics the effects of ablative surgery. The advantages of DBS over ablations include the absence of a permanent lesion and greater flexibility. The functional size of the lesion, and to some extent the actual placement, can be changed. The mild loss of efficacy over time seen with pallidotomy makes these advantages particularly enticing. Several case reports demonstrate the efficacy of DBS when the electrodes are placed in the GPi for dystonia (61,62). Larger trials are currently ongoing. Although DBS has several disadvantages when compared with ablative surgery (higher cost, higher main-

tenance, the risk of equipment failure, risk of infection, and the need for periodic battery replacements), it may eventually replace ablation as the surgical procedure of choice.

REFERENCES

1. Burke R, Fahn S, Jankovic J, et al. Tardive dystonia: late onset and persistent dystonia caused by antipsychotic drugs. *Neurology* 1982;32:1335–1346.
2. Demirkiran M, Jankovic J. Paroxysmal dyskinesia: clinical features and classification. *Ann Neurol* 1995;38:571–579.
3. Ichinose H, Ohye T, Takahashi E, et al. Hereditary progressive dystonia with marked diurnal fluctuation caused by mutations in the GTP cyclohydrolase I gene. *Nat Genet* 1994;8:236–242.
4. Furukawa Y, Shimadzu M, Rajput A, et al. GTP-cyclohydrolase I gene mutations in hereditary progressive and dopa-responsive dystonia. *Ann Neurol* 1996;39:609–617.
5. Ozelius LJ, Hewett JW, Page CE, et al. The early-onset torsion dystonia gene *(DYT1)* encodes an ATP-binding protein. *Nat Genet* 1997;17:40–48.
6. Augood SJ, Penney JB Jr, Friberg IK, et al. Expression of the early-onset torsion dystonia gene *(DYT1)* in human brain. *Ann Neurol* 1998;43:669–673.
7. Warner TT, Jarman P. The molecular genetics of the dystonias. *J Neurol Neurosurg Psychiatry* 1998;64:427–429.
8. Almasy L, Bressman SB, Raymond D, et al. Idiopathic torsion dystonia linked to chromosome 8 in two Mennonite families. *Ann Neurol* 1997;42:670–673.
9. Leube B, Hendgen T, Kessler KR, et al. Evidence for *DYT7* being a common cause of cervical dystonia (torticollis) in Central Europe. *Am J Med Genet* 1997;74:529–532.
10. Quinn NP. Essential myoclonus and myoclonic dystonia. *Mov Disord* 1996;11:119–124.
11. Waters CH, Takahashi H, Wilhelmsen KC, et al. Phenotypic expression of X-linked dystonia-parkinsonism (lubag) in two women. *Neurology* 1993;43:1555–1558.
12. Scott B, Jankovic J. Delayed onset progressive movement disorders. *Neurology* 1996;46:68–74.
13. Jankovic J, Fahn S. Dystonic disorders. In: Jankovic J, Tolosa E, eds. *Parkinson's disease and movement disorders.* Philadelphia: Williams & Wilkins, 1998:513–551.
14. Marsden CD, Obeso JA, Zarranz JJ. The anatomic basis of symptomatic hemidystonia. *Brain* 1985;108:463–483.
15. Jankovic J. Post-traumatic movement disorders: central and peripheral mechanisms. *Neurology* 1994;44:2006–2014.
16. Playford E, Fletcher N, Sawle G, et al. Striatal [18F]dopa uptake in familial idiopathic dystonia. *Brain* 1993;116:1191–1199.
17. Perlmutter JS, Stambuk MK, Markham KT, et al. Decreased [18F]spiperone binding in idiopathic focal dystonia. *J Neurosci* 1997;17:843–850.
18. Papa SM, Chase T. Levodopa induced dyskinesias improved by a glutamate antagonist in parkinsonian monkeys. *Ann Neurol* 1996;39:574–578.
19. Mink JW, Thach WT. Basal ganglia intrinsic circuits and their role in behavior. *Curr Opin Neurobiol* 1993;3:950–957.
20. Vitek JL, Zhang J, Evatt M, et al. Gpi pallidotomy for dystonia: clinical outcome and neuronal activity. *Adv Neurol* 1998;78:211–219.
21. Lenz FA, Mandir AS. Rationales for pallidotomy: what are the mechanisms? In: Jankovic J, Grossman R, Krauss J, eds. *Pallidal surgery for movement disorders.* Philadelphia: Lippincott–Raven, 1997.

22. Ikoma K, Samii A, Mercuri B, et al. Abnormal cortical motor excitability in dystonia. *Neurology* 1996;46:1371–1376.

23. Eidelberg D, Moeller JR, Ishikawa T, et al. Regional metabolic correlations of surgical outcome following unilateral pallidotomy for Parkinson's disease. *Ann Neurol* 1996;39:450–459.

24. Samuel M, Ceballos-Baumann AO, Turjanski N, et al. Pallidotomy in Parkinson's disease increases supplementary motor area and prefrontal activity during performance of volitional movements: a $H_2^{15}O$ PET study. *Brain* 1997;120:1301–1313.

25. Rascol O, Sabatini U, Chollet F, et al. Supplementary and primary sensory motor area activity in Parkinson's disease: regional cerebral blood flow changes during finger movements and the effects of apomorphine. *Arch Neurol* 1992;49:144–148.

26. Jenkins IH, Fernandez W, Playford ED, et al. Impaired activation of the supplementary motor area in Parkinson's disease is reversed when akinesia is treated with apomorphine. *Ann Neurol* 1992;32:749–757.

27. Grafton AT, Waters C, Sutton J, et al. Pallidotomy increases activity of the motor association cortex in Parkinson's disease: a positron emission tomographic study. *Ann Neurol* 1995;37:776–783.

28. Ceballos-Baumann AO. Overactivity of primary and association motor areas in secondary hemi-dystonia (SHD) due to thalamic or basal ganglia lesions: a PET study. *Mov Disord* 1994;[Suppl 1]: P238.

29. Kumar R, Dagher A, Hutchison W, et al. Globus pallidus deep brain stimulation for generalized dystonia: clinical and PET investigation, *Neurology* 1999;53:871–874.

30. Meyers R. Surgical experiments in the therapy of certain extrapyramidal diseases: a current evaluation. *Acta Psychiatr Neurol* 1951;67:1–42.

31. Speigel EA, Wycis HT, Marks M, et al. Stereotaxis apparatus for operations on the human brain. *Science* 1947;106:349–350.

32. Cooper IS. An investigation of neurosurgical alleviation of parkinsonism, chorea, athetosis and dystonia. *Ann Intern Med* 1956;5:381–392.

33. Jankovic J, Schwartz K. Response and immunoresistance to botulinum toxin injections. *Neurology* 1995;45:1743–1746.

34. Favre J, Taba JM, Nguyen TT, et al. Pallidotomy: a survey of current practice in North America. *Neurosurgery* 1996;39:883–892.

35. Krauss JK, Desaloms JM, Lai E, et al. Microelectrode-guided posteroventral pallidotomy for treatment of Parkinson's disease: postoperative magnetic resonance imaging analysis. *J Neurosurg* 1997;87:358–367.

36. Ondo WG, Desaloms JM, Jankovic J, et al. Pallidotomy for generalized dystonia. *Mov Disord* 1998;13:693–698.

37. Burke RE, Fahn S, Marsden CD, et al. Validity and reliability of a rating scale for the primary torsion dystonias. *Neurology* 1985;35:73–77.

38. Comella C, Leurgans S, Chmura T, et al. The unified rating cale: initial concurrent validity testing with other dystonia scales. *Neurology* 1999;[Suppl 2]:A292.

39. Tasker RR. Surgical treatment of the dystonias. In: Gildenberg P, Tasker RR, eds. *Textbook of stereotactic and functional neurosurgery.* New York: McGraw-Hill, 1996:1015–1032.

40. Lozano AM, Kumar R, Gross RE, et al. Globus pallidus internus pallidotomy for generalized dystonia. *Mov Disord* 1997;12:865–870.

41. Lin JJ, Lin SZ, Lin GY, et al. Application of bilateral sequential pallidotomy to treat a patient with generalized dystonia. *Eur Neurol* 1998;40:108–110.

42. Iacono R, Kuniyoshi S, Lonser R, et al. Simultaneous bilateral pallidoansotomy for idiopathic dystonia musculorum deformans. *Pediatr Neurol* 1996;14:145–148.

43. Iacono RP, Kuniyoshi SM, Lonser RR, et al. Experience with stereotactics for dystonia: case examples. *Adv Neurol* 1998;78:221–226.

44. Vitek J, Evatt M, Zhang JU, et al. Pallidotomy and deep brain stimulation as a treatment for dystonia. *Neurology* 1999[Suppl 2]:A294.

45. Kumar R, Lozano AM, Hutchison WD, et al. Pallidal procedures for the treatment of refractory dystonia. *Mov Disord* 1997;12:865–870.

46. Lin JJ, Lin GY, Shih SZ, et al. Benefit of bilateral pallidotomy in the treatment of generalized dystonia. *J Neurosurg* 1999;90:974–976.

47. Justesen CR, Penn RD, Kroin JS, et al. Stereotactic pallidotomy in a child with Hallervorden-Spatz disease. *J Neurosurg* 1999;90:551–554.

48. Bhatia KP, Marsden CD, Thomas DG. Posteroventral pallidotomy can ameliorate attacks of paroxysmal dystonia induced by exercise. *J Neurol Neurosurg Psychiatry* 1998;65:604–605.

49. Cubo E, Shannon KM, Penn DR, et al. Internal globus pallidotomy in dystonia secondary to Huntington's disease. *Mov Disord* 2000;15:1248–1251.

50. Cardosa F, Jankovic J, Grossman RG, et al. Outcome after stereotactic thalamotomy for dystonia and hemiballismus. *Neurosurgery* 1995;36:501–597.

51. Schaltenbrad G, Wahren W. *Atlas for stereotaxy of the human brain,* 2nd ed. Chicago: Year Book, 1977.

52. Tasker RR, Doorly T, Yamashiro K. Thalamotomy in generalized dystonia. In: Fahn S, Marsden CD, Calne DB, eds. *Advanced Neurology.* New York: Raven Press, 1988.

53. Tasker RR, Lenz F, Yamashiro K, et al. Microelectrode techniques in localization of stereotactic targets. *Neurol Res* 1987;9:105–112.

54. Tasker RR, Organ LW, Hawrylyshyn P. *The thalamus and midbrain of man: a physiological atlas using electrical stimulation.* Springfield, IL: Charles C Thomas, 1982.

55. Cooper IS. 20-year follow-up study of the neurosurgical treatment of dystonia musculorum deformans. In: Eldridge R, Fahn S, eds. *Adv Neurol* 1976;14:423–452.

56. Cooper IS. *Involuntary movement disorders.* New York: Harper & Row, 1969:160–292.

57. Kandel EI. *Functional and stereotactic neurosurgery.* [Watts G, trans.] New York: Plenum, 1989.

58. Gros C, Frerebeau PH, Perez-Dominguez E, et al. Long-term results of stereotaxic surgery for infantile dystonia and dyskinesia. *Neurochirurgia (Stuttg)* 1976;19:171–178.

59. Andrew J, Fowler CJ, Harrison MJD. Stereotaxic thalamotomy in 55 cases of dystonia. *Brain* 1983;106:981–1000.

60. Laitinen LV. Short-term results of stereotaxic treatment for infantile cerebral palsy. *Confin Neurol* 1965;26:258–263.

61. Sa D, Teive H, Grande C, et al. Bilateral simultaneous pallidotomy for generalized dystonia. *Neurology* 1999 [Suppl 2]:A521.

62. Vitek J, Evatt M, Zhang JU, et al. Pallidotomy and deep brain stimulation as a treatment for dystonia *Neurology* 1999;52 [Suppl 2]: A294.

Surgery for Parkinson's Disease and Movement Disorders,
edited by J.K. Krauss, J. Jankovic, and R.G. Grossman.
Lippincott Williams & Wilkins, Philadelphia © 2001.

28

DEEP BRAIN STIMULATION IN THE TREATMENT OF DYSTONIA

MITCHELL F. BRIN
ISABELLE GERMANO
FABIO DANISI
DONALD WEISZ
C. WARREN OLANOW

OVERVIEW AND GENERAL CONSIDERATIONS

Dystonia is a neurologic syndrome characterized by involuntary and repetitive muscle contractions of opposing muscles that causes twisting, spasmodic movements, or abnormal postures. The current management of dystonia is symptomatic (16). Because the underlying neurochemical abnormality associated with dystonia is unknown, pharmacotherapeutic programs are empiric. The mainstay of oral pharmacotherapy includes levodopa, anticholinergics, benzodiazepines, and baclofen. The dose is increased until either benefit is observed or intolerable side effects develop. When these drugs fail, dopamine-depleting and dopamine-blocking agents are considered. Out of desperation, clinicians often try other neurochemically active agents. With this approach, some relief may be afforded, but only rarely and often with problematic side effects. Local injections of botulinum toxin (BTX) have emerged as the most efficacious form of therapy for patients with focal dystonia, particularly those with cranial symptoms (16). Nevertheless, at least 15% of patients with focal cranial dystonia lack an adequate response to BTX, and approximately 5% of patients with cervical dystonia develop resistance to therapy. For those with immunoresistance to therapy, BTX type B is effective for cervical dystonia (13,17), and regulatory approval is anticipated soon. Patients with respiratory involvement are not candidates for this therapeutic modality (14), because one cannot routinely inject the diaphragm with BTX. Patients with generalized dystonia may derive regional benefit from BTX treatment; however, their generalized symptoms typically go unabated. Intrathecal baclofen infusion

through an implantable pump has been effective in relieving spastic limbs and bladders associated with demyelinating disease, cerebral or spinal cord trauma, cerebral palsy, transverse myelitis, postencephalitic spasticity, hereditary spasticity, and stiff-person syndrome (3,63,74,85,86). We, and others, have used intrathecal baclofen in treating patients with both idiopathic and secondary dystonia with sporadic instances of benefit (39,80,84,111).

BRAIN SURGERY FOR DYSTONIA

Historical Overview

In the early twentieth century, lesioning of the motor cortex was performed in an effort to ameliorate hyperkinetic movements, including dystonia (48). However, these excisional procedures (18,54), in addition to incising the pyramidal tracts in the upper cervical spinal cord (89,110), often resulted in a spastic hemiparesis as a substitute for the dyskinesia. In 1940, Meyer described pallidotomy for Parkinson's disease (PD) (75,76), and he later demonstrated that dyskinesias can be improved with his procedure without pyramidal tract damage (77). During a surgical procedure in a postencephalitic patient with PD, Cooper accidentally severed the anterior choroidal artery, which feeds the medial globus pallidus (GP) and lateral ventral thalamus, and discovered marked improvement in tremor and rigidity (26, 28). In 1969, Cooper then reported that dystonic posturing in patients with parkinsonism improved with anterior choroidal artery ligation, and he began to operate on patients with primary dystonia.

Thalamotomies were then used with some frequency for selected severe cases (4,24,29–31,100). Nuclear destruction was performed by stereotactically injecting procaine and alcohol (chemopallidectomy, chemothalamectomy) (27), by freezing the tissue with liquid nitrogen delivered by a cannula

M.F. Brin, I. Germano, F. Danisi, and C.W. Olanow: Department of Neurology, Mount Sinai School of Medicine, New York, New York 10029.
I. Germano and D. Weisz: Department of Neurosurgery, Mount Sinai School of Medicine, New York, New York 10029.

(cryothalamotomy) (32), or by electrical coagulation (95). Thalamotomies were the most common procedure for dystonia, although Cooper's early patients underwent pallidotomies. Most authors report that approximately 33% to 70% of patients with dystonia treated with either a unilateral operation or bilateral procedures (predominantly thalamotomies) have significant improvement. However, complications have occurred in 16% to 33% of patients, including dysphagia, dysarthria, cerebral hemorrhage, and death (100).

Lesions of the pallidum in dystonia were made by early stereotactic neurosurgeons (4,23,25,29,44,46,53,98,100). In these series, outcomes of patients were typically lumped with those of patients who underwent thalamotomy. However, the pallidal ablation reports were encouraging, and in Cooper's report, his three patients had a substantial benefit.

Rationale for Functional Neurosurgery in Dystonia

A history of the renaissance of pallidotomy for movement disorders, which established the enthusiasm for subsequent procedures, is reviewed by Krauss and Grossman (56). Along with its use for PD, functional neurosurgery for dystonia enjoyed a resurgence of interest in the 1990s. The reasons are (a) improved neuroimaging for targeting specific brain nuclei, (b) improved microelectrode recording techniques for verifying target by identifying its electrophysiologic signature, (c) improved stereotactic equipment, (d) the development of the deep brain stimulation (DBS) equipment that can provide benefit without necessitating a large lesion, and (e) improvement in the hyperkinetic dyskinetic and dystonic features of patients with PD who are undergoing pallidal procedures, a finding suggesting that these procedures may help patients with dystonia (60,62).

Although there have been major advances in our understanding of the circuitry of the basal ganglia, particularly as it applies to PD, no adequate explanation has been proposed for the role of pallidal or thalamic lesions in the management of dystonia. Indeed, the neuroanatomic consequences of dystonia are largely unknown. Basal ganglia involvement is supported by neuroanatomic studies (10,47,113), response to medications that affect basal ganglia pathways (16), and positron emission tomography studies (1,2,36). Byl and coworkers, in a series of studies (20,21,103), explored the concept that dystonia, in animal models, may be associated with central defocusing or degradation of limb representation in the brain, in particularly the sensory cortex. Microelectrode recording of brain nuclei during surgical intervention has provided additional insights, as reviewed later.

With advances in surgical technique, movement disorder teams have reexplored neurosurgery for dystonia. Pallidotomy for medically intractable dystonia has been reported to have marked benefit (41,51,69,72,83,90,93,96, 102,108,109).

DBS is a surgical technique that simulates the effects of a lesion and is now employed in the management of the motor features of PD and essential tremor. In comparison with pallidotomy, DBS has the following advantages: (a) it is not necessary to make a lesion other than that produced by the placement of the stimulation electrodes, and this accordingly is associated with a decreased risk of adverse effects; (b) stimulation settings and the response to stimulation can be modified at any time postoperatively to maximize symptomatic relief; (c) if there are complications of stimulation, such as paresthesias, dysarthria, and dysphagia, stimulation parameters can be modified or stimulation can be discontinued; and (d) bilateral stimulation can be performed without the risks associated with bilateral lesions. DBS of the ventralis intermedius nucleus has emerged as an effective therapy for tremor relief in patients with PD and essential tremor. In most patients, tremor is totally suppressed (8, 9,11,22,49,55,68,87). When the stimulator is turned on, tremor is suppressed; when the stimulator is turned off, the tremor returns. DBS procedures of the internal segment of the GP (GPi) and subthalamic nucleus have been used in treating patients with PD (9,67,68,88,94). We performed the first DBS procedures on the subthalamic nucleus for PD in the United States (42,78,82). Clinical improvement was observed with stimulation in both the medication-"on" and medication-"off" states. Patients experienced a marked increase in the percentage of "on" time without dyskinesia and a corresponding reduction in the percentage of "off" time.

DBS of the thalamus has been used in a limited number of patients with dystonia (6,7,12,92). The authors reported moderate improvement in contralateral signs and symptoms. These encouraging results have prompted other investigators to explore DBS of thalamus and other nuclei, in particular the GPi.

Deep Brain Stimulation in Dystonia

The following is a description of the technique employed at Mount Sinai School of Medicine in New York.

Magnetic Resonance Imaging Localization of the Internal Segment of the Globus Pallidus

The GPi is localized on 1.5-Tesla magnetic resonance imaging (MRI) scans acquired with contiguous 2-mm sections to increase spatial accuracy. First, the anterior commissure (AC) and posterior commissure (PC) coordinates are obtained. These are then used to localize a tentative target within the GPi using the coordinates of Laitenin et al. (59). The ideal target is 2 to 3 mm anterior, 18 to 22 mm lateral, and 6 mm inferior to the AC-PC line. The target obtained using these coordinates in the projected on the MRI scan. The final location of the target is adjusted based on the recognition of anatomic structures readily visible on the sequences used. These include the internal capsule, located medial to the GPi, and the optic tract, inferior to the GPi. When one is targeting the ventrolateral GPi, the ideal target is 2 mm superior and just lateral to the optic tract, to include the junction of the ansa lenticularis with the GPi.

Deep Brain Stimulation System

We currently use a quadripolar electrode (Medtronic model 3387 DBS lead, Medtronic, Minneapolis) and the ITREL II as the implantable pulse generator (Medtronic model 7424).

Intraoperative Recordings

The techniques and principles of microelectrode recording are detailed in Chapter 6. We record consecutively from the striatum, the external segment of the GP (GPe), the GPi, and the white matter below the GPi (traversing the white matter for no more than 1.0 mm). The shape of each spike's waveform is viewed on a fast time base on one oscilloscope (5-millisecond sweep duration), and the firing patterns are viewed on a slower time base on another (1.0-second sweep duration) (112).

For each cell, a mean firing frequency is determined. In addition, a burst index is determined (50).

Surgical Procedure

After administration of local anesthesia, the patient is placed in a stereotactic frame and is taken to the radiology suite for MRI localization of the target site. The patient is then taken to the operating room and, using standard stereotactic techniques, a guiding cannula is inserted to 10 mm above the target site based on MRI coordinates (45,62,71,81,99, 101). A Teflon-coated tungsten microrecording electrode is inserted into the cannula and is advanced by 0.10-mm increments using a microdriver. Microelectrode recordings are used to confirm the target site in the GPi. Cells in the GPi can be discriminated from neighboring cells and border regions based on their firing rate and pattern. The discharge pattern is normally characterized by a firing frequency of approximately 60 to 80 Hz, but it may be slower in patients with dystonia. Active and passive movements are performed in an attempt to map the motor-sensory area, the desired target site for electrode placement. Cells may respond selectively to movements of a particular limb or joint. The stereotactic coordinates of responsive cells may be used to select the target area in GPi. The simultaneous display of the microelectrode and movement recordings makes it easier to determine whether a relationship exists between the firing pattern and the movements. In the current study, we perform electromyographic studies recording from surface electrodes on the hands, arms, and legs. In the GPi, the firing of approximately 20% of the cells can be modulated by movement (35,37). At least three microelectrode passes

are employed per side to assess the boundaries of the target site. Once the target site has been identified, the permanent electrode is inserted to cover the full extent of the target. Contact sites measure 1.5 mm each and are spaced at 1.5-mm intervals, so the electrical stimulus can be directed over a range of 10.5 mm. In the operating room, a test stimulator (Medtronic model 3625) may be used to evaluate the acute effects of stimulation. The electrode is then secured to the bur-hole ring with a bur-hole cap. A postoperative brain MRI scan is obtained to confirm accurate electrode placement and to evaluate for acute complications intracranial hemorrhage. The implantable pulse generator is then connected to the intracranial electrode by an extension wire and is implanted subcutaneously in the subclavicular area. The procedure may be repeated on the opposite side using an identical procedure either during the same session or at a later time, depending on the judgment of the neurologist and neurosurgeon.

Neuropsychologic Testing

Cognitive change has been observed after ablative stereotaxic procedures such as thalamotomy and pallidotomy (52,61,91). Little is known about the cognitive effects of DBS. Preliminary findings in patients with PD who have undergone DBS have been mixed, with some reporting no effect (5) and others finding both improvement and decline in cognitive functioning (78,105). We recently developed a standardized method for evaluating neuropsychologic changes associated with DBS in patients with PD and in patients with dystonia known as the Program for Neuropsychological Investigation of Deep Brain Stimulation (PNIDBS) (79). Testing in this population addresses (a) the physical limitations of patients who may have abnormal movements that limit their ability to perceive complex visual stimuli and (b) the need to account for test-retest confounds. We performed a feasibility analysis of the PNIDBS in three patients with PD and in two patients with dystonia. The DBS procedure had minimal effect on cognition in any patient (79).

CLINICAL RESULTS

Mount Sinai Experience

At the Mount Sinai School of Medicine, we petitioned the United States Food and Drug Administration (FDA) to allow us to perform DBS in patients with dystonia. Our original research approval permitted us to perform this surgical procedure only unilaterally. These initial four patients form the basis for the following summary of our first four unilateral DBS GPi procedures in patients with dystonia. All patients were recruited from, and were followed in, the movement disorder clinic at Mount Sinai. Figure 28.1 shows a postoperative MRI scan of deep brain electrodes implanted into the

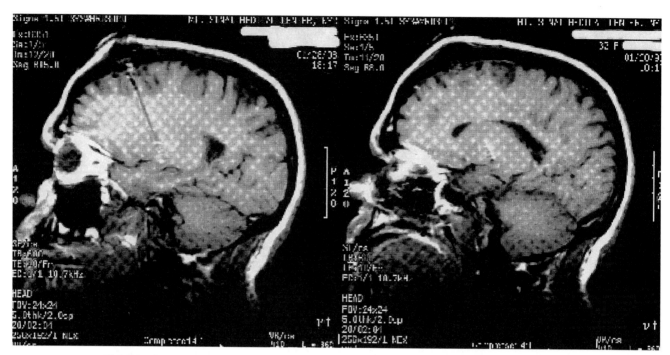

FIGURE 28.1. Postoperative T1-weighted sagittal magnetic resonance imaging of patient 1, a 32-year-old woman with segmental cranial and brachial dystonia. The stimulating electrode is stereotactically placed into the internal segment of the globus pallidus (GPi). The electrode angles from superolateral to inferomedial, so the full length is displayed in two figures. The **left** shows the lateral entry and proximal portion of the electrode. The **right** shows the distal, most medial portion of the electrode in the GPi.

GPi. The procedure was associated with moderate benefit in two of four patients; none worsened (Table 28.1).

The large number of stimulation options, including electrode configuration (unipolar, bipolar, multipolar), amplitude, pulse width, and frequency, makes the task of parameter adjustments complex and lengthy. We proposed a simplified method for identifying the optimal electrode configuration and stimulation settings in patients with PD who are

TABLE 28.1 MOUNT SINAI (NEW YORK) HOSPITAL EXPERIENCE WITH DEEP BRAIN STIMULATION FOR DYSTONIA

Patient	Distribution of Dystonia	Visual Analog Scale[a] (15)		Rating Scale no. 3[b]	Burke-Fahn-Marsden Scale (19)		Long-term Clinical Follow-up
		Baseline	12 mo	Change from Baseline	Baseline	12 mo	
1	Arm, voice	10%	75%	3	19	16	Continued moderate improvement
2	Generalized	35%	65%	2	62	45	Continued moderate improvement
3	Cervical	20%	15%	0	30.5	27.5 (6 mo)	No benefit; device removed
4	Generalized	30%	NA	NA	88	—	Device removed
Mean score		24%	52%	1.67	49.9	29.5	
Median score		25%	65%	2	46.3	27.5	

NA, not available.
[a]Visual analog scale: higher percentage, improved function; 100%, normal function.
[b]Rating scale no. 3:
  -4 = marked worsening in severity of spasm, tremor, or pain and in function
  -3 = moderate worsening in severity of spasm, tremor, or pain and in function
  -2 = moderate worsening in spasm, tremor, or pain, but no change in function
  -1 = mild worsening in spasm, pain, or tremor, but no change in function
  0 = no effect
  $+1$ = mild improvement in spasm, pain, or tremor, but no change in function
  $+2$ = moderate improvement in spasm, tremor, or pain, but no change in function
  $+3$ = moderate improvement in severity of spasm, tremor, or pain and in function
  $+4$ = marked improvement in severity of spasm, tremor, or pain and in function

receiving subthalamic nucleus stimulation (42). However, no such paradigm exists for pallidal stimulation. The problem is accentuated in dystonia because, as in ablative surgery, in which a significant delay exists between the time of intervention and a clinical effect, there is often a latency of hours to days before one appreciates the full impact of each parameter adjustment.

In the foregoing experience, three of the patients experienced wound dehiscence or local irritation of the skin resulting in granuloma; two patients required removal of devices. We performed an investigation to determine the basis of this problem. These problems were observed in patients who underwent surgical treatment at Mount Sinai and in one of the two additional patients who underwent surgical treatment performed by the New York University Medical Center team (not included in this report). None of our patients with PD experienced this complication. During this investigation, we learned that during manufacture by Medtronic, some of the bur-hole caps had been contaminated with 2,4-dichlorobenzoic acid, a substance that is known to be a local irritant. Medtronic subsequently issued a letter to physicians advising them of this contamination and recalled unimplanted devices. In view of the lack of this adverse effect in PD, but the presence of the problem in dystonia, we have considered that it is possible that an interaction occurred between our patients with dystonia and the initial equipment used in this procedure.

The procedures at Mount Sinai were associated with some benefit in two of these four patients who underwent unilateral GPi implantation of DBS equipment. These results are encouraging in view of the finding that the patients selected to participate in these studies had severe and intractable dystonia that could not be improved with traditional medical therapies. We have recently received approval from the FDA to proceed with bilateral procedures and are pursuing this approach.

Microelectrode Recordings

Recently, Lenz et al. reported on thalamic single neuron activity recorded in patients with dystonia during thalamic procedures (65). These investigators showed that patients with dystonia appeared to have increased representations of parts of the body affected by dystonia in the deep sensory thalamic cells. They found that stimulation in the presumed ventralis intermedius nucleus in patients with dystonia produced simultaneous contraction of multiple forearm muscles, similar to the cocontractions observed in dystonia, a finding suggesting that there are altered sensory maps resulting in an overactivation of muscles characteristic of dystonia. In further studies, Lenz and Byl showed that the proportion of the receptive fields to multiple parts of the body was greater in patients with dystonia undergoing thalamic surgery as compared with patients with essential tremor (64).

Vitek et al. reported on sensorimotor pallidal microelectrode recordings in patients with generalized dystonia (107,109). These investigators found overall a decreased mean firing rate as compared with patients with idiopathic PD. These data are supported by other reports (73,97). However, the firing pattern was relatively chaotic, in irregularly grouped discharges separated by pauses.

The results of our preliminary analyses on the patients operated on at Mount Sinai suggest the possibility of small differences in the firing frequencies of cells in the GPi and GPe of dystonic patients when compared with similar values from patients with PD or from nonhuman primates. The mean neuronal firing rates of cells in the GPe and GPi are slightly lower for dystonic patients than the values PD, but they are higher than the values for dystonic patients reported by Vitek et al. (109). Cells recorded from PD have a mean firing frequency of approximately 50 Hz for high-frequency discharge cells in the GPe and approximately 80 Hz for GPi cells (106). Other reports found mean rates of 38 to 46 Hz for high-frequency discharge cells in the GPe and 35 to 58 Hz for cells in the GPi of dystonic patients (58,66,109). Our values of 44.2 Hz for GPe cells and 69.3 Hz for GPi cells are intermediate. Representative neuronal firing patterns from GPi and GPe neurons in our patients are provided in Fig. 28.2. Perhaps the neuronal firing rate in dystonic patients is distributed in a continuum, which correlates with both dystonic symptoms and underlying brain disease. It is also possible that our patient population is different from that studied by Vitek et al. (109). Finally, institution-specific and patient-specific operative conditions (use of anesthesia, other medications) may have an impact on neuronal firing rates.

Summary and Review of Literature

Brain surgery is considered in the management of refractory cases of dystonia. Because these procedures are not without risk, and the benefit is not yet predictable, brain neurosurgical procedures are reserved for patients who fail to respond to other accepted therapies. Many patients benefit from ablative thalamic or other pallidal surgical procedures, and even with the complications reported with thalamic surgery, these patients often state that they do not regret having an ablative procedure. We prefer not to ablate regions of the brain that may hold important neurochemical pathways and receptors for future interventional pharmacotherapy.

Including our own experience, 11 authors (Table 28.2) described 43 patients who underwent DBS procedures for the management of idiopathic or symptomatic dystonia. The results were good to excellent for most patients with idiopathic disease, including patients with generalized and focal (cervical or limb) dystonia. Patients with symptomatic dystonia appeared to experience a more favorable outcome with thalamic stimulation rather than with pallidal stimulation, with the exception of the case reported by Loher et al. (70).

TABLE 28.2 DEEP BRAIN STIMULATION FOR DYSTONIA

Author (ref.)	Nucleus (N)	Unilateral/Bilateral	Characteristics	Reported Outcome
Blond and Siegfried (12)	Thalamus (VPL, n = 4)	Unilateral	"Postapoplectic dystonia"	Successfully controlled in 3, partially in 1
Sellal et al. (92)	Thalamus, VPL nucleus (n = 1)	Unilateral	Delayed-onset symptomatic hemidystonia associated with head injury	Excellent
Benabid et al. (7)	Thalamus (n = 5)	Thalamic	Not specified	None or "less significant"
Fogel et al. (38)	GPi (n = 1)	Bilateral	Idiopathic dystonia	"Remarkable"
Tronnier and Fogel (104)	GPi (n = 3)	Bilateral	Idiopathic in 2; secondary in 1	Very good in 1
Kumar et al. (58)	GPi (n = 1)	Bilateral	Idiopathic dystonia	Excellent
Coubes et al. (33,34)	GPi (n = 15)	Bilateral	Idiopathic dystonia	Excellent in at least 13
Krauss et al. (57)	GPi (n = 3)	Bilateral in 1	Cervical dystonia	Excellent
Loher et al. (70)	GPi (n = 1)	Unilateral	Posttraumatic hemidystonia	Excellent
Ghika et al. (40)	Thalamic (VOA; n = 1) and GPi (n = 4)	Bilateral	Postanoxic dystonia with necrosis of bilateral pallidum	GPi: no benefit in 4; thalamus: excellent in 1
Brin (current series)	GPi (n = 4)	Unilateral	Idiopathic	Moderate in 2; failed in 2

GPi, internal segment of globus pallidus; VPL, lateral ventralis posterior subnucleus; VOA, ventralis oralis anterior.

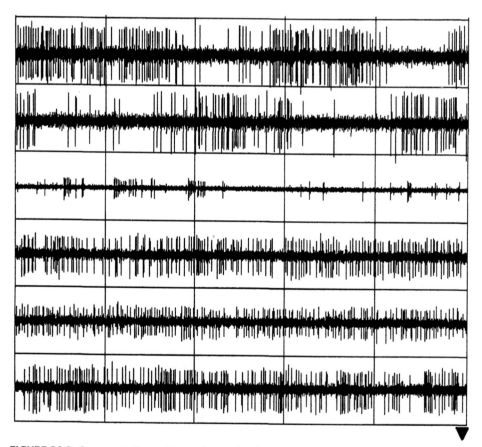

FIGURE 28.2. Representative patterns of neural activity are shown for three high-frequency discharge cells (HFD) from the external segment of the globus pallidus (GPe) (traces 1 and 2), one low-frequency discharge cell (LFD) also from the GPe (trace 3), and three cells from the internal segment of the GP (GPi) (traces 4 to 6). The mean firing frequencies of cells in the GPe and GPi were calculated from three patients studied at the Mount Sinai School of Medicine in New York. The mean frequencies were 44.2 Hz (range, 14 to 67) for 19 HFD cells in the GPe and 69.3 Hz (range, 44 to 98) for 25 GPi cells. *X* axis, 2,000 milliseconds.

With our advancing understanding of the genetics and molecular biology of dystonia, it is hoped that specific therapy either to either halt the progression of or relieve dystonic spasms will be available shortly. Nevertheless, until such time, DBS may replace ablative neurosurgical treatments in patients with intractable disease. It is clear from our experience and that of others, and particularly in view of the strongly positive results from Europe (Table 28.1), that bilateral surgery is probably required in patients with dystonia that either involves or crosses the midline. Additional studies are required to further define the ideal candidate for surgery (idiopathic versus symptomatic, generalized versus focal), to ascertain the preferred target nucleus and region within a nucleus, to determine the relative benefits of DBS versus ablative procedures, and, in the case of DBS, to find an efficient method of optimizing stimulation parameters (43) in the presence of a delayed clinical effect after each stimulation change in patients with dystonia.

Acknowledgment

This work is supported in part by United States Public Health Grant FD-R-001452 and the Bachmann-Strauss Dystonia and Parkinson Foundation.

REFERENCES

1. Fahn S, Marsden CD, Calne DB. *Dystonia 2* (Advances in Neurology, Vol. 50). New York: Raven Press, 1988.
2. Fahn S, Marsden CD, Delong MR. *Dystonia 3* (Advances in Neurology, Vol. 78). Philadelphia: Lippincott-Raven, 1998.
3. Albright AL, Cervi A, Singletary J. Intrathecal baclofen for spasticity in cerebral palsy. *JAMA* 1991;265:1418–1422.
4. Andrew J, Fowler CJ, Harrison MJ. Stereotaxic thalamotomy in 55 cases of dystonia. *Brain* 1983;106:981–1000.
5. Ardouin C, Pillon B, Peiffer E, et al. Lateral stimulation of STN or GPi does not affect cognitive functions in Parkinson's disease. *Mov Disord* 1998;13[Suppl 2]:136.
6. Benabid AL, Pollack P, Limousin P, et al. Chronic stimulation of the ventrolateral thalamic nucleus in dystonia. *Focus Dystonia* 1994;26.
7. Benabid AL, Pollak P, Gao D, et al. Chronic electrical stimulation of the ventralis intermedius nucleus of the thalamus as a treatment of movement disorders. *J Neurosurg* 1996;84:203–214.
8. Benabid AL, Pollak P, Gervason C, et al. Long-term suppression of tremor by chronic stimulation of the ventral intermediate thalamic nucleus. *Lancet* 1991;337:403–406.
9. Benabid AL, Pollak P, Gross C, et al. Acute and long-term effects of subthalamic nucleus stimulation in Parkinson's disease. *Stereotact Funct Neurosurg* 1994;62:76–84.
10. Bhatia KP, Marsden CD. The behavioural and motor consequences of focal lesions of the basal ganglia in man. *Brain* 1994;117:859–876.
11. Blond S, Caparros-Lefebvre D, Parker F, et al. Control of tremor and involuntary movement disorders by chronic stereotactic stimulation of the ventral intermediate thalamic nucleus. *J Neurosurg* 1992;77:62–68.
12. Blond S, Siegfried J. Thalamic stimulation for the treatment of tremor and other movement disorders. *Acta Neurochir Suppl (Wien)* 1991;52:109–111.
13. Brashear A, Lew MF, Dykstra DD, et al. Safety and efficacy of Neurobloc (botulinum toxin type B) in type A–responsive cervical dystonia. *Neurology* 1999;53:1439–1446.
14. Braun N, Abd A, Baer J, et al. Dyspnea in dystonia: a functional evaluation. *Chest* 1995;107:1309–1316.
15. Brin MF. Interventional neurology: treatment of neurological conditions with local injection of botulinum toxin. *Arch Neurobiol* 1991;54:173–189.
16. Brin MF. Treatment of dystonia. In: Jankovic J, Tolosa E, eds. *Parkinson's disease and movement disorders*. New York: Williams & Wilkins, 1998:553–578.
17. Brin MF, Lew, MF, Adler CH, et al. Safety and efficacy of Neurobloc (botulinum toxin type-B) in type–A resistant cervical dystonia (CD) patients. *Neurology* 1999;52[Suppl 2]:A293.
18. Bucy PC, Case JT. Tremor: physiologic mechanism and abolition by surgical means. *Arch Neurol Psychiatry* 1939;41:721–746.
19. Burke RE, Fahn S, Marsden CD, et al. Validity and reliability of a rating scale for the primary torsion dystonias. *Neurology* 1985;35:73–77.
20. Byl N, Wilson F, Merzenich M, et al. Sensory dysfunction associated with repetitive strain injuries of tendinitis and focal hand dystonia: a comparative study. *J Orthop Sports Phys Ther* 1996;23:234–244.
21. Byl NN, Merzenich MM, Cheung S, et al. A primate model for studying focal dystonia and repetitive strain injury: effects on the primary somatosensory cortex. *Phys Ther* 1997;77:269–284.
22. Caparros-Lefebvre D, Blond S, Vermersch P, et al. Chronic thalamic stimulation improves tremor and levodopa induced dyskinesias in Parkinson's disease. *J Neurol Neurosurg* 1993.
23. Caracalos A. Results of 103 cryosurgical procedures in involuntary movement disorders. *Confin Neurol* 1972;34:74–83.
24. Cardoso F, Jankovic J, Grossman RG, et al. Outcome after stereotactic thalamotomy for dystonia and hemiballismus. *Neurosurgery* 1995;36:501–507.
25. Cooper IM, Bravo GM. Alleviation of dystonia musculorum deformans and other involuntary movement disorders of childhood by chemopallidectomy and chemopallido-thalamectomy. *Clin Neurosurg* 1958;5:127–149.
26. Cooper IS. Ligation of the anterior choroidal artery for involuntary movements of parkinsonism. *Psychiatr Q* 1953;27:317–319.
27. Cooper IS. Intracerebral injection of procaine into the globus pallidus in hyperkinetic disorders. *Science* 1954;119:417–418.
28. Cooper IS. Surgical alleviation of parkinsonism: effects of occlusion of the anterior choroidal artery. *J Am Geriatr Soc* 1954;11:691–717.
29. Cooper IS. 20-year followup study of the neurosurgical treatment of dystonia musculorum deformans. *Adv Neurol* 1976;14:423–452.
30. Cooper IS. Dystonia: surgical approaches to treatment and physiologic implications. *Res Publ Assoc Res Nerv Ment Dis* 1976;55:369–383.
31. Cooper IS. Twenty-five years of experience with physiological neurosurgery. *Neurosurgery* 1981;9:190–200.
32. Cooper IS, Gioino G, Terry R. The cryogenic lesion. *Confin Neurol* 1965;26:161–177.
33. Coubes P, Roubertie A, Vayssiere N, et al. Treatment of DYT1-generalised dystonia by stimulation of the internal globus pallidus. *Lancet* 2000;355:2220–2221.
34. Coubes P, Roubertie A, Vayssiere N, et al. Early-onset generalized dystonia: neurosurgical treatment by continuous bilateral stimulation of the internal globus pallidus in 15 patients. *Neurology* 2000;54[Suppl 3]:A220.

35. DeLong MR. Activity of pallidal neurons during movement. *J Neurophysiol* 1971;34:414–427.

36. Eidelberg D. Abnormal brain networks in DYT1 dystonia. *Adv Neurol* 1998;78:127–133.

37. Fetter M, Klockgether T, Schulz JB, et al. Oculomotor abnormalities and MRI findings in idiopathic cerebellar ataxia. *J Neurol* 1994;241:234–241.

38. Fogel W, Tronnier V, Krause M, et al. Bilateral pallidal stimulation in a case of idiopathic torsion dystonia: a new treatment option? *Mov Disord* 1998;13[Suppl 2]:199.

39. Ford B, Greene PE, Louis ED, et al. Intrathecal baclofen in the treatment of dystonia. *Adv Neurol* 1998;78:199–210.

40. Ghika J, Vingerhoets F, Temperli P, et al. Ventrooralis nucleus thalamic deep brain stimulation (Voa-DBS), but not pallidal DBS (GPi-DBS), is effective in generalized postanoxic dystonia with necrosis of bilateral pallida. *Neurology* 2000;54[Suppl 3]:A220.

41. Gibson GJ, Douglas NJ, Stradling JR, et al. Sleep apnoea: clinical importance and facilities for investigation and treatment in the UK. Addendum to the 1993 Royal College of Physicians sleep apnoea report. *J R Coll Physicians Lond* 1998;32:540–544.

42. Gracies JM, Bucobo JC, Danisi FO, et al. Proposal for a method of stimulation parameter adjustment after deep brain stimulation for Parkinson's disease (PD). *Mov Disord* 1998;13[Suppl 2]:50.

43. Gracies JM, Simpson D. Neuromuscular blockers. *Phys Med Rehabil Clin North Am* 1999;10:357–383.

44. Gros C, Frerebeau P, Perez-Dominguez E, et al. Long term results of stereotaxic surgery for infantile dystonia and dyskinesia. *Neurochirurgia (Stuttg)* 1976;19:171–178.

45. Gybels JM, Kupers RC. Brain stimulation in the management of persistent pain. In: Schmidek HH, Sweet WH, eds. *Operative neurosurgical techniques: indications, methods, and results.* Philadelphia: WB Saunders, 1995:1389–1401.

46. Hassler R, Riechert T, Mundinger F, et al. Physiological observations in stereotaxic operations in extrapyramidal motor disturbances. *Brain* 1960;83:337–350.

47. Hedreen JC, Zweig RM, DeLong MR, et al. Primary dystonias: a review of the pathology and suggestions for new directions of study. *Adv Neurol* 1988;50:123–132.

48. Horsley V. The functions of the so-called motor areas of the brain. *BMJ* 1909;124:5–28.

49. Hubble JP, Busenbark KL, Wilkinson S, et al. Effects of thalamic deep brain stimulation based on tremor type and diagnosis. *Mov Disord* 1997;12:337–341.

50. Hutchison WD, Allan RJ, Opitz H, et al. Neurophysiological identification of the subthalamic nucleus in surgery for Parkinson's disease. *Ann Neurol* 1998;44:622–628.

51. Iacono RP, Kuniyoshi SM, Lonser RR, et al. Simultaneous bilateral pallidoansotomy for idiopathic dystonia musculorum deformans. *Pediatr Neurol* 1996;14:145–148.

52. Jurko MF, Andy OJ. Psychological changes correlated with thalamotomy site. *J Neurol Neurosurg Psychiatry* 1973;36:846–852.

53. Kelly PJ. Outcome after stereotactic thalamotomy for dystonia and hemiballismus: comment. *Neurosurgery* 1995;36:507.

54. Klemme RM. Surgical treatment of dystonia, paralysis agitans and athetosis. *Arch Neurol Psychiatry* 1940;44:926.

55. Koller W, Pahwa R, Busenbark K, et al. *High-frequency unilateral thalamic stimulation in the treatment of essential and parkinsonian tremor.* American Neurological Association, 1997.

56. Krauss JK, Grossman RG. Historical review of pallidal surgery for treatment of parkinsonism and other movement disorders. In: Krauss JK, Grossman RG, Jankovic JJ, eds. *Pallidal surgery for the treatment of Parkinson's disease and movement disorders.* New York: Lippincott–Raven, 1998:1–24.

57. Krauss JK, Pohle T, Weber S, et al. Bilateral stimulation of globus pallidus internus for treatment of cervical dystonia [Letter]. *Lancet* 1999;354:837–838.

58. Kumar R, Dagher A, Hutchison WD, et al. Globus pallidus deep brain stimulation for generalized dystonia: clinical and PET investigation. *Neurology* 1999;53:871–874.

59. Laitenin LV, Bergenheim AT, Hariz MI. Leksell's posteroventral pallidotomy in the treatment of Parkinson's disease. *J Neurosurg* 1992;76:53–61.

60. Lang AE. Surgery for levodopa-induced dyskinesias. *Ann Neurol* 2000;47:S193–S199.

61. Lang AE, Lozano A, Tasker R, et al. Neuropsychological and behavioral changes and weight gain after medial pallidotomy. *Ann Neurol* 1997;41:834–835.

62. Lang AE, Lozano AM, Montgomery E, et al. Posteroventral medial pallidotomy in advanced Parkinson's disease. *N Engl J Med* 1997;337:1036–1042.

63. Lazorthes Y, Sallerin-Caute B, Verdie JC, et al. Chronic intrathecal baclofen administration for control of severe spasticity. *J Neurosurg* 1990;72:393–402.

64. Lenz FA, Byl NN. Reorganization in the cutaneous core of the human thalamic principal somatic sensory nucleus (ventral caudal) in patients with dystonia. *J Neurophysiol* 1999;82:3204–3212.

65. Lenz FA, Jaeger CJ, Seike MS, et al. Thalamic single neuron activity in patients with dystonia: dystonia-related activity and somatic sensory reorganization. *J Neurophysiol* 1999;82:2372–2392.

66. Lenz FA, Suarez JI, Metman LV, et al. Pallidal activity during dystonia: somatosensory reorganisation and changes with severity. *J Neurol Neurosurg Psychiatry* 1998;65:767–770.

67. Limousin P, Krack P, Pollak P, et al. Electrical stimulation of the subthalamic nucleus in advanced Parkinson's disease. *N Engl J Med* 1998;339:1105–1111.

68. Limousin P, Pollak P, Benazzouz A, et al. Effect of parkinsonian signs and symptoms of bilateral subthalamic nucleus stimulation. *Lancet* 1995;345:91–95.

69. Lin JJ, Lin GY. Bilateral posteroventral pallidotomy in treatment of generalized dystonia. *Mov Disord* 1998;13[Suppl 2]:68.

70. Loher TJ, Hasdemir MG, Burgunder JM, et al. Long-term follow-up study of chronic globus pallidus internus stimulation for posttraumatic hemidystonia. *J Neurosurg* 2000;92:457–460.

71. Lozano A, Hutchison W, Kiss Z, et al. Methods for microelectrode-guided posteroventral pallidotomy. *J Neurosurg* 1996;84:194–202.

72. Lozano AM, Kumar R, Gross RE, et al. Globus pallidus internus pallidotomy for generalized dystonia. *Mov Disord* 1997;12:865–870.

73. Lozano AM, Kumar R, Gross RE, et al. Globus pallidus internus pallidotomy for generalized dystonia. *Mov Disord* 1997;12:865–870.

74. McLean BN. Intrathecal baclofen in severe spasticity. *Br J Hosp Med* 1993;49:262–267.

75. Meyers R. Surgical procedure for postencephalitic tremor, with notes on the physiology of premotor fibres. *Arch Neurol Psychiatry* 1940;44:455–457.

76. Meyers R. The modification of alternating tremors, rigidity and festination by surgery of the basal ganglia. *Proc Assoc Nerv Ment Dis* 1942;21:602–665.

77. Meyers R. Surgical experiments in therapy of certain "extrapyramidal" diseases: current evaluation. *Acta Psychiatr Neurol Scand Suppl* 1951;67:1–42.

78. Morrison CE, Borod JC, Raskin SA, et al. Cognitive effects of brain surgery and stimulation in Parkinson's disease. *Clin Neuropsychologist* 1998;12:256.

79. Morrison CE, Borod JC, Raskin SA, et al. A program for neuropsychological investigation of deep brain stimulation

(PNIDBS) in movement disorder patients: program development and preliminary data. *Neuropsychiatr Neuropsychol Behav Neurol.*

80. Narayan RK, Loubser PG, Jankovic J, et al. Intrathecal baclofen for intractable axial dystonia. *Neurology* 1991;41:1141–1142.

81. North RB. Spinal cord stimulation for chronic, intractable pain. In: Schmidek HH, Sweet WH, eds. *Operative neurosurgical techniques: indications, methods, and results.* Philadelphia: WB Saunders, 1995:1403–1411.

82. Olanow CW, Germano I, Brin MF, et al. Deep brain stimulation of the subthalamic nucleus for Parkinson's disease. *Mov Disord* 1996;11:598–599.

83. Ondo WG, Desaloms JM, Jankovic J, et al. Pallidotomy for generalized dystonia. *Mov Disord* 1998;13:693–698.

84. Penn RD, Gianino JM, York MM. Intrathecal baclofen for motor disorders. *Mov Disord* 1995;10:675–677.

85. Penn RD, Kroin JS. Long-term intrathecal baclofen infusion for treatment of spasticity. *J Neurosurg* 1987;66:181–185.

86. Penn RD, Mangieri EA. Stiff-man syndrome treated with intrathecal baclofen. *Neurology* 1993;43:2412.

87. Pollak P, Benabid AL, Gervason CL, et al. Long-term effects of chronic stimulation of the ventral intermediate thalamic nucleus in different types of tremor. *Adv Neurol* 1993;60:408–413.

88. Pollak P, Benabid AL, Gross C, et al. Effects of subthalamic nucleus stimulation in Parkinson's disease. *Rev Neurol* 1993;149:175–176.

89. Putnam TJ. Relief from unilateral paralysis agitans by section of the lateral pyramidal tract. *Arch Neurol Psychiatry* 1938;40:1049.

90. Rezak M, Vergenz SM, Eller TW, et al. Successful treatment of segmental idiopathic dystonia with internal segment pallidotomy. *Mov Disord* 1998;13[Suppl 2]:98.

91. Riklan M, Halgin R, Maskin M, et al. Psychological studies of longer range L-DOPA therapy in parkinsonism. *J Nerv Ment Dis* 1973;157:452–464.

92. Sellal F, Hirsch E, Barth P, et al. A case of symptomatic hemidystonia improved by ventroposterolateral thalamic electrostimulation. *Mov Disord* 1993;8:515–518.

93. Shima F, Sakata S, Sun S, et al. The role of the descending pallido-reticular pathway in movement disorders. In: Segawa M, Nomura Y, eds. *Age-related dopamine-dependent disorders.* New York: Karger, 1995:197–207.

94. Siegfried J, Lippitz B. Chronic electrical stimulation of the VL-VPL complex and of the pallidum in the treatment of movement disorders: personal experience since 1982. *Stereotact Funct Neurosurg* 1994;62:71–75.

95. Spiegel AE, Wycis HT. Pallidothalamotomy in chorea. *Arch Neurol Psychiatry* 1950;64:295–296.

96. Sterio D, Beric A, Alterman R, et al. Pallidotomy treatment for torsion dystonia. *Mov Disord* 1998;13[Suppl 2]:198.

97. Suarez JI, Metman LV, Reich SG, et al. Pallidotomy for hemiballismus: efficacy and characteristics of neuronal activity. *Ann Neurol* 1997;42:807–811.

98. Tasker RR. Outcome after stereotactic thalamotomy for dystonia and hemiballismus: comment. *Neurosurgery* 1995;36:507–508.

99. Tasker RR. Stereotactic surgery: movement disorders: role and technique of thalamotomy. In: *11th International Congress of Neurological Surgery,* vols 1 and 2. Bologna: Monduzzi Editore, 1997:261–263.

100. Tasker RR, Doorly T, Yamashiro K. Thalamotomy in generalized dystonia. *Adv Neurol* 1988;50:615–631.

101. Tasker RR, Lang AE, Lozano AM. Pallidal and thalamic surgery for Parkinson's disease. *Exp Neurol* 1997;144:35–40.

102. Teive H, Sa D, Grande CV, et al. Bilateral simultaneous globus pallidus internus pallidotomy for generalized posttraumatic dystonia. *Mov Disord* 1998;13[Suppl 2]:33.

103. Topp KS, Byl NN. Movement dysfunction following repetitive hand opening and closing: anatomical analysis in owl monkeys. *Mov Disord* 1999;14:295–306.

104. Tronnier VM, Fogel W. Pallidal stimulation for generalized dystonia: report of three cases. *J Neurosurg* 2000;92:453–456.

105. Vingerhoets G, Van der Linden C, Caemaert J, et al. Cognitive changes after unilateral stimulation of the globus pallidus internus (GPi) for treatment of refractory Parkinson's disease. *J Int Neuropsychol Soc* 1998;4:63.

106. Vitek JL, Bakay RA, Hashimoto T, et al. Microelectrode-guided pallidotomy: technical approach and its application in medically intractable Parkinson's disease. *J Neurosurg* 1998;88:1027–1043.

107. Vitek JL, Chockkan V, Zhang JY, et al. Neuronal activity in the basal ganglia in patients with generalized dystonia and hemiballismus. *Ann Neurol* 1999;46:22–35.

108. Vitek JL, Evatt M, Zhang J, et al. Pallidotomy as a treatment for medically intractable dystonia. *Ann Neurol* 1997;42:409.

109. Vitek JL, Zhang J, Evatt M, et al. GPi pallidotomy for dystonia: clinical outcome and neuronal activity. *Adv Neurol* 1998;78:211–219.

110. Walker AE. Cerebral pedunculotomy for the relief of involuntary movements. II. Parkinsonian tremor. *J Nerv Ment Disord* 1952;116:766–775.

111. Walker RH, Muralidharan N, Gujjari P, et al. Distribution and immunohistochemical characterization of torsin A-immunoreactive neurons in rat and macaque brain. *Neurology* 2000;54[Suppl 3]:A54.

112. Weisz DJ, Yang B. Intraoperative electrophysiological recording techniques. In: Germano IM, ed. *Neurosurgical treatment of movement disorders.* Park Ridge, IL: American Association of Neurological Surgeons, 1998:207–218.

113. Zweig RM, Hedreen JC, Jankel WR, et al. Pathology in brainstem regions of individuals with primary dystonia. *Neurology* 1988;38:702–706.

Surgery for Parkinson's Disease and Movement Disorders,
edited by J.K. Krauss, J. Jankovic, and R.G. Grossman.
Lippincott Williams & Wilkins, Philadelphia © 2001.

29

INTRATHECAL BACLOFEN FOR TREATMENT OF DYSTONIA

A. LELAND ALBRIGHT

In 1991, Narayan and co-workers were the first to report the use of intrathecal baclofen (ITB) to treat dystonia (1). Their patient was an 18-year-old man whose generalized and axial dystonia had been unresponsive to numerous oral medications but who substantially improved when he was treated with 825 μg ITB per day. Since then, several articles have been published about the use of ITB to treat dystonia. This chapter describes the pharmacology of baclofen and the rationale for its use in dystonia, patient selection, screening trials, pump implantation, results of ITB for dystonia, and complications associated with this form of treatment.

PHARMACOLOGY OF BACLOFEN

Baclofen (β-4-chlorophenyl-γ-aminobutyric acid [GABA]) is a GABA agonist that acts at $GABA_b$ receptors, where it inhibits the release of excitatory neurotransmitters such as glutamate (2,3). It does not bind to $GABA_a$ receptors. In the spinal cord, baclofen acts in the superficial layers (Rexed layers I to III), where GABA is heavily concentrated. GABA levels in the brain are highest in the putamen and the substantia nigra. The use of baclofen in the treatment of dystonia may be related to its effects on GABA, although the role of GABA in dystonia is unclear. However, baclofen affects other areas of the basal ganglia, by increasing serotonin levels and decreasing dopamine release in the striatum, by decreasing firing of noradrenergic neurons in the locus caeruleus, by hyperpolarizing neurons in the substantia nigra pars compacta, and by increasing turnover of the inhibitory neurotransmitter glycine (4–8).

Baclofen has been given orally to treat dystonia since the mid-1970s. In 1992, Greene reviewed the subject and reported that 30% of 31 children and adolescents with idiopathic dystonia improved dramatically, but adults with

focal and cranial dystonia improved less dramatically and less frequently (18%) (9). Greene and Fahn reported that oral baclofen caused substantial improvement in five of 15 children with idiopathic dystonia, moderate improvement in two others, and no improvement in the remainder (10). In children with secondary dystonia associated with cerebral palsy, baclofen has been one of the mainstays of treatment, along with trihexyphenidyl and levodopa.

Oral baclofen doses are rapidly absorbed from the gastrointestinal tract, but baclofen crosses the blood-brain barrier poorly. Oral doses are associated with serum baclofen levels of 275 ng/mL but cerebrospinal fluid (CSF) levels of less than 12 ng/mL (11). ITB infusion, however, results in considerably higher baclofen levels: infusion of 400 μg per day is associated with a CSF level of 396 μg/mL (12). The half-life of ITB doses is approximately 4 hours (13). Bolus doses cause maximal relief of spasticity in 4 hours, and clinical effects clear within 8 to 10 hours (14). Baclofen is cleared at a rate of 30 mL per hour, the rate of CSF clearance, apparently by bulk flow with CSF (15). Injections of baclofen into lumbar CSF are associated with decreasing concentrations cephalad, so concentrations in the upper cervical region are 25% of those in the lumbar region (16).

INTRATHECAL BACLOFEN FOR TREATMENT OF DYSTONIA

Rationales

The mechanism of action by which ITB alters dystonia is unknown, but two sites may be involved, one spinal and the other intracranial. One of the hallmarks of dystonia is muscle cocontraction, which may result from a lack of reciprocal inhibition at the brainstem and spinal cord level, although the primary disturbance is within the cerebral hemispheres (17). ITB is known to act at a spinal level, to inhibit descending excitatory impulses.

A supratentorial site of action for ITB in addition is suggested by the observation that dystonic movements do not

A.L. Albright: Department of Neurosurgery, University of Pittsburgh School of Medicine, and Department of Pediatric Neurosurgery, Children's Hospital of Pittsburgh, Pittsburgh, Pennsylvania 15213.

respond to the 50- to 100-μg bolus doses that provoke a response in spasticity, as well as by the observation that the responses to continuous ITB infusions do not occur within the 4 to 6 hours, as for spasticity, but rather often take 2 to 5 days of infusion, enough for the medication to enter the intracranial subarachnoid spaces. Parenthetically, patients with dystonia who receive 1,000 to 2,000 μg per day usually do not become drowsy, as do patients with spasticity who receive far lower doses. Hallet reported a lack of cortical inhibition in dystonia, leading to hyperexcitable cortex and excessive movement (18). ITB within the subarachnoid space thus may also inhibit the hyperexcitable cortex.

Patient Selection

The use of ITB for dystonia is relatively new, and indications for treatment are evolving. In general, for patients to be considered for treatment with ITB, their dystonia must be severe and inadequately controlled with oral medications. Because the effects of ITB are systemic, it is used predominantly for persons with generalized dystonia, although it has been used in hemidystonia and segmental dystonia. Use of ITB to treat focal dystonias has been very limited. ITB has the particular advantage of being adjustable, so doses can be increased if dystonia worsens.

The indications for treating dystonia are multiple and include increased comfort, increased function, increased ease of positioning, and ease of care. ITB is especially appropriate for patients with mixed dystonia and spasticity.

ITB is administered on a long-term basis through an implanted infusion pump, and patients must obviously be large enough for the pump to be implanted. Current pumps can be implanted in all adults and in children weighing as little as 20 lb, although implantation is easier in those who weight more than 30 lb. Size, not age, is the consideration. Although ITB has been approved for the treatment of spasticity in patients 4 years of age and older, it is occasionally indicated in younger children, to treat either spasticity or dystonia.

Screening Trials

Our work using ITB for dystonia began with a 35-year-old woman who had severe generalized dystonia after a hypoxic episode at age 5 years (19). In the intervening years, she had been relatively unresponsive to oral medications and was taking baclofen, 100 mg per day, when my colleagues and I first saw her. She underwent a double-blind baclofen screening trial consisting of bolus lumbar injections on 6 consecutive days, alternating between placebo and baclofen, 25 μg, 50 μg, and 100 μg. We observed no difference in her dystonia at any dose, but at the end of the trial, when the randomization code was broken, she

had been able to detect whether she received baclofen or placebo on each day. Her oral baclofen dose was increased to 150 mg per day, with minimal improvement, and a pump was inserted for ITB. Within 48 hours postoperatively, her dystonia improved dramatically; it remains improved 7 years later. Since then, we have used continuous infusions when screening patients for responsiveness to ITB.

The goal of screening patients with dystonia is to identify those who will experience a sustained benefit from long-term ITB. The end point in such screening is less clear-cut than when screening patients with spasticity, in whom a one- to two-point decrease in the Ashworth scale is considered to be clinically significant (14). The Ashworth scale evaluates resistance to passive muscle stretch and has no role in screening for dystonia. In screening for dystonia, there is no widely accepted grading scale. Both the Burke-Fahn-Marsden scale and the Barry-Albright dystonia (BAD) scale have been used (20–22). There is no consensus on what constitutes a clinically significant response; we consider a 25% decrease in the BAD scale at two consecutive time intervals to be significant.

Dystonia screening with bolus injections uses baclofen doses of 50 to 200 μg, injected through lumbar punctures, with responses expected within 12 hours, usually within 6 hours. Infusion screening is done through an intrathecal catheter inserted in sterile fashion through a lumbar puncture and advanced cephalad to the C-7–T-2 region. The catheter is tunneled subcutaneously several centimeters, then exits the skin and is connected to an external microinfusion pump that infuses baclofen continuously, beginning at 200 μg per day and increasing by 50 μg every 8 hours or 75 μg every 12 hours until the dystonia is improved, unacceptable side effects develop, or the infusion rate is 900 μg per day with no significant response.

A review of the literature indicates that although bolus lumbar injections of 50 to 100 μg baclofen are highly effective ways to screen for responsiveness of spasticity to ITB, such is not the case when screening patients with dystonia. Of patients with spasticity who receive 50 to 100 μg baclofen screening boluses, 85% to 95% will respond with a clinically significant decrease in muscle tone. Currently available publications indicate a lower response rate for bolus doses in screening dystonia, with 24 of 46 patients (52%) responding (19,24–32). Responses after infusions occurred in 15 of 19 patients (79%) of published cases (33–36). In our unpublished institutional series, 54 of 62 patients (87%) with dystonia, predominantly generalized secondary dystonia, responded to continuous infusion screening.

Operative Technique of Pump Implantation

Pump models currently available are either programmable, powered by batteries that last 7 to 8 years, or nonprogrammable, powered by gas. Because numerous dose adjustments are needed when treating dystonia, programmable

TABLE 29.1. PUBLISHED REPORTS OF THE USE OF INTRATHECAL BACLOFEN IN SEVERE INTRACTABLE DYSTONIA

Author (ref.)	Demographics	Type	Screening	Results	Long-Term Results	Dosings
Narayan et al. (1)	18-yr-old man	Axial dystonia secondary to CP	Continuous 30 µg/d with an implanted pump (Infusaid)	2 d on 100 µg/d decreased muscle contractions	6 mo: decreased dystonia, no decrease in strength, improved walking	Not reported
Silbert and Stewart-Wynne (27)	33-yr-old woman	Generalized dystonia secondary to encephalitis	Bolus of 50 µg	Dystonia increased for 6 h	Not implanted	—
Brin et al. (23)	8 patients	5 patients: generalized primary dystonia; 3 patients: secondary dystonia	Boluses 50–200 µg	1 patient with primary dystonia; 2 patients with secondary dystonia had positive screenings	2 patients had pumps implanted and had "striking" benefit that was sustained	Not reported
Penn et al. (25)	5 patients with dystonia of an 18-patient series: 1. 53-yr-old man 2. 37-yr-old woman 3. 59-yr-old man 4. 40-yr-old man 5. 36-yr-old man	1. Primary generalized dystonia 2. Leg secondary to surgery 3. Focal: left foot 4. Focal: right foot 5. Hemidystonia and spasticity secondary to TBI	Boluses 50–100 µg	Positive results for all but 1 patient, who was not implanted	38–63 mo: 1. Mildly improved (double-blind) 3. Marked improvement pain, spasms 4. Excellent pain relief, less dystonia 5. Decreased dystonia for 6 mo: less spasticity long term	300–900 µg/d
Albright et al. (19)	5-patient series: 1. 36-yr-old woman 2. 7-yr-old boy 3. 10-yr-old boy 4. 19-yr-old man 5. 15-yr-old boy	Generalized dystonia: patients 1–3 secondary to CP Patients 4,5 secondary to Hallevorden-Spatz	Continuous up 50–900 µg/d	Patients 1–3 decreased dystonia Patients 4,5 did not respond	10–19 mo: patients 1–3 implanted with pump, continued reduction in dystonia	1. 556 µg/d 2. 350 µg/d 3. 452 µg/d
Ford et al. (24)	25-patient series pooled by several neurologists: 16–73 yr of age, sex not reported	13 patients: primary dystonia 12 patients: secondary dystonia (7 patients encephalopathy, 5 patients Parkinsonism) Generalized in 21 patients; segmental in 4 patients	Boluses 25–250 µg; some patients also received placebo	13 patients had positive response by neurologist and patient report Blinded assessment of videotapes of 10 patients found no significant change in severity for group as a whole, although mean rating scores improved in 6 of 10 patients	13 patients implanted with pumps; 21 mo mean follow-up on 11 patients implanted >3 mo; 6/11 continued efficacy	400–1,840 µg/d

Study	Patient	Dystonia type	Administration	Response	Outcome	Dose
Latash and Penn (26)	2 patients with dystonia of a 12-patient series: 1. 53-yr-old man 2. 38-yr-old	1. Primary dystonia 2. Right hemidystonia secondary to TBI	Continuous to 360 µg/d placebo for 12 h	Dystonia controlled Dystonia returned	14 mo: dystonia "under good control"; Resumed activities of daily living	825 µg/d
Paret et al. (31)	9-yr-old boy	Primary generalized dystonia (hereditary torsion dystonia)	Boluses 25 to 150 µg over 6 d	Hereditary torsion dystonia arrested at a dose less than 150 µg; recovered Dystonia responded well to boluses	Dystonia controlled but pump removed at 3 wk for infection; after removal, dystonia resolved, normal function returned	Not reported
Diederich et al. (34)	32-yr-old man	Primary generalized dystonia	Continuous 42 µg/h (1,108 µg/d)	Dramatic reduction in dystonia in 12 h; dystonia returned once infusion stopped	32 mo: blinded video evaluation; 13 and 14 mo preimplant: 6,12, 21 mo postimplant; improved turn and legs, but not neck 8/10 at baseline (10 worst), 1/10 at 900 µg/d; able to walk again	900 µg/d
Dressler et al. (33)	49-yr-old woman	Axial tardive dystonia	Continuous 30 µg/d with an implanted pump (Infusaid)	2 days on 100 µg/d decreased muscle contractions	6 mo: decreased dystonia, no decrease in strength, improved walking	Not reported
Albright (32)	12 patients ages 4–42 (Includes patients 1–3 from above study)	Generalized dystonia secondary to CP	Continuous up to 900 µg/d	10/12 patients responded with decreased dystonia as assessed by blinded rate: baseline 22.9, on intrathecal baclofen 15.6 (worst: 32)	11–24 mo: 8/10 implanted with pump; 6/8 continued reduction in dystonia	185 µg/d to 625 µg/d (mean, 441)
Awaad et al. (29)	15-yr-old girl	Generalized dystonia due to chromosome 18p deletion	Boluses 50 and 100 µg	Decreased dystonia, improved range of motion and walking	18 mo: severity 3+ at baseline, 1+ with pump; walking, activities of daily living and social life improved	1,200 µg/d
Dalvi et al. (28)	16-yr-old boy	Generalized primary dystonia	Boluses 50 and 75 µg	50: marked reduction in dystonia 75: similar results but drowsy	Fahn-Marsden scale: severity decreased 22 points, function decreased by 4 points	900 µg/d
Siebner et al. (30)	19-yr-old man	Primary generalized dystonia	"Port-catheter system"	Positive testing (not described)	"Marked lasting improvement of generalized dystonia"	1,400 µg/d

CP, cerebral palsy; TBI, traumatic brain injury.

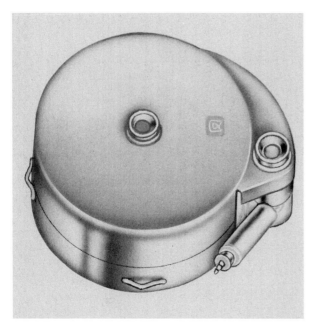

FIGURE 29.1. Programmable pump with an 18-mL reservoir for long-term intrathecal administration of baclofen. (From Medtronic, Inc., Minneapolis, with permission.)

pumps are almost always used (Fig. 29.1). They are inserted while the patient is under general anesthesia in operations that have two main components: insertion of the pump and insertion of the catheters extending from the pump into the spinal fluid. Pumps are implanted subcutaneously, usually in the right lower quadrant (Fig. 29.2). They can be implanted either just superficial to the fascia overlying the rectus abdominis and external oblique muscles or immediately below it. The subfascial placement is associated with less bulge of the pump and better wound healing.

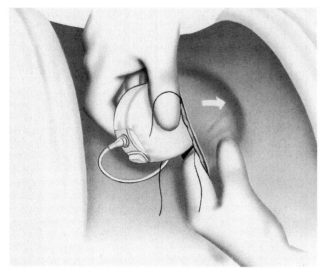

FIGURE 29.2. Subcutaneous implantation of a baclofen pump connected to an intrathecal catheter. (From Medtronic, Inc., Minneapolis, with permission.)

The intrathecal catheter is inserted into the spinal fluid through a Tuohy needle at approximately L2-3 and is advanced cephalad to C-7–T-2 for dystonia, higher than catheters are positioned when one treats spasticity (T4-6). The intrathecal catheter can either be tunneled subcutaneously around to the abdomen where it is attached to the pump, or it can be connected at the back to a larger catheter that is tunneled anteriorly and connected to the pump.

Pumps are programmed postoperatively to fill the catheter and to give a baclofen bolus of 50 to 100 μg, then a constant rate of 200 to 300 μg per day. Rates are increased by approximately 50 μg daily until the dystonia is appreciably improved, usually within 5 days. Most pumps contain 18 mL baclofen and need to be refilled approximately every 3 months. Daily baclofen doses for dystonia range from 200 to 2,000 μg, usually 500 to 1,000 μg, higher than when treating spasticity. Doses are titrated with improving dystonia as the primary end point and improving function as a secondary goal. During long-term ITB therapy, the initial response of the dystonia to ITB lessens in approximately 15% of patients, and increasing doses are given, often 1,000 to 2,000 μg per day. For these patients, it is often helpful to infuse the baclofen not in the customary manner as a constant infusion, but rather as periodic boluses of perhaps 200 to 300 μg every 6 hours with low infusion rates in the intervals between boluses. The pathophysiologic explanation of the better responses after boluses is unknown.

Results

ITB has been reported for treatment of both severe primary dystonia and secondary dystonia, resulting from head injury, cerebral palsy, glutaric aciduria, and tardive dystonia. It has also been used in patients with "dystonic storm." In our series, we have applied it to treat dystonia associated with cerebral palsy, Hallervorden-Spatz disease, glutaric aciduria, Huntington's disease, and posttraumatic dystonia.

After continuous ITB, dystonia improves in all body regions, but it probably improves more in the extremities than in the facial and cervical regions. Sustained improvement in dystonia was reported in 28 of 38 (73.7%) published cases (Table 29.1). Although patients with primary and secondary dystonias have been treated with ITB, insufficient numbers have been reported to determine whether the two groups respond similarly. The responsiveness of patients with hemidystonia and segmental dystonia is anecdotal. The frequency with which improved dystonia is accompanied by improved function is likewise unknown. We have observed improved speech in more than half the patients with generalized dystonia after ITB but have not observed any dramatic improvement in extremity function, as is sometimes seen when treating spasticity. In the experience of Ford et al., function improved in two of 11 patients, although other important aspects of quality of life, such as pain or spasms, improved in others (24). In their series, 54% of patients continued to take oral antidystonic medications.

During the first year of treatment, ITB doses commonly increase, but thereafter they remain relatively stable. As in spasticity in most patients, the need for substantially increased doses should raise the suspicion of a system malfunction.

In our experience with ITB for dystonia since the mid-1990s, approximately 85% of patients who responded to the infusion screening trial have long-term improvement of their dystonia; the other 15% appear to become refractory to treatment. Their doses escalate from levels that provided good relief of dystonia postoperatively to high levels, usually more than than 1,500 μg per day, with diminishing results. The cause of that decline in effect is unknown. Kroin demonstrated downregulation of GABA$_b$ receptors after ITB infusion, but whether that change is associated with the decreased dystonia effect is unknown (35).

For patients who become refractory to ITB, even when it is given in bolus doses, there are no other effective intrathecal medications. For treating spasticity, morphine, midazolam, and clonidine have been infused intrathecally (36,37). Ford et al. treated two patients with dystonia who had become refractory to ITB with intrathecal morphine; one subsequently underwent thalamotomy (24). We treated two patients who had become refractory to ITB with intrathecal clonidine, without significant improvement. Apomorphine has been infused subcutaneously for dystonia, but I am not aware of its intrathecal use (38).

Complications

The complications of treatment of dystonia are similar to those of treating spasticity, although the number of catheter-related problems seems to be higher, perhaps because of the greater amount of trunk movement in dystonia. Complications are related to the infusion system far more often than to the medication itself.

Systemic complications include infections, CSF leaks, and catheter problems. Problems with the pump itself are rare in my experience. Infections usually occur within 1 month of pump implantation, they are almost always caused by staphylococci, and they occur in 5% to 10% of cases. If infection is limited anteriorly at the pump, it can often be cleared by intravenous antibiotics without pump removal. If infection involves both the pump and the CSF, removal of the pump and the intrathecal catheter is usually indicated.

CSF leaks occur at the site where the catheter penetrates the dura. If the dura does not seal around the entry site, CSF leaks along the catheter, accumulating subcutaneously in the lumbar region, then tracking anteriorly to the abdomen, where it accumulates around the pump. The primary consequence of CSF leaks is the risk of CSF leaking through the incisions, thus allowing the introduction of bacteria. To reduce the risk of leaks, a blood patch or fibrin glue

patch can be inserted into the epidural space at the site where the catheter penetrates the dura during pump implantation. Without such patches, CSF leaks occur in at least 10% of patients.

Catheter problems include disconnection, kinking, obstruction, leaking, and breaking. Currently available catheters have a substantially lower risk of such problems than did the catheters available in the mid-1990s.

Acute ITB withdrawal may be a serious medical problem. Symptoms include increased dystonia, itching, agitation, hallucinations or psychosis, fever, diaphoresis, and opisthotonic posturing. (39,40). In my experience, severe symptoms are more likely to develop if ITB is abruptly discontinued, such as by catheter disconnection, than if the pump runs dry. When acute withdrawal occurs, baclofen should be given orally in substantial doses, such as 30 mg three times daily, until the infusion can be resumed.

ITB overdoses in treating either dystonia or spasticity are far more likely to result from iatrogenic programming errors than from an overinfusion of baclofen by the pump itself. Overdoses cause marked hypotonia, respiratory depression, and coma, and they are treated by assisted ventilation, discontinuance of the pump, and withdrawal and barbotage of CSF. Symptoms clear as baclofen is metabolized, and most patients resume the infusion afterward.

CONCLUSIONS

ITB provides an effective method of treating severe generalized dystonia unresponsive to oral medication. The use of ITB to treat dystonia differs in several ways from its use in treating spasticity: patients are more likely to respond to continuous infusion than to bolus doses, they require higher doses than when treating spasticity, they are more likely to become resistant to the treatment, and they are less likely to experience substantial improvement in function. The effects of ITB are systemic and adjustable, and the side effects and complications are acceptable. Long-term effectiveness is being determined.

REFERENCES

1. Narayan RK, Loubser PG, Jankovic J, et al.. Intrathecal baclofen for intractable axial dystonia. *Neurology* 1991;41:1141–1142.
2. Misgeld U, Bijak M, Jarolimek W. A physiological role for GABA$_b$ receptors and the effects of baclofen in the mammalian central nervous system. *Prog Neurobiol* 1995;46:423–462.
3. Davidoff RA. Antispasticity drugs: mechanisms of action. *Ann Neurol* 1985;17:107–116.
4. Nishikawa T, Scatton B, Enomoto T, et al. Modulation of striatal serotonin metabolism by baclofen, a gamma-aminobutyric acid$_b$ receptor agonist. *Tokai J Exp Clin Med* 1989;14:375–380.
5. Guyenet PG, Aghajanian GK. Ach, substance P, and met enkephalin in the locus coeruleus: pharmacological evidence

for independent sites of action. *Eur J Pharmacol* 1979;53:319–328.

6. Seabrook GR, Howson W, Lacey MG. Electrophysiological characterization of potent agonists and antagonists at pre-and postsynaptic GABA$_b$ receptors on neurones in rat brain slices. *Br J Pharmacol* 1990;101:949–957.

7. Bowery NG, Hill DR, Hudson AL. (-) Baclofen decreases neurotransmitter release in the mammalian CNS by an action at a novel GABA receptor. *Nature* 1980;283:92–94.

8. Potashner SJ. Baclofen: effects on amino acid release and metabolism in slices of guinea pig cerebral cortex. *J Neurochem* 1978;32:103–109.

9. Greene P. Baclofen in the treatment of dystonia: review. *Clin Neuropharmacol* 1992;15:276–288.

10. Greene PE, Fahn S. Baclofen in the treatment of idiopathic dystonia in children. *Mov Disord* 1992;7:48–52.

11. Knutsson E, Lindblom U, Martensson A. Plasma and cerebrospinal fluid levels of baclofen (Lioresal) at optimal therapeutic responses in spastic paresis. *J Neurol Sci* 1974;23:473–484.

12. Muller H, Zierski J, Dralle D, et al. Pharmacokinetics of intrathecal baclofen. In: Muller H, Zierski J, Penn R, eds. *Local spinal therapy of spasticity.* Berlin: Springer, 1988:155–214.

13. Penn RD, Kroin JS. Long-term intrathecal baclofen infusion for treatment of spasticity. *J Neurosurg* 1987;66:181–185.

14. Albright AL, Cervi A, Singletary J. Intrathecal baclofen for spasticity in cerebral palsy. *JAMA* 1991;265:1418–1422.

15. Ochs G, Reimann I. *Baclofen intrathekal.* Stuttgart: Thieme, 1995.

16. Kroin JS, Ali A, York M, et al. The distribution of medication along the spinal canal after chronic intrathecal administration. *Neurosurgery* 1993;33:226–230.

17. Hallett M, Toro C. Dystonia and the supplementary sensorimotor area. *Adv Neurol* 1996;70:471–476.

18. Hallett M. The neurophysiology of dystonia. *Arch Neurol* 1998;55:601–603.

19. Albright AL, Barry MJ, Fasick MP, et al. Effects of continuous intrathecal baclofen infusion for symptomatic generalized dystonia. *Neurosurgery* 1996;38:934–939.

20. Burke RE, Fahn S, Marsden CD, et al. Validity and reliability of a rating scale for the primary torsion dystonias. *Neurology* 1985;35:73–77.

21. Albright AL. Intrathecal baclofen in cerebral palsy movement disorders. *J Child Neurol* 1996;11[Suppl 1]:S29–S35.

22. Barry MJ, Van Swearingen JM, Albright AL. Reliability and responsiveness of the Barry-Albright dystonia scale. *Dev Med Child Neurol* 1999.

23. Brin M, Sadiq S, Goodman R, et al. Intrathecal baclofen (IT-B) for dystonia. *Neurology* 1994;44:1141–1142.

24. Ford B, Greene P, Louis ED, et al. Use of intrathecal baclofen in the treatment of patients with dystonia. *Arch Neurol* 1996;53:1241–1246.

25. Penn RD, Gianino JM, York MM. Intrathecal baclofen for motor disorders. *Mov Disord* 1995;10:675–677.

26. Latash ML, Penn RD. Changes in voluntary motor control induced by intrathecal baclofen inpatients with spasticity of different etiology. *Physiother Res Int* 1996:1:229–246.

27. Silbert PL, Stewart-Wynne EG. Increased dystonia after intrathecal baclofen [Letter]. *Neurology* 1992;42:1639–1640.

28. Dalvi A, Fahn S, Ford B. Intrathecal baclofen in the treatment of dystonic storm. *Mov Disord* 1998;13:611–612.

29. Awaad Y, Munoz S, Nigro M. Progressive dystonia in a child with chromosome 18p deletion, treated with intrathecal baclofen. *J Child Neurol* 1999;14:75–77.

30. Siebner HR, Dressnandt J, Auer C, et al. Continuous intrathecal baclofen infusions induced a marked increase of the transcranially evoked silent period in a patient with generalized dystonia. *Muscle Nerv* 1998;21:1209–1212.

31. Paret G, Tirosh R, Ben Zeev B, et al. Intrathecal baclofen for severe torsion dystonia in a child. *Acta Paediatr* 1996;85:635–637.

32. Albright AL, Barry MJ, Painter MJ, et al. Infusion of intrathecal baclofen for generalized dystonia in cerebral palsy. *J Neurosurg* 1996;88:73–76.

33. Dressler D, Oeljeschlager RO, Ruther E. Severe tardive dystonia: treatment with continuous intrathecal baclofen administration. *Mov Disord* 1997;12:585–587.

34. Diederich NJ, Comella CL, Matge G, et al. Sustained effect of high-dose intrathecal baclofen in primary generalized dystonia: a 2-year follow-up study. *Mov Disord* 1997;12:1100–1102.

35. Kroin JS, Bianchi GD, Penn RD. Intrathecal baclofen downregulates GABA$_b$ receptors in the rat substantia gelatinosa. *J Neurosurg* 1993;79:544–549.

36. Siegfried J, Rea L. Intrathecal application of drugs for muscle hypertonia. *Scand J Rehabil Med Suppl* 1988;17:145–148.

37. Middleton JW, Siddall PJ, Walker S, et al. Intrathecal clonidine and baclofen in the management of spasticity and neuropathic pain following spinal cord injury: a case study. *Arch Phys Med Rehabil* 1996;77:824–826.

38. Zuddas A, Pintor M, DeMontis N, et al. Continuous infusion of apomorphine improves torsion dystonia in a boy unresponsive to other dopaminergic drugs. *J Child Neurol* 1996;11:343–345.

39. Rivas DA, Chancellor MB, Hill K, et al. Neurological manifestations of baclofen withdrawal. *J Urol* 1993;150:1903–1905.

40. Kofler M, Kronenberg MF, Rifici C, et al. Epileptic seizures associated with intrathecal baclofen application. *Neurology* 1994;44:25–27.

Surgery for Parkinson's Disease and Movement Disorders,
edited by J.K. Krauss, J. Jankovic, and R.G. Grossman.
Lippincott Williams & Wilkins, Philadelphia © 2001.

30

TREATMENT OPTIONS FOR SURGERY OF CERVICAL DYSTONIA

JOACHIM K. KRAUSS
ROBERT G. GROSSMAN
JOSEPH JANKOVIC

Cervical dystonia (CD) is the most frequent form of focal dystonia seen in movement disorders centers (1,2). Many different surgical approaches have been developed for treatment of this common movement disorder (3).

We prefer using the term "cervical dystonia" rather than the historical expression "spasmodic torticollis" for several reasons. First, few patients present with simple turning of the head. Second, the abnormal movement is not always spasmodic. Third, nondystonic abnormal neck postures have been labeled torticollis as well. CD is characterized by involuntary sustained contractions of cervical muscles that produce abnormal patterned head movements or postures. It is usually associated with neck pain, which may be severe and may further disable the patient. Often, there are also tremulous or jerking movements of the head. According to the involvement of different cervical muscles, various common patterns of CD are recognized. Contemporary nomenclature defines *rotation (torticollis)* as movement of the chin to the opposite shoulder in the horizontal plane, *tilt (laterocollis)* as moving of the ear to the ipsilateral shoulder, and *flexion/extension* in the anteroposterior axis as *anterocollis/retrocollis*. Translation of the axis of the head with regard to the axis of the body is defined as *lateral or sagittal shift*. Most patients present with combined deviations of the head. The individual pattern of CD is determined by the degree of dystonic activity in specific cervical muscles (Fig. 30.1). Rotation of the head, for example, usually involves contraction of the sternocleidomastoid muscle on the side opposite to where the chin is rotated and contraction of the posterior neck muscles ipsilateral to where the chin is rotated.

The goals of treatment of CD are improving the abnormal neck posture and associated pain and preventing secondary complications such as the development of contractures, cervical myelopathy, and radiculopathy. These goals may be achieved either by modification of the central mechanisms involved in the generation of dystonia or by weakening of the dystonic muscles. Medical treatment with anticholinergics and muscle relaxants often has limited benefit, and patients are frequently burdened by side effects. The treatment of choice of CD nowadays is the local injection of botulinum toxin type A into the dystonic muscles (4–10). Most trials report benefit in about 90% of patients, with mild side effects resolving within a few weeks in up to 28% of patients. Improvement occurs about 1 week after injection, and the average duration of optimal benefit is 3 to 4 months. Therefore, the injections have to be repeated indefinitely. The estimated frequency of primary nonresponders to botulinum toxin injections is 6% to 14% of patients with CD, and this approach loses its efficacy with continued use because of the development of immunoresistance in about another 3% to 10% of patients (11).

Surgical treatment options for patients with otherwise intractable CD are gaining increased attention and acceptance (12–14). Surgery can provide permanent relief of this disabling movement disorder and can effectively prevent its secondary complications. Because these procedures are performed on a purely elective basis, the avoidance of operative side effects and of additional disability is of paramount importance. One of the crucial points of contemporary surgery for CD is tailoring the approach to the specific pattern of the individual patient, and this may involve several successive operative steps and the use of different surgical techniques.

HISTORICAL AND METHODOLOGIC ASPECTS

History of Surgical Treatment of Cervical Dystonia

The first operative procedures for treatment of CD were probably performed in ancient Greece (15). In 1641, the

J.K. Krauss: Department of Neurosurgery, University Hospital, Klinikum Mannheim, Mannheim 68167, Germany.
R.G. Grossman: Department of Neurosurgery, Baylor College of Medicine, Houston, Texas 77030.
J. Jankovic: Department of Neurology, Baylor College of Medicine, Houston, Texas 77030.

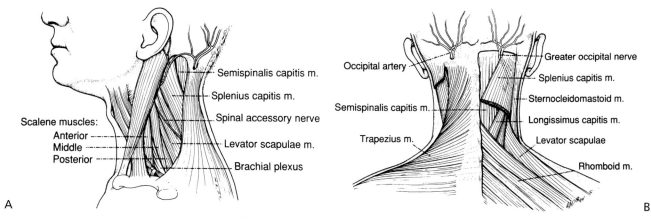

FIGURE 30.1. Topography of cervical muscles frequently involved in cervical dystonia. **A:** Lateral view. **B:** Posterior view. (From Brin MF, Jankovic J, Comella C, et al. Treatment of dystonia using botulinum toxin. In: Kurlan R, ed. *Treatment of movement disorders.* Philadelphia: JB Lippincott, 1995:183–246, with permission.)

German surgeon Minnius sectioned the sternocleidomastoid muscle in a patient with CD (16). Since then, myotomies and myectomies have been performed in varying frequency both as primary surgical procedures or as adjuncts to other types of surgery.

Bujalski is credited for having performed the first denervation of cervical muscles by ligation of the spinal accessory nerve in 1834 (17). Surgical treatment of CD by various approaches became more popular in the late nineteenth and early twentieth centuries. Keen introduced the concept of division of the posterior rami of C1 to C3 in 1891 (18). Intradural procedures initially involved sectioning of the posterior cervical roots (19). Then, attention soon shifted to the anterior roots. In the 1920s, McKenzie developed intradural sectioning of the anterior upper cervical roots in combination with sectioning of the intradural spinal accessory nerve (20). The procedure was further refined by Dandy and by Hamby and Schiffer (21–23). Intradural sectioning of the spinal accessory nerve aimed at sectioning only the fibers to the sternocleidomastoid muscle and leaving the innervation of the trapezius intact. Later, when the operating microscope became available, it was added as a technical aid to the procedure (24). Extradural approaches including posterior ramisectomy and peripheral nerve sectioning were developed and were popularized by Bertrand in the 1970s (25,26). Bertrand emphasized the more selective nature of these procedures and the lower frequency of side effects. Until the early 1990s, intradural anterior cervical nerve roots and spinal accessory nerve sectioning were the most common surgical procedures. Over the past few years, however, extradural denervations have become increasingly popular and have been favored by several surgeons.

There have been occasional reports on the use of ablative surgery of the cerebral cortex and in the subcortical white matter for treatment of CD. Section of frontal capsular pathways involved in adversive head movements were described in a small series of patients (27). Single patients even underwent leukotomies for treatment of their CD (28). In the 1950s and 1960s, functional stereotactic operations targeting the thalamus and various basal ganglia nuclei were performed, with beneficial results in patients with CD (29,30). Such procedures were abandoned almost completely, however, with the decline of functional stereotactic surgery in the 1970s. Iontophoresis, which involves suppression of labyrinthine activity, did not gain widespread acceptance (31). Epidural dorsal column stimulation of the cervical spine was performed in the 1970s for treatment of CD (32,33). It fell out of favor, however, after independent evaluation of outcome could not confirm its therapeutic benefit (34,35). Microvascular decompression (MVD) of the spinal accessory nerve as a therapeutic alternative was added to the armamentarium of surgical treatment options in the early 1980s (36). Despite of several reports of its efficacy, this procedure remained confined to a few centers and did not become widely accepted, mainly because of conceptual difficulties with regard to the pathophysiology of CD.

Evaluation of Surgical Outcome

It is almost impossible to compare any of the various surgical approaches that have been used for treatment of CD with regard to their efficacy and long-term benefits. Furthermore, it is also difficult to appreciate the results of the same procedure from studies by different centers because of the lack of comparable diagnostic standards and methods for assessment of surgical outcome. Many studies used only subjective global outcome scales, and follow-up was evaluated by questionnaires or by chart review only. There is an appreciable lack of prospective studies with independent control of the results. Nevertheless, valuable information on the frequency and severity of intraoperative complications and postoperative side effects can be obtained from these published studies.

Evaluation and comparative assessment at different times of the various aspects of CD including abnormal posture,

TABLE 30.1. TORONTO WESTERN SPASMODIC TORTICOLLIS RATING SCALE (TWSTRS) FOR CLINICAL ASSESSMENT OF PATIENTS WITH CERVICAL DYSTONIA

	Scores[a]
Severity scale	
Rotation	0–4
Laterocollis (Tilt)	0–3
Anterocollis/retrocollis	0–3
Lateral shift	0–1
Sagittal sgift	0–1
Time present	0–5
Effect of sensory tricks	0–2
Shoulder elevation	0–3
Range of voluntary motion	0–4
Time head can be held straight	0–4
Disability scale	
Work	0–5
Activities of daily living	0–5
Driving	0–5
Reading	0–5
Television	0–5
Outside activities	0–5
Social embarrassment	0–5
Pain scale	
Severity of neck pain	Visual analog
Duration of neck pain	0–5
Pain-associated disablity	0–5

[a]Some items have weighted scores.
Modified from Consky ES, Lang AE. Clinical assessments of patients with cervical dystonia. In: Jankovic J, Hallett M, eds. *Therapy with botulinum toxin*. New York: Marcel Dekker, 1994:211–237.

involuntary dystonic movements, accompanying dystonic tremor and myoclonus, limited range of voluntary movement, the effect of sensory tricks, and other aspects are very difficult (37). Along with the assessment of the efficacy of botulinum toxin injections, various rating scales have been introduced. The Toronto Western Spasmodic Torticollis Rating Scale (TWSTRS) is a clinical rating scale adopted by several investigators. The TWSTRS consists of three subscales scoring quantitatively the severity of CD, functional disability, and pain (38). Specific issues are addressed with graded scales for various subcategories within the three main domains (Table 30.1). Modified forms have been used for assessment of surgical outcome (39,40).

Indications for Surgical Treatment of Cervical Dystonia

Currently, surgery is performed mainly in patients who are primary or secondary nonresponders to botulinum toxin injections. Patients with long-standing CD may not respond to the injections because of additional fibrosis or contractures of the dystonic muscles. These patients, however, may be appropriate candidates for selective myectomies. The development of immunoresistance resulting from blocking

antibodies is related to several factors including frequency of administrations, individual and cumulative dosages of toxin, and age at onset of dystonia. Surgical treatment, in general, is indicated in those patients with functional disability caused by the dystonic movement disorder. Restriction of social activities because of embarrassment related to CD is also a major driving force, particularly in young patients, to seek more invasive therapies. Surgical treatment of CD may be an alternative to botulinum toxin injections in some patients, and in others it can be used as an adjunct to conservative treatment to reduce drug dosages. The selection of the operative procedure is largely guided by the personal operative experience of the individual surgeon. The rationales for the choices of the different surgical procedures are discussed in detail later.

Preoperative Assessment and Follow-Up

The selection of patients and the choice of procedure are best discussed by neurologists and neurosurgeons with expertise in the care and management of patients with movement disorders. All patients should have computed tomography or magnetic resonance imaging scans of the head and the cervical spine preoperatively. In patients with phasic dystonic movements, head tremor, or myoclonus, sedation before imaging is advisable. Extension and flexion radiographs of the cervical spine should be obtained in patients with severe neck pain or radicular pain, to detect and plan treatment of coexistent spinal instability or radicular compression. Videotaping according to a standard protocol is important to allow comparison of preoperative and follow-up assessments. Rating scales that are helpful in the further evaluation include the TWSTRS, the Mini-Mental Status Examination, and instruments measuring depression and quality of life. Patients should not have had botulinum toxin injections for at least 3 to 4 months preoperatively.

PRINCIPLES OF SELECTIVE SURGERY FOR CERVICAL DYSTONIA

In the past, operative procedures for treatment of CD were often performed as "standard" procedures, not taking into account the specific pattern of dystonic activity in the individual patient. Thus, for example, some surgeons always performed bilateral intradural sectioning of the anterior upper cervical roots. This technique produced unnecessary weakening of antagonist muscles or other side effects such as dysphagia. It was Bertrand who emphasized that denervation should be selective, and he consequently applied this principle to peripheral denervation (25). Nevertheless, such selectivity should be applied to any surgical procedure used for treatment of CD. We have used and continue to use various surgical options or a combination of procedures to yield optimal benefit in an individual patient (39,41). Instead of performing a standard procedure, we adapt the technique to the pattern of dystonic activity in every patient. The primary rationale for this treatment algorithm is the selective weakening of the muscles that produce dystonia with preservation of normal muscle function and the avoidance of side effects. The procedure can be planned to be performed in successive steps, to avoid postoperative weakness or discomfort in patients when large denervations or myectomies are necessary to provide adequate relief. In our experience, staged procedures are often also necessary to produce satisfactory relief of the dystonia. We have abandoned procedures that are accompanied by a relatively high frequency of side effects such as bilateral anterior rhizotomy.

Preoperative Planning Strategies

The muscles involved in the dystonic activity are best identified during a scrupulous physical examination including palpation of the cervical muscles while the patient holds the head in the position determined by the dystonic activity and also during active as well as passive movement in the direction opposite to the dystonic movements. Such passive movements may induce dystonic tremor, which also can be useful for identifying the muscles that are mainly involved. Hypertrophy of dystonic muscles can be very prominent in some cases and easily discloses the main offenders. Temporary blocks with local anesthetics injected into different muscles can be used to determine the contribution of single muscles to the overall dystonic activity. To differentiate the involvement of various muscles further in patients with complex CD, serial injections into different muscles may be performed at different times. Electromyographic guidance can be useful to elucidate the dystonic pattern further (5,42). Four-channel electromyography routinely should include recording of the sternocleidomastoid, trapezius, splenius, and semispinalis muscles and, in individual cases, also the levator scapulae, scalene, longissimus colli, and paraspinal erector trunci muscles. Activity in different muscles is compared at rest and while the patient turns the head to the right and to the left. Dystonic activity may be rated semiquantitatively.

Clinical Application of Selective Surgery for Cervical Dystonia

Our preoperative planning strategy, including selective targeting of dystonic muscles, staged procedures, and a combination of different techniques, may be best illustrated by the following example. A 44-year-old woman with a 6-year history of CD was referred for evaluation of surgical treatment. In the early course of her disease, she had a good response to botulinum toxin injections into the dystonic cervical muscles. After 4 years of treatment, she developed secondary immunoresistance with loss of efficacy of the injections. At that time, there was also no response to injection of botulinum toxin into the extensor digiti minimi muscle of the right foot. She presented with rotation of her head to the right, tilting of the head to the right, and elevation and anteversion of her right shoulder (Fig. 30.2A and B). Her movement disorder impaired her daily routine, and the dystonia was a source of marked social embarrassment. She also suffered from marked neck pain that was only partially improved by analgetic medication. Surgical treatment options were discussed with her, and a treatment plan was devised including two subsequent operative steps. The patient was entered in a prospective study protocol including assessment with a modified TWSTRS and standardized videotaping. The first operative step consisted of unilateral posterior ramisectomy from C1 to C6 on the right side and peripheral denervation of the left sternocleidomastoid muscle combined with myotomy and partial myectomy. Postoperatively, there was marked improvement of the head rotation and also mild amelioration of the tilting (Fig. 30.2C and D). She was still bothered, however, by the dystonic shoulder elevation and the residual tilting. One year after the first operation, this patient underwent myectomy of the levator scapulae muscle, partial myectomy of the right splenius capitis muscle, and partial myotomy/myectomy of the right trapezius muscle, with an asleep-awake-asleep technique, as described later. After this operation, she had further progressive relief of her CD. One year after the second operation, she had marked relief in the dystonic posture (Fig. 30.2E and F). This was reflected in significant improvement of the TWSTRS subscores for severity of dystonia, functional disability, and pain.

FIGURE 30.2. Sequential video stills of a 44-year-old woman with cervical dystonia preoperatively and at follow-up assessments after combined peripheral denervations and myotomies/myectomies performed in two stages. The patient is wearing a small scarf to allow blinded evaluation of the videotapes. **A** and **B:** Preoperatively, there is rotation of the head to the right, tilting of the head to the right side, and dystonic elevation and anteversion of the right shoulder. **C** and **D:** Three months after the first stage of surgery consisting of posterior ramisectomy from C1 to C6 on the right side and peripheral denervation combined with myotomy and partial myectomy of the left sternocleidomastoid muscle, the patient benefits from marked improvement of the head rotation. There is still, however, tilting of the head and dystonic shoulder elevation. **E** and **F:** The patient is shown at follow-up 2 years after the first operative stage and 1 year after the second operation, which consisted of myotomies/myectomies of the right levator scapulae and splenius capitis muscles and partial myotomy/myectomy of the right trapezius muscle with an asleep-awake-asleep anesthetic technique.

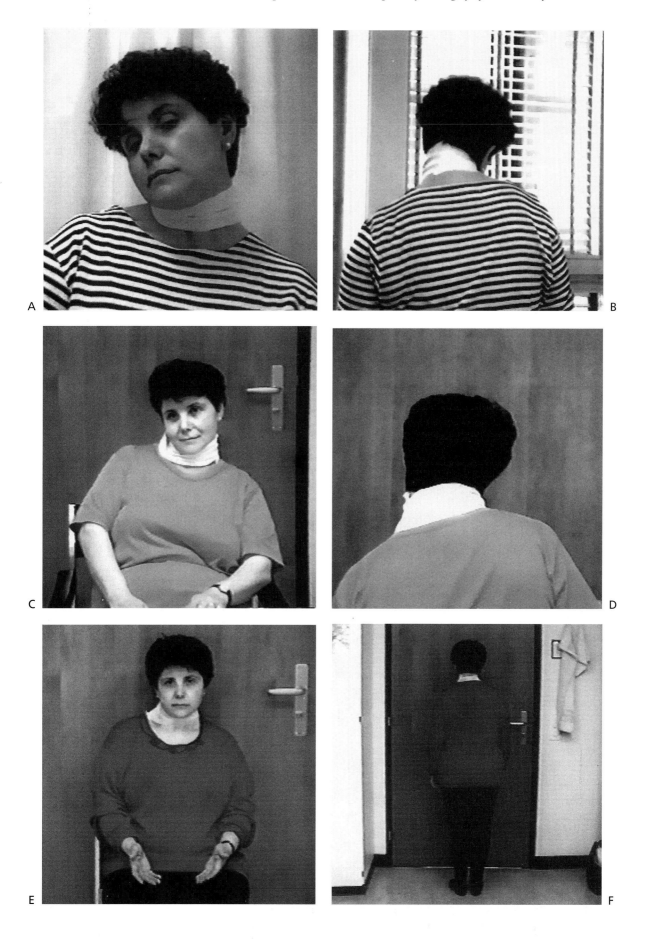

SURGICAL APPROACHES

Operative procedures for treatment of CD are performed while the patient is under general anesthesia, with few exceptions. Some surgeons have used local anesthesia for limited myotomies or myectomies. We recently introduced an asleep-awake-asleep technique that allows partial myotomy/myectomy of the trapezius muscle (43).

In rare instances, CD and segmental craniocervical dystonia are related to mass lesions within the posterior fossa (44,45). These lesions, in general, are extraaxial tumors such as meningiomas or schwannomas. Dystonia may improve after tumor resection, and in rare cases it may remit completely within 1 year.

Myotomy and Myectomy

Although myectomies were used early in the history of treatment of CD, there is limited information on the long-term benefits of this method. Whereas most surgeons have used *myotomies and myectomies* as an adjunct to other surgical procedures, few patients have undergone myectomies exclusively (46–48). It has been stated in some reviews that myectomies would offer only little benefit, and myectomies were abandoned by several surgeons. However, it appears that poor selection of appropriate candidates has produced unsatisfactory results. It is evident that patients with complex CD will not achieve any benefit from unilateral sectioning of single muscles. We perform myotomies and myectomies rarely as a first step in patients with rotational CD, but more frequently we consider it an adjunct to selective denervation or for treatment of dystonic activity in muscles that cannot be denervated completely with ease. Although the posterior neck muscles are denervated adequately by posterior ramisectomies, dystonic activity in the scalene muscles, the levator scapulae, and the omohyoid is not controlled by this approach. In such cases, selective myotomies/myectomies are very useful.

Sectioning of the sternocleidomastoid muscle on the side opposite the direction where the chin is rotated clearly is the simplest choice of surgical treatment of CD. It is suited for those few patients with rotational CD who present with marked dystonic activity in the sternocleidomastoid but minimal dystonia in the contralateral posterior neck muscles. We usually combine this procedure with selective denervation of the peripheral branches of the spinal accessory to the sternocleidomastoid. In patients who present with painful dystonic activity of the trapezius muscle resulting in elevation and anteversion of the shoulder or contributing to ipsilateral head tilt, denervation procedures are not performed because this would result in loss of the ability to elevate the arm above the horizontal plane. These patients can benefit from partial myotomy/myectomy of the upper portion of the trapezius muscle with an asleep-awake-asleep operative technique (43).

Chen has published the largest series on myotomies/myectomies for treatment of CD that were combined with selective peripheral denervations in certain patterns of CD (46). Treatment algorithms included selective resections of dystonic muscles for various patterns of CD such as rotational CD, tilt of the head, anterocollis, and retrocollis. In his series of 60 patients, excellent or marked improvement was described in 83% of patients. Most remarkably, there were no complications. In a series of 15 patients with retrocollis, partial resections of the upper part of the trapezius muscles, splenius, semispinalis capitis, and semispinalis cervicis muscles were performed bilaterally (47). Outcome at follow-up at 3 to 10 years postoperatively was reported as excellent or marked improvement in 87% of patients without persistent side effects. The long-term results of nonselective sternocleidomastoid sectioning in another series of 11 patients, in contrast, were less favorable (48). Good or "fair" outcome was reported in 45% of patients at a mean follow-up of 4 years.

It is difficult to appreciate the contribution of selective myotomy/myectomy when it is used as an adjunct to other surgical procedures (39). Nevertheless, additional amelioration was achieved in our patients who underwent selective sectioning of specific muscles as described earlier. All three patients who underwent partial myectomies of the trapezius muscle benefited from improvement of the dystonic posture of the shoulder and local pain (43).

Techniques

We outline the contours of the dystonic muscles that are to be approached surgically with a marker on the skin while the patient is awake. The choice of the positioning depends mainly on the topography of the muscles that are to be sectioned. Short-acting muscle relaxants are given only for induction of general anesthesia. Skin incisions are made over the belly of the appropriate muscles. During dissection of the subcutaneous tissue, care is taken to preserve sensory nerve branches. Bipolar stimulation forceps are useful to identify fine motor nerve branches and to elicit contractions in the corresponding muscles. This technique also allows us to identify branches to the brachial plexus in performing myectomies of the scalene muscles. The belly of the muscle is cut transversely either with monopolar forceps or sharply with scissors until the posterior sleeve of the muscle fascia is reached. Then, in general, the proximal and distal stumps are cut, with resection of approximately 3 cm of the muscle along its longitudinal axis. The gap is filled with a piece of gelatine foam, which can be soaked in a local anesthetic such as bupivacaine. Postoperatively, patients are administered anti-inflammatory medications.

The asleep-awake-asleep anesthesia to perform myotomy/myectomy of the upper portion of the trapezius muscle as has been described recently allows intraoperative control of the sectioning to avoid postoperative weakness of arm elevation (43). With this technique, the patient wakes up intraoperatively. The anterior rim of the trapezius muscle is sectioned transversely during continuous monitoring of the strength of active arm abduction and elevation.

Intradural Anterior Rhizotomy and Sectioning of the Spinal Accessory Nerve

Several variations of this *intradural approach* have been developed (20–24,49–53). The "standard" procedure includes bilateral intradural sectioning of the C1-3 anterior roots and the caudal rootlets of the spinal accessory nerves. As mentioned earlier, more restricted and selective sectioning is advisable to avoid postoperative side effects. For example, in a patient with rotational CD, unilateral anterior rhizotomy combined with contralateral spinal accessory nerve sectioning may be sufficient (54). In patients with retrocollis, sectioning of the spinal accessory nerves would not be useful. Denervation with this approach, in general, is limited downward to the anterior roots of C3 if it is performed bilaterally. The C4 root may be sectioned on one side, but that approach endangers functioning of the diaphragm. Thus, this intradural approach cannot control dystonic activity mediated by the C4-6 roots.

Both the reported results and the complication rates in different series are highly variable. Most studies claim useful postoperative improvement in 60% to 90% of their patients (23,24,49,50,53). Most often, however, it is unclear whether symptomatic amelioration of the abnormal postures or movements translated to improvement in functional disability with regard to the relatively high number of side effects. In the series of Friedman et al., the head was described to return to a neutral position in 59% of the patients postoperatively (24). The likelihood of the head to return to a normal position postoperatively was inversely related to the duration of CD. Some studies reported only very modest results after anterior intradural rhizotomy (28). Hernesniemi and Keränen, for example, reported no patient with an outcome considered as good based on their patients' self-assessments of the surgical result, extent of disability, and working capacity (48).

Complications of the standard bilateral intradural denervation are frequent and may be persistent and disabling. Mortality with the standard procedure usually ranges between 0% and 1%. However, mortality was as high as 12% in some series (50). Side effects included dysphagia, weakness of the neck, cerebrospinal fluid fistulas, and infection. Weak or unstable neck was estimated to occur in approximately 40% of patients after bilateral rhizotomy (49). Transient dysphagia was thought to occur in approximately 30% of patients. Radiologic swallowing abnormalities were described in as many as 95% of patients postoperatively, frequently representing aggravation of preexisting pharyngeal dysfunction (55).

In rare cases, bilateral infarctions of the medulla oblongata with bilateral Wallenberg's syndrome or ischemia of the upper spinal cord with tetraparesis were reported (56,57). The procedure is much safer and is accompanied by far less morbidity with selective approaches. In our practice, we experienced only one persistent complication consisting of mild difficulty with balance in 37 intradural denervations.

Techniques

Intracranial sectioning of nerve roots is performed with the patient either sitting or in the prone position with the head fixed in a Mayfield head holder. The posterior neck muscles are divided within the ligamentum nuchae in the dorsal midline. A small suboccipital craniotomy widening the posterior rim of the foramen magnum and laminectomies of the three upper cervical vertebrae are performed. After opening of the dura, the upper spinal cord, the medulla oblongata, the cerebellar tonsils, the upper cranial nerve roots, the spinal accessory nerves, and the blood vessels of the cervicomedullary junction and the upper cervical medulla are visualized with the operating microscope (Fig. 30.3). The anterior nerve roots lie ventral to the dentate ligament. Each rootlet is stimulated with a bipolar nerve stimulator and then is divided. Any arterial blood vessels that accompany the nerve roots should be spared. If sectioning is carried out down to the C4 root unilaterally, it is advisable to monitor muscular activity of the diaphragm. When sectioning of the spinal accessory is performed, the nerve is usually cut at the C1 level, where it crosses the upper margin of the dentate ligament. Bipolar stimulation may be used to delineate further the nerve rootlets of the spinal accessory nerve that supply the sternocleidomastoid, trapezius, and pharyngeal muscles. Evoked muscle contractions can also be monitored with surface electrodes. In addition, anastomotic branches between the C1 roots and the spinal accessory nerves should be divided when they are present. Rarely, a more prominent anastomosis, the McKenzie branch, may be found (Fig. 30.3). This branch should also be sectioned when it is encountered.

Microvascular Decompression of the Spinal Accessory Nerve

MVD of the spinal accessory nerve for treatment of CD has been used in analogy to the therapeutic benefit of this procedure in other cranial neuropathies such as hemifacial spasm (58). The existence of two pathogenetically different types of CD has been suggested by proponents of MVD. The first is CD of "central origin," and the second is "spasmodic torticollis of eleventh nerve origin" (58,59). In other cranial neuropathies such as hemifacial spasm or trigeminal neuralgia, clinical symptoms are thought to be related to contact of small blood vessels with the vulnerable root exit zone respectively entry zone, resulting either in ectopic excitation and ephaptic transmission or in nuclear

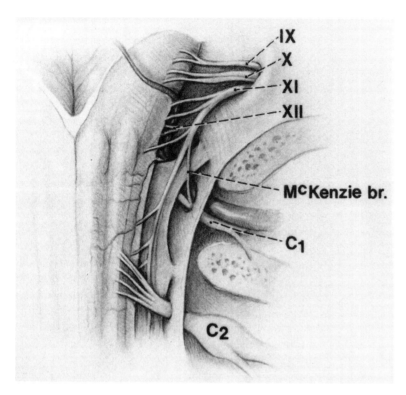

FIGURE 30.3. Anatomic sketch of the cervicomedullary junction showing the caudal cranial nerves, the rootlets of the spinal accessory nerve, the dentate ligament, and the rarely encountered McKenzie branch. (From Friedman AH, Nashold BS Jr, Sharp R, et al. Treatment of spasmodic torticollis with intradural selective rhizotomies. *J Neurosurg* 1993;78:46–53.)

hyperexcitability (60,61). The transition zone between central (oligodendroglia) and peripheral (Schwann glia) myelination is regarded as an area particularly vulnerable to compression. The average extension of glial spread into the facial nerve was found to measure 2.5 mm in one study and to be slightly shorter in another study; however, this segment has been described as very short, less than 0.1 mm, in the spinal accessory nerve (62,63). Thus, it is difficult to understand, how MVD of the spinal accessory nerve should work. Furthermore, with decompression for hemifacial spasm and trigeminal neuralgia, the benefit is apparent immediately after the operation, whereas the improvement after MVD in patients with CD has been described to be delayed. It is even more difficult to understand how CD can be improved by MVD when other muscles than the sternocleidomastoid are involved in dystonic activity.

Surgery in some of the studies that have reported on the benefits of MVD for treatment of CD also involved sectioning of rootlets of the spinal accessory nerve, sectioning of the spinal accessory nerve proper, sectioning of anastomoses between the accessory nerve roots and the posterior C1 and C2 roots, lysis of "cross-sectional adhesions" and "hypertrophied dentate ligaments," and division of the posterior C1 and C2 roots (64–67). The offending arteries usually were described as loops of the posterior inferior cerebellar artery and the vertebral artery and, more rarely, the posterior spinal arteries. Remarkably, Freckmann and associates, who performed MVD of the spinal accessory nerve in 33 patients, thought that postoperative improvement in their patients was not

related to vascular decompression, but to lysis from anastomoses and "adhesions" of the spinal accessory nerve related to "pathogenic factors in the afferent part of head control" (67). Also notably, in another series of 22 patients who underwent "microneural decompression" of the spinal accessory nerve, a compressive vessel was thought to be responsible for CD in only six patients (66). Only in a few studies, such in the series reported by Jho and Jannetta, were no nerve sections performed (58).

Bertrand reported that he performed selective peripheral denervation and posterior ramisectomies in six patients who had undergone prior MVD (26). Apparently, there was marked dystonic activity in the sternocleidomastoid muscle in all these patients. Scarring from the previous laminectomy interfered with the denervation.

Outcome data of MVD for treatment of CD are very limited. It is of particular concern that although the postoperative benefits have been ascribed to MVD, multiple "adhesiolyses" and nerve sectionings were performed in most instances, and these may have contributed to the postoperative benefit. It has been suggested that MVD is more successful in patients with rotational torticollis than in other forms and more complex patterns of CD. In the series of Freckmann and colleagues, five of 33 patients (15%) were reported to have "excellent" results, ten patients (30%) had "good" results, and 12 patients (36%) had less improvement (67). Jho and Jannetta claimed a "cure" of CD in 65% of their patients (13 of 20 patients), significant improvement in four patients (20%), moderate improvement in one patient (5%), and minimal improvement in two patients at long-term follow-up between 5 and 10 years after MVD (58). Most of these patients showed gradual improvement over 2 years. Notably, however, patients in the "cured" group were said to continue to "have some subtle tendency to move their necks to the prior abnormal position when they relax their head in the neutral position."

Postoperative death was reported to result from "medullary symptoms with severe respiratory insufficiency" (67). Surgical morbidity included cerebrospinal fluid leaks, meningitis, and stroke. The frequency of complications was as high as 27% in one series (66).

Posterior Ramisectomy and Selective Peripheral Denervation

Extradural section of the posterior primary divisions of the cervical nerve roots is also known as *ramisectomy*. Bertrand coined the term "selective peripheral denervation" for the combination of sectioning of the peripheral branch of the spinal accessory nerve to the sternocleidomastoid muscle combined with posterior ramisectomy from C1 to C6 (9,25,26). The difference between intradural and extradural denervation of a cervical spinal nerve is outlined in Fig. 30.4. In contrast to anterior rhizotomy, there is no need for laminectomy and opening of the dura in posterior ramisectomy. At the C1 and C2 levels, either extradural rhizotomies or posterior ramisectomies may be performed. Beneficial results with this technique have been reported in 70%

to 90% of patients in surgical series, with few persistent side effects (9,25,26,68,69). Conversely, in a recent retrospective study that investigated the long-term outcome after selective extradural denervation at a mean of 5 years, benefit was more limited (40). In approximately one-third of patients, long-term improvement with a reduction in dystonia by about 30% was present. In most studies, head tremor improved in some patients but increased in other instances postoperatively. The techniques and outcome of selective peripheral denervation are reviewed in Chapter 31.

Chronic Spinal Cord Stimulation

Chronic epidural dorsal column stimulation of the cervical spine has been largely abandoned. With this technique, quadripolar electrodes were placed longitudinally in the epidural space at C4-2. The hypothetic concept for the mechanism of this procedure was based on a modified concept of the "gate theory" suggesting that altered sensory input could modify motor functioning. Stimulation frequencies that were used often were in the range of 500 to 700 Hz.

Beneficial responses were described in several series (32,33). Waltz reported moderate to marked improvement of CD in 69 of 90 patients (76%) (32). Conversely, Fahn reported almost complete lack of benefit on follow-up in a series of 25 patients (34). Four patients had transient mild benefit, and only one patient benefited from long-lasting improvement. In a subsequent double-blind study, Goetz and colleagues found no objective improvement of CD in a series of ten patients (35).

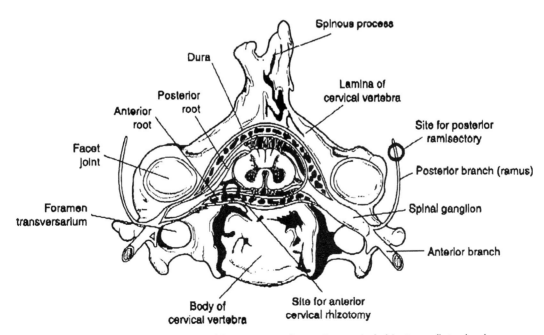

FIGURE 30.4. Schematic topographic anatomy of anterior cervical rhizotomy (intradural approach) and posterior ramisectomy (extradural approach).

Functional Stereotactic Thalamic and Pallidal Surgery

Along with the resurgence of basal ganglia surgery for Parkinson's disease has been considerable renewed interest in *functional stereotactic surgery* for treatment of dystonia. Patients who present with both CD and segmental dystonia or hemidystonia may benefit most from thalamic or pallidal surgery (70,71). Recently, the benefits of *bilateral pallidal deep brain stimulation* for treatment of complex types of CD were demonstrated (72). The history and current perspectives of basal ganglia surgery in the therapy of CD are discussed in Chapter 32.

Combined Approaches

Surgical treatment combining several approaches has been common in the treatment of CD. It has often been difficult to appreciate the contribution of certain procedures to the overall clinical improvement.

We have evaluated the symptomatic and functional outcome in a retrospective series of 46 consecutive patients with independent assessment using the TWSTRS rating scale (39). In this group, 70 procedures were performed, including intradural denervation in 33 instances, extradural denervation in 21 instances, and muscle sections in 22 instances. Global outcome at long-term follow-up at a mean of 6.5 years postoperatively was rated as excellent in 21% of patients, as marked in 27%, as moderate in 21%, as mild in another 21%, and as nil in 11%. Almost all mean TWSTRS subscores for severity of CD, functional disability, and pain were significantly improved. Mild transient side effects were present in 10% of the patients and included swallowing difficulties, severe neck pain or headaches, psychotic decompensation, and cellulitis at the site of the skin incision. A persistent side effect, however, occurred only in one patient after an intradural procedure, as described earlier. There were no significant differences in the distribution of outcome scores between patients with idiopathic and secondary dystonia, nor were significant differences reported between patients who primarily did not respond to botulinum toxin injections and those who had developed secondary immunoresistance. There was a significant difference, however, with regard to the number of procedures performed. Patients with an excellent outcome underwent a higher number of surgical procedures on average than those patients who achieved no benefit.

CONCLUSIONS

Various surgical alternatives for treatment of CD are available. At this time, we recommend selective targeting of dystonic activity that may involve staged procedures and combination of different techniques. Peripheral denervation and posterior ramisectomies are clearly less invasive than intradural procedures and appear to have similar if not better postoperative benefit at much lower complication rates. Myotomies and myectomies are useful adjuncts to other surgical procedures. Patients with complex cases and those with more widespread dystonia may be candidates for functional stereotactic basal ganglia surgery. The indications and results of intrathecal baclofen for treatment of CD with severe generalized dystonia, which can be useful in particular in those patients who also suffer from spasticity, are reviewed in Chapter 29. With the increasing number of patients with CD who are expected to undergo surgical treatment in the future, carefully conducted prospective studies with adequate assessment of postoperative outcome are urgently needed.

REFERENCES

1. Jankovic J, Fahn S. Dystonic disorders. In: Jankovic J, Tolosa E, eds. *Parkinson's disease and movement disorders,* 3rd ed. Baltimore: Williams & Wilkins, 1998:513–551.
2. Jankovic J, Leder S, Warner D, et al. Cervical dystonia: clinical findings and associated movement disorders. *Neurology* 1991;41:1088–1091.
3. Tasker RR. Overview of the surgical treatment of spasmodic torticollis. In: Gildenberg PL, Tasker RR. *Textbook of stereotactic and functional neurosurgery.* New York: McGraw-Hill, 1998:1053–1058.
4. Brin MF, Jankovic J, Comella C, et al. Treatment of dystonia using botulinum toxin. In: Kurlan R, ed. *Treatment of movement disorders.* Philadelphia: JB Lippincott, 1995:183–246.
5. Comella CL, Buchman AS, Tanner CM, et al. Botulinum toxin injection for spasmodic torticollis: increased magnitude of benefit with electromyographic assistance. *Neurology* 1992;42:878–882.
6. Jankovic J, Schwartz K. Botulinum toxin injections for cervical dystonia. *Neurology* 1990;40:277–280.
7. Dauer WT, Burke RE, Greene P, et al. Current concepts on the clinical features, aetiology and management of idiopathic cervical dystonia. *Brain* 1998;121:547–560.
8. Greene P. Medical and surgical therapy of idiopathic torsion dystonia. In: Kurlan R, ed. *Treatment of movement disorders.* Philadelphia: JB Lippincott, 1995:153–181.
9. Odegren T, Hjalatason H, Kaakkola S, et al. A double blind, randomised, parallel group study to investigate the dose equivalence of Dysport and Botox in the treatment of cervical dystonia. *J Neurol Neurosurg Psychiatry* 1998:64:6–12.
10. Brin MF, Lew MF, Adler CH, et al. Safety and efficacy of Neurobloc™ (botulinum toxin type B) in type A–resistant cervical dystonia patients. *Neurology* 1999;53:1431–1438.
11. Hanna PA, Jankovic J. Mouse bioassay versus Western blot assay for botulinum toxin antibodies: correlation with clinical response. *Neurology* 1998:50:1624–1629.
12. Bertrand CM, Lenz FA. Surgical treatment of dystonias. In: Tsui JKC, Calne DB, eds. *Handbook of dystonia.* New York: Marcel Dekker, 1995:329–345.
13. Jankovic J. Re-emergence of surgery for dystonia. *J Neurol Neurosurg Psychiatry* 1998;65:434.
14. Lang AE. Surgical treatment of dystonia. *Adv Neurol* 1998; 78: 185–198.
15. Iskandar BJ, Nashold BS Jr. History of functional neurosurgery. *Neurosurg Clin North Am* 1995;6:1–25.

16. Putnam TJ, Herz E, Glaser GH. Spasmodic torticollis. *Arch Neurol Psychiatry* 1949;61:240–247.

17. Finney JMT, Hughson W. Spasmodic torticollis. *Ann Surg* 1925; 81:255– 269.

18. Keen WW. A new operation for spasmodic wry neck namely, division or exsection of the nerves supplying the posterior rotator muscles of the head. *Ann Surg* 1891;13:44–47.

19. Foerster O. On the indications and results of the excision of posterior spinal nerve roots in men. *Surg Gynecol Obstet* 1913;16:463–474.

20. McKenzie KG. Intermeningeal division of the spinal accessory and roots of the upper cervical nerves for the treatment of spasmodic torticollis. *Surg Gynecol Obstet* 1924;39:5–10.

21. Dandy WE. An operation for the treatment of spasmodic torticollis. *Arch Surg* 1930;20:1021–1032.

22. Hamby WB, Schiffer S. Spasmodic torticollis: results after cervical rhizotomy in 80 cases. *Clin Neurosurg* 1970;17:28–37.

23. Hamby WB, Schiffer S. Spasmodic torticollis: results after surgical rhizotomy in 50 cases. *J Neurosurg* 1969;31:323–326.

24. Friedman AH, Nashold BS Jr, Sharp R, et al. Treatment of spasmodic torticollis with intradural selective rhizotomies. *J Neurosurg* 1993;78:46–53.

25. Bertrand CM. Selective peripheral denervation for spasmodic torticollis: surgical technique, results, and observations in 260 cases. *Surg Neurol* 1993;40:96–103.

26. Bertrand CM. Surgical management of spasmodic torticollis and adult-onset dystonia. In: Schmidek HH, Sweet WH, eds. *Operative neurosurgical techniques,* 3rd ed. Philadelphia: WB Saunders, 1995:1649–1659.

27. Mazars G, Merienne L, Chodkiewicz JP. La chirurgie des dyskinesies d'orientation cephalique. *Neurochirurgie* 1968;14:745–752.

28. Meares R. Natural history of spasmodic torticollis, and effect of surgery. *Lancet* 1971;2:149–150

29. Cooper IS. Effects of thalamic lesions upon torticollis. *N Engl J Med* 1964;270:967–972.

30. Krauss JK, Pohle T. Historical review of functional stereotactic neurosurgery for treatment of cervical dystonia. *Mov Disord* 1998;13[Suppl 2]:134(abst).

31. Svien HJ, Cody DT. Treatment of spasmodic torticollis by suppression of labyrinthine activity: report of a case. *Mayo Clin Proc* 1969;44:825–827.

32. Waltz JM. Chronic stimulation for motor disorders. In: Gildenberg PL, Tasker RR. *Textbook of stereotactic and functional neurosurgery.* New York: McGraw-Hill, 1998:1087–1099.

33. Gildenberg PL. Treatment of spasmodic torticollis by dorsal column stimulation. *Appl Neurophysiol* 1978;41:113–121.

34. Fahn S. Lack of benefit from cervical cord stimulation for dystonia. *N Engl J Med* 1985;313:1229.

35. Goetz CG, Penn RD, Tanner CM. Efficacy of cervical cord stimulation in dystonia. *Adv Neurol* 1988;50:645–649.

36. Freckmann N, Hagenah R, Herrmann HD, et al. Treatment of neurogenic torticollis by microvascular lysis of the accessory nerve roots: indication, techniques and first results. *Acta Neurochir (Wien)* 1981;59:167–175.

37. Lindeboom R, De Haan RJ, Aramideh M, et al. Treatment outcomes in cervical dystonia: a clinimetric study. *Mov Disord* 1996;11:371–376.

38. Consky ES, Lang AE. Clinical assessments of patients with cervical dystonia. In: Jankovic J, Hallett M, eds. *Therapy with botulinum toxin.* New York: Marcel Dekker, 1994:211-237.

39. Krauss JK, Toups EG, Jankovic J, et al. Symptomatic and functional outcome of surgical treatment of cervical dystonia. *J Neurol Neurosurg Psychiatry* 1997;63:642–648.

40. Ford B, Louis ED, Greene P, et al. Outcome of selective ramisectomy for botulinum toxin resistant torticollis. *J Neurol Neurosurg Psychiatry* 1998;65:472–478.

41. Krauss JK, Grossman RG. Surgery for hyperkinetic movement disorders. In: Jankovic J, Tolosa E, eds. *Parkinson's disease and movement disorders,* 3rd ed. Baltimore: Williams & Wilkins, 1998: 1017–1047.

42. Russo LS Jr, Arce C. Simultaneous four-channel electromyography as an adjunct to selective denervation in the treatment of spasmodic torticollis. *Ann Neurol* 1990;28:266(abst).

43. Krauss JK, Koller R, Burgunder JM. Partial myotomy/myectomy of the trapezius muscle with an asleep-awake-asleep anesthetic technique for treatment of cervical dystonia. *J Neurosurg* 1999;91:889–891.

44. Krauss JK, Seeger W, Jankovic J. Cervical dystonia associated with tumors of the posterior fossa. *Mov Disord* 1997;12:443–447.

45. Pohle T, Krauss JK, Burgunder JM. Petroclival meningioma as a cause of ipsilateral cervicofacial dyskinesias. *J Neurol Neurosurg Psychiatry* 2000;68:113–114.

46. Chen X. Selective resection and denervation of cervical muscles in the treatment of spasmodic torticollis: results in 60 cases. *Neurosurgery* 1981;8:680-688.

47. Chen XK, Ji SX, Zhu H, et al. Operative treatment of bilateral retrocollis. *Acta Neurochir (Wien)* 1991:113:180–183.

48. Hernesniemi J, Keränen T. Long-term outcome after surgery for spasmodic torticollis. *Acta Neurochir (Wien)* 1990;103:128–130.

49. Colbassani HJ Jr, Wood JH. Management of spasmodic torticollis. *Surg Neurol* 1986;25:153–158.

50. Arseni C, Maretsis M. The surgical treatment of spasmodic torticollis. *Neurochirurgia* 1971;14:177–180.

51. Fabinyi G, Dutton J. The surgical treatment of spasmodic torticollis. *Aust NZ J Surg* 1980;50:155–157.

52. Gauthier S, Perot P, Bertrand G. Role of surgical anterior rhizotomies in the management of spasmodic torticollis. *Adv Neurol* 1988;50:633–635.

53. Speelman JD, van Manen J, Jacz K, et al. The Foerster-Dandy operation for the treatment of spasmodic torticollis. *Acta Neurochir Suppl (Wien)* 1987;39:85–87.

54. Grossman RG, Hamilton WJ. Surgery for movement disorders. In: Jankovic J, Tolosa E, eds. *Parkinson's disease and movement disorders,* 2nd ed. Baltimore: Williams & Wilkins, 1993:531–548.

55. Horner J, Riski JE, Ovelmen-Levitt J, et al. Swallowing in torticollis before and after rhizotomy. *Dysphagia* 1992;7:117–125.

56. Scoville WB. Motor tics of the head and neck: surgical approaches and their complications. *Acta Neurochir (Wien)* 1978;45:338.

57. Sweet WH. What should the neurosurgeon do when faced with a malpractice suit? *Clin Neurosurg* 1975;23:112–124.

58. Jho HD, Jannetta PJ. Microvascular decompression for spasmodic torticollis. *Acta Neurochir* 1995;134:21–26.

59. Shima F, Fukui M, Kitamura K, et al. Diagnosis and surgical treatment of spasmodic torticollis of 11th nerve origin. *Neurosurgery* 1988;22:358–363.

60. Nielsen VK. Electrophysiology of the facial nerve in hemifacial spasm: ectopic/ephaptic excitation. *Muscle Nerve* 1985;187:161–164.

61. Wilkins RH. Hemifacial spasm: a review. *Surg Neurol* 1991; 36:251–277.

62. Lang J. Ueber Bau, Länge und Gefässbeziehungen der "zentralen" und "peripheren" Strecken der intrazisternalen Hirnnerven. *Zentralbl Neurochir* 1982;43:217–255.

63. Skinner HA. Some histologic features of the cranial nerves. *Arch Neurol Psychiatry* 1931;25:356–372.

64. Shima F, Fukui M, Matsubara T, et al. Spasmodic torticollis caused by vascular compression of the spinal accessory root. *Surg Neurol* 1986;26:431–434.

65. Pagni CA, Naddeo M, Faccani G. Spasmodic torticollis due

to neurovascular compression of the 11th nerve. *J Neurosurg* 1985;63:789–791.

66. Aksik I. Microneural decompression operations in the treatment of some forms of cranial rhizopathy. *Acta Neurochir (Wien)* 1993;125:64–74.

67. Freckmann N, Hagenah R, Herrmann HD, et al. Bilateral microsurgical lysis of the spinal accessory nerve roots for treatment of spasmodic torticollis. *Acta Neurochir (Wien)* 1986;83:47–53.

68. Braun V, Richter HP. Selective peripheral denervation for the treatment of spasmodic torticollis. *Neurosurgery* 1994;35:58–63.

69. Davis DH, Ahlskog JE, Litchy WJ, et al. Selective peripheral denervation for torticollis: preliminary results. *Mayo Clin Proc* 1991;66:365–371.

70. Krauss JK, Mohadjer M, Braus DF, et al. Dystonia following head trauma: a report of nine patients and review of the literature. *Mov Disord* 1992;7:263–372.

71. Ondo WG, Desaloms JM, Jankovic J, et al. Pallidotomy for generalized dystonia. *Mov Disord* 1998;13:693–698.

72. Krauss JK, Pohle T, Weber S, et al. Bilateral deep brain stimulation of the globus pallidus internus for treatment of cervical dystonia. *Lancet* 1999:354:837–838.

Surgery for Parkinson's Disease and Movement Disorders,
edited by J.K. Krauss, J. Jankovic, and R.G. Grossman.
Lippincott Williams & Wilkins, Philadelphia © 2001.

31

SELECTIVE PERIPHERAL DENERVATION AND POSTERIOR RAMISECTOMY IN CERVICAL DYSTONIA

VEIT BRAUN
HANS-PETER RICHTER

No therapy is currently available for treatment of the cause of *cervical dystonia* (CD). Conservative methods including various medications, psychotherapy (1), and physical therapy are highly unsuccessful. Therefore, botulinum toxin injections are widely accepted as the best therapeutical option. This symptomatic treatment unifies low risk and promising results. Unfortunately, a few patients do not profit from such injections. Most of them respond well primarily, but they develop antibodies to the toxin as a result of repeated applications. These patients are therefore called *secondary nonresponders*. For unknown reasons, a smaller group of CD patients—the so-called *primary nonresponders*—will not profit from botulinum toxin. For both groups, more invasive treatment has to be considered.

SELECTIVE PERIPHERAL DENERVATION: OVERVIEW

Neurosurgical procedures used for treatment of CD include anterior upper cervical rhizotomy, myotomies, microvascular decompression, and functional stereotactic basal ganglia surgery (2–6). In 1891, Keen inaugurated a peripheral neurosurgical procedure for CD (7). This method was refined by Bertrand et al. (8), which they called *selective peripheral denervation*. It is highly successful and without major risks (9,10). We started performing this operation in 1988 and subsequently modified Bertrand's technique (11,12). The following chapter presents not only our own experience but also published results with this neurosurgical method and discusses its value for patients suffering from CD.

PERSONAL EXPERIENCE
Patients and Methods

From June 1988 to February 1999, 133 patients with CD (65 men, 68 women) were operated on in our department. Twenty were operated on two different occasions because of recurrence of symptoms. In 15 patients, we targeted the same muscles as in the first procedure. In five patients, other muscles had to be denervated during the second procedure because the dystonia had progressed. Finally, five patients were surgically treated by selective peripheral denervation in other hospitals and were operated on once more in our department. Surgical treatment was performed an average of 8.3 years after the onset of symptoms (range, 0.5 to 30 years). The mean age of the patients at onset of dystonia was 39.6 years (range, 17 to 66 years). A patient was considered to be a candidate for surgery when symptoms had been present for at least 1 year (13) and conservative methods had failed. Since 1990, we have operated exclusively on patients who have undergone botulinum toxin therapy. Meanwhile, we have treated 96 patients who are botulinum toxin nonresponders, 36 primary and 60 secondary nonresponders. A computed tomographic or magnetic resonance imaging scan of the brain is routinely performed to rule out the presence of a space-occupying mass.

The involved muscles are identified by clinical examination and a multichannel electromyographic recording (9–11). A simultaneous record from both sternocleidomastoid and capitis muscles is mandatory and, if necessary, from both trapezius muscles as well. The dystonia is documented on videotape. Most of our patients have had combined involvement of ipsilateral or contralateral splenius capitis and sternocleidomastoid muscles. The involvement of only the sternocleidomastoid muscle is an exception. In October 1996, we started to assess our patients' symptoms and functional disability additionally with the *Toronto Western Spasmodic Torticollis Rating Scale (TWSTRS)*.

V. Braun and H-P. Richter: Department of Neurosurgery, University of Ulm, 89312 Günzburg, Germany.

Surgical Technique

All patients are operated on while they are under general anesthesia and in a half-sitting position with their head fixed in a Mayfield clamp, with a right atrial catheter, precordial or transesophageal Doppler ultrasound examination, and the recording of end-expiratory partial carbon dioxide pressure. Muscle relaxants are not given because the different nerve branches have to be identified by monopolar stimulation. We have not seen an air embolism during this procedure. For the denervation of the sternocleidomastoid muscle, its motor point is first identified transcutaneously by a supramaximal electrical stimulation with 2 Hz. Using a 5-cm skin incision on the posterior margin of this muscle, we first identify the trapezius branch of the spinal accessory nerve in the lateral neck triangle. With the help of the surgical microscope, this structure is followed proximally, thus avoiding an injury of the greater auricular nerve, which crosses the operative field. On reaching the main trunk of the spinal accessory nerve, the branches to the sternocleidomastoid muscle are detected by electrical stimulation (Radionics RFG-3B and TEC Ganglion Gasseri electrode [Radionics Co., Burlington Ma.]) of 0.6 to 2 v with a 2-millisecond duration. Then these branches are sectioned and resected. Because the sternocleidomastoid muscle may also be innervated by branches of the spinal roots C-l and C-2 or by recurrent nerves branching from the trapezius branch of the spinal accessory nerve, the procedure is terminated only by resecting these branches as well.

With the exception of the trapezius muscle, the posterior neck muscles receive their innervation from the posterior branches of C-l–T-l (14). Among these, those from C-l to C-6 are the most important contributions. For sufficient denervation, they all have to be resected. The selective peripheral denervation of the neck muscles can be done superselectively, with any muscle (e.g., splenius capitis, semispinalis capitis or cervicis, inferior oblique muscles) approached separately. Taking into account that injection of botulinum toxin into the splenius capitis muscle may also weaken the deeper ipsilateral muscles (by passive diffusion of the toxin), we recommend not only denervation of the splenius capitis muscle, but also denervation of the deeper cervical muscles on the same side. As mentioned earlier, this is done by the complete resection of the posterior branches of C-1 to C-6. By sparing the trapezius muscle, the risk of no head instability is diminished, even if bilateral neck denervation is performed.

The posterior branches can be best identified extraspinally, lateral to the joint facets, thus leaving the anterior branches (innervating the muscles for shoulder and arm movement) intact. These branches are approached by a midline skin incision in the neck running from the external occipital protuberance down to the spinous process of C-6, to allow operation on both left and right sides (Fig. 31.1). As with cranial procedures, we do not routinely shave the patient's hair. After disinfection with a regular undyed isopropanol/dibrom/propyleneglycol solution, the wet hair is

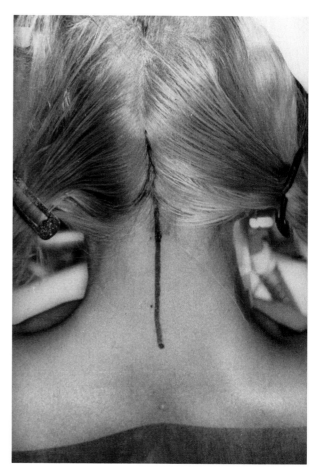

FIGURE 31.1. Skin incision from the occipital protuberance down to the spinous process of C-6 for denervation of the posterior neck muscles.

parted with a sterilized metal comb. The hair is then dried with sterilized towels and is fixed with drapes. Having reached the spinous processes of C2-6, we enter the plane of cleavage between the more superficially located semispinalis capitis and the more deeply located semispinalis cervicis and multifidus muscles on the involved side (Fig. 31.2). The inferior oblique capitis muscle is detached from its origin at the spinous process of C-2. We then proceed laterally to the articular facets and the multifidus muscle. In this area, the posterior branches are easily identified by monopolar stimulation. In addition, we routinely use the surgical microscope for identification, dissection, and resection of the nerve branches. The easiest nerve to locate is the greater occipital nerve arising from the posterior branch of C-2. It is found beneath the inferior oblique muscle, which is either mobilized cranially or is sectioned (Fig. 31.3).

The most difficult nerve to locate is the suboccipital nerve or posterior branch of C-1; however, it is regularly identified between the arch of the atlas and the vertebral artery (Fig. 31.4), 1.5 to 2 cm lateral to the midline. After dissection of the arch of the atlas, this nerve is found within the vertebral sulcus, regularly surrounded by the enormous suboccipital

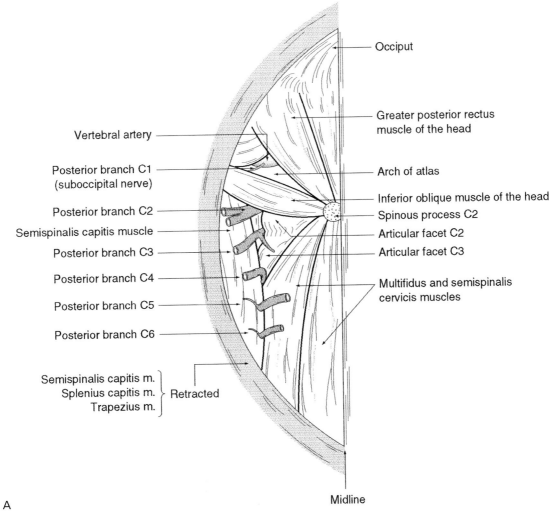

A

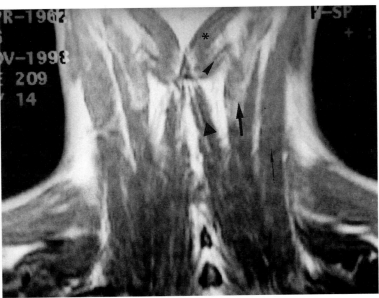

B

FIGURE 31.2. A: To reach the posterior branches of C1-6, the surgeon can use the natural plane of cleavage between the more superficial semispinalis capitis muscle and the deeper multifidus and semispinalis cervicis muscles. **B:** Horizontal magnetic resonance scan of the posterior neck muscles: *thin arrow,* splenius capitis m.; *thick arrow,* semispinalis capitis m.; *triangle,* semispinalis cervicis m.; *arrowhead,* inferior oblique capitis m.; *,* rectus capitis m.

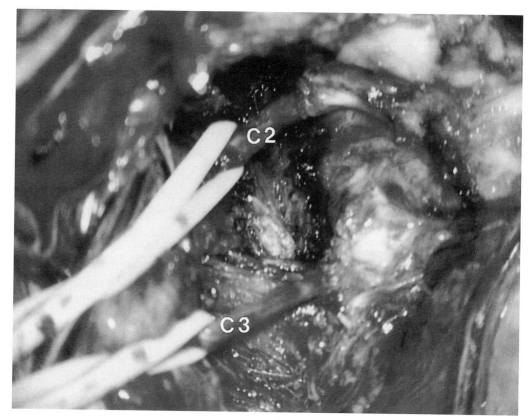

FIGURE 31.3. Posterior branch of C-2 and C-3 on the left. (See Color Figure 31.3.)

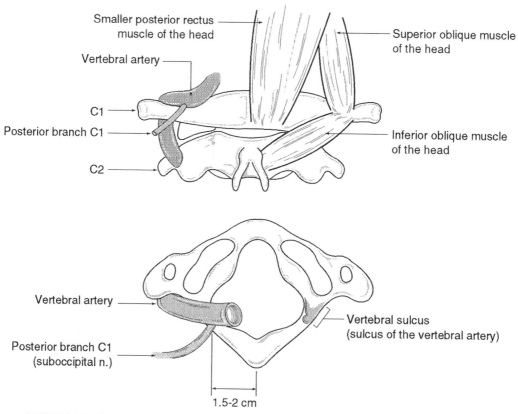

Smaller posterior rectus muscle of the head

Superior oblique muscle of the head

Vertebral artery

C1

Posterior branch C1

C2

Inferior oblique muscle of the head

Vertebral artery

Posterior branch C1 (suboccipital n.)

Vertebral sulcus (sulcus of the vertebral artery)

1.5-2 cm

FIGURE 31.4. The posterior branch most difficult to identify is the posterior branch of C-1, which lies between the vertebral artery and the arch of the atlas in the region of its vertebral sulcus about 1.5 to 2 cm from the midline. **A:** Posterior (surgeon's) view. **B:** View from above.

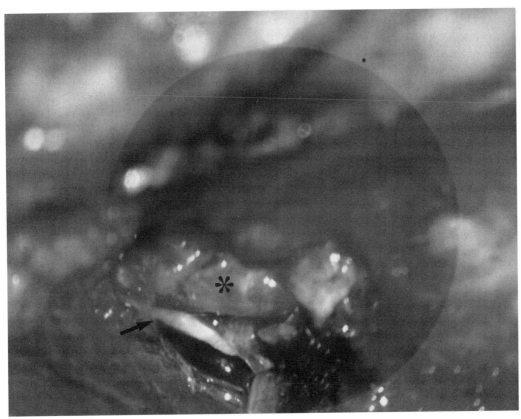

FIGURE 31.5. Intraoperative view of C-1 *(arrow)* on the left side, beneath the vertebral artery (*).
(See Color Figure 31.5.)

venous plexus. When the patient is in the prone position, this plexus tends to bleed heavily, thus making its identification nearly impossible. Because air embolism did not occur during our 153 procedures, we strongly recommend the half-sitting position. The suboccipital nerve emerges from below the vertebral artery, runs laterally to the neck muscles, and can easily be identified by monopolar stimulation (Fig. 31.5).

All the posterior branches of C2-6 are located in a perpendicular plane between the lateral margin of the semispinalis cervicis muscle and the medial margin of the semispinalis capitis muscle. Whereas the posterior branches of C2-4 are easily identified lateral to the facets, the very tiny branches of C-5 and C-6 can be found medially, on the surface of the semispinalis cervicis muscle (Fig. 31.6). All posterior branches of C1-6 that are identified are resected. Specimens are sent for histopathologic examination (15). We then stimulate the entire region lateral to the articular facets, to look for any further muscle contraction. Often, additional posterior branches can be found in the multifidus layer, and these are also resected. Bertrand (personal communication) sees some risk of the disappearance of the muscle response resulting from overdistraction when a vertical incision is used and therefore recommends a skin incision in the form of an inverted L, to detach the trapezius muscle from the occiput. We have not seen this problem, even with mild electrical

stimuli. Furthermore, our modification has the advantage of reduced oozing from the muscles, thus minimizing the risk of missing any tiny branch because of impaired visibility. The denervation is considered complete only when no further muscle contraction can be evoked. All proximal and distal nerve stumps are extensively coagulated. Contrary to Bertrand, we do not use hemostatic clips to prevent nerve regeneration. Postoperatively, almost all patients are sent to another institution for physical therapy (15). Usually, patients continue physical therapy for at least 1 year postoperatively.

Results

To evaluate the results of selective peripheral denervation, we have relied primarily on estimates provided by the patients themselves. Patients have also specified whether they would choose the selective peripheral denervation again as treatment for their dystonia. As mentioned earlier, we have also tried to establish an objective method using TWSTRS. To date, we have evaluated 49 patients preoperatively and 12 patients postoperatively with this scale. Our preliminary results with TWSTRS do not differ substantially from results of the self-assessment score. On the contrary, two patients who regarded the operation as a failure improved

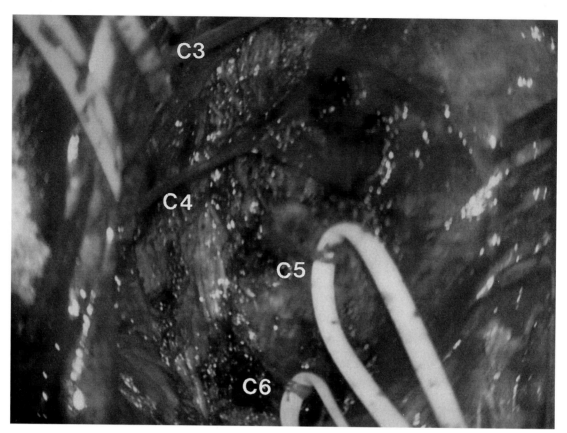

FIGURE 31.6. Posterior branches of C3-6 on the left side. (See Color Figure 31.6.)

significantly from 63 to 37 points and from 55 to 29 points, respectively.

To date, results from 112 patients are available, with the mean follow-up period ranging from 3 to 96 months (average, 22.5 months). Of these patients, 14% (16 patients) noticed complete relief of their symptoms, 33% (37 patients) had significant improvement, and 24% (27 patients) had moderate improvement of their dystonia. Conversely, 12% (13 patients) reported only minor improvement, and 17% (19 patients) had no improvement from the operation. In summary, 71% regarded the operation as successful and would choose it again as treatment for their

TABLE 31.1. OPERATIVE RESULTS OF PRIMARY AND SECONDARY NONRESPONDERS TO BOTULINUM TOXIN

Result	Primary Nonresponder	Secondary Nonresponder
Complete relief	4	9
Significant improvement	8	16
Moderate improvement	2	15
Minor improvement	6	1
No improvement	8	7
No long-term result available yet	8	12

CD. Twenty-nine percent of our patients did not benefit from the procedure.

Our results differed remarkably with regard to the prior response to botulinum toxin injections. As mentioned earlier, 96 of our surgically treated patients had botulinum toxin injections before they underwent surgical treatment. Sixty of these patients (63%) had a good initial response. They subsequently developed antibodies (secondary nonresponders) proven either by laboratory examinations or by test injections into the small muscles of the thumb or foot. Thirty-six of these 96 patients, conversely, had not benefited from botulinum toxin injections and were considered primary nonresponders. Table 31.1 shows the detailed results within these two subgroups. Overall, 83% of the secondary nonresponders were satisfied with the surgical result, whereas only 50% of the primary nonresponders found the operation helpful. Results differed even more markedly in patients with more widespread dystonia also involving the extremities and the trunk. None of these seven patients had improvements in dystonic symptoms.

Complications

Since 1990, we have not seen any major complications after selective peripheral denervation. None of our patients complained of head or neck instability. Because the procedure does not touch the brain or spinal cord, no paresis of the limbs or mental disturbance is anticipated. Injury to the vertebral artery during dissection of the dorsal branch C-1 (suboccipital nerve) is theoretically possible, but it did not occur in our patients. Although we routinely refrained from shaving the patient's hair, no wound infection occurred. The following untoward sequelae were found. All patients had a variable sensory deficit in the area of the greater occipital nerve. This could not be avoided because this nerve arises from the posterior branch of C-2, which has to be severed; we regularly observed muscular contractions when we stimulated the greater occipital nerve after resection of the anterior part of the posterior branch C-2.

Three patients complained of occipital neuralgia after the greater occipital nerve (dorsal branch of C-2) was severed. All three patients spontaneously recovered within 3 months. Six patients complained of a temporary hypesthesia in the region of the greater auricular nerve, probably from a stretch injury of this nerve.

During our first 19 procedures, we inadvertently sectioned the trapezius branch of the spinal accessory nerve in two patients. In both cases, this nerve was very superficial and had already been injured during skin incision. It was sutured immediately, and both patients fully recovered. Subsequently, we modified our technique using the surgical microscope right from the beginning, and we have not seen this complication since then. In two other patients, the development of excessive postoperative scar tissue led to compression of the trapezius branch of the spinal accessory nerve and subsequently to paresis of the trapezius muscle. In one patient, neurolysis had to be performed. With continuous physical therapy, only mild residual weakness (4 of 5 paresis score) remained in both patients. In three patients, a postoperative hemorrhage in the area of the sternocleidomastoid muscle had to be managed. Finally, four patients reported prolonged (up to 3 months) dysphagia. Its cause remained unclear. In two other patients, the tremor component of the dystonia was intensified postoperatively.

Histopathologic Findings

The resected nerves were examined histologically (15). Many different pathologic changes were found (17). Frequently, signs of chronic, sometimes severe, compression neuropathy were evident. Furthermore, Renaut's bodies, endoneural edema, and atrophy or a significant reduction of myelin sheath of the nerve fibers were noted. Not all the resected nerves were equally involved. Normal posterior branches next to severely altered nerves were seen in the same patient. Some nerve branches showed signs of spontaneous regeneration. These histologic findings are even more surprising in patients who had to be operated on twice. In at least three patients, spontaneous functional motor nerve regeneration after surgical resection of the posterior branches was shown, and in nine other patients functional recovery occurred in the presence of nerve fibers, which obviously were overlooked during the first procedure.

DISCUSSION

Nowadays, the symptomatic treatment of choice for CD is the selective weakening of the involved muscles. Although botulinum toxin blocks the neuromuscular transmission, selective peripheral denervation reaches this goal by severing the nerve supply close to the effectors. At present, botulinum toxin injections are regarded as the treatment of first choice. Selective peripheral denervation is indicated mainly in patients who have not responded to prior botulinum toxin therapy, either primary or secondary nonresponders.

Although both methods aim to paralyze the involved muscles, botulinum toxin injections are less specific than the operation. The toxin is injected at one or two sites within the muscle and spreads by diffusion. Therefore, adjacent muscles may be paralyzed as well, sometimes causing dysphagia. In contrast, the operation focuses only on those muscles receiving their innervation from the resected nerves. To date, it is not clear what mechanism is responsible for the primary failure of botulinum toxin observed in a small group of patients. Preexisting immunoresistance is a probable explanation. In our opinion, multiple muscle involvement can sometimes be responsible in primary nonresponders. This assumption is supported by the observation that a few patients noticed some effect of botulinum toxin on their dystonia only when simultaneous untoward side effects such as head instability were obvious. In such cases, only widespread denervation would lead to significant improvement of the dystonia, with the possible consequence of permanent instability of the head. Nevertheless, 50% of our primary nonresponders were satisfied with the result of the operation, although no complete relief could be seen in this group. To date, we do not know why some patients respond to surgery but not to botulinum toxin injections. Preexisting antibodies may be an explanation. Previous inapparent infection with *Clostridium botulinum* seems to be very unlikely. With regard to these considerations, we think that surgical treatment is also indicated in primary nonresponders who wish to be operated on despite their lower chances of postoperative improvement.

The situation is different for patients with complex generalized dystonia. Although selective peripheral denervation may improve the CD, patients usually do not benefit from the procedure, because CD represents only one facet in the overall syndrome. We have therefore stopped operating on this group of patients.

Secondary nonresponders to botulinum injections are the most likely to benefit from surgical treatment. The explanation for the good outcome in primary responders in general could be that muscles that had been denervated by botulinum toxin injections (sternocleidomastoid and splenius capitis muscles) are suitable targets for selective peripheral denervation as well. Within this group of patients, only those with major involvement of the trapezius or levator scapulae muscles failed to achieve benefit. At this time, we recommend selective peripheral denervation only after prior botulinum toxin injections. The injections provide the surgeon with additional information about which muscles should be denervated.

Because of the good results and the low rate of untoward side effects, selective peripheral denervation is a very useful tool in the surgical treatment of CD. We modified the technique of Bertrand et al. (8) in some aspects: the skin incision in the neck is a straight vertical one; the natural planes of cleavage between the neck muscles are used in our approach to the posterior branches; we reduce oozing from the muscles and therefore have better visibility. By the additional use of the surgical microscope, the risk of overlooking small rootlets is decreased.

To date, few centers have reported their experience with selective peripheral denervation (10,17,18). In Bertrand's series, 88% of patients showed excellent or good results. The data from other surgeons are promising as well. So far, no fatality has been reported. Both therapeutic options (botulinum toxin and selective peripheral denervation) brought considerable progress in the treatment of spasmodic torticollis in the 1990s. It is hoped that the search for the origin of the dystonia will keep pace, and a more causally based treatment will be established one day.

REFERENCES

1. Mitscherlich M. Die Psychosomatik des Torticollis spasticus: Ergebnisse einer psychoanalytischen Untersuchung an 95 Patienten. *Fortschr Myol* 1980;6:210–212.
2. Mundinger F, Riechert T, Disselhoff J. Long-term results of stereotaxic treatment of spasmodic torticollis. *Confin Neurol* 1972; 34:4146.
3. Freckmann N, Hagenah R, Hermann HD, et al. Bilateral microsurgical lysis of the spinal accessory nerve roots for treatment of spasmodic torticollis. *Acta Neurochir (Wien)* 1986;83:47–53.
4. Jho HD, Jannetta PJ. Microvascular decompression for spasmodic torticollis. *Acta Neurochir (Wien)* 1995;134:21–26.
5. Hassler R, Dieckmann G. Die stereotaktische Behandlung des Torticollis aufgrund tierexperimenteller Erfahrungen über die richtungsbestimmenden Bewegungen. *Nervenarzt* 1970;41:473–487.
6. Hamby WB, Schiffer A. Spasmodic torticollis: results after cervical rhizotomy in 80 cases. *Clin Neurosurg* 1970;17:29–37.
7. Keen WW. A new operation for spasmodic wry neck: namely, division or exsection of the nerves supplying the posterior rotator muscles of the head. *Ann Surg* 1891;13:44–47.
8. Bertrand C, Molina-Negro P, Martinez SN. Technical aspects of selective peripheral denervation for spasmodic torticollis. *Appl Neurophysiol* 1982;45:326–330.
9. Bertrand C, Molina-Negro P, Bouvier G, et al. Observations and analysis of results in 131 cases of spasmodic torticollis after selective peripheral denervation. *Appl Neurophysiol* 1987;50:319–323.
10. Bertrand CM. Selective peripheral denervation for spasmodic torticollis: surgical technique, results, and observations in 260 cases. *Surg Neurol* 1993;40:96–103.
11. Braun V, Richter HP. Selective peripheral denervation in patients with spasmodic torticolhs. *Stereotact Funct Neurosurg* 1991;57: 113–122.
12. Braun V, Richter HP. Selective peripheral denervation for the treatment of spasmodic torticollis. *Neurosurgery* 1994;35:58–63.
13. Friedman A, Fahn S. Spontaneous remissions in spasmodic torticollis. *Neurology* 1986;36:398–400.
14. Sorensen BF, Hamby WB. Spasmodic torticollis: results in 71 surgically treated patients. *Neurology* 1966;16:867–878.
15. Peterson E. Ergebnisse der Kombinationsbehandlung von Operation und Physiotherapie des Torticollis spasmodicus. In: Richter HP, Braun V, eds. *Schiefhals, Behandlungskonzepte des Torticollis spasmodicus.* Berlin: Springer, 1993:79–97.
16. Schröder JM, Huffmann B, Braun V, et al. Spasmodic torticollis: severe compression neuropathy in rami dorsales of cervical nerves C l-6. *Acta Neuropathol (Berl)* 1992;84:416–424.
17. Davis DH, Ahlskog JE, Litchy WJ, et al. Selective peripheral denervation for torticollis: preliminary results. *Mayo Clin Proc* 1991; 66:365–371.
18. Arce C, Russo J. Selective peripheral denervation: a surgical alternative in the treatment for spasmodic torticollis: review of 55 patients. *Mov Disord* 1982:1[Suppl]:178.

Surgery for Parkinson's Disease and Movement Disorders,
edited by J.K. Krauss, J. Jankovic, and R.G. Grossman.
Lippincott Williams & Wilkins, Philadelphia © 2001.

32

FUNCTIONAL STEREOTACTIC SURGERY FOR TREATMENT OF CERVICAL DYSTONIA

JOACHIM K. KRAUSS
THOMAS POHLE
ALEXANDER STIBAL
THOMAS LOHER
JEAN-MARC BURGUNDER

Contemporary surgical treatment of *cervical dystonia* (CD) includes several procedures such as selective peripheral denervation, extradural posterior ramisectomy, intradural anterior rhizotomy, and myotomy (1–6). These treatment options, which are reviewed elsewhere in this volume, are appropriate in most patients who are considered surgical candidates. Functional stereotactic surgery for treatment of CD was performed in several centers in the past (7). With the refinement of peripheral surgical techniques and the widespread use of botulinum toxin injections, however, this treatment modality was largely abandoned. The experience with pallidal surgery for dyskinesias and dystonia in patients with Parkinson's disease, the beneficial effect in dystonic movement disorders, and review of the history of functional stereotactic surgery for CD prompted us to reevaluate the potentials of pallidal surgery for treatment of CD. We recently reported on our experience with chronic bilateral deep brain stimulation (DBS) of the internal segment of the globus pallidus (GPi) in selected patients with complex CD (8). In this chapter, we summarize the historical experience with functional stereotactic surgery for treatment of CD, review the possible role of basal ganglia dysfunction in CD, and discuss the preliminary contemporary clinical results and the indications for pallidal surgery in patients with CD.

HISTORICAL REVIEW

The effect of functional stereotactic surgery on CD was first reported in 1954 by Hassler and Riechert, who described their results on generalized dystonia and athetosis (9). Although there was marked improvement of the appendicular dyskinesias after pallidotomy, only a minor impact on CD was achieved in their first case. When the target was modified, however, phasic dystonic movements of the cervical muscles contralateral to the side of the surgical procedure were noted to be considerably reduced in a patient with generalized dystonia who presented with prominent CD. Two years later, the first patient with isolated CD underwent thalamotomy with targets in the ventrooral thalamic nuclei (10–12). Over the next 3 decades, functional stereotactic operations targeting various structures were performed worldwide by several neurosurgeons (13–32). In contrast to the experience with Parkinson's disease, however, functional stereotactic surgery for treatment of CD was not appreciated by a wider community.

Historical Nomenclature of Cervical Dystonia

The term *torticollis spasmodicus* was suggested by Hassler, and it soon replaced the earlier term *torticollis spasticus.* To characterize the movement disorder further, designations such as *torticollis dystonicus, torticollis rigidus,* and *torticollis crampiformis* were used.

The deviation of the head with regard to the axis of the body was categorized by different terminologic systems. The system that gained most widespread acceptance was based on the classification by Hassler (11,12). *Horizontal*

J.K. Krauss: Department of Neurosurgery, University Hospital, Klinikum Mannheim, Mannheim 68167, Germany.

T. Pohle and A. Stibal: Department of Neurosurgery, Inselspital, University of Bern, Switzerland.

T. Loher and J-M. Burgunder: Department of Neurology, Inselspital, University of Bern, Switzerland.

torticollis was defined as "a turning movement in the horizontal plane exclusively to one side with impairment of an active turning to the other side"; *rotatory torticollis* was defined as "a tilting or rotating movement around the anteroposterior axis so that one ear approaches the ipsilateral shoulder with impairment of the active tilting to the other side"; and *retrocollis* and *anterocollis* were defined according to "extension or flexion movement along the horizontal axis." This nomenclature was not used consistently by other authors, and in particular the definition of rotation appeared to be a source of confusion.

Remarkably, the nomenclature we use nowadays differs from Hassler's concept. The *Toronto Western Spasmodic Torticollis Rating Scale (TWSTRS)* (33), for example, defines turning of the head as "rotation" and tilting of the head as "laterocollis" (Hassler's *rotatory torticollis*).

Historical Pathophysiologic Concepts and Choice of Surgical Targets

The historical pathophysiologic models were based primarily on pathoanatomic investigations of single cases and on the analysis of animal experiments. In 1953, Hassler reviewed the cinematographic data and the histologic serial cuts of Hess' famous experiments in cats (34). Based on the effects of stimulations and coagulations in various diencephalic and mesencephalic structures, Hassler proposed an elaborated model to explain the deviation of the head along different axes as described earlier (11,12).

Horizontal torticollis was thought to be related with dysfunction of the GPi. The interstitial nucleus of Cajal was considered to be involved in the development of *rotatory torticollis*. *Retrocollis* and *anterocollis* were regarded to be associated with dysfunction of the "nucleus praecommissuralis" and the "nucleus praestitialis."

The choice of the surgical target was based on hypothetic concepts that in general followed the trait of thoughts of Hassler, or the targets were chosen empirically by trial and error. The question whether bilateral or unilateral procedures should be performed was not unequivocally answered. Furthermore, there was controversy about which side of the brain should be selected for operation in a particular type of CD. Various targets were used by different surgeons including the GPi, different thalamic nuclei, the subthalamic region, and the upper brainstem (Table 32.1).

Results of Clinical Series

The analysis of the postoperative results of most historical series is limited with regard to several aspects. There are considerable differences and inconsistencies both in the patients' assessment and in the evaluation of follow-up. Lesioning techniques included radiofrequency coagulation, the injection of chemicals, and the use of cryogenic probes. Lesions were placed either contralateral or ipsilateral to the direction

TABLE 32.1. TARGETS USED IN HISTORICAL SERIES OF FUNCTIONAL STEREOTACTIC SURGERY FOR TREATMENT OF CERVICAL DYSTONIA

Globus pallidus (internal segment)
Nucleus ventralis oralis anterior (thalami)
Nucleus ventralis oralis posterior (thalami)
Nucleus ventralis oralis internus (thalami)
Centrum medianum (thalami)
Nucleus ventralis posteromedialis and posterolateralis (thalami)
Nucleus ventralis intermedius (thalami)
Pulvinar thalami
Zona incerta
Forel's fields H1 and H2
Nucleus ruber
Interstitial nucleus of Cajal

in which the head was rotated. Peripheral surgical procedures were performed in many patients in addition to functional stereotactic surgery. Between 1960 and the early 1980s, approximately 300 patients with CD were reported to have undergone functional stereotactic surgery (11–32). Overall, postoperative improvement was achieved in about 50% to 70% of patients in most studies. A delay in improvement varying between a few weeks and 2 years postoperatively was often described. Side effects were similar to those seen in patients with Parkinson's disease, with a similar incidence of postoperative dysphonia or dysarthria after bilateral lesioning. During the first decade, the oral part of the ventrolateral thalamus was lesioned most often. Less frequently, the GPi was targeted. Hassler and Dieckmann pioneered lesioning of different nuclei in individual patients according to their pathophysiologic concept by taking into account the specific phenomenology of CD (11,12). Frequently, these investigators used subthalamic targets such as the zona incerta and the fields of Forel H1 and H2. Early examples of DBS with thalamic targets for treatment of CD were reported by Mundinger and by Andy (31,32). Mundinger described the benefits of intermittent unilateral or bilateral DBS with chronically implanted electrodes in the oroventral thalamus and the subthalamic region in seven patients with CD (31). Intermittent stimulation over 30 to 40 minutes resulted in improvement of CD over 3 to 4 hours. Andy subsequently reported on chronic unilateral thalamic stimulation in two other patients (32).

The experience with thalamic radiofrequency lesioning for treatment of CD at the Department of Functional and Stereotactic Neurosurgery at the University of Freiburg, Germany, was summarized in a doctoral thesis that was accepted by the Medical Faculty of the Albert-Ludwigs-University in Freiburg in 1990 (35). The retrospective follow-up study concerned a total of 162 patients with CD who underwent thalamic radiofrequency lesioning between 1972 and 1986. Most procedures were performed by Mundinger. Because it appeared that little interest existed in functional stereotactic surgery for CD when the study was completed, the results were not submitted for publication. Data on long-term outcome of 111 patients were obtained by a questionnaire-based survey. Unilateral procedures were performed in 92 patients and bilateral procedures were done in 19 patients. It was appreciated that bilateral procedures had a greater potential for inducing postoperative improvement. However, with regard to the greater risks of adverse effects, unilateral procedures were preferred primarily, and several patients underwent staged procedures. Different nuclei or combinations of nuclei were chosen according to an algorithm similar to Hassler's concept. Targets included the zona incerta alone (27%) or in combination with the ventrooral nuclei (56%) in most instances. Other structures that were targeted were the pulvinar thalami and the nucleus interstitialis Cajal. Overall, CD improved in 63% of patients in the postoperative course. Only 27% of patients had immediate amelioration postoperatively, and improvement was delayed in the remainder. On long-term follow-up, 52% of patients had sustained improvement, which was described as excellent or good in 30%. No useful long-term benefit, however, was achieved in the other 48% of patients. Adverse side effects were noted in 68% of patients with bilateral procedures and in 40% with unilateral procedures. Although in most instances side effects were considered minor, the occurrence of dysarthria was noted in 15% of patients.

CONTEMPORARY BASAL GANGLIA SURGERY

Ablative Functional Stereotactic Surgery

Although functional stereotactic surgery for isolated CD was abandoned in the 1980s and 1990s, patients with more generalized dystonia still underwent surgical treatment. Thalamotomy has been considered a valuable treatment option for patients who present with hemidystonia or more generalized dystonia and CD. Thalamotomy targeting the thalamic ventralis oralis posterior nucleus and the zona incerta contralateral to the hemidystonia, for example, rendered excellent improvement of CD in a 14-year-old patient with posttraumatic dystonia secondary to severe craniocerebral trauma (36). The beneficial result was sustained over 14 years of follow-up. Because the pallidum was rediscovered as a target to treat dystonia, it has been used more and more often in patients with generalized dystonia (37–41). Marked amelioration of CD was achieved in a 56-year-old man with peripherally induced segmental posttraumatic dystonia after unilateral GPi pallidotomy (39). In several other contemporary studies, improvement of CD was reported along with amelioration of other dystonic symptoms after unilateral or bilateral pallidotomy. CD was not associated with other manifestations of dystonia and was the primary indication for pallidotomy in only one recent report (40). A 47-year-old woman with an 18-year history of CD was

reported "showing gradual improvement of 70% over 4 weeks" subsequent to "contralateral pallidotomy."

Rationales for Bilateral Basal Ganglia Surgery

The pathophysiology of CD still is poorly understood. It is generally thought nowadays that analogous to morphologic findings in patients with secondary dystonia, dysfunction of the basal ganglia or of the brainstem is responsible for the development of CD (42). This concept is also supported by the results of functional neuroimaging investigations. Positron emission tomography studies have shown that glucose metabolism is increased bilaterally in the lentiform nucleus in patients with CD as compared with control subjects (43). There was no correlation between the increase of glucose metabolism and the direction of abnormal head posture. With regard to these findings, investigators suggested that the direction of head turning in patients with CD resulted from individual differences in the susceptibility of neck muscles in the presence of bilateral cerebral disease. Dopaminergic dysfunction in the striatum was demonstrated in a single photon emission computed tomography study in patients with CD (44). Binding of iodine-123 (^{123}I)-epidepride, which is a high-affinity marker of D_2 receptors, was significantly reduced bilaterally in the striatum of patients with CD. Striatal ^{123}I–βCIT uptake, in contrast, did not differ from uptake in control subjects. These and other findings have been thought to indicate involvement of the indirect striatopallidothalamocortical motor circuit underlying the pathologic mechanisms of CD. In addition, transcranial magnetic stimulation studies have confirmed that the corticomotor projection to the sternocleidomastoid muscle involves both contralateral and ipsilateral pathways (45).

Bilateral Pallidal Deep Brain Stimulation

We usually offer peripheral surgical techniques to patients with disabling CD refractory to medical treatment and injections of botulinum toxin. Several patients with CD, however, are not suited ideally for peripheral techniques. Such patients include those with marked translation of the head in the sagittal or lateral axis in relation to the trunk, patients with prominent retrocollis or anterocollis, and patients with continuous phasic dystonic movements and dystonic head tremor. We thought that under such circumstances, functional stereotactic surgery targeting the basal ganglia would have certain advantages. With regard to the findings described earlier, we considered bilateral targeting of the GPi most appropriate. Pallidal surgery has become increasingly accepted as a treatment for dystonic movement disorders (5,37,46). Pallidal DBS has the advantage of being principally reversible and allowing stepwise adjustment of parameters. Thus, it can be performed bilaterally in one session without the inherent risks of bilateral lesioning.

TABLE 32.2. PATTERN OF CERVICAL DYSTONIA AND SUBSCORES OF THE MODIFIED TWSTRS SCALE BEFORE BILATERAL CHRONIC GLOBUS PALLIDUS INTERNAL SEGMENT STIMULATION, AT 3 MONTHS POSTOPERATIVELY AND AT RECENT FOLLOW-UP IN THREE PATIENTS WITH SEVERE CERVICAL DYSTONIA

Patient	Pattern of Cervical Dystonia	TWSTRS Total Severity Score				TWSTRS Total PainScore				TWSTRS Total Functional Disability Score				RFU (mo)
		Max	Pre	3 mo	RFU	Max	Pre	3 mo	RFU	Max	Pre	3 mo	RFU	
1	Retrocollis plus torticollis	32	22	13	13	8	7	2	3	60	44	13	9	15
2	Marked sagittal shift plus retrocollis	32	20	13	10	8	8	6	6	60	46	27	21	12
3	Marked lateral shift plus lateral tilt	32	19	11	9	8	6	4	4	60	35	20	18	6

Max, maximum possible score; Pre, preoperative score; RFU, recent follow-up; TWSTRS, Toronto Western Spasmodic Torticollis Rating Scale; 3 mo, 3-month postoperative score.
From Krauss JK, Pohle T, Weber S, et al. Bilateral stimulation of globus pallidus internus for treatment of cervical dystonia. *Lancet* 1999;354, 837–838, with permission.

We recently presented the first study on the efficacy of bilateral chronic GPi stimulation in patients with severe complex CD (8). Continuous DBS yielded remarkable improvement of CD, dystonia-associated pain, and functional disability.

Three patients, aged 42 to 53 years, two women and one man, with disease duration of 5 to 7 years, were selected for this prospective study. Medical treatment and repeated botulinum toxin injections had not provided long-term relief. All three patients had severe complex CD that was a source of marked disability and severe neck pain. Regarding the dystonic pattern and the presence of continuous phasic movements, these patients were not considered good candidates for peripheral surgical procedures (Table 32.2). The standardized assessment included the Mini-Mental Status Examination, the Hamilton Depression Scale, a modified TWSTRS, and a standard videotaping protocol. All formal assessments were performed by the neurologic team members. The study protocol was approved by the local ethics committee.

Quadripolar electrodes were implanted bilaterally into the posteroventral lateral GPi under stereotactic guidance according to the operative principles described previously (47,48). With the patient's head fixed in the stereotactic ring, it was not possible to assess the effects of intraoperative stimulation on the patients' movement disorders. Intraoperative stimulation was used, however, to determine thresholds for responses from the optic tract and the internal capsule. The electrodes were connected to programmable impulse generators in the subclavicular subcutaneous tissue after induction of general anesthesia in the same operative session. There were no adverse intraoperative events, and the postoperative course was unremarkable. Postoperative 1-mm computed tomography scans demonstrated appropriate localization of the electrodes in the posteroventral lateral GPi (Fig. 32.1). Mild amelioration of dystonia was observed immediately postoperatively. The programmable impulse generators were programmed percutaneously on the first

postoperative day, starting with amplitudes between 0.5 and 1.5 v at a pulse width of 210 microseconds and a frequency of 130 Hz. The second and third electrode contacts were used for bipolar stimulation. During the next 3 to 4 months, the stimulation parameters were gradually adjusted at regular intervals. Parallel to the increase of the amplitudes, further improvement of CD was observed. At each step of the programming, different sets of stimulation parameters were tried. During these sessions, difficulty in talking and a sensation of tightness of the cheeks and pharyngeal muscles could be evoked with higher amplitudes. Amplitudes at which these unwanted effects were not present were then programmed, respectively. At the 3-month assessment, patients had marked amelioration in the TWSTRS total severity score, which was accompanied by improvement in the total functional disability and pain scores. There was some further improvement in all patients during later follow-up evaluations. Figure 32.2 shows our first patient, a 53-year-old woman, preoperatively and 3 months postoperatively. The TWSTRS scores at follow-up at 6 months, 12 months, and 15 months, respectively, are also shown in Table 32.2. Stimulation parameters at the last follow-up were: frequency, 130 to 160 Hz; pulse width, 210 microseconds; and amplitude, between 3.1 and 5.0 v (mean, 4.0 v).

Chronic DBS probably induces a functional ablation of neuronal activity in the GPi with subsequent changes in pallidothalamic outflow. In patients with generalized dystonia, single-unit recordings revealed highly irregular spontaneous neuronal activity in the GPi occurring in intermittent grouped discharges at a mean frequency that was markedly lower than in patients with Parkinson's disease (49). Investigators have suggested that the beneficial effect of pallidotomy disrupts the transmission of abnormal patterns of neuronal activity in the GPi in generalized dystonia. This may also be true for the effects of functional ablation of the GPi in patients with CD. The delayed improvement may be explained by a process of gradual readaptation of the thalamocortical circuitry after removal of the pallidal input.

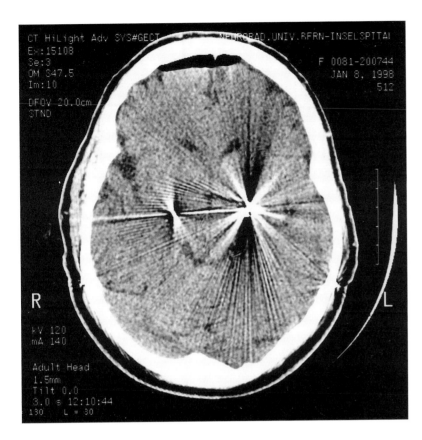

FIGURE 32.1. Axial computed tomography scans obtained on the second postoperative day demonstrate the position of the electrodes in the posteroventral lateral internal segment of the globus pallidus (patient 1).

Postoperative selection and adjustment of the optimal stimulation parameters in pallidal DBS for treatment of CD can be time consuming. In particular, in the upper range of the voltage used, the therapeutic window for optimal benefit without evoking unwanted effects becomes smaller.

Therefore, multiple postoperative visits are necessary to increase the stimulation amplitudes in small increments. A thorough understanding of the inherent difficulties by the patient, the patient's family, and the treating physicians is an absolute prerequisite. We reserve chronic bilateral GPi DBS

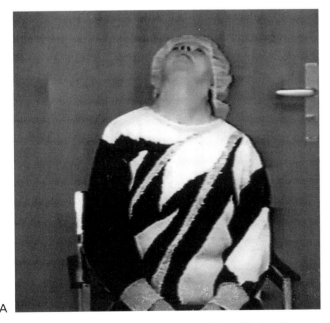

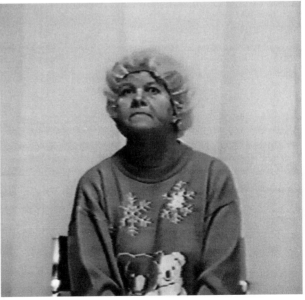

A   B

FIGURE 32.2. Upper: Video still of a 53-year-old woman with severe retrocollis and rotation of the chin to the right preoperatively. **Below:** There is marked improvement of the cervical dystonia 3 months after bilateral chronic stimulation of the internal segment of the globus pallidus.

only for fully cooperative patients. More experience and randomized studies are needed to compare the efficacy of pallidal DBS with that of other surgical procedures available for CD.

REFERENCES

1. Krauss JK, Toups EG, Jankovic J, et al. Symptomatic and functional outcome of surgical treatment of cervical dystonia. *J Neurol Neurosurg Psychiatry* 1997;63:642–648.
2. Bertrand CM, Lenz FA. Surgical treatment of dystonias. In: Tsui JKC, Calne DB, eds. *Handbook of dystonia.* New York: Marcel Dekker, 1995:329–345.
3. Bertrand CM. Selective peripheral denervation for spasmodic torticollis: surgical technique, results, and observations in 260 cases. *Surg Neurol* 1993;40:96–103.
4. Braun V, Richter HP. Selective peripheral denervation for the treatment of spasmodic torticollis. *Neurosurgery* 1994;35:58–63.
5. Lang AE. Surgical treatment of dystonia. *Adv Neurol* 1998; 78:185–198.
6. Krauss JK, Koller R, Burgunder JM. Partial myotomy/myectomy of the trapezius muscle with an asleep-awake-asleep anesthetic technique for treatment of cervical dystonia. *J Neurosurg* 1999;91:889–891.
7. Krauss JK, Pohle T. Historical review of functional stereotactic neurosurgery for treatment of cervical dystonia. *Mov Disord* 1998;13[Suppl 2]:134.
8. Krauss JK, Pohle T, Weber S, et al. Bilateral stimulation of globus pallidus internus for treatment of cervical dystonia. *Lancet* 1999;354:837–838.
9. Hassler R, Riechert T. Indikationen und Lokalisationsmethode der gezielten Hirnoperationen. *Nervenarzt* 1954;25:441–447.
10. Mundinger F, Riechert T. Ergebnisse der stereotaktischen Hirnoperationen bei extrapyramidalen Bewegungsstörungen auf Grund postoperativer und Langzeituntersuchungen. *Dtsch Z Nervenheilkd* 1961;182:542–576.
11. Hassler R, Dieckmann G. Die stereotaktische Behandlung des Torticollis aufgrund tierexperimenteller Erfahrungen über die richtungsbestimmten Bewegungen. *Nervenarzt* 1970;41:473–487.
12. Hassler R, Dieckmann G. Stereotactic treatment of different kinds of spasmodic torticollis. *Confin Neurol* 1970;32:135–143.
13. Handa H, Araki C, Mori K, et al. Spasmodic torticollis treated by chemothalamotomy and chemopallidotomy. *Confin Neurol* 1962;22:393–396.
14. Yasargil MG. Die Ergebnisse der stereotaktischen Operationen bei Hyperkinesen. *Schweiz Med Wochenschr* 1962;92:1550–1565.
15. Cooper IS. Effects of thalamic lesions upon torticollis. *N Engl J Med* 1964;270:967–972.
16. Sano K, Yoshioka M, Mayanagi Y, et al. Stimulation and destruction of and around the interstitial nucleus of Cajal in man. *Confin Neurol* 1970;32:118–125.
17. Mundinger F, Riechert T, Disselhoff J. Long-term results of stereotactic treatment of spasmodic torticollis. *Confin Neurol* 1972; 34:41–46.
18. Sano K, Sekino H Tsukamoto Y, et al. Stimulation and destruction of the region of the interstitial nucleus in cases of torticollis and see-saw nystagmus. *Confin Neurol* 1972;34:331–338.
19. Mazars G, Merienne L, Chodkiewicz JP. La chirurgie des dyskinesies d'orientation cephaliques. *Neurochirurgie* 1968;14:745–752.
20. Caracalos A. Results of 103 cryosurgical procedures in involuntary movement disorders. *Confin Neurol* 1972;34:74–81.
21. Andrew J, Rice Edwards JM, Rudolf N de M. The placement of stereotaxic lesions for involuntary movements other than in Parkinson's disease. *Acta Neurochir Suppl (Wien)* 1974;21:39–47.
22. Laitinen L. Stereotaxic treatment of spasmodic torticollis. *Acta Neurol Scand Suppl* 1963;39:231–236.
23. Hernesniemi J, Laitinen L. Résultats tardifs de la chirurgie dans le torticolis spasmodique. *Neurochirurgie* 1977;2:123–131.
24. Cooper IS. Neurosurgical treatment of the dyskinesias. *Clin Neurosurg* 1977;24:367–390.
25. Bertrand C, Molina-Negro P, Martinez SN. Combined stereotactic and peripheral surgical approach for spasmodic torticollis. *Appl Neurophysiol* 1978;41:122–133.
26. Dieckmann G. Traitement stéréotaxique du torticolis extrapyramidal. *Neurochirurgie* 1976;22:568–571.
27. Goldhahn G, Goldhahn WE. Die Ergebnisse stereotaktischer Hirnoperationen beim Torticollis spasmodicus. *Zentralbl Neurochir* 1977;38:87–96.
28. Andrew J, Fowler CJ, Harrison MJG. Stereotaxic thalamotomy in 55 cases of dystonia. *Brain* 1983;106:981–1000.
29. Stejskal L, Vladyka V, Tomanek Z. Surgical possibilities for alleviation of axial dyskinesias: comparison with forced movements of the head and eyes. *Appl Neurophysiol* 1981;44:320–329.
30. Von Essen C, Augustinsson LE, Lindqvist G. VOI thalamotomy in spasmodic torticollis. *Appl Neurophysiol* 1980;43:159–163.
31. Mundinger F. Neue stereotaktisch-funktionelle Behandlungsmethode des Torticollis spasmodicus mit Hirnstimulatoren. *Med Klin* 1977;72:1982–1986.
32. Andy OJ. Thalamic stimulation for control of movement disorders. *Appl Neurophysiol* 1983;46:107–111.
33. Consky ES, Lang AE. Clinical assessments of patients with cervical dystonia. In: Jankovic J, Hallett M, eds. *Therapy with botulinum toxin.* New York: Marcel Dekker, 1994:211–237.
34. Hassler R, Hess WR. Experimentelle und anatomische Befunde über die Drehbewegungen und ihre nervösen Apparate. *Arch Psychiatr Nervenkr* 1954;192:488–526.
35. Hiltl A. *Torticollis spasmodicus: Langzeitergebnisse nach stereotaktischer Operation.* Dissertation, Albert-Ludwigs-Universität, Freiburg, Germany, 1990.
36. Krauss JK, Mohadjer M, Braus DF, et al. Dystonia following head trauma: a report of nine patients and review of the literature. *Mov Disord* 1992;7:263–372.
37. Vitek JL, Lenz FA. Pallidal surgery: a new option for surgical treatment of dystonia. In: Krauss JK, Grossman RG, Jankovic J, eds. *Pallidal surgery for the treatment of Parkinson's disease and movement disorders.* Philadelphia: Lippincott–Raven, 1998:121–133.
38. Vitek JL, Zhang J, Evatt M, at al. Gpi pallidotomy for dystonia: clinical outcome and neuronal activity. *Adv Neurol* 1998;78:211–219.
39. Ondo WO, Desaloms JM, Jankovic J, et al. Pallidotomy for dystonia. *Mov Disord* 1998;13:693–698.
40. Iacono RP, Kuniyoshi SM, Schoonenberg T. Experience with stereotactics for dystonia: case examples. *Adv Neurol* 1998;78: 221–226.
41. Lozano AM, Kumar R, Gross RE, et al. Globus pallidus internus pallidotomy for generalized dystonia. *Mov Disord* 1997;12:865–870.
42. Dauer WT, Burke RE, Greene P, et al. Current concepts on the clinical features, aetiology and management of idiopathic cervical dystonia. *Brain* 1998;121:547–560.
43. Magyar-Lehmann S, Antonini A, Roelcke U, et al. Cerebral glucose metabolism in patients with spasmodic torticollis. *Mov Disord* 1997;12:704–708.
44. Naumann M, Pirker W, Reiners K, et al. Imaging the pre- and postsynaptic side of striatal dopaminergic synapses in idiopathic

cervical dystonia: a SPECT study using [^{123}I] epidepride and [^{123}I] beta-CIT. *Mov Disord* 1998;13:319–323.

45. Thompson ML, Thickbroom GW, Mastaglia FL. Corticomotor representation of the sternocleidomastoid muscle. *Brain* 1997;120:245–255.

46. Jankovic J. Re-emergence of surgery for dystonia. *J Neurol Neurosurg Psychiatry* 1998;65:434.

47. Krauss JK, Grossman RG. Operative techniques for pallidal surgery. In: Krauss JK, Grossman RG, Jankovic J, eds. *Pallidal surgery for the treatment of Parkinson's disease and movement disorders.* Philadelphia: Lippincott–Raven, 1998:121–133.

48. Krauss JK, Grossman RG. Surgery for hyperkinetic movement disorders. In: Jankovic J, Tolosa E, eds. *Parkinson's disease and movement disorders,* 3rd ed. Baltimore: Williams & Wilkins, 1998:1017–1047.

49. Vitek JL, Chockkan V, Zhang JY, et al. Neuronal activity in the basal ganglia in patients with generalized dystonia and hemiballismus. *Ann Neurol* 1999;46:22–35.

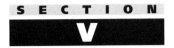

OTHER MOVEMENT DISORDERS

Surgery for Parkinson's Disease and Movement Disorders,
edited by J.K. Krauss, J. Jankovic, and R.G. Grossman.
Lippincott Williams & Wilkins, Philadelphia © 2001.

33

NEURAL TRANSPLANTATION FOR TREATMENT OF HUNTINGTON'S DISEASE

ANNE E. ROSSER
STEPHEN B. DUNNETT

HUNTINGTON'S DISEASE: CLINICAL AND PATHOLOGIC FEATURES

Huntington's disease (HD) is an inherited neurologic disorder characterized by progressive degeneration of the basal ganglia (in particular the caudate and putamen) caused by a single autosomal dominant gene. It affects approximately 6,000 patients in the United Kingdom (1), but with many more gene-carriers destined to develop the condition. The normal version of the Huntington gene *(IT15)* is expressed widely in both neural and nonneural tissues. The gene product is known as huntingtin (from the association of the mutated form with HD), although its function in normal cells is still little understood. The normal gene contains a repeat of the nucleotides CAG, encoding a polyglutamine ("polyQ") stretch at the N-terminus end of the associated protein, which is typically six to 20 repeats in length and always less than 36 to 37 repeats in the normal brain. By contrast, repeat lengths of more than 38 to 39 are associated with HD, and most patients have repeat lengths in the range of 40 to 50 (2). A clear inverse relationship exists between repeat length and disease onset on a population basis, with longer repeat lengths associated with earlier-onset disease. Patients with very early-onset disease tend to have more rigidity or dystonia and less in the way of chorea, and this is particularly true of juvenile, or Westphal variant, HD. However, there is no clear cutoff between early-onset and adult-onset disease, and the relationship between repeat length and age of onset is not precise enough to allow prediction of onset on an individual basis. The way in which the abnormal gene results in disease

is also not yet established, although there are several theories (3). Cellular inclusions were observed in both HD transgenic animals (4) and postmortem brains (5). A relationship between the disease state and the inclusions seems likely, but the precise nature of this relationship and, indeed, whether the inclusions are part of the process of cell dysfunction and death or are simply an associated epiphenomenon are as yet unclear.

HD is a progressive disorder usually starting in midlife and leading to complete dependence and death over a period of approximately 15 years (1). It comprises progressive motor, cognitive, and psychiatric symptoms, although in the early stages of the condition, any one of these set of symptoms may predominate. The onset and duration of the presymptomatic phase are notoriously difficult to estimate clinically, particularly when psychiatric symptoms, such as depression, precede motor or cognitive symptoms. Depression is common in the general population, and there are no clear specific features of depression associated with HD, so proving that a bout of depression signaled the onset of the disease is usually not possible. Evidence also indicates that subtle cognitive decline may precede the clear onset of motor symptoms by several years (6).

Since the mid-1980s, much work has been done to characterize the motor, cognitive, and psychiatric features of HD. The most obvious and best-known motor feature of the disease is choreiform movement, but other motor abnormalities are equally prominent and may be responsible for as much, if not more, disability (7). These include rigidity, bradykinesia, postural instability, and speech and swallowing disorders. The cognitive deficits in HD are characterized by a dysexecutive syndrome, memory deficits, impaired attention, and reduced psychomotor speed (8,9), and the most common psychiatric manifestations are depression, irritability, uncontrolled rage, and lack of motivation (1). The psychiatric manifestations are unpredictable in their appearance, and, as

A.E. Rosser: Centre for Brain Repair, University of Cambridge; Department of Neurology, Addenbrooke's Hospital, Cambridge CB2 1QQ, United Kingdom.

S.B. Dunnett: Centre for Brain Repair, University of Cambridge, Cambridge CB2 1QQ; School of Biosciences, Cardiff University, Museum Avenue, Cardiff CF10 3US, United Kingdom.

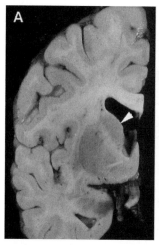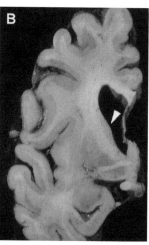

FIGURE 33.1. Postmortem brain slices of a neurologically normal patient **(A)** and of a patient with Huntington's disease (HD) **(B)**. Note the atrophy of the basal ganglia, in particular the caudate nucleus *(arrowhead),* the enlargement of the lateral ventricles, and the thinning of the neocortex in HD. (Courtesy of Professor John Hodges, Cambridge, United Kingdom.)

with the preclinical phase, it can be difficult to know (even in retrospect) whether a bout of depression or another symptom is "reactive" or is specifically caused by the neurodegeneration. The psychiatric and cognitive aspects of this condition make this a particularly expensive disease in both economic and social terms.

At the macroscopic level, the lateral ventricles become enlarged as the striatum degenerates, and this can be easily detected in brain scans, such as magnetic resonance imaging (MRI), as well as at postmortem examination (Fig. 33.1). The two main nuclei of the neostriatum (the caudate and the putamen) both show progressive shrinkage and atrophy as the disease progresses, although of the two, the caudate nucleus is affected earlier and to a greater extent than the putamen. The progression of shrinkage has been categorized into a series of stages, graded from 0 to 4 by Vonsattel et al. (10), which provides a system that is very widely used for descriptive and neuropathologic staging of the disease. At the microscopic level, the greatest cell loss is of the "medium spiny" population of neurons, which constitute the major input and output neurons of the striatum and use the inhibitory amino acid γ-aminobutyric acid (GABA) as their primary neurotransmitter. By contrast, the interneurons of the striatum are characterized by larger spiny and aspiny morphologic features and use somatostatin, neuropeptide Y, and other peptides as neurotransmitters, and they are strikingly less affected by the disease.

POTENTIAL TREATMENT STRATEGIES

Currently, treatment of this devastating and relentless condition is extremely limited. Certain drugs may reduce the

severity of the choreiform movements, but the parkinsonian symptoms are refractory to treatment, except perhaps for a limited and transient response to L-dopa in a few patients in whom these symptoms are particularly marked. However, this response is almost always unsatisfactory and is not comparable to that seen in Parkinson's disease (PD). Moreover, at the time of writing, no intervention can arrest the progression of the disease. Ultimately, a full understanding of the genetics and the pathways involved in cell death and dysfunction may lead to a cure (11), but no such intervention is currently on the horizon, and the most likely feasible alternative in the foreseeable future is cell transplantation, either to replace lost neurons that can restore circuitry or to provide growth factors or other agents support that could slow progression of the degenerative disease process. Of course, these two alternatives are not mutually exclusive, and ultimately various combinations of protection and repair may be required to yield optimal benefit for affected patients.

Some alternative approaches are currently under investigation for modifying the course of HD, although none have yet been proven in clinical trials. For example, it may be possible to slow the process of cell death with agents such as free radical scavengers. Small trials have demonstrated safety but not (as yet) efficacy. Two such drugs, coenzyme Q and remacemide (an inhibitor of glutamate), have been found to be safe in small-scale studies (12,13), and these agents are now undergoing much larger-scale trial in the United States. The finding that small trials did not reveal effects makes a dramatic response to these drugs unlikely, but the possibility remains that they will have a more subtle effect on disease progression.

A second approach is to seek to alter the course of the disease by the presence of growth factors. For example ciliary neurotrophic factor (CNTF), glial cell line–derived growth factor, and nerve growth factor have all been proposed to modulate striatal cell death after lesions. CNTF has been demonstrated to ameliorate neurodegeneration caused by progressive metabolic toxic lesions of the striatum in experimental animals (14), and clinical safety trials of CNTF in a small number of HD patients are now under way. These types of approaches may ultimately depend on transplantation technology for delivery of the active substances.

RATIONALE AND PRINCIPLES OF NEURAL TRANSPLANTATION

The rationale for exploring neural transplantation in HD in the early to moderate preclinical phase is based on several testable premises, which are outlined in detail by Peschanski et al. (15). In summary, these are as follows: (a) the experimental models of HD are valid in the sense of being suitable for the testing of reconstruction of striatal circuitry; (b) HD can be ameliorated by reconstruction of this circuitry, that is, degeneration in other regions such as cortex does not play a major role in the evolution of the clinical feature, at least not in the early stages; and (c) the pathologic process is directly related to the finding that the degenerate neurons carry the abnormal gene, that is, the transplanted neurons will not be subject to the same degenerative process. A large body of evidence suggests that the animal models carry a significant degree of validity (premise a): in these animal models, striatal grafts reliably restore corticobasal ganglia circuitry, and the grafts are associated with significant alleviation of cognitive as well as motor deficits (see the experimental studies described later). Premises b and c are ultimately only testable in clinical models. There will always be a debate about how much experimental information is required before progression to the clinic (15–18), but the growing consensus is that most of the fundamental questions that can be addressed in animal models have been addressed, and the outstanding issues will be resolved only by well-designed clinical trials.

HD is likely to represent a greater challenge than PD for the capacity of grafted cells actually to repair damaged neuronal circuits. In PD (both in humans and in animal models), transplants of developing nigral tissue may act by a combination of diffuse dopamine release from the grafted cells into the host brain and local connections between the transplanted tissue and host (19). This situation contrasts with most other neurodegenerative diseases, including HD, in which it is likely that the functional impact of the grafts on the host (whether experimental animal or patient) will depend critically on the capacity of the transplanted cells to restore afferent connections with the host brain and to become integrated within the host neuronal circuitry. Thus, clinical trials of neural transplantation in HD not only are important to evaluate the benefit of this approach in this devastating incurable disease (17,20–23), but also they provide a prototype for other neurodegenerative conditions (24).

STRIATAL LESIONS IN ANIMALS

The development of neural transplantation strategies has relied on animal models of HD to test the efficacy and principles of neural transplantation. Mechanical injury to the striatum almost always disrupts adjacent structures and fibers *en passage* in addition to the intrinsic cells of this structure. Moreover, these lesions are nonselective in terms of the cell types destroyed. However, the neuropathologic, neurochemical, and behavioral features of HD can be reproduced in experimental animals by the injection of excitotoxins, such as kainic acid (25,26), or metabolic toxins, such as 3-nitroproprionic acid (3-NP) (27,28). The most extensive experience has been with the excitotoxic agents kainic acid, quinolinic acid, and ibotenic acid. Intrastriatal injections of these substances produce neuronal death with preferential loss of GABAergic neurons, sparing cholinergic neurons (as in HD) and fibers of passage (29). Although kainic acid was the first excitotoxin to achieve widespread use, both quino-

linic acid and ibotenic acid induce profiles of cell loss that are closer to that seen in HD, as well as producing fewer side effects than kainic acid (30). Moreover, evidence indicates that metabolic toxins such as 3-NP induce cell death by a process that may more accurately mimic the neuropathogenic process in the human disease (31), and 3-NP can be given by peripheral injection, a feature that has distinct practical advantages in some situations over central injection of the excitotoxins. However, 3-NP requires repeated administration over long and variable periods to yield lesions, and there is typically considerable variability in toxicity from animal to animal. Consequently, because studies of transplant repair first and foremost require a reliable and stable pathologic process, ibotenic and quinolinic acids have been the excitotoxins of choice for modeling the striatal neuropathologic profile of HD.

More recently, transgenic models have been reported in the literature. The best described of these is the R6/2 mouse (32) in which the exon 1 of the human mutant gene carrying approximately 145 CAG repeats is present. The R6/2 mouse develops a progressive illness with locomotor deterioration, weight loss, premature death, and some evidence of cognitive abnormalities. However, its validity as a model of HD remains in question because, in spite of exhibiting overt neurologic deficits, there is little in the way of striatal disease even by the time the animal dies (32,33). Other transgenic models created more recently go some way to addressing these issues (34–38), but functional characterization and selectivity of profiles of cell dysfunction and death remain poorly understood. Although these various models are proving invaluable for investigation of the pathogenesis of HD, including the study of the role of neuronal intranuclear inclusions in the development of disease, their utility for exploration of neural transplantation or other therapies remains to be clarified. Using excitotoxins to make selective lesions within the brain reveals that damage of intrinsic striatal neurons can produce motor, cognitive, and motivational impairments akin to all main classes of symptoms manifested by patients with HD (39,40).

Cognitive Impairments

Bilateral excitotoxic lesions of the neostriatum in rats produce deficits in a range of cognitive tasks, including tests of maze learning, spatial navigation, delayed response, and temporal sequencing of behaviors in operant paradigms (41,42).

Motor Impairments

The deficits induced by striatal lesions include locomotor hyperactivity, disruption of performance of skilled motor tasks, impaired reaction times, and aspects of sensorimotor inattention and neglect. More detailed analyses have suggested that the impairment involves selection and initiation of voluntary or goal-directed behaviors, rather than an inability to execute particular movements *per se* (39,43,44).

Motivational Impairments

Although psychiatric deficits are more difficult to evaluate in animals, rats with striatal lesions exhibit impairments in the motivational control of behavior. For example, striatal lesions disrupt the rats' ability to detect and adapt their response to changes in the value of reward, and these lesions change the animals' reactivity to aversive stimuli (45,46).

From the specific studies of the effects of striatal lesions in rats and monkeys, some general principles arise. Many of the deficits observed after striatal lesions are similar to those described after damage in the cortex. Thus, lesions in the head of the caudate in rats and monkeys produce deficits in a range of cognitive tasks (such as delayed response and spatial alternation) that were first described in the context of damage in the prefrontal cortex. Rosvold and Szwarcbart first recognized that because the caudate nucleus is a major output projection of the prefrontal cortex, the similarity of deficits seen after lesioning in each of these areas suggests that they form part of a distinct "prefrontal system" (47,48). Lesions within the caudate nucleus disrupt the major neocortical outflows, and they are typical of what Geschwind termed a "disconnection syndrome" (49,50), in which cortical plans of action are separated from the downstream motor systems necessary for their execution. In fact, it turns out that a substantial degree of topography is maintained in

each projection within Rosvold's system. In the same way that the neocortical mantle is heterogeneous, with distinctive architectonic areas having different functions, so it is for the related subcortical structures of the thalamus and neostriatum, which are interlinked to the cortex in the form of corticostriatal loops, each of which has a distinctive function (51). The main development since Rosvold's original conception of this topographic organization is one of extent. Corticostriatal loops apply throughout the whole neocortical mantle (all association and motor areas rather than prefrontal cortex alone) as well as the complete striatum (putamen and ventral striatum as well as caudate nucleus), and they apply to all aspects of neocortical/striatal function (including motor and sensorimotor as well as purely cognitive) function (51,52).

STRIATAL GRAFTS IN ANIMALS

The techniques of transplanting striatal cells into the excitotoxically lesioned neostriatum are essentially identical to those already described for grafting embryonic dopamine cells, and the same principles apply (53) (Fig. 33.2). Because of the deep site, most studies have used stereotactic injection of dissociated cell suspensions rather than any of the various solid graft techniques. To be effective, the grafted tissue needs to be taken from the developing embryo at a gestational age of E14 to E16 days in rats, at which stage the developing cells of the neostriatum are differentiating and migrating from the

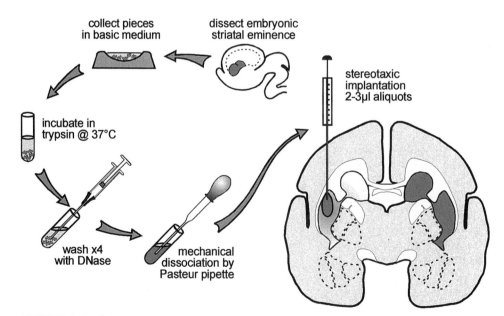

FIGURE 33.2. Schematic illustration of the methods for dissecting embryonic ganglionic eminence and preparing embryonic cells as a dissociated "striatal" cell suspension for stereotactic injection into the basal ganglia of the host, here illustrated for the marmoset brain. (From Kendall AL, Rayment FD, Torres EM, et al. Functional integration of striatal allografts in a primate model of Huntington's disease. *Nat Med* 1998;4:727–729, with permission.)

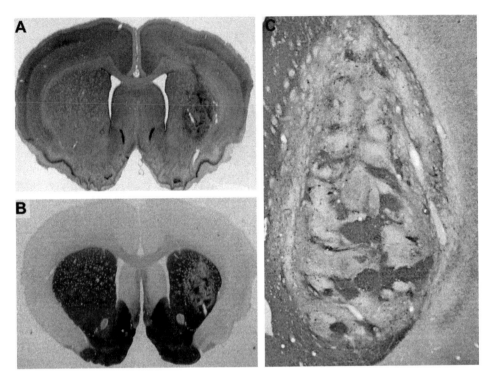

FIGURE 33.3. Photomicrographs of a striatal graft in the unilaterally lesioned neostriatum. **A:** Acetylcholinesterase stain, which labels striatal neuropil. **B:** Tyrosine hydroxylase stain, which labels host-derived dopamine fibers growing into the grafts. **C:** High-power photomicrograph of the graft showing the "patchy" organization of the graft, reflecting zones of striatal-like cells interspersed with zones of nonstriatal-like cells (e.g., neocortex) derived from the multipotential embryonic ganglionic eminence. (Courtesy of Drs. Colin Watts and Stephanie Thian, Cambridge, U.K.)

overlying germinal cell layer of the "ganglionic eminence" in the floor of the lateral ventricles. In contrast to the relatively poor survival that has characterized studies of nigral grafts, striatal grafts survive well, and typically only a single deposit from one striatal primordium is required per grafted animal. On subsequent histologic analysis, the grafts are seen to undergo extensive growth to form a "ministriatum" containing all major cell types and biochemical markers of the normal striatum in a patchy, rather than homogeneous, arrangement (54) (Fig. 33.3).

The anatomy and biochemistry of these grafts are described in more detail later. However, first let us consider the consequences of such grafts on the behavioral deficits induced by experimental striatal lesions, because those data provide a functional framework for the levels of repair that have to be explained.

FUNCTIONAL STUDIES OF STRIATAL GRAFTS

Locomotor Hyperactivity

The first functional studies of striatal grafts revealed that these grafts are capable of reversing the hyperactivity seen with striatal lesions compared to control levels (55,56). In a subsequent study, this effect of the grafts was found to be most marked at night, when normal activity and lesion-induced hyperactivity both reach their heights (57). Moreover, this latter study showed that the grafts were only effective when they were placed homotopically into the striatum and not when they were placed ectopically into the globus pallidus, a finding suggesting that afferent connectivity of the grafts, rather than simply reinnervation of their target, may be important in their functional effects.

Delayed Alternation

In that same study, Isacson et al. considered not only locomotor activity, but also the animals' ability to learn a delayed spatial alternation task in a raised T-maze (57). Striatal lesions totally abolished the ability to learn the alternation task, and all animals of the lesioned group stayed at a chance level of performance throughout the 8 weeks of training. The animals with striatal grafts showed a substantial improvement, and although they were slower to learn than the intact control animals, all but two of them reached an asymptotic level of performance above the 90% criterion by the end of testing. Again, although the group with striatal grafts implanted in the globus pallidus showed a small improvement, they did not differ as a group from the lesion-alone control group, and no animals in the group with ectopic grafts reached criterion.

Rotation

Bilateral lesions in the neostriatum induce a hyperactivity syndrome, whereas the motor asymmetry induced by unilateral lesions can lead to rotation when the animal is activated, including pharmacologic challenges with apomorphine and amphetamine. Striatal grafts can reverse both amphetamine- and apomorphine-induced rotation in striatally lesioned rats (58), although the pattern of reversal is different from that seen in rats with nigrostriatal lesions. Because excitotoxic lesions of the striatum remove postsynaptic neurons of the nigrostriatal dopamine projection on the lesioned side, there can be no postsynaptic receptor supersensitivity. Thus, in striatal lesioned rats, rotation can be induced by apomorphine only at doses (0.5 to 1.0 mg/kg) that act on normal receptors. Moreover, in contrast to the contralateral rotation seen in dopamine-depleted rats, apomorphine-induced rotation in rats with striatal lesions is in the ipsilateral direction, in agreement with preferential drug-induced activation of striatal outputs on the intact but not lesioned side. The demonstration that striatal grafts can reverse apomorphine rotation and with the demonstration from receptor binding studies (see later) that neurons in striatal grafts carry functional dopamine receptors suggest that the grafts are able to restitute balance between the output pathways on the two sides of the brain.

The loss of intrinsic neurons with striatal lesions and the corresponding asymmetry of functional outputs mean that rats with striatal lesions will rotate in the same direction with the same dose of amphetamine challenges as seen in the nigrostriatally lesioned rat. Amphetamine does not act directly on striatal neurons but indirectly by stimulating dopamine release from dopamine nerve terminals in the striatum, which then produces its effect through postsynaptic (i.e., striatal) dopamine receptor activation. Moreover, host dopamine fibers do grow into striatal grafts to make contact with the striatal output neurons (see later) and by so doing promote recovery of amphetamine-induced rotation. This finding suggests that the host dopaminergic inputs to the striatal grafts are functional and can interact with the graft regulation of striatal outputs to restore balance between the two sides. Although rotation is an artificial behavioral test, these observations provided the first clear suggestion that information could be relayed from host through the graft back to the host, that is, a functional incorporation of the grafted neurons into the neural circuitry of the host brain.

Skilled Paw Reaching

A more interesting set of tests to compare the skilled motor capacity of rats with nigral and striatal grafts is provided by tests of skilled paw reaching. Unilateral nigrostriatal lesions produce marked deficits in the coordination and accuracy with which a rat can use the contralateral paw to reach for and retrieve food pellets. This has always been one of the deficits resistant to alleviation by grafts of embryonic nigral tissue or other dopamine-secreting tissues. By contrast, several studies have shown a significant alleviation of the paw reaching deficit induced by excitotoxic lesions of the neostriatum in rats with striatal grafts (58–60).

The clearest demonstration of this efficacy of striatal grafts is provided by the fully counterbalanced study of Montoya et al. (60), in which these investigators compared the effects of nigral and striatal grafts in rats with either 6-hydroxydopamine lesions of the nigrostriatal pathway or ibotenic acid lesions of intrinsic striatal neurons. Neither nigral nor striatal tissue grafts alleviated the nigrostriatal deficit when these grafts were implanted into the dopamine-depleted striatum. By contrast, although *a priori* the striatal lesion may be considered to produce more extensive damage of multiple pathways than lesions of nigrostriatal inputs alone, this deficit was alleviated by striatal grafts implanted into the same striatal site. In this case, the graft was homotopic, in contrast to the situation with nigrostriatal lesions, in which both types of graft are ectopic to the loss induced by this lesion. The specificity of the striatal graft action is confirmed by the finding that nigral grafts were without effect.

EVIDENCE OF STRIATAL CIRCUIT RECONSTRUCTION

It appears that placement of striatal grafts into a homotopic rather than ectopic site is important for their functional efficacy. Investigators have proposed that the reason for the failure of recovery in rats with nigrostriatal lesions and nigral grafts on some tasks may be that although nigral grafts restore a diffuse dopaminergic activation of the striatum, they do not reconstruct the damaged nigrostriatal pathway (19,61). Consequently, although performance on tests that reflect dopaminergic activation and net striatal output may be restored (such as locomotor activity, rotation, somatosensory neglect, posture, and side biases), performance remains impaired on other tests involving complex coordinated action (such as skilled paw reaching, disengagement behavior, food hoarding, or the aphagia/adipsia syndrome) because of a failure to reconstruct the damaged nigrostriatal circuitries and thus to restore the input and output of patterned information. Recovery in tests such as T-maze alternation, skilled paw reaching, and aspects of rotation in rats with intrinsic striatal lesions and homotopic striatal grafts suggests on functional grounds alone that a degree of circuit reconstruction must be taking place in this model system. Certain other observations converge to support that hypothesis, as described in the following paragraphs.

First, although the recovery in locomotor activity may be attributable to a downregulation of striatal overactivity at the level of striatal terminals in the globus pallidus, the T-maze alternation task provides a long-established test sensitive to disturbance of corticostriatal integrity. Therefore, a deficit in

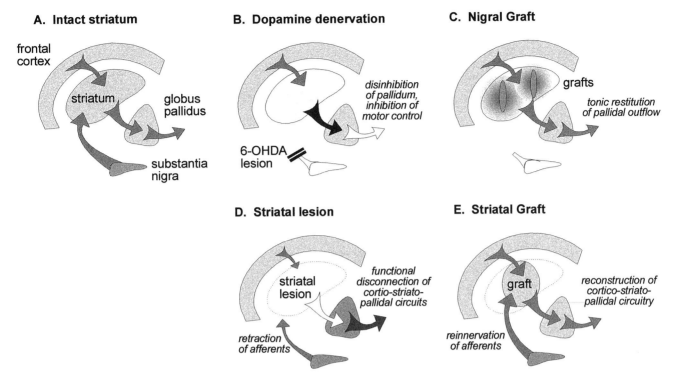

FIGURE 33.4. Schematic diagram of the circuit reconstruction provided by striatal grafts. **A:** The principal striatal input and output circuits between the striatum and the frontal cortex, globus pallidus, and substantia nigra. **B:** After a 6-hydroxydopamine (6-OHDA) lesion to the median forebrain bundle, the dopaminergic input to the striatum from the substantia nigra is selectively destroyed. This results in disinhibition of the pallidum and thus inhibition of motor control. **C:** Implantation of embryonic nigral tissue into the ectopic position of the striatum allows normal inhibition of the pallidum and restitution of motor control. **D:** After a striatal lesion, cortical and substantia nigra inputs are disconnected from outputs to the globus pallidus (and brainstem) leading to disinhibition of motor control. **E:** Implantation of embryonic striatal tissue allows reconstitution of corticostriatal circuitry and restores control over descending motor pathways.

this test and its recovery with homotopic striatal grafts indicate a reversal of the lesion-induced disconnection syndrome isolating the neocortex from its motor targets in the globus pallidus and beyond.

Second, no pharmacologic treatments have been found to overcome the cognitive impairments of the prefrontal type after intrinsic striatal damage, whether caused by neurodegenerative disease as in HD or after experimental lesions in animals. Striatal grafts can therefore be seen to work not in a purely pharmacologic way, but in terms of circuit reconstruction.

Third, in some tests, striatal grafts were ineffective when they were implanted into the main output target of the neostriatum, namely, the globus pallidus. This finding is important because it indicates that the striatal grafts reconstruct the circuitry appropriate to this structure, and attempts to use striatal grafts to mimic the circumstances in which nigral grafts are effective, namely, ectopic placement in the primary target area, are unsuccessful.

The contrast between nigral grafts, which have their limited effect primarily when they are placed into the ectopic site, and striatal grafts, which have a more extensive effect

when they are implanted into the homotopic site, suggests that quite different mechanisms of action must apply in the two models: diffuse reinnervation of denervated targets, tonic release of deficient neurochemicals, and trophic actions on the host brain in the case of nigral grafts versus a hypothesized reconstruction of damaged neuronal circuitry in the case of striatal grafts (Fig. 33.4).

This strong hypothesis turns out to be difficult to demonstrate directly. However, since the mid-1990s, a newly invigorated research effort has been oriented toward identifying principles of circuit reconstruction, and the results continue to support the hypothesis. The anatomic, biochemical, and physiologic studies that give the hypothesis credence are briefly considered.

Internal Organization of Striatal Grafts

The first grafts of striatal tissue into the kainic acid–lesioned or ibotenic acid–lesioned striatum were seen to survive well (see earlier). In postmortem histologic examination, the grafts were primarily composed of neurons when they were stained with simple cell body stains as well as a by certain simple markers of striatal tissue, such as the enzyme acetylcholinesterase. However, from the earliest studies, it became clear that stains characteristic of the normal neostriatum show a distinctly patchy pattern (Fig. 33.3). Moreover, when stains for different markers of striatal tissue are used on adjacent sections, the patchy zones are aligned. Thus, it turns out that "striatal" grafts contain patches—the so called "P zones" (62)—containing all the cell types, neurotransmitters, enzymes, and receptors of the normal striatum (54,63).

This, then, begs the question: So what are all the cells seen in the intervening areas of the grafts, the so called "NP zones"? The NP zones are also rich in neurons, but with the characteristics of nonstriatal populations of cells such as those found in the neocortex and globus pallidum (62, 64,65).

Striatal grafts therefore contain both striatal-like and nonstriatal-like populations of cells. It is not possible to separate these populations at the time of graft dissection because they all originate from the same germinal cell layer in the embryonic ganglionic eminence. The nonstriatal cells then migrate through the deeper striatal layers to reach their ultimate targets. Nor is it possible with present techniques to separate the different populations of cells in suspension before implantation. The problem is that although the fate of the cells is largely determined at the time of dissection, they are all small, round, relatively undifferentiated cells at this stage and are not yet expressing the differences in cell size or distinctive molecular markers on the cell surface that could be used for cell sorting.

Although the grafts contain a mixture of striatal and nonstriatal cells, the important feature for their function is that the cells organize themselves into distinct striatal-like P zones as the grafts develop. It remains unknown how this is achieved. Do the striatal and nonstriatal cells migrate and self-aggregate into clusters of cells of similar types? Is there selective cell death of neurons whose neighbors are of a dissimilar type, resulting in a selective survival of similar cells together? Is the phenotype of each cell itself modified or regulated by its neighbors? Whichever is the process, by what mechanisms do the different cells recognize their neighbors? These issues are difficult to resolve in the absence of suitable markers to track the fate of different populations of migrating cells at this very early stage in their phenotypic development. Although we have no answers to these theoretic issues, the practical fact is that the cells in striatal grafts contain the developmental programs to organize and reorganize themselves into structures akin to the normal neostriatum, which is almost certainly necessary if they are to be engaged in any meaningful functional processing of their inputs and to relay sensible output information to their targets.

Anatomic Connections of the Grafts

As well as reorganizing itself as a new "ministriatum," a striatal graft would need to develop appropriate input and output connections with the host brain if it is to be functionally effective. The extent and specificity of the reciprocal connections that are seen to form between graft and host are perhaps the most remarkable features of this model system (54).

The outputs of a graft have been visualized anatomically in several different ways. Retrograde tracers can be injected in the host brain; anterograde tracers can be injected into the grafts, and xenografts of human or mouse striatal tissues have been implanted in the rat striatum and their connections demonstrated using species-specific antibodies. All have shown extensive axon outgrowth from striatal grafts coursing in a caudal direction toward the globus pallidus, which is reinnervated in most cases. Furthermore, in many cases, the axon outgrowth is seen to extend even further caudally to reach the other major output nucleus of the basal ganglia, the substantia nigra pars reticulata (Fig. 33.5B). Retrograde tracing from the putamen and substantia nigra shows that these outputs all originate from the striatal-like P zones of the grafts. Similarly, the inputs to the grafts can be visualized using anterograde and retrograde tracers as well as markers for the afferent dopaminergic input from the substantia nigra (Fig. 33.5A).

Excitotoxic lesions of the striatum destroy intrinsic neurons but leave the terminals of the input axons intact. These terminals eventually die back, but for several months they are able to sprout into any appropriate new target tissue. Striatal grafts provide a very effective stimulus for inducing this sprouting and by so doing allow ingrowth of all the normal major inputs to the striatum, including cortical and thalamic, both serotonergic and dopaminergic projections. As one could expect from the nature of the grafted tissue, some inputs (such as those from the neocortex) grow into both the P zones and the NP zones of the grafts, whereas other inputs (such as the dopamine inputs) preferentially innervate the P zones in a manner that one would expect developmentally.

Perhaps the most dramatic demonstration of reconstruction of striatal circuits in striatal grafts is provided by the electron microscope studies of Debby Clarke and Stephen Dunnett (66). With the electron microscope, the actual form of the synaptic contacts can be observed. Initially, Golgi staining and glutamic acid decarboxylase immunohistochemistry were used to identify cells in the grafts that were GABAergic and of the medium spiny neuron type. Then, a combination of other techniques was used to show the connections of these cells (Fig. 33.6). First, the retrograde tracer horseradish peroxidase was injected into the globus pallidus: the presence of horseradish peroxidase crystals in the cells of the graft showed that the medium spiny neurons gave rise to the pallidal outputs. Second, lesions were made in the neocortex: degenerating terminals of corticostriatal axons were seen making contact with the same medium spiny neurons in the grafts. Third, the sections were further stained with a tyrosine hydroxylase antibody: this showed that dopamine inputs to the grafts made synaptic terminals

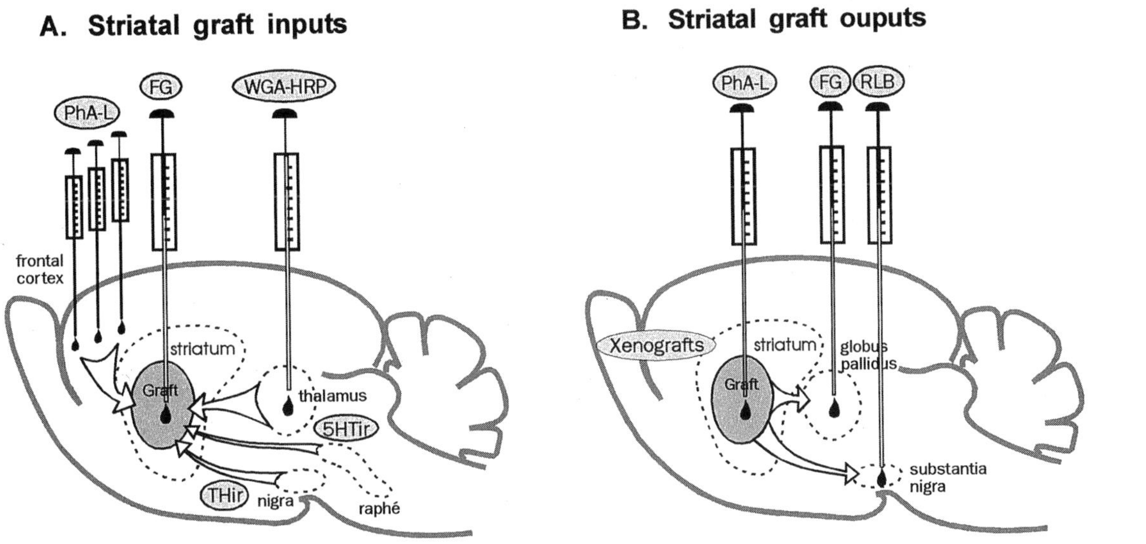

A. Striatal graft inputs

B. Striatal graft ouputs

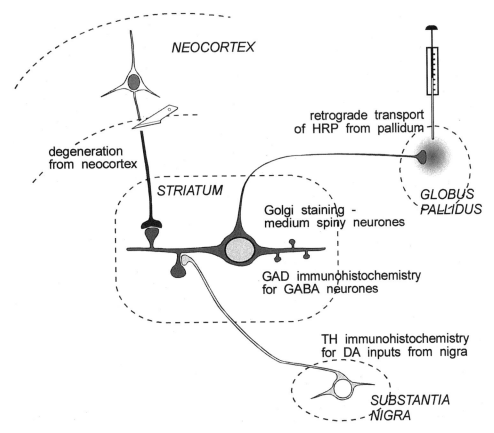

FIGURE 33.5. Schematic illustration of anatomic tracing and selective staining strategies for identifying afferent **(A)** and efferent **(B)** connections of striatal grafts. (From Wictorin K. Anatomy and connectivity of intrastriatal striatal transplants. *Prog Neurobiol* 1992;38:611–639.)

FIGURE 33.6. Schematic illustration of circuit reconstruction at the ultrastructural level. Neurons in striatal grafts are identified as having a medium spiny morphology by Golgi staining, as using γ-aminobutyric acid (GABA) as their transmitter based on immunoreactivity for glutamic acid decarboxylase (GAD), as projecting to the globus pallidus based on back labeling with wheat-germ agglutinin-horseradish peroxidase conjugate (WGA-HRP), as receiving projections from host dopamine systems based on tyrosine hydroxylase (TH) immunoreactivity, and as receiving projections from neocortex by visualization of degenerating terminals after a cortical lesion.

onto the dendritic spines of GABA medium spiny neurons. Indeed, in some cases, the corticostriatal and dopaminergic nigrostriatal inputs were seen to converge onto the same output neurons.

From these various anatomic studies, we now have convincing evidence that striatal grafts do have the capacity to reconstruct striatal input and output circuits through the grafts. Indeed, the evidence of circuit reconstruction is perhaps now stronger for this model system than for any other. The more difficult issue is to determine the association between the structural and functional levels of analysis—just because grafts do reconstruct a damaged circuit does not mean that this is the basis for their functional effect.

Physiologic and Biochemical Indices of Circuit Reconstruction

How are we to determine whether the observed anatomic connections are in any way functional? One approach has been electrophysiologic. This has so far been little investigated, but two studies have shown that stimulation in the host cortex or thalamus can be detected by recording electrodes placed within striatal grafts (67,68). Moreover, the recorded cellular firing patterns exhibit the characteristics of monosynaptic inputs, a finding suggesting that the projections from the host brain to the grafts have the capacity to relay basic patterned electrical information.

A second approach is to monitor changes in gene expression in cells in responses to changes in their inputs. In the normal striatum, the level of expression of two peptides colocalized in the medium spiny output neurons, enkephalin and substance P, is regulated by the dopamine input to the striatum. If the nigrostriatal inputs are lesioned, expression of enkephalin increases, whereas expression of substance P decreases. Similarly, in striatal grafts, normal levels of enkephalin and substance P expression are seen within the P zones, whereas after lesioning or blockade of the dopaminergic inputs, enkephalin expression again increases, and substance P expression decreases (69). Thus, the levels of expression of genes related to peptide neurotransmitters in the grafts are regulated by the host dopaminergic input in exactly the same manner as in the normal striatum.

A third approach is to use *in vivo* measurements of neurotransmitter turnover to monitor the activity of inputs and outputs of the grafts. For example, the graft projection to the globus pallidus is GABAergic. Sirinathsinghji and colleagues used a push-pull perfusion cannula to monitor GABA release in the globus pallidus of control, striatal-lesion only; and grafted striatal-lesion rats (70). The lesions produced a 97% loss of GABA release in the ipsilateral globus pallidus, which was restored to approximately 30% of normal levels in the graft-reinnervated pallidum. Of particular interest in this study was the observation that activation of dopamine inputs to the normal striatum induced a large, brief surge of GABA release in the pallidum. This response was completely abolished in the pallidum ipsilateral to a striatal lesion, but it was restored after reinnervation by a striatal graft.

These various approaches all suggest that the reformed host cortical, thalamic, and dopamine inputs making direct synaptic connections with GABA output neurons are indeed capable of relaying functional information from the host brain to neurons of the graft. Furthermore, the grafts can transduce that information to exert a reciprocal influence back onto the appropriate neuronal circuits within the host brain.

ETHICAL ISSUES FOR CLINICAL NEURAL TRANSPLANTATION

The ethical issues relate both to the collection of human fetal tissue and to safeguarding the recipient.

Collection of Human Fetal Tissue

In many countries in which induced abortion is legal, it is considered ethical to collect tissues for the purpose of wide-ranging research, some of which has contributed to the protection and safety of intrauterine life. The main thrust of recent debate has therefore not been the use of the tissue *per se,* but it has centered on the possibility that such use could influence the decision to proceed with an abortion and the methods by which this may take place. This debate is discussed more fully elsewhere (71), but in essence, in most European countries, the grounds for approving each individual case of induced abortion involve a process balancing the interests and well-being of the woman against that of the intrauterine life. Needless to say, views differ on how this balance should be weighted. Concern is centered around the possibility that a woman who is ambivalent about termination of pregnancy could be influenced to proceed with it were she to perceive that it would aid other patients. More extreme extensions of this idea are that a woman who is inclined to continue a pregnancy could be influenced to have an abortion as part of a selfless act of donation and that women would conceive to donate tissue for a relative. Thus, most current guidelines on the collection and use of human fetal tissue are centered on the separation of the decision to terminate a pregnancy from the decision to donate tissue and the separation of the management of the woman from the use of such tissue (71,72).

Issues Relating to the Recipient

As with any experimental procedure, it is essential that the intervention is optional and that the patient is fully informed and consenting. The consenting procedure requires special attention in conditions such as HD in which cognitive decline is part of the disease. It is thus important that the patient's mental and cognitive status is carefully assessed and that the physician in charge is fully convinced that the patient is capable of making an informed decision. For this reason, the multicenter European groups contributing to the development of a Core Assessment Protocol for Transplantation in Huntington's Disease (CAPIT-HD) elected to restrict experimental trials of neural transplantation in this disease to early to moderate disease states (23).

Certain other, more general ethical issues relate to experimental interventions in humans, including the need for the study to be carefully designed and controlled so that meaningful data can eventually be extracted; and the requirement for a process of independent supervision to monitor adverse effects and to ensure unbiased assessment and analyses.

ASSESSMENT ISSUES FOR NEURAL TRANSPLANTATION

Central to the investigation of any experimental therapy are the proper design and application of an assessment tool. There are special problems associated with surgical interventions, and in particular interventions such as neural transplantation, in which practical constraints dictate that only small numbers of patients can be assessed in any one center. Thus, to acquire large enough numbers for meaningful analysis, multicenter trials are required. Assessment protocols must be standardized so comparisons can be made across time and among examiners. Such an approach has an inherent problem in that variability often exists among different examiners. To minimize such variability, standardized protocols have now been developed and validated. Training videotapes can further help to standardize the assessment procedure.

To this end, all major European centers involved in cell transplantation for movement disorders have cooperated under the auspices of the European Network for Clinical Transplantation and Restoration, to develop, validate, and publish protocols for the assessment of neural transplants and other neurosurgical interventions in PD and HD (23,73). The elements that make up the research protocol must be relatively easy to apply and to quantify, and they must be sensitive to the core pathogenic events as well as the therapeutic intervention. The tests that form the core assessment program need to be applied longitudinally in patients while minimizing any practice effect. The initial assessment requires a relatively long pre-intervention period for a stable baseline to be obtained, given that most patients with neurologic disorders show day-to-day variability. Furthermore, the tests should be given under similar conditions if possible. Ideally, the complete assessment protocol should be done using a series of different approaches including historical information, clinical examination with neuropsychologic and neuropsychiatric assessments when appropriate, imaging, and neurophysiologic measures.

The adoption of assessment protocols for interventional therapy requires that clear end points are defined. These are encompassed by the core assessment protocols in the form of primary end points and a series of secondary, less important end points. In such circumstances, the need for control patients requires consideration, given the placebo effect of such therapies and the variable natural history of the untreated condition, although there is currently considerable debate about what constitutes a proper ethical control for a surgical intervention such as intracerebral transplantation (74–77). Finally, the assessments need to include measures of activities of daily living as well as quality of life, because there is only limited use in assessing the effect of treatments on clinical measures if this does not translate into a functionally meaningful impact on the patients life.

For HD, one well validated tool is the Unified Huntington's Disease Rating Scale (UHDRS) (78). It has been used for assessment in reported studies of drug intervention in HD (79,80), as well as studies of the natural history of the condition (81). The UHDRS comprises four domains of clinical performance in HD: motor performance, functional capacity, cognitive functions, and psychiatric abnormalities (Table 33.1).

The UHDRS is also part of a larger battery, initially developed for assessment of patients undergoing neural transplantation—CAPIT-HD (23). The way in which answers are recorded (yes/no or a number on a scale) makes transfer of information to a computerized database straightforward. Although this and similar test batteries (such as the Unified Parkinson's disease rating scale) were originally designed to provide minimum standards for the longitudinal assessment of patients receiving intrastriatal neural transplants of human fetal tissue, they are also suitable for other surgical interventions (82–84).

The CAPIT-HD battery consists of the following: the UHDRS, described earlier, which is largely concerned with motor and functional assessment with minimal cognitive and behavioral testing; an extensive battery of neuropsychologic tests; comprehensive neuropsychiatric tests; and imaging. The imaging comprises mandatory positron emission tomography (PET) and MRI scans immediately preoperatively and at 2 years, and ideally also 12 months preoperatively. This imaging is used to study the anatomic integrity of the graft (MRI) as well as functional measures such as the extent of dopamine receptor binding (e.g., raclopride binding on PET scanning). This latter measure is especially helpful because it gives an *in situ* measure of the functional capacity of the graft to restore and to repair neuropharmacologic systems, features that in the case of PD have been shown to correlate well with functional recovery as assessed clinically.

The major aspects of the CAPIT-HD, including the timing, are shown in Fig. 33.7. These batteries comprise an agreed international minimum, and many centers also employ additional tests.

TABLE 33.1. STRUCTURE OF THE UNIFIED HUNTINGTON'S DISEASE RATING SCALE (UHDRS)[a]

Section	Contents
Structured history	Demographicdata, past and current general health status, brief psychiatric history, family history, and onset of symptoms. This is usually taken once, at the first visit.
Drug history	Drugs are prescribed, including doses, at each visit.
Genetic analysis	Details of genetic analysis and whether the patient and family are aware of results are determined.
Cognitive assessment	Verbal fluency, symbol digit modalities test, and Stroop interference test. Results are entered as raw scores.
Behavioral assessment	Moodsymptoms, especially those relating to HD such as depression and obsessive-compulsive behavior, are assessed by the rater according to clinical impression from the patients and informants reports. Symptoms are rated on a scale of 1 to 4 as follows: 0, absent; 1, slight; questionable; 2, mild; 3, moderate; 4, severe. The rater is also asked to comment on whether the patient is confused, demented, and depressed, and requires pharmacotherapy for depression.
Motor assessment	Examinationof ocular pursuit, saccade initiation, saccade velocity, dysarthria, tongue protrusion, finger taps, pronation-supination hand taps, the Luria tristep test, arm rigidity, overall bradykinesia, maximal dystonia, maximal chorea, gait, tandem walking, and the retropulsion pull test. The rater is required to estimate severity on a precisely defined five-point scale of 0 to 4 for each of the above.
Functional scales	Three scales are completed. a. Functionalassessment: 25 yes-no questions assessing the ability to perform a range of activities of daily living, from the ability to continue in employment and to drive to getting out of bed without help. b. Shoulsonand Fahn independence scale rating current level of independence from 100 (indicating no special care) to 10 (indicating tube feeding and total bed care). c. Functionalcapacity assessing ability to function normally at work, to handle personal financial matters, domestic chores, activities of daily living, and the overall care level.

[a]Every section of the UHDRS requires identification of the rater, because in large multidisciplinary clinics, more than one person may complete the assessment. For example, the cognitive assessment may be performed by a psychologist, and the motor assessment may be done by a neurologist. Rater identification is important in the estimation of tool reliability in each center.

SURGICAL CONSIDERATIONS FOR NEURAL TRANSPLANTATION

Tissue Collection

Human fetal tissue is collected according to the ethical guidelines discussed earlier. The practicalities of collections vary from place to place according to local arrangements and constraints. However, a common requirement is for the removal of tissue by low-pressure aspiration (in contrast to high-pressure aspiration, which is the more usual operative procedure in many centers), to minimize tissue disruption and to allow a confident identification of the relevant CNS region (85,86). This has been our own experience also, in that collection using high-pressure aspiration significantly reduces the potential to identify reliably specific brain regions such as striatum and ventral mesencephalon compared with collection using low-pressure aspiration (Table 33.2). It has also been our experience, and that of others (M. Peschanski,

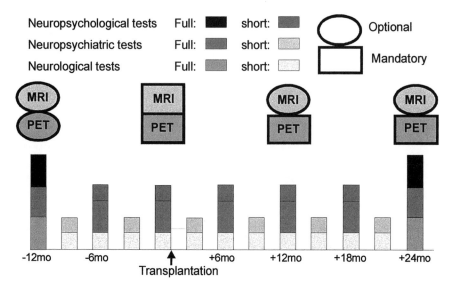

FIGURE 33.7. Schematic depiction of the timing of short and full versions of the neuropsychologic, neuropsychiatric, and neurologic tests and of positron emission tomography and magnetic resonance imaging scans in the modified Core Assessment Protocol for Transplantation in Huntington's disease (CAPIT-HD) assessment battery.

TABLE 33.2. RECOVERY OF FETAL TISSUES FROM ROUTINE (HIGH-PRESSURE) VERSUS ULTRASOUND-GUIDED LOW-PRESSURE TERMINATIONS

Fetal Age[a](d)	Total No. Examined	Fetal Parts (%)	Brain Tissue (%)	Striatum (%)	Brainstem[b] (%)	Spinal Cord (%)	Cerebellum[c]
Routine (High-Pressure) Terminations							
<42	5	2(40%)	2(40%)	0 / 0	1(20%)	2(40%)	nd
42–48	23	12(52%)	8(35%)	0	5(22%)	7(30%)	nd
49–55	34	15(44%)	12(35%)		7(21%)	10(29%)	nd
56–62	24	10(42%)	11(46%)	1(4%)	7(29%)	11(46%)	nd
63–69	14	11(79%)	9(64%)	0 / 0	3(21%)	7(50%)	nd
70–76	7	6(86%)	6(86%)	0	0	4(57%)	nd
>76	4	3(75%)	2(50%)		1(25%)	3(57%)	nd
Totals	111	59(53%)	50(45%)	1(1%)	24(22%)	44(40%)	
Ultrasound-Guided Low-Pressure Terminations							
<42	0	—	—	—	—	—	—
42–48	0	—	—	—	—	—	—
49–55	7	4(57%)	3(43%)	1(14%)	1(14%)	4(57%)	2(28%)
56–62	9	6(67%)	5(56%)	5(56%)	5(56%)	6(67%)	5(56%)
63–69	5	5(100%)	3(60%)	3(60%)	3(60%)	4(80%)	2(40%)
70–76	6	4(67%)	3(50%)	3(60%)	2(33%)	2(31%)	2(33%)
>76	2	1(50%)	1(50%)	1(50%)	1(50%)	1(50%)	1(50%)
Totals	29	20(69%)	15(52%)	13(45%)	12(41%)	17(59%)	12(41%)

nd, not determined.
[a]Fetal age is determined by *in utero* ultrasound measurements, available for all specimens.
[b]The poor morphologic preservation of tissue obtained by high-pressure aspiration precluded identification of ventral mesencephalon based on anatomic criteria, and data are given for gross brainstem. By contrast, identification was possible in specimens obtained by low-pressure aspiration and could be subsequently confirmed by tyrosine hydroxylase immunohistochemistry.
[c]The cerebellar anlage in the rhomencephalic lip was not specifically sought in specimens obtained by high-pressure aspiration.

personal communication), that the use of pelvic ultrasound greatly improves the efficiency of this procedure, although this imaging is not believed to be mandatory by all groups (85). A further constraint is the experience of certain groups (M. Peschanski, A. Björklund, personal communications) that successful aspiration of tissues suitable for transplantation depends on one or more committed obstetricians who are willing to become familiar with the low-aspiration technique, because a period of learning is required. In our own center, after collection, fetal tissues are placed immediately into tissue hibernation medium at 4°C for transportation to the laboratory, where dissection and tissue preparation take place. Once in the laboratory, tissues are dissected under sterile conditions in a tissue culture hood.

Striatal Identification

When the fetal central nervous system is intact, the striatum can clearly be seen as a swelling arising from the lateral wall of the basal telencephalon (Fig. 33.8), although the anatomic landmarks for dissection of the striatal primordium are present only in embryos of crown rump length 20 mm or larger (87). In more fragmented tissue, it still may be possible to identify the striatum attached to a cortical flap; however, in this case, it is essential that members of the dissecting team become familiar with this appearance and verify the presence of striatal tissue by techniques such as cell culture and staining for a specific striatal marker, such as DARPP-32, or histologic analysis and staining for acetylcholinesterase.

Optimum Gestational Age

The optimum gestational age for collection of human fetal striatum for the purposes of transplantation in HD has not been determined empirically, and ultimately clinical studies will be required to determine this age. However, animal models can be used to produce an estimate of the optimum age, as was achieved in animal models of PD and then used to guide clinical studies (88). There is now general acceptance of the principle that the optimal donor stage for transplantation is during embryonic development, when the most relevant cell is in the process of differentiation but has not begun axonal development (89). In the rat, Fricker et al. demonstrated that optimal recovery on certain behavioral tests in an HD rat model is produced after transplantation of E14 striatal tissue (Carnegie stage 18) (59). These grafts contained the highest proportion of striatal-like tissue (see later). In the marmoset, functional recovery was demonstrated with tissue of 13- 16-mm crown rump length, that is, 73 to 75 days

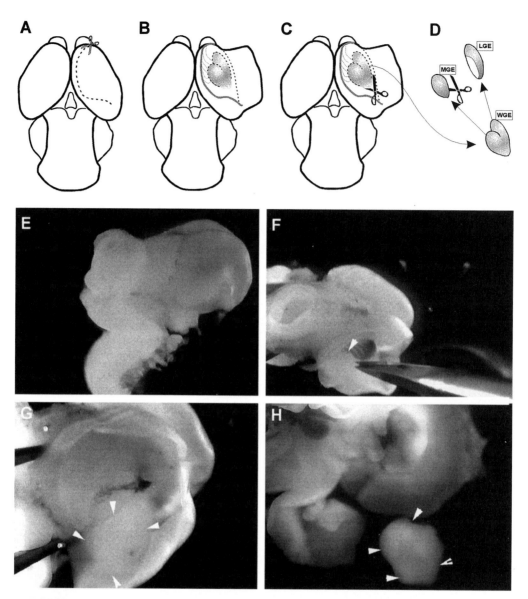

FIGURE 33.8. A–D: Schematic dissection of whole, lateral, and medial ganglionic eminence from the developing embryonic forebrain. **E–H:** Photomicrographs of this procedure in a fetus 8 weeks after conception. The borders of the ganglionic eminence are indicated by *arrowheads.* **E:** Lateral view of the brain. **F:** View of the ganglionic eminence through an incision in the developing cerebral hemisphere. **G:** Exposure of striatum *in situ.* **H:** Whole striatal eminence is dissected free from the basal forebrain. (**A–D,** from Watts C, Brasted PJ, Eagle DM, et al. Embryonic donor age and dissection influence striatal graft development and functional integration in a rodent model of Huntington's disease. *Exp Neurol* 2000;163:85–97.)

of gestation (again, Carnegie stage 18 to 21) (90). Thus, work using two species points to a Carnegie stage of approximately 18 to 21 as optimal; the human corollary is an embryo with a crown rump length of 13 to 24 mm, that is, 44 to 53 days after conception. However, because the striatal anlage is dissectible in human material only from 20 mm, this window of opportunity may turn out to be at slightly later Carnegie stages in humans. This issue has not been addressed directly in animal models using human fetal tissue as the donor tissue, although the few studies to date using human tissue have suggested an extended window of oppor-

tunity: surviving grafts have been reported from embryos of 21 to 30 mm (87), 35 mm (91), and 110 mm (92). In the last study, reduction of apomorphine-induced rotation was also reported (93). Our own preliminary studies of human fetal tissue transplanted into the excitotoxically lesioned rat striatum have suggested a window of approximately 65 and 80 days after conception as optimal in terms of graft volume (Fig. 33.9) (94). However, it is clear that further empiric studies are required to define this time window properly. A consistent feature of all these reports is the extended period of maturation required for human fetal tissue such that

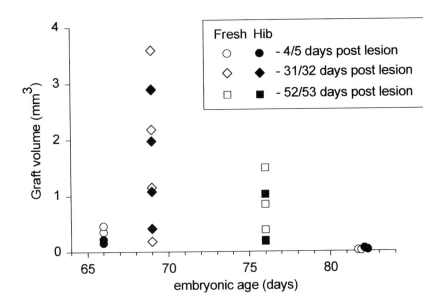

FIGURE 33.9. Survival and growth of human striatal grafts (based on the whole ganglionic eminence dissection; Fig. 33.8) derived from embryos of four different developmental ages and implanted either fresh *(open symbols)* or after 24-hour hibernation *(filled symbols).* (From Hurrelbrink CB, Armstrong RJE, Barker RA, et al. Hibernated human fetal striatal tissue: successful transplantation in a rat model of Huntington's disease. *Cell Transplant* 2000;9:743–749.)

maturation is still ongoing at 4 months after transplantation, and this complicates further the investigation of this issue by extending the survival times required.

Staging of human fetal gestational age can be estimated in various ways. Estimated time from the last menstrual period (LMP) is the most commonly used and widespread method, but it is known to be subject to errors including inaccuracy of recording by the maternal donor and variation in cycle length, so the relation of LMP to the actual time of conception is variable. Ultrasound provides a more reliable method, although this, too, is subject to a certain amount of error, which tends to be greater the younger the fetus. A further method of dating tissues between 4 and 12 weeks after conception has been suggested by Evtouchenko et al. (86), based on certain easily measured morphometric characteristics of retrieved tissue, and this may provide a more reliable way of determining gestational age. Using this as a reference, our own studies (R.J.E. Armstrong, S.B. Dunnett, and A.E. Rosser, unpublished data) have confirmed that ultrasound data provide a far more consistent correlation with morphologic indices of development than does LMP, a finding reinforcing the perspective that this may provide a more accurate index for embryonic staging (Fig. 33.10). In light of experimental evidence suggesting the critical importance of embryonic age in graft viability, it becomes imperative to refine criteria for accurate staging of embryos to be used for transplant donation and not simply to use the most readily available.

Tissue Dissection

Another important issue is whether to transplant the whole striatal ganglionic eminence (WGE) or to perform a selective dissection into lateral and medial eminences (LGE and MGE, respectively). Because the LGE is the major source of DARPP-32–positive medium spiny neurons, the principal cell population lost in HD, there has been interest in whether a selective dissection may provide superior tissue for transplantation in HD. Studies of selective implantation of embryonic rat LGE or MGE into rat models of HD demonstrated that laterally derived implants have a much higher proportion of striatal-like tissue compared with medial dissections (95–97). However, there were no functional measures in these studies and no comparison to WGE. The major drawback of comparing LGE with MGE alone is that it ignores the contribution that MGE cells may make to the final cell composition and development of LGE tissue, and indeed cholinergic neurons have been isolated from MGE, but not from LGE (96,98,99). Watts et al. suggested that the presence of MGE potentiates the maturation of LGE, and this effect may be more significant when early donors are used (98). Using human donor tissue implanted into the excitotoxically lesioned striata of immunosuppressed rats, Grasbon-Frodl et al. suggested that LGE resulted in more striatal-like tissue than MGE (87), although in a separate study, the same group also suggested that graft survival was enhanced by the presence of MGE (100). Clarification of these issues is awaited, and in particular the influence of selective dissection on functional recovery.

To date, clinical practice has varied among the few groups of investigators who have proceeded to neural transplantation in humans (see later), with some groups choosing to transplant WGE and others LGE. Our own choice is to transplant WGE (possibly enriched with LGE when collections provide sufficient tissue) until such a time as these issues are more completely resolved, because this is the one dissection for which functional efficacy has been demonstrated in the primate (90), as well as in the rat.

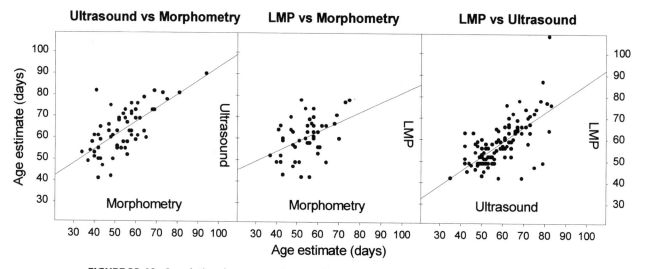

FIGURE 33.10. Correlations between estimates of human fetal age as determined by three different methods: measurement of morphometric parameters postmortem according to the formula of Studer et al., *in utero* measurement of crown rump length by ultrasound, and calculations based on last menstrual period using Nägele's rule. R, Pearson's coefficients of product-moment correlations.

Tissue Preparation

Graft tissue survives preparations involving either dicing the tissue into small pieces or preparing it as a cell suspension. Few studies to date have compared these approaches in animal models of HD (101), although a recent study using rodent embryonic tissue suggested that there is little to choose between them in terms of graft morphology (102).

Again, there is uncertainty about the amount of tissue to be transplanted, and indeed this information will presumably emerge from clinical transplantation studies. However, rodent studies have suggested that little is to be gained by grafting more than 500,000 cells as a single implant (approximately equivalent to one fetal striatum) (103). In this study, the proportion of striatal cells increased to 35% with single implants of 500,000 cells, and remained constant thereafter. Moreover, the proportion of striatal cells surviving implantation increased up to 500,000 cells and then diminished slightly with greater numbers. Two primate studies demonstrated functional recovery after transplantation, and these used between one striatum and two striata per implanted side (90,104).

Tissue Hibernation

The requirement for fresh human tissue in neural transplantation presents considerable logistical difficulties in terms of the timing of surgery. The procurement of viable tissue is unreliable, making the coordination of tissue collection and preparation of the patient on the same day problematic. In particular, the short period between collection and transplantation to obtain acceptable grafts has meant that physicians were required to start preparing patients for surgery,

including the fitting of a stereotactic frame, before the collection of sufficient viable tissue could be confirmed. Thus, investigators have searched for ways to circumvent this problem by using tissue storage protocols. Storage of tissue brings with it other advantages such as the ability to collect from more than one surgical list, the facility to transport tissue between centers, and the opportunity to undertake more detailed safety screening of the donor tissue itself. One obvious method of storage would be cryopreservation, but unfortunately this so reduces the viability of the tissue as to render this approach untenable in practice. However, it is possible to reduce tissue metabolism by a process termed *hibernation* (105), in which tissue is stored in a medium specifically designed to shut down metabolism, after which the tissue can be washed and transferred into a conventional medium for transplantation. This approach has been shown to be effective for storage of embryonic rat ventral mesencephalic cells for several days without an adverse effect on cell viability (106–108), and it has been confirmed for human ventral mesencephalic cells transplanted into rodent models of PD and has been employed in clinical studies (109,110). Similarly, rat striatal tissue can be successfully hibernated before transplantation in rat models of HD (111). Dong et al. demonstrated *in vitro* that human striatal tissue can be successfully hibernated (112), and our own studies confirmed that human striatal tissue survives transplantation in the rat excitotoxic striatal lesion model of HD after hibernation (94). In this last study, we confirmed little difference in graft survival between hibernated tissue and fresh tissues derived from embryos at various stages of development, although, as expected, the age of the embryos did themselves confirm a critical time window for effective grafts (Fig. 33.9).

Graft Placement

In human disease, grafts need to be placed in both the caudate and the putamen if the intention is to improve both cognition and motor deficits, because the putamen is known to have most of the motor connections and the caudate most of the cognitive connections. The animal model data to confirm this are discussed earlier in this chapter, for example, the evidence that a striatal graft needs to be placed into the denervated striatum to be functionally viable, whereas implantation into a pallidal target site is without functional effect (57). The optimum placement of grafts within these structures is unclear, although Kendall et al. found that greatest motor improvement was found when graft placement was more laterally within the putamen (90).

Timing of Surgery in Relation to the Course of the Disease

It is unknown to what extent the severity of the host disease influences the graft development, and thus there is no clear answer to the question at which stage of the disease transplantation should take place. Experimental animal studies using excitotoxic lesions show that grafts remain small and have less striatal tissue than in the nonlesioned compared with the lesioned striatum, but grafts placed into severely atrophic lesions also do less well than those in smaller lesions (113–115). From a clinical perspective, there are two further reasons for wanting to perform transplantation in early rather than late disease. First, in advancing disease, cortical atrophy increases. Currently, it is not known whether this represents a primary process or is largely the result of deafferentation of the cortex as the striatum degenerates. If the latter turns out to be the case, then it is important that transplantation occurs in relatively early disease, to have a chance of stopping this process. Second, with such experimental therapy, patients need to be able to consent fully to the procedure. In a disease such as HD in which cognitive decline is a major feature, this limits the procedure to the early stages of the disease until the procedure is established.

REVIEW OF PRELIMINARY CLINICAL STUDIES

Very little published literature pertains to the results of clinical neural transplantation in HD, although a few centers worldwide have embarked on clinical studies. At the time of writing, there are published reports of neural transplantation in patients with HD from four centers: in the United States, in Mexico, in Cuba, and in Czechoslovakia. All record some benefit (20,116–119). However, all these reports are based on what we would consider inadequate assessment protocols, that is, limited clinical and scanning data for inadequate periods, so proper evaluation of efficacy is difficult. The clinical details are particularly scant in the two earlier reports (117,119), and in the later single case report, although a much greater range of tests was administered, the motor tests were given a maximum of 25 weeks preoperatively and 29 weeks postoperatively, and neuropsychologic evaluation done was 2 months before and 4 months after surgical treatment. Variability of patient performance and possible perioperative artifacts (underlined in this report in which improvement at 3 days was reported, a time at which transplanted tissue could not have reconstructed circuitry) have led many investigators to conclude that much longer assessment times are required, as discussed in more detail earlier.

Other centers involved in neural transplantation trials at the time of writing include a group of investigators in Los Angeles who produced the 1998 single case report, a group in Tampa, Florida (120); and a multicenter European consortium in which the two most active groups are in Créteil, France, (121) and a multicenter United Kingdom group of investigators who have completed the first phase of their safety trial (121a,121b), and a further group of investigators in Kings College, London, who have also recently launched an independent program. An initial safety evaluation has been published on the first three patients from the Los Angeles team. Each patient received bilateral grafts in a single-stage operation from multiple donors. The grafts survived in all patients, as assessed by MRI, and grew within the implanted striatum without causing any displacement of surrounding tissue over a 1-year follow-up period. No patients demonstrated any adverse effects of the operation or the associated cyclosporine immunosuppression, nor did any patient exhibit clinical deterioration after the procedure. The authors concluded that "the limited experience provided by these three patients indicates that fetal tissue transplantation can be performed in HD patients without unexpected complications" (116).

Porcine xenotransplants have been performed in Boston in both HD and PD. A preliminary report of postmortem data from one PD patient has been published (122). However, we do not consider the immunosuppression regimens adopted for this xenotransplantation trial to be adequate, and survival of tissue was correspondingly poor.

SUMMARY

There is a sound basis of experimental animal model work on which to base the progression to clinical transplantation of human fetal tissue in HD. However, such clinical studies are extremely early in their genesis, and as yet there is no clear indication of the extent to which the procedure will prove clinically useful or whether it will produce unforeseen side effects. Indeed, many issues pertaining to the details of the approach are yet to be fully resolved, and many of these issues will be resolved only with further careful experimental animal and clinical studies. The importance at this stage of adequate patient assessment cannot be overemphasized if progress is to be made.

So the question "does neural transplantation have a place in HD?" is yet to be answered. If the answer is yes, then the future will lie in the identification of alternative sources of tissue for transplantation, because the ethical and practical constraints of using human fetal tissue are likely to limit its widespread application. Certain alternatives are being explored experimentally, including the use of xenograft tissue (most likely porcine), stem cells including neural stem cells and embryonic stem cells (ES cells), and genetically modified neural and nonneural tissue. Although various of lines of data suggest optimism for each of these approaches, each also has as yet unsolved problems, and none are yet ready for clinical application.

REFERENCES

1. Harper PS, ed. *Huntington's disease.* London: WB Saunders, 1996.
2. Huntington's Disease Collaborative Research Group. A novel gene containing a trinucleotide repeat that is expanded and unstable on Huntington's disease chromosomes. *Cell* 1993;72:971–983.
3. Jones AL. The Huntington's disease gene and its protein product. In: Harper PS, ed. *Huntington's disease.* London: WB Saunders, 1996:293–316.
4. Davies SW, Turmaine M, Cozens BA, et al. Formation of neuronal intranuclear inclusions (NII) underlies the neurological dysfunction in mice transgenic for the HD mutation. *Cell* 1997;90:537–548.
5. DiFiglia M, Sapp E, Chase KO, et al. Aggregation of huntingtin in neuronal intranuclear inclusions and dystrophic neurites in brain. *Science* 1997;277:1990–1993.
6. Lawrence AD, Hodges JR, Rosser AE, et al. Evidence for specific cognitive deficits in preclinical Huntington's disease. *Brain* 1998;121:1329–1343.
7. Van Vugt JP, Van Hilten BJ, Roos RA. Hypokinesia in Huntington's disease. *Mov Disord* 1996;11:384–388.
8. Brandt J, Butters N. Neuropsychological characteristics of Huntington's disease. In: Grant I, Adams KM, eds. *Neuropsychological assessment of neuropsychiatric disorders.* Oxford: Oxford University Press, 1996:321–341.
9. Lawrence AD, Sahakian BJ, Robbins TW. Cognitive functions and corticostriatal circuits: insights from Huntington's disease. *Trends Cogn Sci* 1998;2:379–388.
10. Vonsattel JP, Myers RH, Stevens TJ. Neuropathologic classification of Huntington's disease. *J Neuropathol Exp Neurol* 1985;44:559–577.
11. Haque NSK, Borghesani P, Isacson O. Therapeutic strategies for Huntington's disease based on a molecular understanding of the disorder. *Mol Med Today* 1997;3:175–183.
12. Feigin A, Kieburtz K, Como P, et al. Assessment of coenzyme Q10 tolerability in Huntington's disease. *Mov Disord* 1996;11:321–323.
13. Kieburtz K, Feigin A, McDermott M, et al. A controlled trial of remacemide hydrochloride in Huntington's disease. *Mov Disord* 1996;11:273–277.
14. Emerich DF, Winn SR, Hantraye P, et al. Protective effect of encapsulated cells producing neurotrophic factor CNTF in a monkey model of Huntington's disease. *Nature* 1997;386:395–399.
15. Peschanski M, Cesaro P, Hantraye P. Rationale for intrastriatal grafting of striatal neuroblasts in patients with Huntington's disease. *Neuroscience* 1995;68:273–285.
16. Brundin P, Fricker RA, Nakao N. Paucity of P-zones in striatal grafts prohibit commencement of clinical trials in Huntington's disease. *Neuroscience* 1996;71:895–897.
17. Shannon KM, Kordower JH. Neural transplantation for Huntington's disease: experimental rationale and recommendations for clinical trials. *Cell Transplant* 1996;5:339–352.
18. Peschanski M, Césaro P, Hantraye P. What is needed versus what would be interesting to know before undertaking neural transplantation in patients with Huntington's disease. *Neuroscience* 1996;71:899–900.
19. Dunnett SB, Björklund A. Mechanisms of function of neural grafts in the injured brain. In: Dunnett SB, Björklund A, eds. *Functional neural transplantation.* New York: Raven, 1994:531–567.
20. Kopyov OV, Jacques S, Kurth M, et al. Fetal transplantation for Huntington's disease: clinical studies. In: Freeman TB, Kordower JH, eds. *Cell transplantation for neurological disorders.* Totowa, NJ: Humana, 1998:95–134.
21. Sanberg PR, Borlongan CV, Wictorin K, et al. Fetal tissue transplantation for Huntington's disease: preclinical studies. In: Freeman TB, Kordower JH, eds. *Cell transplantation for neurological disorders.* Totowa, NJ: Humana, 1998:77–93.
22. Lindvall O. Prospects of transplantation in human neurodegenerative diseases. *Trends Neurosci* 1991;14:376–384.
23. Quinn NP, Brown R, Craufurd D, et al. Core assessment programme for intracerebral transplantation in Huntington's disease (CAPIT-HD). *Mov Disord* 1996;11:143–150.
24. Barker RA, Dunnett SB. *Neural repair, transplantation and rehabilitation.* Hove, UK: Psychology Press, 1999.
25. Coyle JT, Schwarcz R. Lesions of striatal neurones with kainic acid provides a model for Huntington's chorea. *Nature* 1976;263:244–246.
26. Ferrante RJ, Kowall NW, Cipolloni PB, et al. Excitotoxin lesions in primates as a model for Huntington's disease: histopathologic and neurochemical characterization. *Exp Neurol* 1993;119:46–71.
27. Sladek JR, Shoulson I. Neural transplantation: a call for patience rather than patients. *Science* 1988;240:1386–1388.
28. Palfi SP, Ferrante RJ, Brouillet E, et al. Chronic 3-nitropropionic acid treatment in baboons replicates the cognitive and motor deficits of Huntington's disease. *J Neurosci* 1996;16:3019–3025.
29. McGeer EG, Olney JW, McGeer PL. *Kainic acid as a tool in neurobiology.* New York: Raven, 1978.
30. Schwarcz R, Foster AC, French ED, et al. Excitotoxic models for neurodegenerative disorders. *Life Sci* 1984;35:19–32.
31. Beal MF, Brouillet EP, Jenkins BG, et al. Neurochemical and histologic characterization of striatal excitotoxic lesions produced by the mitochondrial toxin 3-nitropropionic acid. *J Neurosci* 1993;13:4181–4192.
32. Mangiarini L, Sathasivam K, Seller M, et al. Exon 1 of the HD gene with an expanded CAG repeat is sufficient to cause a progressive neurological phenotype in transgenic mice. *Cell* 1996;87:493–506.
33. Davies SW, Turmaine M, Cozens BA, et al. From neuronal inclusions to neurodegeneration: neuropathological investigation

of a transgenic mouse model of Huntington's disease. *Philos Trans R Soc Lond B Biol Sci* 1999;354:971–979.

34. Goldberg YP, Kalchman MA, Metzler M, et al. Absence of disease phenotype and intergenerational stability of the CAG repeat in transgenic mice expressing the human Huntington disease transcript. *Hum Mol Genet* 1996;5:177–185.

35. Martindale D, Hackam AS, Wieczorek A, et al. Length of huntingtin and its polyglutamine tract influences localization and frequency of intracellular aggregates. *Nat Genet* 1998;18:150–154.

36. Reddy PH, Williams M, Charles V, et al. Behavioural abnormalities and selective neuronal loss in HD transgenic mice expressing mutated full-length HD cDNA. *Nat Genet* 1998;20:198–202.

37. Schilling G, Becher MW, Sharp AH, et al. Intranuclear inclusions and neuritic aggregates in transgenic mice expressing a mutant N-terminal fragment of huntingtin. *Hum Mol Genet* 1999;8:397–407.

38. Wheeler VC, Auerbach W, White JK, et al. Length-dependent gametic CAG repeat instability in the Huntington's disease knock-in mouse. *Hum Mol Genet* 1999;8:115–122.

39. Sanberg PR, Coyle JT. Scientific approaches to Huntington's disease. *CRC Crit Rev Clin Neurobiol* 1984;1:1–44.

40. Divac I, öberg RGE, eds. *The neostriatum.* Oxford: Pergamon, 1979.

41. Divac I, Markowitsch HJ, Pritzel M. Behavioural and anatomical consequences of small intrastriatal injections of kainic acid in the rat. *Brain Res* 1978;151:523–532.

42. öberg RGE, Divac I. "Cognitive" functions of the neostriatum. In: Divac I, öberg RGE, eds. *The neostriatum.* Oxford: Pergamon, 1979:291–313.

43. Brasted P, Humby T, Dunnett SB, et al. Unilateral lesions of the dorsal striatum in rats disrupt responding in egocentric space. *J Neurosci* 1997;17:8919–8926.

44. Mittleman G, Brown VJ, Robbins TW. Intentional neglect following unilateral ibotenic acid lesions of the striatum. *Neurosci Res Commun* 1988;2:1–8.

45. Eagle DM, Humby T, Howman M, et al. Differential effects of ventral and regional dorsal striatal lesions on sucrose drinking and affective contrast in rats. *Psychobiology* 1999;27:267–276.

46. Eagle DM, Humby T, Dunnett SB, et al. Effects of regional striatal lesions on motor, motivational and executive aspects of progressive ratio performance in rats. *Behav Neurosci* 1999;113:716–731.

47. Rosvold HE, Szwarcbart MK. Neural structures involved in delayed response performance. In: Warren JM, Akert K, eds. *The frontal granular cortex and behavior.* New York: McGraw-Hill, 1964:1–15.

48. Rosvold HE. The frontal lobe system: cortical-subcortical interrelationships. *Acta Neurobiol Exp* 1972;32:439–460.

49. Geschwind N. Disconnexion syndromes in animals and man. I. *Brain* 1965;88:237–294.

50. Geschwind N. Disconnexion syndromes in animals and man. II. *Brain* 1965;88:585–644.

51. Alexander GE, DeLong MR, Strick PL. Parallel organization of functionally segregated circuits linking basal ganglia and cortex. *Annu Rev Neurosci* 1986;9:357–381.

52. Alexander GE, Crutcher MD. Functional architecture of basal ganglia circuits: neural substrates of parallel processing. *Trends Neurosci* 1990;13:266–271.

53. Schmidt RH, Björklund A, Stenevi U. Intracerebral grafting of dissociated CNS tissue suspensions: a new approach for neuronal transplantation to deep brain sites. *Brain Res* 1981;218:347–356.

54. Wictorin K. Anatomy and connectivity of intrastriatal striatal transplants. *Prog Neurobiol* 1992;38:611–639.

55. Deckel AW, Robinson RG, Coyle JT, et al. Reversal of long-term locomotor abnormalities in the kainic acid model of Huntington's disease by day 18 fetal striatal implants. *Eur J Pharmacol* 1983;92:287–288.

56. Isacson O, Brundin P, Kelly PAT, et al. Functional neuronal replacement by grafted striatal neurons in the ibotenic acid lesioned rat striatum. *Nature* 1984;311:458–460.

57. Isacson O, Dunnett SB, Björklund A. Graft-induced behavioral recovery in an animal model of Huntington disease. *Proc Natl Acad Sci USA* 1986;83:2728–2732.

58. Dunnett SB, Isacson O, Sirinathsinghji DJS, et al. Striatal grafts in rats with unilateral neostriatal lesions. III. Recovery from dopamine-dependent motor asymmetry and deficits in skilled paw reaching. *Neuroscience* 1988;24:813–820.

59. Fricker RA, Torres EM, Hume SP, et al. The effects of donor stage on the survival and function of embryonic striatal grafts. II. Correlation between positron emission tomography and reaching behaviour. *Neuroscience* 1997;79:711–722.

60. Montoya CP, Astell S, Dunnett SB. Effects of nigral and striatal grafts on skilled forelimb use in the rat. *Prog Brain Res* 1990;82:459–466.

61. Dunnett SB, Whishaw IQ, Rogers DC, et al. Dopamine-rich grafts ameliorate whole body motor asymmetry and sensory neglect but not independent limb use in rats with 6- hydroxy-dopamine lesions. *Brain Res* 1987;415:63–78.

62. Graybiel AM, Liu FC, Dunnett SB. Intrastriatal grafts derived from fetal striatal primordia. 1. Phenotypy and modular organization. *J Neurosci* 1989;9:3250–3271.

63. Björklund A, Campbell K, Sirinathsinghji DJS, et al. Functional capacity of striatal transplants in the rat Huntington model. In: Dunnett SB, Björklund A, eds. *Functional neural transplantation.* New York: Raven, 1994:157–195.

64. Clarke DJ, Wictorin K, Dunnett SB, et al. Internal composition of striatal grafts: light and electron microscopy. In: Percheron G, McKenzie JS, Féger J, eds. *The basal ganglia. IV. New ideas on structure and function.* New York: Plenum, 1994:189–196.

65. Sirinathsinghji DJS, Mayer E, Fernandez JM, et al. The localisation of CCK mRNA in embryonic striatal tissue grafts: further evidence for the presence of non-striatal cells. *Neuroreport* 1993;4:659–662.

66. Clarke DJ, Dunnett SB. Synaptic relationships between cortical and dopaminergic inputs and intrinsic GABAergic systems within intrastriatal striatal grafts. *J Chem Neuroanat* 1993;6:147–158.

67. Rutherford A, Garcia-Muñoz M, Dunnett SB, et al. Electrophysiological demonstration of host cortical inputs to striatal grafts. *Neurosci Lett* 1987;83:275–281.

68. Xu ZC, Wilson CJ, Emson PC. Synaptic potentials evoked in spiny neurons in rat neostriatal grafts by cortical and thalamic stimulation. *J Neurophysiol* 1991;65:477–493.

69. Campbell K, Wictorin K, Björklund A. Differential regulation of neuropeptide mRNA expression in intrastriatal striatal transplants by host dopaminergic afferents. *Proc Natl Acad Sci USA* 1992;89:10489–10493.

70. Sirinathsinghji DJS, Dunnett SB, Isacson O, et al. Striatal grafts in rats with unilateral neostriatal lesions. II. *In vivo* monitoring of GABA release in globus pallidus and substantia nigra. *Neuroscience* 1988;24:803–811.

71. Boer GJ. Ethical guidelines for the use of human embryonic or fetal tissue for experimental and clinical neurotransplantation and research. *J Neurol* 1994;242:1–13.

72. Polkinghorne J. *Review of the guidance on the research use of*

fetuses and fetal material. London: Her Majesty's Stationery Office, 1989.

73. Langston JW, Widner H, Goetz CG. Core assessment program for intracerebral transplantation (CAPIT). *Mov Disord* 1992;7: 2–13.

74. Albanese A, Aebischer P, Annett LE, et al. NIH neural transplantation funding [Letter]. *Science* 1994;263:737.

75. Freeman TB, Vawter D, Goetz CG, et al. The use of cosmetic surgical placebo controlled trial in the treatment of Parkinson's disease. *Soc Neurosci Abstr* 1995;21:1756.

76. Freeman TB, Vawter D, Goetz CG, et al. Fetal mesencephalic transplants in Parkinson's disease: indications for the use of a cosmetic surgical placebo-controlled protocol. *Exp Neurol* 1995;135:164–164.

77. Peschanski M, Defer G, Dethy S, et al. Towards a phase III multicenter study of fetal ventral mesencephalic transplants in patients with late-stage Parkinson's disease. In: Freeman TB, Widner H, eds. *Cell transplantation for neurological disorders.* Totowa, NJ: Humana, 1998:31–43.

78. Kieburtz K, Penney JB, Como P, et al. Unified Huntington's disease rating scale: reliability and consistency. *Mov Disord* 1996;11:1360–142.

79. Shoulson I, Penney JB, Kieburtz K, et al. Safety and tolerability of the free-radical scavenger OPC-14117 in Huntington's disease. *Neurology* 1998;50:1366–1373.

80. Van Vugt JP, Siesling S, Vergeer M, et al. Clozapine versus placebo in Huntington's disease: a double blind randomised comparative study. *J Neurol Neurosurg Psychiatry* 1997;63:35–39.

81. Siesling S, Van Vugt JPP, Zwinderman KAH, et al. Unified Huntington's disease rating scale: a follow up. *Mov Disord* 1998;13:915–919.

82. Shannon KM, Penn RD, Kroin JS, et al. Stereotactic pallidotomy for the treatment of Parkinson's disease: efficacy and adverse effects at 6 months in 26 patients. *Neurology* 1998;50:434–438.

83. Kazumata K, Antonini A, Dhawan V, et al. Preoperative indicators of clinical outcome following stereotaxic pallidotomy. *Neurology* 1997;49:1083–1090.

84. Duff J, Sime E. Surgical interventions in the treatment of Parkinson's disease (PD) and essential tremor (ET): medical pallidotomy in PD and chronic deep brain stimulation (DBS) in PD and ET. *Axone* 1997;18:85–89.

85. Nauert GM, Freeman TB. Low-pressure aspiration abortion for obtaining embryonic and early gestational fetal tissue for research purposes. *Cell Transplant* 1994;3:147–151.

86. Evtouchenko L, Studer L, Spenger C, et al. A mathematical model for the estimation of human embryonic and fetal age. *Cell Transplant* 1996;5:453–464.

87. Grasbon-Frodl EM, Nakao N, Lindvall O, et al. Phenotypic development of the human embryonic striatal primordium: a study of cultured and grafted neurons from the lateral and medial ganglionic eminence. *Neuroscience* 1996;73:171–183.

88. Brundin P. Dissection, preparation, and implantation of human embryonic brain tissue. In: Dunnett SB, Björklund A, eds. *Neural transplantation: a practical approach.* Oxford: IRL Press, 1992:139–160.

89. Björklund A, Stenevi U. Intracerebral neural implants: neuronal replacement and reconstruction of damaged circuitries. *Annu Rev Neurosci* 1984;7:279–308.

90. Kendall AL, Rayment FD, Torres EM, et al. Functional integration of striatal allografts in a primate model of Huntington's disease. *Nat Med* 1998;4:727–729.

91. Naimi S, Jeny R, Hantraye P, et al. Ontogeny of human striatal DARPP-32 neurons in fetuses and following xenografting to the adult rat brain. *Exp Neurol* 1996;137:15–25.

92. Pundt LL, Kondoh T, Conrad JA, et al. Transplantation of human striatal tissue into a rodent model of Huntington's disease: phenotypic expression of transplanted neurons and host-to-graft innervation. *Brain Res Bull* 1996;39:23–32.

93. Pundt LL, Kondoh T, Conrad JA, et al. Transplantation of human fetal striatum into a rodent model of Huntington's disease ameliorates locomotor deficits. *Neurosci Res* 1996;24:415–420.

94. Hurrelbrink CB, Armstrong RJE, Barker RA, et al. Hibernated human fetal striatal tissue: successful transplantation in a rat model of Huntington's disease. *Cell Transplant* 2000;9:743–749.

95. Pakzaban P, Deacon TW, Burns LH, et al. Increased proportion of acetylcholinesterase-rich zones and improved morphological integration in host striatum of fetal grafts derived from the lateral but not the medial ganglionic eminence. *Exp Brain Res* 1993;97:13–22.

96. Olsson M, Campbell K, Wictorin K, et al. Projection neurons in fetal striatal transplants are predominantly derived from the lateral ganglionic eminence. *Neuroscience* 1995;69:1169–1182.

97. Deacon TW, Pakzaban P, Isacson O. The lateral ganglionic eminence is the origin of cells committed to striatal phenotypes: neural transplantation and developmental evidence. *Brain Res* 1994;668:211–219.

98. Watts C, Torres EM, White DJG, et al. Implantation of embryonic porcine nigral and striatal tissues into rat models of Parkinson's and Huntington's diseases: graft-host interactions. *Exp Neurol* 1999.

99. Watts C, Dunnett SB, Rosser AE. Effect of embryonic donor age and dissection on the DARPP-32 content of cell suspensions used for intrastriatal transplantation. *Exp Neurol* 1997;148:271–280.

100. Grasbon-Frodl EM, Nakao N, Lindvall O, et al. Developmental features of human striatal tissue transplanted in a rat model of Huntington's disease. *Neurobiol Dis* 1997;3:299–311.

101. Fricker RA, Barker RA, Fawcett JW, et al. A comparative study of preparation techniques for improving the viability of striatal grafts using vital stains, *in vitro* cultures and *in vivo* grafts. *Cell Transplant* 1996;5:599–611.

102. Watts C, Brasted PJ, Dunnett SB. The morphology, integration and functional efficacy of striatal grafts differs between cell suspensions and tissue pieces. *Cell Transplant* 2000;9:395–407.

103. Watts C, Dunnett SB. The development of intrastriatal striatal grafts is influenced by the numbers of LGE cells implanted. *Cell Transplant* 1999.

104. Palfi S, Condé F, Riche D, et al. Fetal striatal allografts reverse cognitive deficits in a primate model of Huntington's disease. *Nat Med* 1998;4:963–966.

105. Kawamoto JC, Barrett JN. Cryopreservation of primary neurons for tissue culture. *Brain Res* 1986;384:84–93.

106. Thajeb P, Ling ZD, Potter ED, et al. The effects of storage conditions and trophic supplementation on the survival of fetal mesencephalic cells. *Cell Transplant* 1997;6:297.

107. Nikkhah G, Eberhard J, Olsson M, et al. Preservation of fetal ventral mesencephalic cells by cool storage: *in vitro* viability and TH-positive neuron survival after microtransplantation to the striatum. *Brain Res* 1995;687:22–34.

108. Sauer H, Brundin P. Effects of cool storage on survival and function of intrastriatal ventral mesencephalic grafts. *Restor Neurol Neurosci* 1991;2:123–135.

109. Freeman TB, Olanow CW, Hauser RA, et al. Fetal nigral

transplantation into the postcommissural putamen in Parkinson's disease: the USF experience. *J Neurosurg* 1995;82:A354.

110. Kordower JH, Freeman TB, Snow BJ, et al. Neuropathological evidence of graft survival and striatal reinnervation after the transplantation of fetal mesencephalic tissue in a patient with Parkinson's disease. *N Engl J Med* 1995;332:1118–1124.

111. Grasbon-Frodl EM, Nakao N, Brundin P. The lazaroid U-83836E improves the survival of rat embryonic mesencephalic tissue stored at 4°C and subsequently used for cultures or intracerebral transplantation. *Brain Res Bull* 1996;39:341–347.

112. Dong JF, Detta A, Hitchcock ER. Susceptibility of human fetal brain tissue to cool storage and freeze storage. *Brain Res* 1993;621:242–248.

113. Labandeira-Garcia JL, Wictorin K. Development and integration of intrastriatal striatal grafts implanted into long-term ibotenate lesions. *J Neural Transplant Plast* 1992;3:181–182.

114. Labandeira-Garcia JL, Wictorin K, Cunningham ET, et al. Development of intrastriatal striatal grafts and their afferent innervation from the host. *Neuroscience* 1991;42:407–426.

115. Watts C, Dunnett SB. Effects of severity of host striatal damage on the morphological development of intrastriatal transplants in a rodent model of Huntington's disease: implications for timing of surgical development. *J Neurosurg* 1998;89:367–374.

116. Kopyov OV, Jacques S, Lieberman A, et al. Safety of intrastriatal neurotransplantation for Huntington's disease patients. *Exp Neurol* 1998;119:97–108.

117. Madrazo I, Franco-Bourland RE, Castrejon H, et al. Fetal striatal homotransplantation for Huntington's disease: first two case reports. *Neurol Res* 1995;17:312–315.

118. Philpott LM, Kopyov OV, Lee AJ, et al. Neuropsychological functioning following fetal striatal transplantation in Huntington's chorea: three case presentations. *Cell Transplant* 1997;6:203–212.

119. Sramka M, Rattaj M, Molina H, et al. Stereotactic technique and pathophysiological mechanisms of neurotransplantation in Huntington's chorea. *Stereotact Funct Neurosurg* 1992;58:793.

120. Freeman TB, Hauser RA, Willing AE, et al. Transplantation of human fetal striatal tissue in Huntington's disease: rational for clinical studies. *Neural transplantation in neurodegenerative disease: Novartis symposium no. 231.* London: Novartis Foundation, 2000.

121. Bachoud-Lévy AC, Bourdet C, Brugières P, et al. Safety and tolerability assessment of intrastriatal neural allografts in Huntington's disease patients. *Exp Neurol* 2000;161:194–202.

121a. Bachoud-Lévi A, Bourdet C, Brugiéres P, et al. Safety and tolerability assessment of intrastriatal neural allografts in five patients with Huntington's disease. *Exp Neurol* 2000;161(1): 194–202.

121b. Bachoud-Lévi AC, Remy P, Ngayen JP, et al. Motor and cognitive improvements in patients with Huntington's disease after neurol transplantation. *Lancet* 2000;356(9246):1975–1979.

122. Deacon T, Schumacher J, Dinsmore J, et al. Histological evidence of fetal pig neural cell survival after transplantation into a patient with Parkinson's disease. *Nat Med* 1997;3:350–353.

123. Watts C, Brasted PJ, Eagle DM, et al. Embryonic donor age and dissection influence striatal graft development and functional integration in a rodent model of Huntington's disease. *Exp Neurol* 2000;163:85–97.

Surgery for Parkinson's Disease and Movement Disorders,
edited by J.K. Krauss, J. Jankovic, and R.G. Grossman.
Lippincott Williams & Wilkins, Philadelphia © 2001.

34

MICROVASCULAR DECOMPRESSION FOR TREATMENT OF HEMIFACIAL SPASM

DANIEL K. RESNICK
PETER J. JANNETTA

Hemifacial spasm (HFS) is a condition characterized by spasmodic, intermittent, uncontrolled contraction of the facial muscles on one side of the face. Symptoms usually occur in a middle-aged or older adult, although pediatric cases have been reported (1). Symptoms are almost invariably limited to one side; however, bilateral HFS has been documented in a few patients (2). Women are more frequently afflicted than men (3,4). The typical presentation is one of a rostrocaudal progression of spasms from the upper face to the lower face, although the reverse may be seen in up to 10% of patients (5,6). The disorder is uncommon, with an estimated prevalence of approximately 7 in 100,000 men and 14 in 100,000 women (7). Those affected may be severely distressed by the recurrent, uncontrolled, and occasionally disfiguring spasms. HFS may also be associated with underlying facial weakness, especially in patients who manifest a tonus phenomenon. The widespread use of botulinum toxin may temporarily exacerbate this underlying weakness.

HISTORICAL BACKGROUND

Multiple procedures were proposed earlier for the treatment of HFS; however, none except microvascular decompression (MVD) demonstrated long-term efficacy, and all involved the purposeful production of facial paresis. These techniques generally involved partial or complete ablation of the facial nerve as it emerged from either the stylomastoid foramen or the parotid gland. German described a partial section technique that led to less severe facial paresis, but this investigator was not able to demonstrate efficacy beyond 1 to 2 years (8). Alcohol injections at the stylomastoid foramen were also

attempted. This procedure produced complete facial paralysis, followed by a gradual return of function and spasm over 4 to 6 months (9). Ehni and Woltman carried out neurolysis of the facial nerve in its bony canal, but they abandoned this procedure when they recorded an 80% failure rate (4). Bragdon was the first to attempt treatment of HFS by an intracranial route. He crushed the facial nerve within the cerebellopontine angle with a hemostat. This maneuver resulted in lasting relief from spasm, as well as permanent facial palsy (10).

The intracranial portion of the facial nerve was further implicated in the pathogenesis of HFS by the observations of Cushing, Dandy, Laine, and Campbell. In 1917, Dandy reported the occurrence of HFS in four of 30 patients with tumors of the cochlear nerve (11). Dandy also described some cases of HFS associated with tumors of the cerebellopontine angle (12). Laine reported HFS in a patient with a cirsoid aneurysm of the basilar artery (13). Campbell and Keedy reported the same vascular disease in two patients with a combination of HFS and trigeminal neuralgia (14).

The first vascular decompression procedure aimed at the intracranial portion of the facial nerve was reported by Gardner, in 1960. Gardner described a 36-year-old woman with typical HFS. Exploration of the facial nerve in the cerebellopontine angle revealed compression of the nerve by a loop of the internal auditory artery. The loop was mobilized away from the nerve (which appeared normal) and was held away with a small piece of gelatin foam (Gelfoam). This patient's symptoms were markedly improved and remained improved through a 5-year follow-up period (15). Gardner continued to explore the cerebellopontine angle in patients with HFS and ultimately reported his findings and results in 19 patients. Gardner found vascular compression by a redundant anterior inferior cerebellar artery in seven patients and by the internal auditory artery in one patient (other findings included cirsoid aneurysms of the basilar artery in three patients, arteriovenous malformations in three, and

D.K. Resnick: Department of Neurological Surgery, University of Wisconsin Medical School, Madison, Wisconsin 53792.

P.J. Jannetta: Department of Neurological Surgery, University of Pittsburgh School of Medicine, Pittsburgh, Pennsylvania 15213.

displacement of the pons in one). In four patients, Gardner was unable to find a causative lesion. Gardner decompressed all cases of vascular compression and manipulated the nerve in each case. His overall results were 12 patients with an immediate cure, five patients with delayed improvement, and two patients with no improvement. There were no failures and no recurrences in the group of patients who were found to have vascular compression and who underwent a decompressive procedure (3).

Jannetta introduced the operating microscope into the treatment of cranial rhizopathies (16). Using the microscope, Jannetta was able to demonstrate vascular compression in virtually all patients explored for HFS and was able both to improve cure rates and to reduce morbidity significantly. In the first 47 patients treated, Jannetta was able to identify a compressive vessel in 46 (one patient had a small cholesteatoma). Of 45 patients with typical HFS, excellent results were obtained in 38 (no spasm), and good results were noted in two (trace spasm). One patient developed permanent facial weakness, and three patients developed hearing loss as a result of the operation (17). Progressive improvements in operative technique and in facial and cochlear nerve monitoring have led to further gains in the safety and efficacy of the procedure (see later). At present, MVD remains the only effective long-term treatment for HFS.

MICROVASCULAR DECOMPRESSION
Patient Selection and Preoperative Evaluation

Virtually all patients with HFS may be considered candidates for operation. The only absolute contraindication for MVD in these patients is prohibitive anesthetic risk. There is no effective medical treatment for HFS, and the cumulative cost of multiple botulinum toxin injections is likely not significantly different from that of a single operative procedure. Severe contralateral hearing loss may be considered a relative contraindication, because there is still a 1% to 4% risk of hearing loss even when the procedure is performed by the most experienced surgeons (5). These patients are probably best managed by referral to a center with an active cranial rhizopathy practice.

All patients with HFS should undergo magnetic resonance imaging to rule out pathologic lesions that may first manifest as HFS. Tumors, aneurysms, and arteriovenous malformations have all been reported to present with HFS as their first symptom (17–19). The pathologic lesion likely causes vascular compression of the facial nerve by distorting the local arterial anatomy. It is also important to rule out malformations of the skull base, because these can influence the operative procedure. For example, patients with Chiari I malformations should undergo posterior fossa decompression before retromastoid craniectomy because the abnormally small posterior fossa makes the usual approach

for MVD much more difficult and hazardous. The magnetic resonance imaging scan can also document dolichoectatic arteries in the region of interest. Recognition of these arteries aids in the surgeon's preoperative planning. Finally, plain skull radiographs or computed tomography scans with bone reconstruction can be helpful by delineating the posterior extension of the mastoid air cells.

Operative Technique

The patient is anesthetized while supine on the operating table. Pneumatic compression stockings, appropriate intravenous and intraarterial lines, and monitoring electrodes are placed. A three-point head holder is affixed to the skull, and the patient is rolled into the lateral "park bench" position. An axillary roll and a pillow between the legs aid in the prevention of compression neuropathies. It is important to secure the patient to the table with tape, to allow rotation of the table during the approach and the decompression. The head is placed in a military position of "attention," with extension of the neck and capital flexion. For MVD of the facial nerve, the vertex of the head is tilted downward 5 to 10 degrees. The anteroposterior axis of the head should be level with the floor (Fig. 34.1). A strip of hair behind the ear, beginning just above the pinna and approximately 3 cm in width, is shaved, and the area is prepared. Before draping, the mastoid process and the level of the external auditory canal are marked. The intersection of the sinuses occurs at or near the intersection of a vertical line along the posterior border of the mastoid process and a line drawn from the external auditory canal to the inion (Fig. 34.2). The incision for MVD of the facial nerve begins just behind the hairline, just caudal to the top of the pinna, and extends caudally and posteriorly, staying just behind the hairline, for a distance of 5 to 8 cm. The field is draped, and the incision is made sharply. Subcutaneous tissues are divided with electrocautery. Caution should be exercised during the deep muscle dissection caudally, because the vertebral artery lies close to the plane of dissection.

The dissection continues caudally until the floor of the posterior fossa is encountered. This is marked by the acute angulation of the skull base toward the foramen magnum. The dissection usually requires the division of the occipital artery; however, efforts should be made to preserve the occipital nerve when possible. An adequate dissection exposes the asterion, the root of the mastoid process, and the beginning of the digastric groove. The initial bur hole is placed 4 to 5 cm posterior to the external auditory meatus along an extension of an imaginary line connecting the lateral canthus to the external auditory meatus. This places the bur hole away from the sinuses. Bone rongeurs or a high-speed drill is used to complete the craniectomy. When the procedure is complete, the edge of the sigmoid sinus is exposed from its junction with the transverse sinus to the jugular bulb.

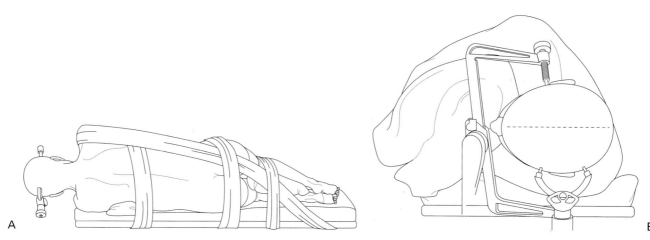

FIGURE 34.1. Operative positioning. Posterior **(A)** and rostral **(B)** views of patient in "park bench" position. The vertex is parallel to the floor or is tilted slightly downward. The anteroposterior plane of the head should be parallel to the floor.

A crescent-shaped dural opening is created, based laterally with the rostral end at the junction of the sinuses and the caudal end approaching the jugular bulb. Dural tack-up sutures are placed close to the base of the flap to provide crucial millimeters of exposure. The operative microscope is brought into play, and a rubber dam and cottonoid are placed over the exposed cerebellum. A malleable, self-retaining retractor is used for elevation of the cerebellum off the skull base. The retractor should be bent approximately 70 degrees, and the distal blade should be kept straight so as not to avoid "toeing in" of the retractor against the cerebellum or brainstem. The

tip of the retractor should be tapered so the tip is approximately 2 mm across. The initial angle of approach is slightly caudal to direct lateral and is aimed at the caudal cranial nerves (IX to XI). Rotating the patient away from the surgeon at the beginning of the approach allows visualization of the petrous bone. As the dissection continues, the patient is rotated progressively toward the surgeon to minimize retraction of the cerebellum. The arachnoid over the caudal nerves is opened sharply, and the retractor is used to elevate the cerebellum gently off the caudal cranial nerves, thus exposing the choroid plexus as it exits the foramen of Luschka.

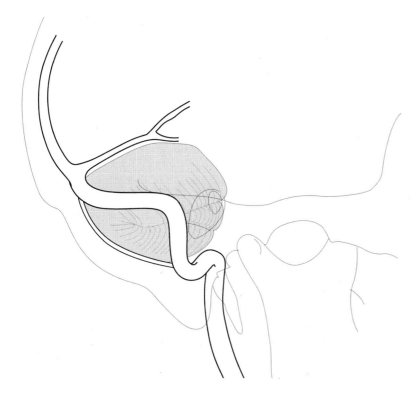

FIGURE 34.2. Incision planning. The mastoid process is palpated and marked, and a line connecting the external auditory meatus to the inion is drawn. The intersection of this line with the posterior border of the mastoid process marks the confluence of the sinuses.

The retractor blade is now adjusted to assume a caudal to rostral orientation with the tip of the retractor blade lying just in front of or on the choroid plexus. It is often helpful to rotate the patient 15 to 20 degrees toward the surgeon to facilitate visualization of the facial nerve as it runs from the pontomedullary junction toward the vestibulocochlear nerve.

Intraoperative Clinicopathologic Correlation

In typical (or classic) HFS, the causative vessel is usually found to be compressing the nerve from a caudal and anterior direction. The site of compression is the root entry zone as the facial nerve exits the pons. Figure 34.3 illustrates the usual site of compression in typical HFS. Figures 34.4 and 34.5 are operative photographs from two patients with typical HFS. The causative vessel is usually the posterior inferior cerebellar artery; however, the anterior inferior cerebellar artery may be involved in more than one-third of cases. Only rarely are unnamed small arteries or veins alone responsible for the compressive lesion (fewer than 6% of cases). The vertebral artery itself may contribute to the compression, especially in older patients and on the left side (Fig. 34.5) (5).

The nature of compression in atypical HFS (progression of the spasm from the lower face to the upper face) is different. In these patients, the site of compression is rostral and posterior to the nerve at the root entry zone. Figure 34.6 illustrates the findings in cases of atypical HFS. In either typical or atypical HFS, it is imperative to have a clear understanding of the expected pathologic features before operative

correction is attempted. The surgeon must be skilled, well prepared, and determined to locate and treat the pathologic vessels.

Decompression Technique

In cases of typical HFS, the compressing vessel is anterior and caudal to the pontine portion of the facial nerve. It is usually possible to mobilize the offending vessel off the nerve (Figs. 34.5B and 34.6). Extreme care must be taken to preserve branches that enter the pons, because these branches may be considered end arteries, and any vessel sacrificed may result in a brainstem infarction. Once the artery is mobilized, shredded Teflon felt is placed to move the vessel away from the facial nerve. Small veins should be coagulated and divided. It is important to divide the vessel completely, because recanalization does occur and may lead to a recurrence of symptoms.

The pathologic process of atypical HFS differs from that of typical HFS. In atypical spasm, in which the spasms start in the buccal muscles and work their way rostrally, the blood vessel is almost always rostral and posterior to the nerve as it exits the pons. The exposure should be more rostral, but the usual caudal extent should be maintained. A caudal vessel may loop up onto the rostral side of the nerve, and this can be mobilized in the usual fashion. If the vessel is a vein, it should be coagulated and divided in multiple locations. If an artery is running between the facial and the vestibulocochlear nerves (Fig. 35.6), a serious problem will exist because this anterior inferior cerebellar artery branch usually has one perforator to the brainstem. The artery must be separated from the

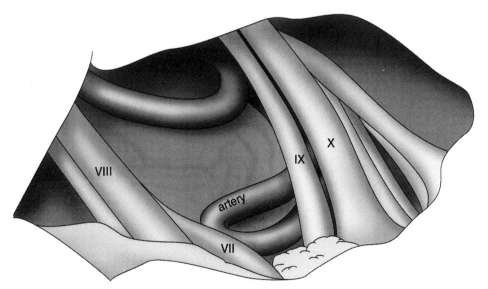

FIGURE 34.3. This figure illustrates the usual site of compression seen in typical hemifacial spasm (on the right side). The arterial loop (usually the anterior or posterior inferior cerebellar artery) compresses the facial nerve as it emerges from the pons on its caudal and lateral aspect. This figure is based on the operative photograph shown in Fig. 34.4.

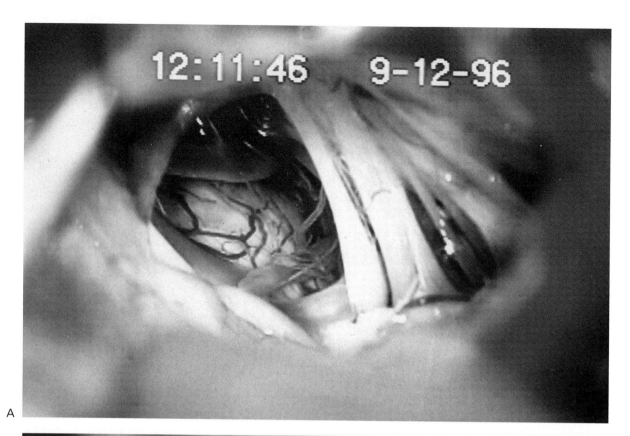

A

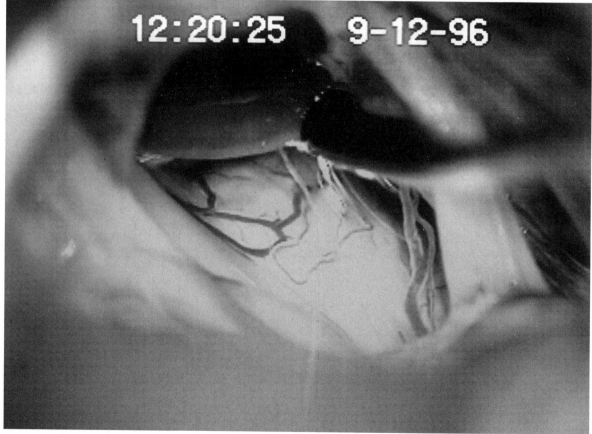

B

FIGURE 34.4. A: This is an operative photograph from a patient with typical right-sided hemifacial spasm. Note the arterial loop compressing the nerve as it emerges from the pons on its caudal and lateral aspect. **B:** The vessel can be mobilized away from the root entry zone with gentle manipulation. A piece of Teflon felt is then placed under the artery to hold it away from the facial nerve. Care must be taken not to damage any perforating vessels in this region. (See Color Figure 34.4.)

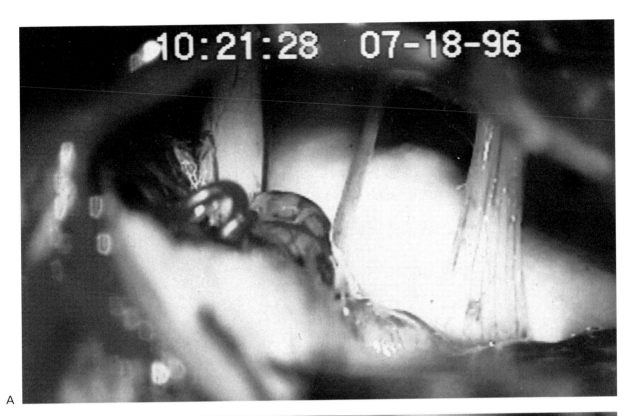

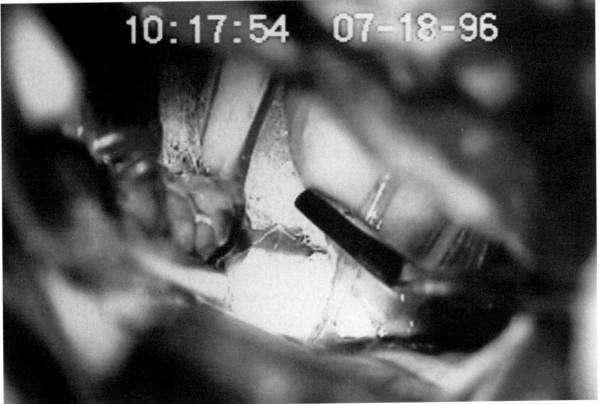

FIGURE 34.5. A: This photograph, also from a patient with typical hemifacial spasm, demonstrates compression of the nerve by an ectatic vertebral artery. **B:** Decompression in this case is accomplished by gradual mobilization of the vessel beginning caudal to the lower cranial nerves and moving progressively rostrally. Felt is used to lift the artery gradually and carefully off the facial root entry zone. (See Color Figure 34.5.)

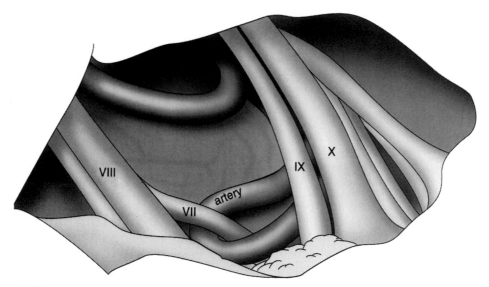

FIGURE 34.6. The site of compression seen in atypical hemifacial spasm. Here, the vessel runs medial and rostral to the facial nerve. Mobilization of this vessel is hampered by its close relation to the cochlear and vestibular nerves. Compare this situation with the usual case, illustrated in Fig. 34.3.

brainstem rostrally and off the facial nerve caudally. Small wisps of Teflon felt are placed between the nerve and artery progressively, beginning at the brainstem, with care taken not to tear the perforator. If there is no perforator, the artery should be moved as far distally as possible away from the root entry zone. There is an increased risk of hearing loss with atypical HFS, and the patient needs to be forewarned.

In either typical or atypical HFS, intraoperative neurophysiologic monitoring is extremely useful. Changes (delays of wave V or loss of amplitude) in intraoperative brainstem auditory evoked potentials are an indication of impending damage to the cochlear nerve and brainstem nuclei and should prompt the surgeon immediately to lessen the amount of cerebellar or brainstem retraction used. Facial nerve monitoring is also extremely useful, because the loss of lateral spread on mobilization of a blood vessel provides reliable feedback to the surgeon that the pathologic vessel has been identified and treated. We believe that the information gained from such monitoring is so useful that we ask patients who have undergone recent botulinum toxin injections to delay the operation for 6 months, to allow for adequate facial nerve monitoring (botulinum toxin injection interferes with neuromuscular transmission and hides the lateral spread phenomenon).

Results

MVD is an effective treatment for HFS. In the most recently published series of 703 patients reported by Barker and Jannetta et al., more than 90% of patients operated on for typical HFS had immediate relief of their spasm on recovery from anesthesia. After 1 year, 86% of these patients reported an excellent outcome, and 5% reported significant improvement. At 10 years after operation, 79% of patients still reported excellent results, and 5% report partial success. Eleven patients who failed to improve immediately underwent reexploration within 30 days of the surgical procedure, and 10 of these patients achieved excellent long-term results (5). Most recurrences occurred within the first few years after operation, and recurrences after 10 years were extremely uncommon. Operative results for patients operated on for late recurrences (more than 30 days after the initial operation) were not as good as for the early reoperation group. In the series of Barker and Jannetta et al., of the 49 patients who underwent late reoperation, 61% reported excellent long-term relief.

The pattern of spasm was an important predictor of operative success. Overall, only 70% of patients with atypical HFS had an immediate relief of spasm. Overall, long-term (more than 10 years) cure rates for patients with a typical HFS were also less gratifying than the results for patients with typical symptoms. At 10 years postoperatively, only 59% of patients reported excellent relief of symptoms (5).

Other factors associated with outcome were the patient's sex and the operative findings. Men fared significantly better than women. Finally, when operative findings were limited to small, unnamed vessels (arteries or veins), then the results of surgical treatment were worse (5).

In another large series, Huang et al. reported their results in 310 patients with typical HFS. The mean follow-up period was 4.3 years, and the operative findings were very similar to those described earlier of Barker and Jannetta et al. Huang et al. reported an 88% excellent immediate outcome rate, with an additional 5.2% of patients who had a delayed improvement of their symptoms after MVD (20).

Complications

MVD of the facial nerve is a procedure that demands exceptional attention to detail and excellent operative technique. Despite the technical difficulties associated with the operation, complication rates are low when the procedure is performed by experienced surgeons.

In the series reported by Barker and Jannetta et al. of more than 700 patients who underwent MVD for HFS at the University of Pittsburgh, there was one operative death in a patient who was referred for reoperation for recurrent HFS. This patient also had a Chiari malformation. She developed progressive brainstem signs immediately after the procedure and was brought back to the operating room for an emergency suboccipital craniectomy. After this procedure, she was extubated, but she later suffered respiratory arrest (perhaps from narcotic administration) and ultimately died. Other complications noted in this series were brainstem infarction (0.3%), facial weakness (3.2%, transient; 1.8%, mild permanent; 2.4%, moderate or severe permanent), hearing loss (2.7%, deaf ear), and cerebrospinal fluid leak (2.4%) (5). Intraoperative monitoring of facial nerve function (performed since 1980) has dramatically decreased the incidence of postoperative facial weakness. In the foregoing series, only two cases of facial weakness occurred in the last 480 operative procedures. Electrophysiologic monitoring has also resulted in a substantially lower incidence of hearing loss. The rate of hearing loss before the use of monitoring was 4.8%. Since the introduction of routine brainstem auditory evoked response monitoring in 1980, the incidence of hearing loss has been reduced to 1.9% (5).

CONCLUSION

Vascular compression of the facial nerve as it exits the brainstem underlies the pathophysiology of HFS. There is no effective medical treatment for HFS. Botulinum toxin injections provide temporary relief of symptoms. The site of vascular compression determines the nature of the symptoms, with compression from a caudal and anterior vector causing typical spasms and compression from a rostral and posterior vector causing atypical spasms. The operating surgeon must have a clear idea of the expected pathologic features to perform the decompression procedure effectively. Outstanding technical skills and adequate neurophysiologic monitoring are essential for the safe and efficacious application of this technique. When used correctly, MVD results in long-term cure in more than 80% of patients, with a low morbidity rate. If patients fail to show improvement in their symptoms within the first 48 to 72 hours postoperatively, early reexploration is recommended.

REFERENCES

1. Levy EI, Resnick DK, Jannetta PJ, et al. Pediatric hemifacial spasm: the efficacy of microvascular decompression. *Pediatr Neurosurg* 1998;27:238–241.
2. Tan EK, Jankovic J. Bilateral hemifacial spasm: a report of 5 cases and a literature review. *Mov Disord* 1999;14:345–349.
3. Gardner WJ, Sava GA. Hemifacial spasm: a reversible pathophysiological state. *J Neurosurg* 1962;19:240–247.
4. Ehni, G, Woltman HW. Hemifacial spasm: review of 106 cases. *Arch Neurol Psychiatry* 1945;53:205–211.
5. Barker FG, Jannetta PJ, Bissonette DJ, et al. Microvascular decompression for hemifacial spasm. *J Neurosurg* 1995;82:201–210.
6. Wang A, Jankovic J. Hemifacial spasm: clinical correlates and treatments. *Muscle Nerve* 1998;21:1740–1747.
7. Auger RG, Whisnant JP. Hemifacial spasm in Rochester and Olmstead County, Minnesota, 1960 to 1984. *Arch Neurol* 1990; 47:1233–1234.
8. German WJ. Surgical treatment of spasmodic facial tic. *Surgery* 1942;11:912–914.
9. Greenwood J. The surgical treatment of hemifacial spasm. *J Neurosurg* 1946;3:506–510.
10. Bragdon FH. Intracranial crushing of facial nerve for hemifacial spasm. Paper presented at the 46th Annual Clinical Congress of the American College of Surgeons, San Francisco, 1960.
11. Cushing H. *Tumors of the nervus acusticus and the syndrome of the cerebellopontile angle.* Philadelphia: WB Saunders, 1917.
12. Revilla AG. Neurinomas of the cerebellopontine recess: a clinical study of one hundred and sixty cases including operative mortality and end results. *Johns Hopkins Hosp Bull* 1947;80:254–296.
13. Laine E, Nayrac P. Hémispasme facial guéri par intervention sur la fosse postérieure. *Rev Neurol (Paris)* 1948;80:38–40.
14. Campbell E, Keedy C. Hemifacial spasm: a note on the etiology in two cases. *J Neurosurg* 1947;4:342–347.
15. Gardner WJ. Five year cure of hemifacial spasm. *CleveClin Q* 1960; 27:219–221.
16. Jannetta PJ. Microsurgical exploration and decompression of the facial nerve in hemifacial spasm. *Curr Top Surg Res* 1970;2:217–220.
17. Jannetta PJ, Abbasy M, Maroon JC, et al. Etiology and definitive microsurgical treatment of hemifacial spasm. *J Neurosurg* 1977;47:321–328.
18. Maroon JC, Lunsford LD, Deeb ZL. Hemifacial spasm due to aneurysmal compression of the facial nerve. *Arch Neurol* 1978;35:545–546.
19. Glocker FX, Krauss JK, Deuschl G, et al. Hemifacial spasm due to posterior fossa tumors: the impact of tumor location on electrophysiological findings. *Clin Neurol Neurosurg* 1998;100:104–111.
20. Huang CI, Chen IH, Lee LS. Microvascular decompression for hemifacial spasm: analyses of operative findings and results in 310 patients. *Neurosurgery* 1992;30:53–56.

Surgery for Parkinson's Disease and Movement Disorders,
edited by J.K. Krauss, J. Jankovic, and R.G. Grossman.
Lippincott Williams & Wilkins, Philadelphia © 2001.

35

SURGICAL TREATMENT
OF BLEPHAROSPASM

IVAN P. HWANG
RICHARD L. ANDERSON
DAVID R. JORDAN

Essential blepharospasm is a condition defined by involuntary spasm of the orbicularis oculi, the corrugator, and the procerus muscles around the eyelids (1) (Fig. 35.1). The occurrence of contractions of these muscles may be intermittent, progressive, or persistent. Blepharospasm may be isolated in the eyelid region, but more commonly it is part of a spectrum of dystonic movements involving facial, oral, mandibular, pharyngeal, or cervical muscles (2).

If there are associated intermittent midfacial movements with blepharospasm, the disorder is referred to as *Meige's syndrome* (also called orofacial dystonia or spasm facial median), which was described by Henry Meige in 1910 (3) (Fig. 35.2). The involvement of lower facial, mandibular, and cervical muscles in association with blepharospasm is termed oromandibular dystonia syndrome or *Brueghel's syndrome* (4) (Fig. 35.3). This designation is in reference to a painting by the sixteenth-century Flemish artist Brueghel that depicts a person with grotesque facial and eyelid spasms, the first record of blepharospasm with marked lower facial dystonia (Fig. 35.4).

Another important condition associated with essential blepharospasm is apraxia of eyelid opening. Patients with blepharospasm with apraxia of eyelid opening are unable to open their eyes even with maximal effort in the absence of blepharospasm (5,6) (Figs. 35.5 and 35.6). Jordan, Anderson, and Digre reported a 7% incidence of apraxia of eyelid opening in patients with essential blepharospasm (7). In our experience, approximately 50% of our referred patients in whom botulinum A toxin therapy failed demonstrated apraxia of eyelid opening. Therefore, recognition of the common association of blepharospasm with apraxia of eyelid opening is important to proper medical and surgical treatment of the patient. Other syndromes associated with

blepharospasm include idiopathic torsion dystonia, segmental cranial dystonia (or craniocervical dystonia), nuchal dystonia, and spastic dyspnea (8).

Although essential blepharospasm is often associated with other movement disorders, the greatest disability is related to the muscle contracture around the eyelids that, at times, may cause severe functional visual impairment. In our experience, the disability from blepharospasm not only limits a person's occupational performance, but also affects a person's daily function on an intermittent and often continuous basis. The unpredictable nature of the spasms also creates a tremendous amount of stress and frustration for a person suffering from blepharospasm. It is not unusual in advanced stages of blepharospasm for patients to be functionally blind and to become socially reclusive and unable to care for themselves. Therefore, any therapy that can alleviate the blepharospasm and can improve functional vision is greatly appreciated by these patients.

HISTORY AND DEVELOPMENT
OF SURGICAL TREATMENT

Since the early twentieth century, multiple procedures have been proposed for the treatment of blepharospasm including alcohol injection of the facial nerve, neurotomy, neurectomy, and selective facial nerve avulsion (9–17). These early treatments were directed at the innervation of the contracting muscles in essential blepharospasm (cranial nerve VII). Although destruction of the facial nerve was a logical approach to the problem of blepharospasm, the consequence of destroying the facial nerve carried a high recurrence rate (18), as well as severe side effects, as reported by Henderson in 1956 (19). These side effects included aggravation of brow ptosis, blepharoptosis, dermatochalasis, and eyelid malposition, most of which are usually already present in patients with blepharospasm (Fig. 35.7). Other side effects included lip paresis, drooping of the mouth, sequestration of saliva in

I.P. Hwang: California Eye Clinic, Antioch, California 94509.
R.L. Anderson: Salt Lake City, Utah 84102.
D.R. Jordan: Eye Institute, University Of Ottawa, Ottawa, Ontario, Canada K2P 1A4.

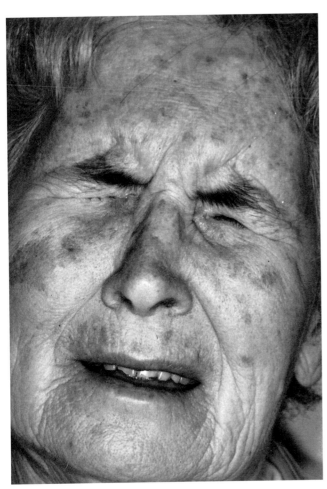

FIGURE 35.1. Essential blepharospasm with involuntary contraction of the orbicularis oculi, the corrugator, and the procerus muscles around the eyelids.

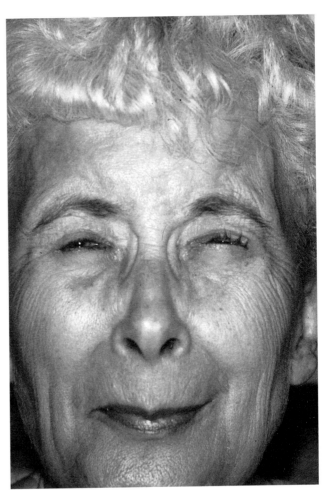

FIGURE 35.2. Meige's syndrome demonstrating eyelid spasm with midfacial contractions.

the parotid gland, loss of facial expression, and the inability to close the eyes (lagophthalmos). Lagophthalmos after facial nerve destruction can lead to chronic corneal exposure and can exacerbate one of the most common causes of blepharospasm, reflex irritation of the eyes (20).

Bates et al. found that 42% of patients undergoing facial nerve avulsion also needed concurrent reconstructive eyelid procedures (21). Grandas et al. reported that 22 of 27 (81.5%) patients developed a recurrence of blepharospasm within 1 year of bilateral facial nerve avulsion (22). McCord et al. (23) noted that patients who had undergone facial nerve avulsion (Reynold's procedure) had a 4.5 times higher frequency of requiring a secondary procedure than patients who had undergone myectomy (Anderson's procedure) (18,21,24,25–32).

Having been displeased with the complications and high recurrence rate of neurectomy, Anderson et al. began their early surgical "myectomy procedures" initially in 1974 (18), and Gillum and Anderson published the first description of the myectomy operation in 1981 (24). Since this publication, articles describing and updating the myectomy procedures have been reported (21,23,25–32).

The "full myectomy" procedure described by Anderson et al. requires the complete removal of the protractor muscles of eyelid closure (the orbicularis oculi, the corrugator, and the procerus muscles). Some surgeons have considered this procedure a neuromyectomy, but the peripheral nerves do regenerate, whereas the protractor muscles of eyelid closure do not. In a survey of 1,653 patients, Anderson et al. found that 1,455 of 1,653 (88%) patients in whom medical and botulinum A toxin therapy had failed and who had undergone the full myectomy procedure noted marked improvement (18).

The full myectomy is a technically demanding and difficult procedure requiring anatomic and surgical expertise. Favorable results are directly related to the meticulous removal of the protractor muscles of eyelid closure. Complication rates vary and are related to the initial surgical procedure and the experience in postoperative management. The surgical approach and treatment algorithm are discussed later in the chapter.

In the 1980s, the discovery of botulinum A toxin treatments for essential blepharospasm was described by Scott et al. after initially reporting its use for correcting

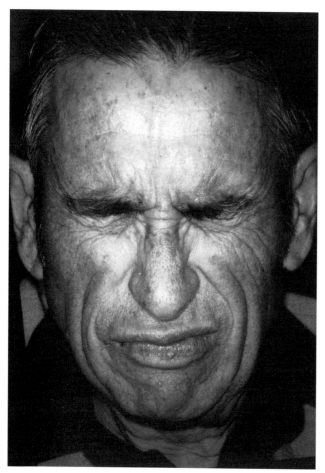

FIGURE 35.3. Brueghel's syndrome showing blepharospasm with associated spasms in the lower face and neck regions.

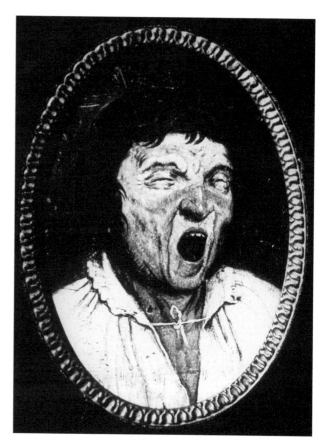

FIGURE 35.4. *De Gaper* by the sixteenth-century Flemish painter Pieter Brueghel the Elder that depicts the oromandibular dystonia syndrome or Brueghel's syndrome.

strabismus (33,34). In 1989, botulinum A toxin was approved by the United States Food and Drug Administration, and since then, the treatment of essential blepharospasm has changed dramatically. Botulinum A toxin has become one of the main nonsurgical treatment for patients with essential blepharospasm. Now, extended limited myectomy and full myectomy are reserved for patients in whom medical treatment or botulinum A toxin therapy fails or provides inadequate relief.

ETIOLOGY

The pathophysiology of essential blepharospasm remains elusive. Although the theory that blepharospasm is the result of a single defective locus within the central nervous system may be valid, postmortem neuropathologic studies have been unsuccessful in localizing the pathologic features (1,23). Postmortem regional neurochemical examinations, however, have detected areas of adrenergic preponderance and depletion (35,36). It also has been reported that a genetic predisposition is identifiable in 33% of patients with essential blepharospasm (26).

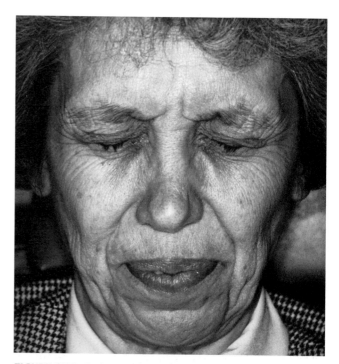

FIGURE 35.5. Patient with blepharospasm and associated apraxia of eyelid opening during eyelid spasm. During eyelid spasm, the diagnosis of apraxia of eyelid opening is not apparent and cannot be made.

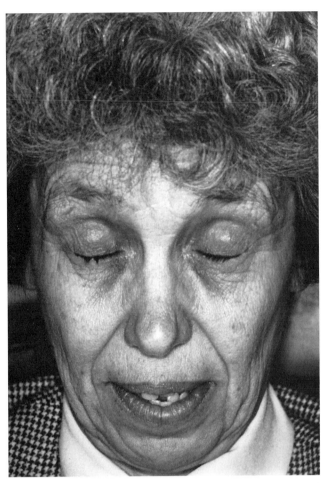

FIGURE 35.6. The same patient as Fig. 35.5, now without eyelid spasm. Despite the lack of eyelid spasm, note the inability to raise the eyelids even with maximal eyelid elevation effort as evidenced by the maximally elevated eyebrows.

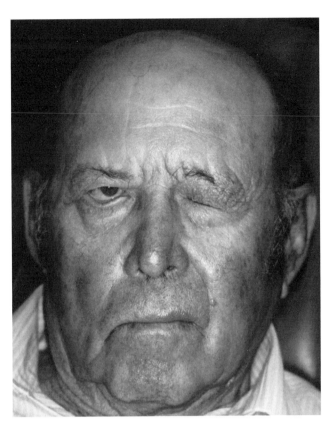

FIGURE 35.7. A patient after selective facial neurectomy. Notice the aggravation of brow ptosis, blepharoptosis, lower lid retraction, lower lid ectropion, and facial palsy on the "successful" right side of the face and the recurrence of blepharospasm on the unsuccessful left side of the face.

We propose that essential blepharospasm is the result of a "vicious cycle" consisting of three main subunits: the afferent limb, the central processing unit, and the efferent limb (Fig. 35.8). The afferent limb provides the initial stimulus of the vicious cycle, which is multifactorial and may consist of light, corneal irritation, eyelid inflammation, periocular irritation, emotional instability, psychiatric instability, and internal stress. The central processing unit lies within the central nervous system and may exist within the basal ganglia, midbrain, or brainstem (1,35,37–40). The efferent limb consist of the facial nucleus, facial nerve, and the protractor muscles of eyelid closure.

Patients with essential blepharospasm may have a predisposition in the central processing unit to develop a neurochemical imbalance as a result of an overwhelming stimulus or a combination of strong stimuli leading to increased output to the efferent limb and resulting in uncontrollable eyelid spasms. The amount, type, and timing of the stimulus that can create such a situation varies tremendously from patient to patient, as suggested by clinical testimony. However, once a stimulus or a combination of stimuli creates the imbalance or overrides the ability of the central processing unit to mod-

ulate the input from the afferent limb to the output of the efferent limb, the cycle can no longer be properly regulated. The result is a vicious cycle in which the output from the efferent limb increases the input from the afferent limb with an overwhelmed central processing unit that clinically translates to a gradual and persistent worsening of eyelid spasms. This cycle may also affect other regulatory movement systems, as evidenced by the development of other associated dystonias in up to 80% of patients with essential blepharospasm (8).

Keeping this simple algorithm in mind, it is logical that therapy must be directed to all three components of the vicious cycle (Fig. 35.8), to alleviate the symptoms of the patient and possibly to slow the progression of the disease. Therefore, expedient and proper clinical diagnosis of essential blepharospasm is essential to maximize the benefits to the patient.

CLINICAL PRESENTATION

The diagnosis of essential blepharospasm is based on clinical judgment, and there is currently no specific laboratory diagnostic test. Because the clinical presentations and the history of the illness usually vary and are often indistinct, proper diagnosis may be challenging. In the survey of

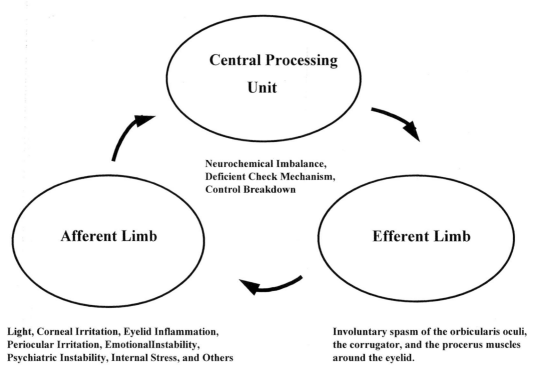

Central Processing Unit

Neurochemical Imbalance,
Deficient Check Mechanism,
Control Breakdown

Afferent Limb

Efferent Limb

Light, Corneal Irritation, Eyelid Inflammation,
Periocular Irritation, EmotionalInstability,
Psychiatric Instability, Internal Stress, and Others

Involuntary spasm of the orbicularis oculi,
the corrugator, and the procerus muscles
around the eyelid.

FIGURE 35.8. The vicious cycle of essential blepharospasm.

1,653 patients with essential blepharospasm by Anderson et al. (18), patients reported visiting an average of five physicians before receiving the correct diagnosis, with a range of one to 75 physicians. Fifty-nine percent of the patients reported a cost greater than $1,000 before they obtained the proper diagnosis, and 1% of the patients reported a cost exceeding $50,000.

The mean age of onset for essential blepharospasm has been reported to be approximately 56 years (18,19). Female-to-male ratio is 3:1 (2,4,19,41). Often, patients present with variable episodes of increased blinking lasting from seconds to minutes. As the term "vicious cycle" suggests, the increased blinking typically progresses to involuntary eyelid spasms and eyelid closure causing severe functional disability. Factors that commonly aggravate and precipitate blepharospasm include sunlight, stress, fatigue, driving, reading, and watching television. Often, patients do not know what event triggers the eyelid spasms.

Fortunately, many patients with blepharospasm have developed abilities, habits, or "tricks" to alleviate or temporarily halt the cycle of essential blepharospasm. These tricks include humming, singing, whistling, yawning, coughing, opening the mouth, chewing gum, pinching the nose, wiping across the eyes, continuously talking, applying pressure to parts of the face, concentrating on other problems, playing games, and even playing piano.

Although essential blepharospasm is typically bilateral, the disease may present in the beginning as unilateral or predominantly unilateral. With time, blepharospasm gradually becomes bilateral and may be more involved on one side

compared with the other. Occasionally, the patient with essential blepharospasm may only report unilateral symptoms, but careful observation will reveal bilateral eyelid spasms to the observer.

When suspecting the diagnosis of essential blepharospasm, one must keep in mind several other entities in the differential diagnosis (Table 35.1). Corneal irritation from keratitis sicca, spastic entropion, eyelash abnormalities (such as trichiasis or distichiasis), blepharitis, and other irritating

TABLE 35.1. DIFFERENTIAL DIAGNOSIS OF ESSENTIAL BLEPHAROSPASM

Essential blepharospasm[a]
Meige's syndrome (idiopathic orofacial dystonia)[a]
Breughel's syndrome (oromandibular facial dystonia)[a]
Segmental cranial dystonia[a]
Reflex or secondary blepharospasm
Hemifacial spasm
Parkinson's disease
Progressive supranuclear palsy
Huntington's chorea
Apraxia of eyelid opening
Drugs (antihistamines, levodopa-induced dyskinesia)
Tardive dyskinesia
Myokymia
Tics
Hysteria
Wilson's disease
Encephalitis

[a]These phenomenologic entities may all be manifestations of primary or secondary dystonia.

conditions of the eyelid may cause reflex blepharospasm. Intraocular conditions such as anterior uveitis and posterior subcapsular cataracts can be associated with photophobia and ocular pain and cause reflex blepharospasm. Examples of other conditions that may mimic essential blepharospasm are hemifacial spasm and orbicularis myokymia (8).

TREATMENT OF ESSENTIAL BLEPHAROSPASM

Treatment of the Afferent Limb

Treatment for essential blepharospasm can be directed to each arm of the vicious cycle (i.e., afferent limb, central processing unit, and efferent limb). With regard to the afferent component of the disease, any process that leads to irritation of the eyelids and ocular surface (e.g., blepharitis, meibomianitis, trichiasis, distichiasis, entropion) should be treated and, if possible, eliminated. Keeping the eyelids clean can significantly reduce eyelid margin inflammation as well as provide a healthy tear film in patients with blepharitis and meibomianitis. Eliminating misdirected eyelashes and correcting eyelid position decrease ocular irritation in patients with trichiasis, distichiasis, and entropion. Dry and irritated ocular surfaces can be alleviated with artificial tear supplements in the day and lubricating tear ointment at night before sleeping. Keeping the relative room humidity higher than 40% with humidifiers (we prefer heat-generated models) in the home environment is often helpful for patients with dry eye. Many patients with essential blepharospasm report painful light sensitivity (oculophotodynia), which may be improved significantly with tinted eyeglasses. In our experience, the afferent limb of the vicious cycle can nearly always be improved and is very important to the treatment of essential blepharospasm.

Treatment of the Central Processing Unit

Treatment of the central processing unit is also important in the vicious cycle model of essential blepharospasm. Therapies include group support and education, professional psychiatric counseling, and systemic drug therapy.

The Benign Essential Blepharospasm Research Foundation was founded by Mattie Lou Koster in 1981. Koster and her daughter, Mary Lou Thompson, have provided tremendous support and relief for patients with essential blepharospasm. The organization has continued to improve awareness of essential blepharospasm, to organize support groups for patients and families around the United States, and to fund research to understand the origin of the disease and to improve treatment. All patients diagnosed with essential blepharospasm need to be informed of this organization and should be encouraged to contact it because it provides education, group support, and treatment (Benign Essential Blepharospasm Research Foundation, Inc., P.O. Box 12468, Beaumont, TX 77726-2468; telephone: 409-832-0890).

Many patients with essential blepharospasm are strong "type A" personalities. They tend to become more frustrated and stressed with the inability to control the opening of their eyelids than the average population. This, in turn, may cause a worsening of the ability of the central processing unit to regulate the information flow from the afferent limb to the efferent limb. In another words, the check mechanism of the central processing unit becomes faulty and can no longer regulate or control the output to the efferent limb; the result is uncontrollable squeezing of the eyelids. Perhaps, as the central processing unit deteriorates further during the progression of essential blepharospasm, other related dystonias manifest themselves as a spillover effect from the inability of the central processing unit to maintain appropriate output signals to the other efferent units along the facial nerve. Therefore, in some cases, professional psychiatric counseling may be beneficial to patients with essential blepharospasm patient in helping them to understand their personality and to control their stress and frustrations. In this way, the central processing unit may be prevented from deteriorating in the cycle of blepharospasm.

Systemic pharmacologic therapy of this condition is currently a "shotgun" approach directed at the central processing unit because we do not yet understand the cause or location of the central processing unit in the brain. The medications used to treat essential blepharospasm are based on three unproved theories of cholinergic excess, γ-aminobutyric acid (GABA)hypofunction, and dopamine excess (18). In our experience, the most effective medications appear to be the anticholinergic drugs, followed by GABAergic drugs and systemic sedative drugs. Results often vary tremendously from patient to patient, and systemic side effects can be intolerable to most patients' lifestyles. The duration and the degree of improvement also can be discouraging. We usually use systemic medications only as an adjunct to botulinum A toxin in a limited number of patients.

Treatment of the Efferent Limb

Treatment of the efferent limb of the vicious cycle of blepharospasm is aimed at decreasing the function of the protractor muscles of eyelid closure (the orbicularis oculi, the corrugator, and the procerus muscles). At present, botulinum A toxin offers the most effective initial treatment for protractor muscle spasm.

Subcutaneous injections of the botulinum toxin into the upper eyelids, lower eyelids, brows, and glabellar regions provide effective temporary relief to patients with eyelid spasms (Fig. 35.9). Care must be taken not to inject the area above the central upper eyelid, to avoid affecting the levator muscle and to prevent ptosis. If the botulinum A toxin diffuses into the deeper tissue around the eye, extraocular muscles may be affected, and binocular diplopia can result. In our experience, the complications associated with diffusion of botulinum A toxin into adjacent tissues can be minimized

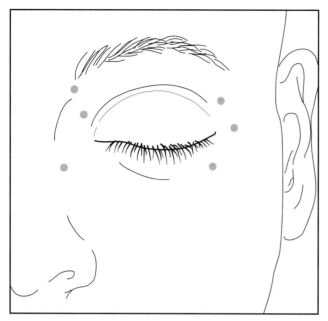

FIGURE 35.9. Illustration of injection sites for the subcutaneous injection of botulinum A toxin.

by using a concentration of 10 units of botulinum A toxin to 0.1 mL of sterile 0.9% sodium chloride.

Common side effects of botulinum A toxin include dry eye symptoms, the inability to close the eyelid (lagophthalmos) completely, and exposure keratitis. We recommend preservative-free artificial tear supplements during the daytime and preservative-free artificial tear ointments before bedtime as long as the patient has dry eye symptoms (ocular foreign body sensations, burning, and blurry vision). Generally, systemic side effects such as nausea and general weakness are rare, usually transient, and well tolerated by these patients.

The duration of relief from botulinum A toxin varies and has been reported to range from 6 to 28 weeks (42). In our experience, botulinum A toxin injections are effective in most patients for 12 to 16 weeks. Most of these patients return for repeat injections at 12-week intervals.

The exact quantity of injection and the maximally effective sites for injection may vary among patients and should be carefully documented and customized to each individual patient. An increased frequency and higher doses of botulinum A toxin injections may be needed with time in some patients because they develop resistance to the agent. Binding of botulinum A toxin to large protein chains and antitoxins and regrowth of motor end plates have been suggested to be the cause of resistance (34,43–46).

Botulinum A toxin injections offer symptomatic relief to most patients. In a survey of 1,083 patients who received botulinum A toxin injections, Anderson et al. reported that 86% of these patients reported improvement in blepharospasm symptoms (18). Sixty-six percent of these patients reported that the duration of relief was longer than

3 months. This finding demonstrates the high level of patient satisfaction, long duration, and general effectiveness of botulinum A toxin injections for essential blepharospasm.

Despite the effectiveness of botulinum A toxin, however, many patients are not adequately relieved by the injections alone. Some are primary treatment failures, and others develop resistance with repeated injections of the botulinum A toxin. Those patients who obtain adequate protractor muscle weakening with botulinum A toxin but who also suffer from apraxia of eyelid opening will not benefit from further weakening of the protractor muscles of eyelid closure. We often see patients with apraxia of eyelid opening who continue to receive higher and higher doses of botulinum A toxin despite a satisfactory weakening of the squeezing muscles around the eyelid. Increasing the dosage of botulinum A toxin in this situation could lead to an increased risk of ptosis as a result of paralyzing the levator muscle and could exacerbate the patient's inability to open the eyelids. Patients with apraxia of eyelid opening need surgical treatment to advance the levator aponeurosis, to correct functional brow and eyelid abnormalities, and to remove the upper eyelid orbicularis muscle (limited myectomy).

Many patients with essential blepharospasm demonstrate brow ptosis, dermatochalasis, and lower eyelid laxity that may be aggravated by botulinum A toxin injections. Patients with continual tight squeezing of the eyelids, brows, and periocular tissue over a long period often develop tissue laxity resulting from stretching of the elastic connective tissue. Once the squeezing muscles are weakened by botulinum A toxin injections, these functional structural abnormalities manifest themselves and may require surgical treatment. Correction of these problems will improve the patients' ability to open the eyelids and, ultimately, will enlarge the visual field and thus aid the ability to see. Therefore, brow position, eyelid position, and periocular tissue laxity are very important in the assessment for surgical treatment of essential blepharospasm. Clinically significant eyelid and periocular abnormalities should be surgically corrected for maximal visual benefit and symptomatic relief.

CONTEMPORARY SURGICAL TREATMENT OF BLEPHAROSPASM

We generally identify two groups of patients with essential blepharospasm in whom botulinum A toxin treatments fail. The first group of patients comprises those who do not obtain functionally adequate relief from their eyelid squeezing. The second group of patients comprises those who obtain adequate relief of the squeezing around their eyelids, but they also suffer from apraxia of eyelid opening, as previously discussed. For these patients, surgical removal of the protractor muscles of eyelid closure is the next best option.

Currently, we offer the extended limited myectomy procedure (with botulinum A toxin injection as an adjunct if

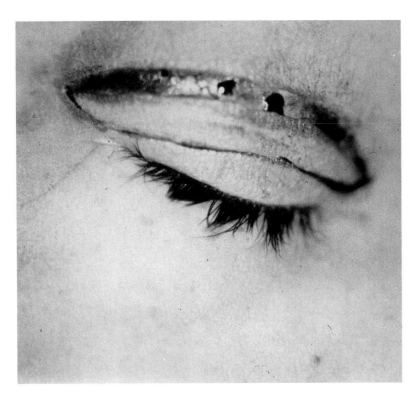

FIGURE 35.10. The extended limited myectomy procedure is performed through an upper eyelid crease incision.

needed) as the first step when considering the myectomy operation. If this does not provide the patient adequate symptomatic relief, we proceed to the full myectomy procedure.

Extended Limited Myectomy

The extended limited myectomy procedure is performed through an eyelid crease incision and involves the removal of the pretarsal orbicularis muscle, the preseptal orbicularis muscle, part of the orbital orbicularis muscle, and part of the corrugator superciliaris muscle (Fig. 35.10). The levator aponeurosis is often also tightened to correct upper eyelid position because it is frequently stretched as a result of long-term forceful eyelid squeezing. Excess skin and fat are also removed with tightening of the lateral canthal tendon to reconstruct the proper anatomy and elasticity of the eyelids. The orbicularis muscle around the lateral raphe and the temporal portion of the lower eyelids are also removed. In conjunction, we raise the suborbicularis oculi fat temporally to fill the hollow left after myectomy in this region. Frequently, to correct mild to moderate brow ptosis, we release the aponeurotic attachments to the brow and improve functional and aesthetic results.

In our experience, after extended limited myectomy procedures, patients recover much faster, with less lymphedema, ecchymosis, supraorbital anesthesia, or hypesthesia, compared with patients after the full myectomy procedure. Because the procedure involves less protractor muscle removal, patients who undergo extended limited myectomy also tend to have fewer corneal surface exposure problems and dry eyes than patients who undergo full myectomy initially. Patients commonly report an improvement in the intensity of squeezing of the protractor muscles that allows them to open their eyelids and to tolerate the remaining residual amount of squeezing. With botulinum A toxin as an effective adjunct to the extended limited myectomy procedure, almost all patients report a significant improvement in eyelid squeezing.

Often, patients in whom botulinum A toxin injections failed before extended limited myectomy respond to botulinum A toxin after the procedure. Therefore, we recommend retreatment with botulinum A toxin after extended limited myectomy even if this treatment had previously failed.

Full Myectomy

Patients in whom extended limited myectomy and adjunct botulinum A toxin fail should undergo full myectomy (Fig. 35.11). The full myectomy procedure involves the removal of as much of the remaining orbicularis oculi muscles as possible (including the lower eyelids) with removal of all the procerus and the corrugator muscles as well. The second full myectomy procedure is performed through a brow incision above and a blepharoplasty incision in the lower eyelids. After the orbicularis oculi muscle is removed from the lower eyelids, the lateral canthal tendon is again tightened, and the suborbicularis oculi fat and midface are lifted to prevent a "step-off" effect in the lower eyelid to midface area.

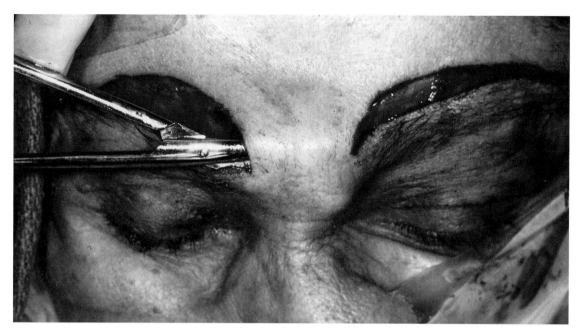

FIGURE 35.11. The full myectomy procedure is performed through a brow incision, and the remaining orbicularis oculi muscle, corrugator, and procerus muscles are removed.

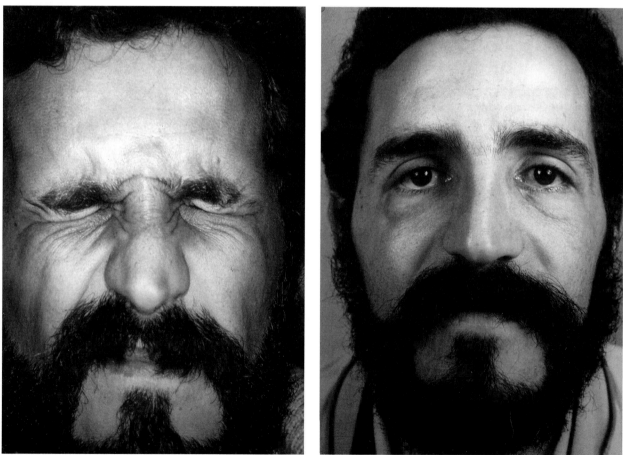

FIGURE 35.12. A: Preoperative view of a patient with essential blepharospasm with severe uncontrollable squeezing of the eyelids and part of the midface. **B:** The same patient postoperatively after the full myectomy procedure.

The reason to perform full myectomy as the second procedure is that postoperative hematoma and lymphedema after the full myectomy procedure do not migrate down to the patient's upper eyelids because of tissue adhesion from the previous extended limited myectomy procedure. This situation allows the patient to have significantly less upper eyelid lymphedema after the full myectomy procedure, with a minimal decrease in functional vision. Upper eyelid lymphedema is of utmost importance and concern because it may last for weeks, months, and even years. Patients with significant upper eyelid edema cannot open their eyelids because of mechanical resistance, and it can be a very difficult problem to resolve. The goal of surgical treatment is to improve eyelid opening, and therefore, avoiding long-term upper eyelid edema is an important consideration in the postoperative care of the patient with essential blepharospasm.

Other potential complications of the myectomy procedures include infection, hematoma, brow hair loss, skin damage from tissue ischemia, upper eyelid retraction, lower eyelid retraction, trichiasis, lateral canthal deformity, and visual loss. Fortunately, in our experience of more than 800 procedures, there has not been a case of visual loss after the myectomy procedures. Our experience is similar to that of others, including the long-term follow-up of a large number of patients treated with protractor myectomy at the Mayo Clinic (47).

CONCLUSIONS

In conclusion, treatment of essential blepharospasm aims at decreasing the stimuli to the three components of the vicious cycle. The afferent limb treatment includes eliminating all stimuli that lead to irritation of the eyelids and ocular surface. Group support, professional counseling, and systemic drug therapy are treatment options for the central processing unit. The efferent limb can be alleviated with botulinum A toxin injections and the myectomy procedures (Fig. 35.12). Therefore, a clear understanding and a systematic approach to the treatment and management of essential blepharospasm are important in the treatment of the debilitating problems associated with this disease.

REFERENCES

1. Jankovic J. Clinical features, differential diagnosis, and pathogenesis of blepharospasm and cranial-cervical dystonia. In: Bosniak SG, Smith BC, eds. *Advances in ophthalmic plastic and reconstructive surgery: blepharospasm.* New York: Pergamon, 1985:67–93.
2. Patrinely JR, Anderson RL. Essential blepharospasm: a review. *Geriatr Ophthalmol* 1986;2:27–33.
3. Meige H. Les convulsion de la face: une forme clinique de convulsion faciale, bilateral et médiane. *Rev Neurol (Paris)* 1970;10:437–443.
4. Marsden CD. Blepharospasm: oromandibular dystonia syndrome (Brueghel's syndrome): a variant of adult-onset torsion dystonia. *J Neurol Neurosurg Psychiatry* 1976;39:1204–1209.
5. Goldstein JE, Cogan DG. Apraxia of lid opening. *Arch Ophthalmol* 1965;73:155–159.
6. Lepore FE, Duvoisin RC. "Apraxia" of eyelid opening: an involuntary levator inhibition. *Neurology* 1985;35:423–427.
7. Jordan DR, Anderson RL, Digre KB. Apraxia of lid opening in blepharospasm. *Ophthalmic Surg* 1990;21:331–334.
8. Jordan DR, Patrinely JR, Anderson RL, et al. Essential blepharospasm and related dystonias. *Surv Ophthalmol* 1989;34:123–132.
9. Fumagalli A. La injesioni sottocutanee de alcool nella cure de blepharospasmo e del'entropion spastico. *Ann Ottal* 1909;38:163.
10. Gurdijian ES, Williams HW. The surgical treatment of intractable blepharospasm. *JAMA* 1928;91:2053.
11. Dvorak M, Nemec J. Beitrag zur neurochirurgischen Therapie der hartnackigen Blepharospasmus. *Opthalmologica* 1964;148:130.
12. Reynolds DH, Smith JL, Walsh TJ. Differential section of the facial nerve for blepharospasm. *Trans Am Acad Ophthalmol Otolaryngol* 1967;71:656–664.
13. Callahan A. Blepharospasm with resection of part of orbicularis supply. *Arch Ophthalmol* 1963;70:508–511.
14. Callahan A. Surgical correction of intractable blepharospasm: technical improvements. *Am J Ophthalmol* 1965;60:788–791.
15. Frueh BR, Callahan A, Dortzbach RK, et al. The effects of differential section of the VIIth nerve on patients with intractable blepharospasm. *Trans Am Acad Ophthalmol Otolaryngol* 1976;81:595–602.
16. Weingarten CZ, Putterman AM. Management of patients with essential blepharospasm. *Eye Ear Nose Throat* 1976;55:8–24.
17. Dortzbach RK. Complications in surgery of blepharospasm. *Am J Ophthalmol* 1973;75:142–147.
18. Anderson RL, Patel BCK, Holds J, et al. Blepharospasm: past, present, future. *Ophthal Plast Reconstr Surg* 1998;14:305–317.
19. Henderson JW. Essential blepharospasm. *Trans Am Ophthalmol Soc* 1956;54:453–520.
20. Duke ES. The movements of the eyelids. In: Duke ES, ed. *System of ophthalmology,* vol 12. London: Henry Kimpton, 1976:890–914.
21. Bates AK, Halliday BL, Bailey CS, et al. Surgical management of essential blepharospasm. *Br J Ophthalmol* 1991;75:487–490.
22. Grandas F, Elston J, Quinn N, et al. Blepharospasm: a review of 264 patients. *J Neurosurg Psychiatry* 1988;51:767–772.
23. McCord CD, Coles WH, Shore JW, et al. Treatment of essential blepharospasm. I. Comparison of facial nerve avulsion and eyebrow-eyelid muscle stripping procedure. *Arch Ophthalmol* 1984;102:266–268.
24. Gillum WN, Anderson RL. Blepharospasm surgery: anatomic approach. *Arch Ophthalmol* 1981;99:1056–1062.
25. Anderson RL. Myectomy for blepharospasm and hemifacial spasm. In: Bosniak SG, Smith BC, eds. *Advances in ophthalmic plastic and reconstructive surgery: blepharospasm.* New York: Pergamon, 1985:313–332.
26. Patrinely JR, Anderson RL. Essential blepharospasm: a review. *Geriatr Ophthalmol* 1986;2:27–33.
27. Anderson RL. Myectomy for blepharospasm. In: May M, ed. *The facial nerve.* New York: Thieme, 1986:535–545.
28. Anderson RL, Patrinely JR, Anderson RL, et al. Surgical management of blepharospasm. *Adv Neurol* 1988;49:501–520.
29. Jordan DR, Patrinely JR, Anderson RL, et al. Essential blepharospasm and related dystonias. *Surv Ophthalmol* 1989;34:123–132.
30. Frueh BR, Musch DC, Bersani TA. Effects of eyelid protractor excision for the treatment of benign essential blepharospasm. *Am J Ophthalmol* 1992;113:681–686.

31. Patel BCK, Anderson RL. Diagnosis and management of essential blepharospasm. *Ophthalmic Pract* 1993;11:293–302.
32. Patel BCK, Anderson RL. Blepharospasm and related facial movement disorders. *Curr Opin Ophthalmol* 1995;5:86–99.
33. Scott AB. Botulinum toxin injection of eye muscles to correct strabismus. *Trans Am Ophthalmol Soc* 1981;79:734–770.
34. Scott AB, Kennedy RA, Stubbs HA. Botulinum-A toxin injection as a treatment for blepharospasm. *Arch Ophthalmol* 1985;103:347–350.
35. Jankovic J. Blepharospasm associated with brain stem lesions. *Neurology* 1983;33:1237–1240.
36. Guyton AC, MacDonald MA. Physiology of botulinum toxin. *Arch Neurol Psychiatry* 1947;57:578–592.
37. Aramideh M, Bour LJ, Koelman JH, et al. Abnormal eye movements in blepharospasm and involuntary levator palpebrae inhibition. *Brain* 1994;117:1457–1474.
38. Hotson JR, Boman DR. Memory-contingent saccades and the substantia nigra postulate for essential blepharospasm. *Brain* 1991;114:295–307.
39. Creel DJ, Holds JB, Anderson RL. Auditory brain-stem responses in blepharospasm. *Electrocephalogr Clin Neurophysiol* 1993;86:138–140.
40. Persing JA, Muir A, Becker DG, et al. Blepharospasm-oromandibular dystonia associated with a left angle meningioma. *J Emerg Med* 1990;8:571–574.
41. Jankovic J, Ford J. Blepharospasm and orofacial cervical dystonia: clinical and pharmacological findings in 100 patients. *Ann Neurol* 1983;13:402–408.
42. Maurillo JA. Treatment of benign essential blepharospasm and hemifacial spasm with botulinum toxin: a preliminary study of 68 patients. In: Bosniak SG, Smith BC, eds. *Advances in ophthalmic plastic and reconstructive surgery: blepharospasm.* New York: Pergamon, 1985:283–289.
43. Sellin LC. Botulinum: an update. *Mil Med* 1984;148:12–16.
44. Drachman DB. The role of acetylcholine as a neurotrophic transmitter. *Ann NY Acad Sci* 1974;228:160–176.
45. Duchen LW. The changes in the electron microscopic structure of slow and fast skeletal muscle fibers of the mouse after the local ingestion of botulinum toxin. *J Neurol Sci* 1971;14:61–74.
46. Elston JS, Russell RW. Effective treatment with botulinum toxin on neurogenic blepharospasm. *BMJ* 1985;290:271–281.
47. Chapman KL, Bartley GB, Waller RR, et al. Follow-up of patients with essential blepharospasm who underwent eyelid protractor myectomy at the Mayo Clinic from 1980 through 1995. *Ophthal Plast Reconstr Surg* 1999;15:106–110.

Surgery for Parkinson's Disease and Movement Disorders,
edited by J.K. Krauss, J. Jankovic, and R.G. Grossman.
Lippincott Williams & Wilkins, Philadelphia © 2001.

36

SURGICAL TREATMENT OF STIFF MAN SYNDROME WITH INTRATHECAL BACLOFEN

HANS-MICHAEL MEINCK
VOLKER TRONNIER
GERHARDT MARQUARDT

Stiff man syndrome (SMS), an uncommon neurologic disorder, is characterized by progressive and fluctuating muscle rigidity combined with painful spasms. Both rigidity and spasms involve the trunk and proximal limb muscles, the legs more often than the arms, and usually spare the face. With the exception of brisk reflexes, the neurologic examination is usually normal. Some patients, however, show additional, often transient neurologic symptoms such as ocular motor or sensory disturbances, vertigo, ataxia, a positive Babinski sign, or neuropsychologic deficits. Such cases most likely represent a "plus" variant of SMS, which has been tentatively labeled *progressive encephalomyelitis with rigidity and myoclonus* (PERM) (1–3). In SMS and PERM, both rigidity and spasms can be severe enough to cause incapacitating orthopedic complications such as joint ankylosis, dislocations, and even fractures. Rigid muscles are as hard as a board. Spasms may appear as slowly increasing and decreasing contractions or as myoclonic, most often bilateral jerks (the latter are most often associated with a history of uncontrolled falls). These spasms may occur spontaneously, or they may be provoked by unexpected acoustic or sensory stimuli, active or passive movements, or emotional upset. They can last for seconds or minutes and may recur for hours on end, and they sometimes are extremely painful and frightening. Such attacks are frequently accompanied by vegetative symptoms such as widened pupils or profuse sweating, as well as by serious tachycardia, arterial hypertension, laryngospasm, or apnea. About 10% of patients with SMS or PERM unexpectedly die of acute autonomic failure or from trauma caused by uncontrolled falls (1–3).

H.-M. Meinck: Department of Neurology, University of Heidelberg, D 69120 Heidelberg, Germany.

V. Tronnier: Department of Neurosurgery, University of Heidelberg, D 69120 Heidelberg, Germany.

G. Marquardt: Department of Neurosurgery, University of Frankfurt, D 60528 Frankfurt, Germany.

PATHOGENESIS

Patients with SMS or PERM have a high prevalence of various recognized autoimmune diseases such as type 1 diabetes mellitus, Hashimoto's thyroiditis, or the autoimmune polyendocrine syndrome. Moreover, 60% to 80% of patients (as compared with 1% of control subjects) have autoantibodies directed against the enzyme glutamic acid decarboxylase (GAD). Such prevalence not only is helpful for diagnosis, but also it suggests pathogenetic relevance: GAD catalyzes the conversion of glutamate to γ-aminobutyric acid (GABA), the major inhibitory neurotransmitter of the central nervous system. Therefore, an autoimmune pathogenesis is suspected, possibly directed against GABAergic inhibitory neurons (4,5).

DIAGNOSIS AND DIFFERENTIAL DIAGNOSIS

The diagnosis of SMS or PERM is often difficult, and symptomatic cases must be excluded by neuroimaging and cerebrospinal fluid analysis. A battery of electromyographic tests demonstrates tonic firing of otherwise normal motor units in rigid muscles and abnormally increased cutaneomuscular reflex excitability with latencies less than 80 milliseconds as the pathophysiologic basis of stimulus-sensitive myoclonic spasms (3,6). In most cases, GAD autoantibodies are present in serum or cerebrospinal fluid, or both. Although rare, the paraneoplastic association of SMS with breast cancer deserves particular attention (in such cases, autoantibodies are directed against amphiphysin, a synaptic vesicle protein).

The differential diagnosis of SMS includes many different neuromuscular disorders such as the rigid spine syndrome or neuromyotonia, syndromes with exaggerated startle such as acquired or hereditary hyperekplexia, extrapyramidal movement disorders such as axial dystonia, tetanus, and strychnine poisoning (2,7). However, the main differential diagnosis of SMS is psychogenic movement disorder. In fact, many patients with SMS or PERM have an agoraphobic fear of freely walking or standing that leads to the initial misdiagnosis of a psychogenic movement disorder (8).

MEDICAL AND SURGICAL TREATMENT

Symptomatic treatment is targeted at maintaining free mobility, suppressing painful spasms and uncontrolled falls, and preventing ankylosing joint deformities. Both stiffness and spasms are reduced or even disappear during sleep or administration of neuromuscular blocking agents, and they can be abolished completely with the GABA neuromodulator diazepam (2,3). Consequently, the standard symptomatic therapy for patients with SMS or PERM is diazepam. Oral baclofen or other antispastic or anticonvulsant drugs in most cases are less effective. Initial results with oral drugs (e.g. diazepam 20–40 mg per day) are usually good, but adaptation and disease progression make increasing doses (up to 400 mg diazepam per day) necessary. The subsequent side effects (sedation, dysarthria, vertigo, or ataxia) and the risk of addiction limit the applicability of high-dose oral therapy. Intrathecal drug administration allows high concentrations in the thoracolumbar cerebrospinal fluid and thereby increases efficacy while reducing the incidence of side effects of systemic application (9). In addition to symptomatic therapy with oral medications, attempts have been made to treat SMS with immunosuppressant therapy, but the results are inconclusive, and the treatment is cumbersome and risky (2,10,11,13).

CLINICAL RESULTS

About 50 patients with SMS or PERM have been followed-up at various German centers in cooperation with the Heidelberg Department of Neurology. Among these, eight patients, four with SMS and four with PERM, were treated with intrathecal baclofen over a period of up to 10 years. Reports on a total of 15 patients receiving intrathecal baclofen were mainly nonblinded retrospective studies (14–19). In all, attempts with oral medications (diazepam, clonazepam, tetrazepam, baclofen, tizanidine, carbamazepine, or valproic acid) proved unsatisfactory because of prohibitive side effects, poor therapeutic response, or rapid adaptation to initially effective dosages. Four patients received only intrathecal test boluses (50 to 100 μg baclofen), but no pump system was implanted (15–18).

As in antispastic therapy, patients received one or more intrathecal test boluses before pump implantation. Effective test boluses varied between 40 and 200 μg baclofen, and responses consisted of alleviated pain, reduced frequency or intensity of spasms, normalization of muscle tone, and increase of overall mobility; even three of the four patients tested but not implanted with a pump showed reduced stiffness in response to test boluses of 50 to 100 μg (18). In general, test boluses were well tolerated. However, one patient with SMS had a brief coma after a test bolus of 40 μg (19). In future *de novo* patients, testing of the drug response with an external pump could prevent such adverse events. Most patients were initially implanted with the SynchroMed (Medtronic, Inc., Minneapolis) pump system. Starting doses ranged from 50 to 240 (on average, 170) μg per day, but within a few months, most patients required increasing amounts (Fig. 36.1). Maintenance doses varied among

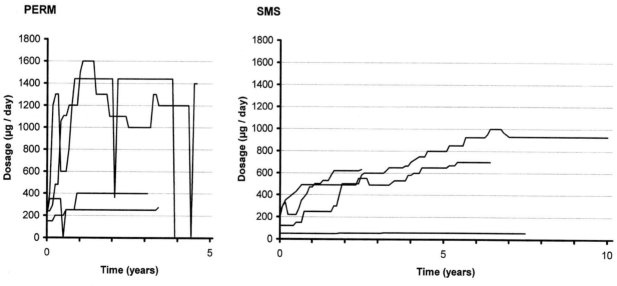

FIGURE 36.1. Dosage over time in patients with stiff man syndrome **(right)** or progressive encephalomyelitis with rigidity and myoclonus **(left)** receiving intrathecal baclofen.

patients between 58.5 and 1,400 μg per day. In two patients with PERM, requirements increased rapidly (within the first year from approximately 200 to about 1,500 μg per day), and dosage would have been increased even more had complaints of sedation not limited applicability (19). Two patients with SMS also required similarly high amounts, but dosages increased over a longer period (14,19). Daily doses in the remaining patients were kept between 58 and 630 μg. In some patients, however, dosages were intentionally maintained at moderate levels to avoid the consequences of reaching the upper dosage limit (i.e., fewer medication alternatives and increased danger of accidental withdrawal, as discussed later).

The dosage was titrated according to both clinical response and suppression of tendon jerks in the lower extremities. Recurrence of deep tendon reflexes in the legs was found to be a reliable sign of adaptation to the myorelaxant effect. No significant reflex changes were noted in the upper extremities. Although orthopedic complications of SMS and PERM such as lower limb ankylosis in five patients made functional assessment difficult, intrathecal baclofen therapy resulted in long-lasting improvement of symptoms: muscle stiffness was significantly reduced, as were the frequency and severity of spasms, and general mobility improved significantly. Before intrathecal baclofen, 11 patients were either wheelchair bound or bedridden; while receiving this therapy, only three patients remained in this condition. Five patients walked with crutches, whereas three no longer required them. Symptoms of autonomic dysfunction, occurring either spontaneously or after acute withdrawal, were also alleviated after administration of intrathecal baclofen. Six patients, however, required antispastic medication simultaneously, to facilitate the therapeutic response or to avoid side effects.

SIDE EFFECTS AND COMPLICATIONS

The side effects (somnolence, weakness, nausea) are similar to but generally milder than those observed with high-dose oral medication. Some complications resemble those of common intrathecal antispastic therapy (e.g., postoperative infection, leakage of the pump system, improper fitting of the pump, catheter obstruction, pump malfunction). However, intrathecal baclofen therapy for patients with SMS or PERM differs from patients with spasticity in several ways. Spastic patients are usually clinically stable at doses lower than 500 μg per day and show only moderate adaptation in the first year (20,21). In five of 11 patients with SMS or PERM, much higher dosages were required, and many patients adapted to intrathecal baclofen necessitating increasing dosage (Fig. 36.1). Moreover, even those patients with SMS or PERM who required comparably low doses had more frequent side effects. In one patient, an increase to more than 58.5 μg per day resulted in severe sedation (19). More dangerous, however, are the complications of sudden cessation of intrathecal baclofen (e.g., rupture of the catheter caused by a severe spasm, erroneous programming, or refilling of the pump). Although otherwise rare in spasticity (20–22), drug withdrawal was reported in three of 11 patients with SMS or PERM, and it ended fatally in one patient (14,16,19). In this situation, only hours after drug administration is reduced or stopped, spasms develop associated with massive vegetative symptoms (diaphoresis, tachycardia, tachypnea, and hyperthermia). Clinically, the picture may resemble that of myocardial infarction or gram-negative sepsis (16). Imminent acute autonomic failure may be prevented by high doses of intravenous benzodiazepines (which also alleviate spasms) and intensive care therapy. Readministration of intrathecal baclofen is necessary, but it may require some time to enter the system.

Because of these risks, intrathecal baclofen is a last-resort alternative to the symptomatic treatment of SMS and PERM with oral antispastic drugs. Patients with SMS or PERM are in danger of acute autonomic failure (23). We recommend that patients carry a card to inform others of the care needed in such an event.

REFERENCES

1. Moersch FP, Woltman HW. Progressive and fluctuating muscle rigidity and spasm (stiff man syndrome): report of a case and some observations in 13 other cases. *Mayo Clin Proc* 1956;31:421–427.
2. Stayer C, Meinck HM. Stiff-man syndrome: an overview. *Neurologia* 1998;13:83–88.
3. Barker RA, Revesz T, Thom M, et al. Review of 23 patients affected by the stiff man syndrome: clinical subdivision into stiff trunk (man) syndrome, stiff limb syndrome, and progressive encephalomyelitis with rigidity. *J Neurol Neurosurg Psychiatry* 1998;65:633–640.
4. Solimena M, DeCamilli P. Autoimmunity to glutamic acid decarboxylase in stiff-man syndrome and insulin-dependent diabetes mellitus. *Trends Neurosci* 1991;14:452–457.
5. Dinkel K, Meinck HM, Jury KM, et al. Inhibition of γ-aminobutyric acid synthesis by glutamic acid decarboxylase autoantibodies in stiff-man syndrome. *Ann Neurol* 1998;44:194–201.
6. Meinck HM, Ricker K, Hülser PJ, et al. Stiff-man syndrome: neurophysiological findings in eight patients. *J Neurol* 1995;242:134–142.
7. Thompson PD. Stiff muscles. *J Neurol Neurosurg Psychiatry* 1993;56:121–124.
8. Henningsen P, Clement U, Küchenhoff J, et al. Psychological factors in the diagnosis and pathogenesis of stiff-man syndrome. *Neurology* 1996;47:38–42.
9. Knutsson E, Lindblom U, Martensson A. Plasma and cerebral spinal fluid levels of baclofen (Lioresal) at optimal therapeutic responses in spastic paresis. *J Neurol Sci* 1974;23:473–484.

10. Blum P, Jankovic J. Stiff-person syndrome: an autoimmune disease. *Mov Disord* 1991;6:12–20.

11. Amato AA, Cornman EW, Kissel JT. Treatment of stiff-man syndrome with intravenous immunoglobulin. *Neurology* 1994; 44: 1652–1654.

12. Dinkel K, Meinck H-M, Jury KM, et al. Inhibition of γ-aminobutyric acid synthesis by glutamic acid decarboxylase autoantibodies in stiff-man syndrome. *Ann Neurol* 1998;44:194–201.

13. Shaw PJ. Stiff-man syndrome and its variants. *Lancet* 1999; 353:86–87.

14. Penn RD, Mangieri EA. Stiff-man syndrome treated with intrathecal baclofen. *Neurology* 1993;43:2412.

15. Ford B, Fahn S. Intrathecal baclofen [Letter]. *Neurology* 1994; 44:1367–1368.

16. Meinck HM, Tronnier V, Rieke K, et al. Intrathecal baclofen treatment for stiff-man syndrome: pump failure may be fatal. *Neurology* 1994;44:2209–2210.

17. Seitz RJ, Blank B, Kiwit JCW, et. al. Stiff-person syndrome with anti-glutamic acid decarboxylase autoantibodies: complete remission of symptoms after intrathecal baclofen administration. *J Neurol* 1995;242:618–622.

18. Silbert PL, Matsumoto JY, McManis PG, et al. Intrathecal baclofen therapy in stiff-man syndrome: a double-blind, placebo-controlled trial. *Neurology* 1995;45:1893–1897.

19. Stayer C, Tronnier V, Dressnandt J, et al. Intrathecal baclofen therapy for stiff-man syndrome and progressive encephalomyelopathy with rigidity and myoclonus. *Neurology* 1997;49:1519–1597.

20. Ochs G, Struppler A, Meyerson BA, et al. Intrathecal Baclofen for long-term treatment of spasticity: a multi-center study. *J Neurol Neurosurg Psychiatry* 1989;52:933–939.

21. Penn RD. Intrathecal baclofen for spasticity of spinal origin: seven years of experience. *J Neurosurg* 1992;77:236–240.

22. Siegfried RN, Jacobson L, Chabal C. Development of an acute withdrawal syndrome following the cessation of intrathecal baclofen in a patient with spasticity. *Anesthesiology* 1992;77:1048–1050.

23. Mitsumoto H, Schwartzmann MJ, Estes ML, et al. Sudden death and paroxysmal autonomic dysfunction in stiff-man syndrome. *J Neurol* 1991;238:91–96.

Surgery for Parkinson's Disease and Movement Disorders,
edited by J.K. Krauss, J. Jankovic, and R.G. Grossman.
Lippincott Williams & Wilkins, Philadelphia © 2001.

37

SURGICAL TREATMENT OF HEMIBALLISM AND HEMICHOREA

JOACHIM K. KRAUSS
FRITZ MUNDINGER

Hemiballism and *hemichorea* are relatively rare movement disorders (1–4). Nevertheless, although these hyperkinesias are seen infrequently, their occurrence has stimulated clinical and experimental neuroanatomic and neurophysiologic research (5,6). Particularly, investigations on the pathophysiology of hemiballism and hemichorea in experimental studies have contributed significantly to our current understanding of the functional organization of the basal ganglia (7).

Ballism and *chorea* are differentiated by phenomenologic qualitative and quantitative criteria (1,8). Experimental data and clinical observations, however, indicate that these two entities are part of a spectrum of hyperkinetic movement disorders. Ballism is characterized by vigorous, poorly patterned, rapidly executed, nonadaptive, high-amplitude involuntary movements affecting predominantly the proximal limbs resulting in large rotatory excursions. The involuntary movements of chorea predominantly affect the distal parts of the limbs and are simpler, more fragmentary, and asynergic. *Hemiballism* refers to involvement of the limbs of one side of the body. In bilateral ballism, both sides are affected (9). The term *hemichorea-hemiballism* is applied to movement disorders with features of choreic as well as ballistic hyperkinesias. The violent hyperkinesias of hemiballism can be very disabling and often interfere markedly with normal motor performance. The uncontrolled movements may lead to multiple injuries and lacerations of the involved extremities. Hemiballism follows a benign course in many instances and may resolve spontaneously or may improve with a regimen of dopamine antagonist therapy (10,11). However, there have also been descriptions of patients who have died of progressive exhaustion and cardiac failure (12). 2 Choreatic hyperkinesias may occur with various neurodegenerative disorders or metabolic diseases (4). Hemichorea and hemiballism are related to vascular disease or stroke in

most cases (12,13). Hemiballism has long been known as the *syndrome of the corpus of Luys* (14). In most patients, hemiballism is secondary to a lesion of the contralateral subthalamic nucleus (STN) (12,15). Ballism has also been described in patients with lesions of the pallidothalamic pathways, the striatum, and the pallidum (4,16). Both hemichorea and hemiballism can be associated with ipsilateral STN lesions, in particular in patients with hemiparesis contralateral to the lesion (17). With regard to experimental studies, it is thought that for hemiballism to occur, more than 20% of STN must be destroyed (12). Less frequently, hemiballism can result from nonvascular disease including neurodegenerative disorders, mass lesions, infectious diseases, and head trauma (4,13,15,18). Hemiballism has been observed in patients with acquired immunodeficiency syndrome (AIDS) and infectious diseases of the basal ganglia (19–21). In the early days of functional stereotactic surgery, hemiballism was a feared complication of thalamic lesioning seen in 0.3% to 9% of patients in the early postoperative period (15,22–26). Postoperative hemiballism, in general, is not a problem in contemporary movement disorders surgery. The issue of targeting the STN for treatment of parkinsonian motor symptoms is discussed in Section II.

INDICATIONS FOR SURGICAL TREATMENT

Data on the prognosis of hemiballism are conflicting (1,2,10,12). Hemiballism secondary to stroke most often has a favorable prognosis, with spontaneous improvement over a few weeks. Medical treatment primarily consists of dopamine antagonists and sodium valproate (2,8). The best responses are usually achieved with low doses of haloperidol. Persistent hemiballism is well recognized (15,16). It has been thought to occur more frequently in patients with lesions outside the STN, but several instances with STN lesions have also been described. With regard to the tendency for spontaneous improvement, surgical treatment should not be considered earlier than 6 months after the onset of the

J.K. Krauss: Department of Neurosurgery, University Hospital, Klinikum Mannheim, Mannheim 68167, Germany.
F. Mundinger: Department of Functional and Stereotactic Neurosurgery, St. Josefs-Krankenhaus, Freiburg, Germany.

movement disorder. Surgery may be indicated earlier, however, in patients who do not tolerate medical therapy or who suffer from very violent hyperkinesias.

Functional stereotactic surgery, in general, is not indicated for choreic dyskinesias in patients with Huntington's disease. Most patients tend to be more disabled by their behavioral and cognitive problems than by the choreic movement disorder. Several patients with Huntington's disease underwent pallidotomies in the 1950s and 1960s. Frequently, beneficial results with regard to the movement disorder were achieved. For example, Spiegel and Wycis reported improvement in choreic dyskinesias in three of four patients at follow-up of up to 10 years after pallidotomy (27). However, symptomatic improvement often was not paralleled by similar functional improvement, and functional stereotactic surgery was subsequently abandoned (28). Laitinen and Hariz reported on a 40-year-old man with Huntington's chorea who underwent a left posteroventral pallidotomy (29). Postoperatively, the patient had complete relief of his incapacitating right-sided hemichoreoathetosis. Nevertheless, there was little overall benefit because of the accompanying dementia.

Nowadays, functional stereotactic surgery targeting the thalamus or the pallidum is used almost exclusively for surgical treatment of hemiballism. Only exceptionally are other surgical procedures considered. Severe disabling hemiballism secondary to toxoplasmosis affecting the basal ganglia that persisted despite antibiotic treatment and antidopaminergic medication was relieved by high cervical cordotomy in a 32-year-old man with AIDS (20). Such operations, however, should be considered a last resort. Patients with hemiballism or hemichorea secondary to cerebral tumors or cysts may benefit from removal of the mass (15). Hemichorea-hemiballism was reported to resolve completely within 2 months after resection of a cavernoma in the contralateral head of the caudate in an 11-year-old boy (30). In another patient, a 66-year-old woman, hemichorea-hemiballism developed secondary to an ipsilateral intraventricular cyst after resection of a meningioma of the lateral ventricle (31). Drainage of the cyst relieved the compression and distortion of the upper brainstem and diencephalon that had affected the contralateral STN. The movement disorder disappeared within days.

HISTORICAL ASPECTS OF SURGICAL TREATMENT OF HEMIBALLISM

Early surgical treatment of hemiballism included several drastic measures. Peripheral operations targeting the affected extremities were performed in the 1930s. In desperate cases, limbs were amputated or paralyzed by alcohol injections in the brachial plexus or "stretching" of the brachial plexus (32–34).

In the next generation of surgeons, there was a change of surgical strategies. The attention shifted to surgical manipulations of the motor cortex and the corticospinal tract.

Bucy performed ablations of the contralateral motor and premotor cortex for treatment of severe disabling movement disorders (35). With this technique, hemiballism was relieved, however, at the cost of enduring hemiparesis. Meyers introduced sectioning of the subcortical U-fibers between the motor and premotor cortex in 1950 (36). With this technique, he achieved improvement of the hyperkinesias in most instances, apparently with only transient hemiparesis. Pedunculotomy or crusotomy was inaugurated by Walker (37). The midbrain peduncle was incised to a depth of 6 to 7 mm through a subtemporal approach. Again, this procedure was beneficial for alleviation of the movement disorder but only with resultant hemiparesis. To reduce the motor deficit, Brown and Walsh presented an alternative method in 1954 (38). Ventrolateral cordotomy ipsilateral to the movement disorder was performed in the cervical spine. With this technique, the hyperkinesias were either fully abolished or markedly reduced, with the resultant hemiparesis less severe or even absent as compared with manipulation at higher levels of the corticospinal tract (38,39).

The first functional stereotactic procedure was performed by Spiegel and Wycis in a patient with Huntington's disease in 1948 (27,40). Their goal was to reduce the choreic hyperkinesias by diminishing "afferent stimuli and emotional reactions." In the 1950s, when functional stereotactic operations for treatment of movement disorders became increasingly popular, they soon were applied in patients of hemiballism. Over the next decades, pallidal and thalamic surgery became the surgical treatment of choice for patients with persistent disabling hemiballism. More recently, the technical advances of deep brain stimulation created further treatment options in patients with disabling hyperkinesias.

RATIONALES FOR BASAL GANGLIA SURGERY FOR HEMIBALLISM

According to the current neurobiologic model of basal ganglia function, hemiballism is the consequence of reduced activity of the internal segment of the globus pallidus (GPi) secondary to decrease of excitatory glutaminergic input from the STN (6,44). Chorea, conversely, is thought to be associated with dysfunction of the striatum and the external segment of the GP (GPe) and secondary involvement of the STN (6,44). Because the pallidothalamic pathway is inhibitory, hypoactivity of the GPi, in turn, should result in decreased inhibition of the pallidal relay nuclei of the thalamus. The motor manifestations of hyperkinetic disorders would be the result of disinhibition of corticothalamocortical loops with subsequent increased drive of the thalamocortical outflow. The findings of microelectrode recordings in human patients with hemiballism demonstrating decreased mean discharge rates support the concept of hypoactivity of the GPi (42,43).

Consistent improvement of hemiballism has been found after functional stereotactic surgery targeting the GPi, the ventrolateral thalamus, and the subthalamic region (41–43).

TABLE 37.1. FUNCTIONAL STEREOTACTIC SURGERY FOR HEMIBALLISM: LITERATURE REVIEW

Author, Year	No. of Cases	Stereotactic Targets	Technique	Improvement in Hemiballism (Early Postoperative)	Improvement in Hemiballism (Follow-up >1 yr)	Complications
Talairach et al., 1950	1	GP, IC, CP, AL	EC	1/1	1/1	1/1
Roeder and Orthner, 1956	1	GPi, AL	EC	1/1	a	0/1
Gurny et al., 1957	1	GP	Chem	1/1	a	a
Velasco-Suarez, 1957	1	GP, IC	Chem, mech	0/1	a	1/1
Martin and McCaul, 1959	1	VL	Chem	1/1	a	1/1
Andy, 1962	4	GPi, IC, SR	EC	4/4	1/1	2/4
Yasargil, 1962[b]	3	GPi, or VL, IC	EC	3/3	a	a
Spiegel et al., 1963	1	SN	EC	1/1	a	a
Gioino et al., 1966	5	GPi, or VL, SR	Chem	5/5	3/3	3/5
Cooper, 1969[b,c]	(4 + 5) 9	GPi, or VL, SR	Chem	b	b	a
Mundinger et al., 1970[b]	11	GPi, or VL, ZI	RF	a	7/11	a
Tsubokawa and Moriyasu, 1975	2	GPe	RF, chem	2/2	2/2	a
Kandel, 1982[b]	3	GPi, or VL, SR	Cryo	a	a	a
Lévesque and Markham, 1992	1	VL	RF	1/1	a	1/1
Siegfried and Lippitz, 1994	1	VIM	DBS	1/1	1/1	a
Tsubokawa et al., 1995	2	VL, VIM	DBS	2/2	2/2	0/2
Cardoso et al., 1995	2	VL, VIM	RF	2/2	1/1	2/2
Krauss and Mundinger, 1996	14	VL, ZI, or GPi	RF	13/14	12/13	3/13
Suarez et al., 1997	1	GPi	RF	1/1	a	1/1
Vitek et al., 1999	1	GPi	RF	1/1	1/1	0/1

Stereotactic targets: AL, ansa lenticularis; CP, caudate and putamen; GP(e,i), globus pallidus (external, internal segments); IC, internal capsule; SN, substantia nigra; SR, subthalamic region; VIM, ventralis intermedius thalami; VL, ventrolateral thalamus; ZI, zona incerta. Technique: Chem, injection of toxin; Cryo, cooling by inserted probe; DBS, chronic deep brain stimulation; EC, electrocoagulation; Mech, mechanical lesion; RF, radiofrequency lesioning.
[a]Information not available.
[b]Only summarized; no detailed information available.
[c]The series of Cooper includes the cases of Gioino et al.
Adapted from Krauss JK, Mundinger F. Functional stereotactic surgery for hemiballism. *J Neurosurg* 1996;85:278–286, with permission.

The current basal ganglia model appears to offer little to explain improvement of hemiballism after posteroventral GPi pallidotomy, which is similar to the difficulty explaining amelioration of levodopa-induced dyskinesias after pallidotomy (44). Probably, the modulation of patterned pathologic neuronal activity is pivotal for the clinical effect of pallidotomy on hemiballism (42). Reduction of the net outflow of the pallidum would not reverse the reduced inhibition of the thalamus. The effective mechanisms of thalamotomy on alleviation of hemiballism are more consistent with reduction of excessive thalamocortical outflow. Improvement of hemiballism after lesioning the zona incerta and the subthalamic region may involve modulation of the activity of neurons of the zona incerta and of neural transmission through afferent and efferent pallidal and thalamic pathways. The functional roles of the zona incerta and its pathways are only poorly understood in humans (45,46). Lesions of the zona incerta affect also pathways of the basal ganglia circuitry in Forel's field H1 and, to a lesser extent, in the H and H2 fields (47–49).

STEREOTACTIC BASAL GANGLIA SURGERY FOR HEMIBALLISM

Functional stereotactic surgery for treatment of hemiballism has been performed in a limited number of patients. We

have identified a total of 60 patients reported between 1950 and 1999 (22,41–43,50–65). The data are summarized in Table 37.1. In several other reports on surgical treatment, some patients were labeled as having "ballism" or "ballistic hyperkinesias." With regard to the clinical descriptions, however, there were concerns about accepting these cases as verifiable presentations of ballism. The simple criterion of the "violence" of a movement disorder occasionally appears to have led to the diagnosis of hemiballism. In particular, severe kinetic posttraumatic tremors were said to remind some clinicians of hemiballism (66).

Early Clinical Studies on Ablative Surgery

Many targets were used for ablative surgery in the early period of surgical treatment of hemiballism (22,50–59). Targets included the anterior pallidum, the GPi, the ansa lenticularis, the caudate, the putamen, the substantia nigra, the subthalamic region, the zona incerta, the ventrolateral thalamus, and the internal capsule. There were also marked variations with regard to surgical technique and the methods for placement of the lesion. The first case published by Talairach and colleagues in 1950 involved extensive lesioning of diverse basal ganglia nuclei in addition to frontal cortectomy (50). Four series published in the 1960s and 1970s provided only summarized data on symptomatic outcome of hemiballism. In most of the early reports, no long-term follow-up was available. In several of the earliest cases, improvement of hemiballism was achieved at the cost of postoperative hemiparesis. In some reports, it was unclear whether postoperative weakness was present. The intentional placement of lesions in the internal capsule was the common practice of several surgeons in the early phase of stereotactic surgery. Overall, taking these limitations into account, the findings of the reports published between 1950 and 1970 can be summarized as follows: immediate postoperative improvement of hemiballism was present in all reported cases except one; there was a high frequency of side effects with subsequent hemiparesis in about two-thirds of patients; long-term improvement was achieved in more than half of the patients.

More Recent Clinical Studies on Ablative Surgery

When the number of functional stereotactic operations for treatment of Parkinson's disease declined in the 1970s, basal ganglia surgery was also less frequently performed in patients with hemiballism. Several surgeons, however, continued to improve surgical techniques that resulted in better control of the movement disorder and less surgical morbidity. Since the 1980s, only thalamic and pallidal targets have been used in functional stereotactic surgery for treatment of hemiballism (41–43,60–65).

Tsubokawa and Moriyasu reported on two patients with hemiballism who benefited from GPe pallidotomy (60). Intraoperative low-frequency stimulation of the GPe induced contralateral involuntary movements that were similar to the patient's hemiballistic hyperkinesias. The authors hypothesized that lesions of the GPe could control hemiballism secondary to lesions not involving the STN, which, under such circumstances, would be overinhibited because of disinhibition of the GPe. Cardoso and colleagues reported excellent control of hemiballism in two patients after ventrolateral thalamotomy at a follow-up of 2 and 17 months, respectively (65). Both patients had persistent mild side effects.

We analyzed symptomatic and functional outcome in a series of 14 patients with persistent disabling and medically refractory hemiballism (41). In seven patients (50%), concomitant hemichorea was present. These patients were operated on over a period of 25 years between 1965 and 1990. Radiofrequency lesions were placed in the contralateral zona incerta combined with lesions in the base of the ventrolateral thalamus (ventrooralis anterior and posterior) in 13 patients. In two patients, the GPi was targeted. In one instance, the GPi was the primary target, whereas the other patient underwent pallidotomy after thalamotomy failed to provide consistent relief. Hemiballism was abolished or was considerably improved in the early postoperative period after 14 of the 15 procedures. Lasting improvement at a mean of 11 years

postoperatively was found in 12 of 13 patients (92%) available for long-term follow-up. Seven of these patients (54%) were free of any hyperkinesias, and five (39%) had minor residual predominantly hemichoreic hyperkinesias. In the six patients who had presented preoperatively with hemichorea in addition to hemiballism, hemichorea was completely abolished in three patients in the long term, whereas mild choreic movements persisted in the other three patients. The patient who did not benefit from surgical treatment in the long term was a 59-year-old man who had presented with monoballism of the left leg preoperatively. He was free of any abnormal movements for several months after combined lesioning in the zona incerta and the ventrolateral thalamus on the right side. However, he did not benefit in the long term because he developed a "probable" psychogenic movement disorder, according to the criteria of Fahn and Williams (67), manifesting as hemiballism. Early postoperative side effects were present after seven of the 15 procedures (47%). In general, these side effects were mild and included lateropulsion on walking, increase of preoperative hemiparesis, and confusion. Persistent morbidity was found in three patients. Two patients had mild dystonia in the extremity that had been affected by hemiballism previously, and one patient had mild hemiparesis. There was a highly significant reduction of functional disability at long-term follow-up. The Huntington's Disease Activities of Daily Living scale was reduced from a preoperative mean of 83% of maximum disablity to a mean of 30% (68,69). Residual disability was most often related to cardiovascular disease in older patients. There was no significant difference in outcome with regard to the origin of hemiballism.

Bilateral ballism may be completely incapacitating and may require bilateral basal ganglia surgery. We described our experience with this unusual movement disorder in two children (9). One of these patients, a 9-year-old boy with bilateral ballism subsequent to meningoencephalitis, benefited from staged bilateral thalamotomy, with additional lesions in the zona incerta at a follow-up of 6 years, although there was some recurrence of the hyperkinesias.

Microelectrode-guided pallidotomies were reported in two patients with hemiballism. In the patient of Suarez et al., a 68-year-old man, hemiballism disappeared after posteroventral GPi pallidotomy, but the patient had mild hemiparesis (42). Moreover, in the patient of Vitek et al., a 70-year-old man, hemiballism was relieved immediately intraoperatively with sustained resolution of the involuntary movements over a follow-up period of 3.5 years (43,70).

Overall, the results of ablative surgery for hemiballism published since 1975 differ markedly from results in the earlier period between 1950 and 1970: the frequency of side effects has been reduced to approximately less than one-third of patients; persistent side effects have been less severe and, in general, associated with less disability than earlier; long-term improvement has been achieved in almost all patients. The question which is the best target for hemiballism, the pallidum, the subthalamic region including the zona incerta, or the thalamus, cannot be settled with the available data.

Deep Brain Stimulation for Treatment of Hemiballism

Deep brain stimulation has been reported in only single patients with hemiballism. Siegfried and Lippitz mentioned a patient who benefited from thalamic ventralis intermedius deep brain stimulation at a follow-up of 1 year (63). Tsubokawa et al. reported on two patients with complete control of hemiballism by contralateral chronic thalamic stimulation (64). The best clinical response was seen at stimulation frequencies between 50 and 150 Hz with 0.2- to 0.3-millisecond pulses at an intensity of 4 to 7 v. Stimulation at higher voltages, in contrast, increased the hyperkinesias. During the initial 3 weeks of stimulation, improvement of hemiballism was incomplete. On disconnection of the extension lead in one patient 10 months postoperatively, hemiballism reappeared. There were no reported side effects in these few patients with deep brain stimulation.

Technical Considerations

Like patients with other movement disorders, patients with ballism are operated on, in general, under local anesthesia.

General anesthesia may be necessary, however, in some patients for fixation of the frame, for stereotactic imaging, or intermittently during the procedure when the vigorous movements impede the operative intervention. When sedation is required only intermittently, short-acting benzodiazepines are advantageous.

Usually, improvement or disappearance of hemiballism is achieved intraoperatively. Sometimes, a *setzeffekt* with temporary suppression of the movement disorder after placement of the electrode in the target can be observed (41). The size of the lesion necessary to control hemiballism remains unclear. Most authors have used composite lesions with up to six smaller lesions at different sites within the target.

Microelectrode Recording

There is little experience with single-unit recording in patients with hemiballism. Suarez and colleagues reported mean lower discharge rates in both pallidal segments in their patient as compared with findings in patients with Parkinson's disease (42). This finding was confirmed recently by Vitek et al. in a 70-year-old man with hemiballism (43,70). Mean discharge rates in the GPi were similar to those in patients with dystonia, whereas discharge rates in the GPe were significantly slower (Fig. 37.1). The discharge pattern both in

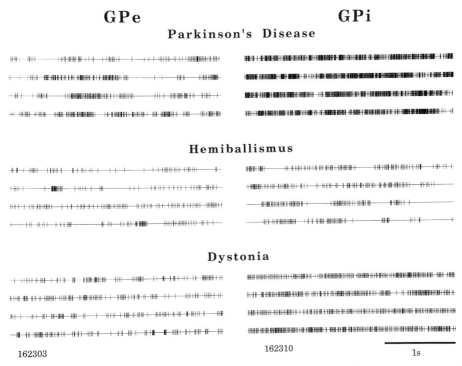

FIGURE 37.1. Microelectrode recording traces displaying the patterns of spontaneous neuronal activity of neurons in the internal (GPi) and external (GPe) segments of the pallidum from patients with Parkinson's disease, hemiballism, and dystonia. (From Vitek JL, Zhang J, Evatt M, et al. Gpi pallidotomy for dystonia: clinical outcome and neuronal activity. *Adv Neurol* 1998;78:211–219, with permission.)

the GPi and in the GPe was characterized by irregular groups of discharges and intermittent pauses. Only one of 34 GPi cells responded to passive movements of the limbs. Pauses of neuronal activity occurred coincidentally with increase of electromyographic activity in the contralateral biceps muscle resulting from involuntary movement.

CONCLUSIONS

Functional stereotactic surgery is a rewarding treatment modality in patients with persistent disabling hemiballism. Contemporary experiences with pallidal and thalamic ablative surgery have shown lasting symptomatic and functional improvement at a low frequency of mostly mild side effects. More data on the results of deep brain stimulation are awaited.

REFERENCES

1. Meyers R. Ballismus. In: Vinken PJ, Bruyn GW, eds. *Handbook of clinical neurology,* vol 6. Amsterdam: North Holland, 1968:476–490.
2. Koller WC, Weiner WJ, Nausieda PA, et al. Pharmacology of ballismus. *Clin Neuropharmacol* 1979;4:157–174.
3. Shannon KM. Hemiballismus. *Clin Neuropharmacol* 1990;13:413–425.
4. Dewey RB Jr, Jankovic J. Hemiballism-hemichorea: clinical and pharmacologic findings in 21 patients. *Arch Neurol* 1989;46:862–867.
5. Crossman AR, Sambrook MA, Jackson A. Experimental hemichorea/hemiballismus in the monkey. *Brain* 1984;107:579–596.
6. Albin RL. The pathophysiology of chorea/ballism and parkinsonism. *Park Rel Disord* 1995;1:3–11.
7. DeLong MR. Primate models of movement disorders of basal ganglia origin. *Trends Neurosci* 1990;13:281–285.
8. Buruma OJS, Lakke JPWF. Ballism. In: Vinken PJ, Bruyn GW, Klawans HL, eds. *Handbook of clinical neurology,* vol 49. Amsterdam: Elsevier, 1986:369–380.
9. Krauss JK, Mohadjer M, Nobbe F, et al. Bilateral ballismus in children. *Childs Nerv Syst* 1991;7:342–346.
10. Klawans HL, Moses H, Nausieda PA, et al. Treatment and prognosis of hemiballismus. *N Engl J Med* 1976;295:1348–1350.
11. Muenter MD. Hemiballismus. *Neurology* 1984;34[Suppl 1]:129.
12. Whittier JR. Ballism and the subthalamic nucleus (nucleus hypothalamicus; corpus Luysi). *Arch Neurol Psychiatry* 1947;58:672–692.
13. Vidakovic A, Dragasevic N, Kostic VS. Hemiballism: report of 25 cases. *J Neurol Neurosurg Psychiatry* 1994;57:945–949.
14. Martin JP. Hemichorea resulting from a local lesion of the brain (the syndrome of the body of Luys). *Brain* 1927;50:35–45.
15. Krauss JK, Borremans JJ, Nobbe F, et al. Ballism not related to vascular disease: a report of 16 patients and review of the literature. *Park Rel Disord* 1996;2:35–45.
16. Lang AE. Persistent hemiballismus with lesions outside the subthalamic nucleus. *Can J Neurol Sci* 1985;12:125–128.
17. Krauss JK, Pohle T, Borremans JJ. Hemichorea and hemiballism associated with contralateral hemiparesis and ipsilateral basal ganglia lesions. *Mov Disord* 1999;14:497–501.
18. Hyland HH, Forman DM. Prognosis in hemiballismus. *Neurology* 1957;7:381–391.
19. Nath A, Jankovic J, Pettigrew LC. Movement disorders and AIDS. *Neurology* 1987;37:37–41.
20. Krauss JK, Collard M, Mohadjer M, et al. Hemiballismus as the first symptom of AIDS. *Nervenarzt* 1990;61:510–515.
21. Nath A, Hobson DE, Russell A. Movement disorders with cerebral toxoplasmosis and AIDS. *Mov Disord* 1993;8:107–112.
22. Gioino GG, Dierssen G, Cooper IS. The effect of subcortical lesions on production and alleviation of hemiballic or hemichoreic movements. *J Neurol Sci* 1966;3:10–36.
23. Brion S, Guiot G, Derome P, et al. Hémiballismes postopératoires au cours de la chirurgie stéréotaxique. *Rev Neurol (Paris)* 1965;112:410–443.
24. Hopf A, Woringer E, Hamou I. Postoperativer Hemiballismus. *Neurochirurgia* 1968;11:1–18.
25. Hughes B. Involuntary movements following stereotactic operations for parkinsonism with special reference to hemichorea (ballismus). *J Neurol Neurosurg Psychiatry* 1965;28:291–303.
26. Modesti LM, Van Buren JM. Hemiballismus complicating stereotactic thalamotomy. *Appl Neurophysiol* 1979;42:267–283.
27. Spiegel EA, Wycis HT. Thalamotomy and pallidotomy for treatment of choreic movements. *Acta Neurochir (Wien)* 1952;2:417–422.
28. Mundinger F, Riechert T. Die stereotaktischen Hirnoperationen zur Behandlung extrapyramidaler Bewegungsstörungen (Parkinsonismus und Hyperkinesen) und ihre Resultate. *Fortschr Neurol Psychiatr* 1963;31:1–66, 69–120.
29. Laitinen LV, Hariz MI. Movement disorders. In: Youmans JR, ed. *Neurological surgery,* 4th ed. Philadelphia: WB Saunders, 1996:3575–3609.
30. Carpay HA, Arts WF, Kloet A, et al. Hemichorea reversible after operation in a boy with cavernous angioma in the head of the caudate nucleus. *J Neurol Neurosurg Psychiatry* 1994;57:1547–1548.
31. Borremans JJ, Krauss JK, Fanardjian RV, et al. Hemichoreahemiballism associated with an ipsilateral intraventricular cyst after resection of a meningioma. *Park Rel Disord* 1996;2:155–159.
32. Jermutowicz W. Un cas d'hémiballisme partiellement amélioré après intervention périphérique. *Rev Neurol (Paris)* 1931;55:374.
33. Kulenkampff D. Ueber die sogenannte Hemichorea posthemiplegica (Hemiballismus) und die Bedeutung der Pyramidenbahn. *Zentralbl Chir* 1938;65:2466–2470.
34. Schaller WF. Discussion of paper by PC Bucy and T Case. *Arch Neurol Psychiatry* 1937;37:983.
35. Bucy PC. *The precentral motor cortex.* Urbana, IL: University of Illinois Press, 1944.
36. Meyers R, Sweeney DB, Schwidde JT. Hemiballismus: aetiology and surgical treatment. *J Neurol Neurosurg Psychiatry* 1950;13:115–126.
37. Walker AE. Cerebral pedunculotomy for the relief of involuntary movements, hemiballismus. *Acta Psychiatr Neurol* 1949;24:723–729.
38. Brown MH, Walsh MN. The effect of ventral quadrant section of the cervical cord on hemiballismus. *J Neurosurg* 1954;11:409–412.
39. Strain RE, Perlmutter I. Hemiballismus relieved by ventral quadrant section of the cervical spinal cord without paralysis. *J Neurosurg* 1957;14:332–336.
40. Krauss JK, Grossman RG. Historical review of pallidal surgery for treatment of parkinsonism and other movement disorders. In: Krauss JK, Grossman RG, Jankovic J. *Pallidal surgery for the treatment of Parkinson's disease and movement disorders.* Philadelphia: Lippincott–Raven, 1998:1–23.
41. Krauss JK, Mundinger F. Functional stereotactic surgery for hemiballism. *J Neurosurg* 1996;85:278–286.

42. Suarez JI, Metman LV, Reich SG, et al Pallidotomy for hemiballismus: efficacy and characteristics of neuronal activity. *Ann Neurol* 1997;42:807–811.
43. Vitek JL, Chockkan V, Zhang JY, et al. Neuronal activity in the basal ganglia in patients with generalized dystonia and hemiballismus. *Ann Neurol* 1999;46:22–35.
44. Albin RL. Pathophysiology of parkinsonism and dyskinesias. In: Krauss JK, Grossman RG, Jankovic J. *Pallidal surgery for the treatment of Parkinson's disease and movement disorders.* Philadelphia: Lippincott–Raven, 1998:41–54.
45. Roger M, Cadusseau J. Afferents to the zona incerta in the rat: a combined retrograde and anterograde study. *J Comp Neurol* 1985;241:480–492.
46. Shammah-Lagnado SJ, Negrao N, Ricardo JA. Afferent connections of the zona incerta: a horseradish peroxidase study in the rat. *Neuroscience* 1985;15:109–134.
47. Hassler R, Mundinger F, Riechert T. *Stereotaxis in Parkinson syndrome.* Berlin: Springer, 1979.
48. Mundinger F. Stereotaxic interventions on the zona incerta area for treatment of extrapyramidal motor disturbances and their results. *Confin Neurol* 1965;26:222–230.
49. Riechert T, Hassler R, Mundinger F, et al. Pathologic-anatomical findings and cerebral localization in stereotactic treatment of extrapyramidal motor disturbances in multiple sclerosis. *Confin Neurol* 1975;37:24–40.
50. Talairach J, Paillas JE, David M. Dyskinésie de type hémiballique traitée par cortectomie frontale limitée, puis par coagulation de l'anse lenticulaire et de la portion interne du globus pallidus. *Rev Neurol (Paris)* 1950;83:440–451.
51. Roeder F, Orthner H. Erfahrungen mit stereotaktischen Eingriffen. *Dtsch Z Nervenheilk* 1956;175:419–434.
52. Gurny J, Kaplan AD, Lambre J, et al. Treatment of Parkinson's disease and other extrapyramidal disorders by chemopallidectomy using Fenelon's technique. In: van Bogaert L, Radermecker J, eds. *Proceedings of the first International Congress of Neurological Science.* London: Pergamon, 1957:116–118.
53. Velasco-Suarez MM. Pallidotomy in the treatment of some dyskinesias. In: van Bogaert L, Radermecker J, eds. *Proceedings of the first International Congress of Neurological Science.* London: Pergamon, 1957:151–159.
54. Martin JP, McCaul IR. Acute hemiballismus treated by ventrolateral thalamolysis. *Brain* 1959;82:104–108.

55. Andy OJ. Diencephalic coagulation in the treatment of hemiballismus. *Confin Neurol* 1962;22:346–350.
56. Yasargil MG. Die Ergebnisse der stereotaktischen Operationen bei Hyperkinesien. *Schweiz Med Wochenschr* 1962;92:1550–1565.
57. Spiegel EA, Wycis HT, Szekely EG, et al. Campotomy in various extrapyramidal disorders. *J Neurosurg* 1963;20:871–884.
58. Cooper IS. Hemiballismus and hemichorea. In: Cooper IS, ed. *Involuntary movement disorders.* New York: Hoeber, 1969:293–315.
59. Mundinger F, Riechert T, Disselhoff J. Long term results of stereotaxic operations on extrapyramidal hyperkinesia (excluding parkinsonism). *Confin Neurol* 1970;32:71–78.
60. Tsubokawa T, Moriyasu N. Lateral pallidotomy for relief of ballistic movement: its basic evidences and clinical application. *Confin Neurol* 1975;37:10–15.
61. Kandel EI. Treatment of hemihyperkinesias by stereotactic operations on basal ganglia. *Appl Neurophysiol* 1982;45:225–229.
62. Lévesque MF, Markham CH. Ventral intermediate thalamotomy for posttraumatic hemiballismus. *Stereotact Funct Neurosurg* 1992;58:26–29.
63. Siegfried J, Lippitz B. Chronic electrical stimulation of the VL-VPL complex and of the pallidum in the treatment of movement disorders: personal experience since 1982. *Stereotact Funct Neurosurg* 1994;62:71–75.
64. Tsubokawa T, Katayama Y, Yamamoto T. Control of persistent hemiballismus by chronic thalamic stimulation. *J Neurosurg* 1995;82:501–505.
65. Cardoso F, Jankovic J, Grossman RG, et al. Outcome after stereotactic thalamotomy for dystonia and hemiballismus. *Neurosurgery* 1995;36:501–508.
66. Bullard DE, Nashold BS Jr. Stereotaxic thalamotomy for treatment of posttraumatic movement disorders. *J Neurosurg* 1984;61:316–321.
67. Fahn S, Williams D. Psychogenic dystonia. *Adv Neurol* 1988;50:431–455.
68. Folstein SE. *Huntington's disease: a disorder of families.* Baltimore: John Hopkins University Press, 1989.
69. Bylsma FW, Rothlind J, Hall MR, et al. Assessment of adaptive functioning in Huntington's disease. *Mov Disord* 1993;8:183–190.
70. Vitek JL, Zhang J, Evatt M, et al. Gpi pallidotomy for dystonia: clinical outcome and neuronal activity. *Adv Neurol* 1998;78:211–219.

Surgery for Parkinson's Disease and Movement Disorders,
edited by J.K. Krauss, J. Jankovic, and R.G. Grossman.
Lippincott Williams & Wilkins, Philadelphia © 2001.

38

SURGICAL TREATMENT OF TOURETTE'S SYNDROME AND TICS

G. REES COSGROVE
SCOTT L. RAUCH

Tourette's syndrome (TS) is a neuropsychiatric condition characterized by multiple motor and vocal tics. The condition, first reported by Itard in 1825, was later better defined by Gilles de la Tourette in 1885, when he described nine patients with the unusual symptom complex of multiple tics, echolalia, and coprolalia (1). Although initially believed to be a rare psychogenic condition, it is now accepted as a distinct neuropsychiatric diagnosis. The current prevalence of TS is estimated to be as high as 0.5%, with males affected approximately three times more often than females (2,3). Detailed genetic studies in afflicted families, twin studies, and segregation analyses have shown that in more than half of all cases, TS may be a hereditary disorder (4–7). The gene for TS is most likely inherited as an autosomal dominant trait with variable penetrance or as a trait with intermediate inheritance in which some heterozygotic persons manifest the disease.

The clinical manifestations of TS can cause significant dysfunction, personal suffering, and social embarrassment. In the most severe cases, deleterious self-injurious behavior may result. Usually, TS can be successfully treated with pharmacologic and behavioral therapy. Surgical treatment remains very controversial, but it may be considered in those patients with severe and disabling TS that is otherwise refractory to conventional treatment.

CLINICAL PICTURE AND PATHOBIOLOGY

Clinical Features

The characteristic clinical features of TS consist of multiple motor and vocal tics that wax and wane over time. To satisfy the criteria for TS defined by the fourth edition of the *Diagnostic and Statistical Manual of Mental Dis-*

orders (DSM IV), a patient has to have multiple motor and vocal tics lasting longer than 1 year and beginning before 21 years of age (8). Tics in patients with TS are typically preceded by a feeling of internal tension building up over time that is then released by the movement or vocalization. Tics can often be suppressed by the patient for many minutes or hours, depending on the severity of the illness and the patient's particular social situation. Factors that typically aggravate the tics include anxiety, stress, and fatigue, whereas alcohol, relaxation, or distraction may lead to a lessening of the movements (9).

Motor tics are involuntary, brief, jerky movements that can affect any part of the body. They can generally be divided into simple or complex types. *Simple motor tics* involve simple movements such as head nodding, eye blinking, eye rolling, or shoulder shrugging. *Complex motor tics* refer to semipurposeful movements such as touching or striking oneself or other people or objects, jumping, or skipping. At times, the tics may be very prolonged, and this may make them appear to be an unusual episodic dystonic movement. Vocal tics can also be divided into simple and complex types. *Simple vocal tics* include throat clearing, grunting, and sniffing, whereas *complex vocal tics* include echolalia, coprolalia, and palilalia.

In most patients, tics begin between the ages of 5 and 10 years old. Motor tics typically begin in the head and neck with eyelid blinking, head jerking, and eye rolling. Vocal tics usually follow the onset of motor tics within several years, but they can be the presenting symptoms in some patients (10).

Tics vary in severity from patient to patient, and they wax and wane over the course of time in the same patient. The location of the tics also changes from month to month, affecting one body part for many weeks or months and then gradually abating, only to reappear in another location or form. In the most severe cases, tics may become self-injurious, with resultant self-mutilation (11). It is in these severe cases that surgery is sometimes considered.

The clinical course of TS can be variable, although it is generally believed to be an incurable and lifelong illness. On occasion, complete remission in adulthood may be

G.R. Cosgrove: Department of Neurosurgery, Massachusetts General Hospital, Boston, Massachusetts 02114.

S.L. Rauch: Department of Psychiatry, Massachusetts General Hospital, East, Charlestown, Massachusetts 02129.

observed, but most patients with TS continue to experience tics throughout their lives. Very few longitudinal studies have been performed, but many experienced clinicians believe that motor and vocal tics are most severe during adolescence and improve throughout adulthood. More recent evidence suggests that the rates of spontaneous remission or improvement may be greater than originally thought. However, it is generally believed that the more severe the tics are in adolescence, the more severe the tics will be in adulthood (10,12).

TS is also frequently associated with other psychiatric or behavioral abnormalities including *obsessive-compulsive disorder* (OCD). Obsessions are defined as unwanted, intrusive thoughts, and compulsions refer to the repetitive or ritualistic activity often in response to an obsession that is designed to produce or prevent a future event and to relieve the patient's anxiety. Obsessive-compulsive behavior is increased in patients with TS, with a reported frequency varying from 45% to 63% or higher (13,14). In some patients, it is extremely difficult to distinguish between complex motor tics and compulsive behavior. In several population studies, patients diagnosed with OCD were demonstrated to have a much higher than expected frequency of tics. These observations suggest that obsessive-compulsive symptoms may be an integral part of TS and may occur either in isolation or in combination with tics (15). Investigators have also observed that patients with OCD and tics tend to have a greater incidence of aggressive symptoms and compulsions.

Another associated abnormality frequently seen in patients with TS is attention-deficit disorder (8). Symptoms of attention-deficit disorder include hyperactivity, decreased concentration, inattention, and impulsivity. These symptoms are seen in many children with TS and may be evident several years before the onset of motor or vocal tics (16).

Most patients with TS have a completely normal neurologic examination, except for the presence of the tics (1). Nonspecific electroencephalographic (EEG) abnormalities can be seen in almost half of all patients, but no specific paroxysmal EEG activity that correlates with either the motor tics or the vocal tics has ever been detected. Visual-evoked and somatosensory-evoked potentials are generally normal as well (12).

Neuroimaging has been performed in many patients with TS, but computed tomography scans are generally reported as completely normal (12). Similarly, no consistent abnormality has been seen on standard magnetic resonance imaging (MRI) scans. However, volumetric MRI studies in both children and adults with TS have shown that the left lenticular region is reduced in volume as compared with neurologically normal control groups (17–19).

Etiology and Pathogenesis

The underlying pathophysiology of TS remains poorly understood because routine postmortem and biochemical studies of the brains of patients with TS have been unrevealing, and no adequate animal model of TS exists. Despite the lack of experimental evidence, two major hypotheses have been promulgated. The first is that TS is a result of an abnormality in the cerebral dopaminergic system. A second, less favored view, is that TS may result from an abnormality in the endogenous opioid system (20).

Several lines of evidence suggest that tics may be mediated by intrinsic cerebral dopaminergic systems and their interactions with the basal ganglia. The first is that dopamine antagonists are often effective therapies for TS, and dopamine agonists typically exacerbate TS (21–24). Reduced levels of homovanillic acid have also been identified in the cerebrospinal fluid of several patients (25). In addition, postmortem analysis demonstrated an increased number of dopamine uptake receptors in the striatum in at least one study (26). Functional neuroimaging studies have also begun to yield new insights into the underlying mechanisms of TS. Positron emission tomography (PET) studies showed normal striatal dopaminergic and D_2 receptor function in a small series of patients (27–29). Single photon emission computed tomography studies demonstrated increased density of dopamine transporter sites in the caudate and putamen of patients with TS and increased striatal D_2 receptor binding in the more severely affected of monozygotic twins with TS (19). Although these investigations provide circumstantial evidence that the dopaminergic system is indeed involved in TS, all these observations should be interpreted with caution because so few patients have been studied.

In support of the opioid theory of TS, investigators have observed that withdrawal of opiate therapy may cause an increase in tics in certain patients (30). Administration of opiates can also result in improvement in some patients with TS, particularly in self-injurious patients (31). In one postmortem study of five patients with TS, there was decreased staining for dynorphin in the globus pallidus, with normal staining for enkephalin (32).

The role of the basal ganglia in mediating cognitive, affective, and motor function is consistent with the notion that it could be the site of the pathologic process in TS. Basal ganglia disease has been well established in a variety of other movement disorders (i.e., Parkinson's disease, Huntington's disease) and suggests that it may be the site of disease in TS as well. Brainstem dopaminergic projections may not be limited to nigrostriatal tracts, but they may also project to limbic structures including mesial limbic and mesial cortical projections (33). PET studies have shown hypermetabolism in the basal ganglia of patients with TS as well as in the frontal cortex and temporal lobes bilaterally. Other PET studies have supported the theory that cortical striatal circuits including the sensorimotor cortex, putamen, and ventral striatum play a role in the pathophysiology of TS. The most widely accepted model of OCD acknowledges involvement of all these structures and emphasizes the frontal striatothalamocortical loops as a possible framework on which both TS and OCD could be explained.

TREATMENT

Medical Treatment

Pharmacologic therapy has always been the primary form of treatment for TS. Traditionally, neuroleptics such as haloperidol have been used successfully to control tics (34,35). Other antidopaminergic agents such as pimozide have also been successful along with clonidine and clonazepam (36). Benzodiazepines have also been useful, especially if the tics are exacerbated by stressful situations. Although not considered first-line treatment, some opiates as well as naloxone have been reported as beneficial in controlling tics.

In general, all these medications are used for as short a term as possible, with gradual tapering after months or years, provided the tics do not recur. In many of the most severe cases, however, long-term treatment with these medications is required. None of the current selective serotonin reuptake inhibitors have been shown to have any beneficial effect on tics, although they can be extremely useful for obsessive-compulsive symptoms.

Surgical Treatment

Historically, various neurosurgical procedures have been performed in an attempt to treat the most severe cases of TS.

Psychiatric Surgery

Various targets for the surgical treatment of TS have also been explored in the frontal lobes. Stevens reported major improvement in a single patient with TS who underwent a bilateral frontal lobotomy, although the postoperative course was complicated by significant weight gain resulting in severe obesity (37). Bimedial frontal leukotomy was reported by Baker in 1962 in a single patient, who had significant improvement in tics and panic attacks (38). Bilateral anterior cingulotomy has also been performed in various patients with TS in whom the primary indication for surgery was severe and intractable OCD with TS as a secondary comorbid condition (39). In each of these patients, although the OCD was substantially better after surgical treatment, there was no improvement in motor or vocal tics. Indeed, in one case, it was believed that the tics were minimally worse after surgical treatment (40). Limbic leukotomy was also performed in two patients, with satisfactory results. Robertson et al. reported the first case in 1990, with complete and sustained resolution of the patient's self-destructive behavior and a 75% reduction in tics (41). Sawle et al. also reported an impressive resolution of the signs of TS in a patient who underwent limbic leukotomy (42).

Functional Stereotactic Surgery Targeting the Thalamus

Most of the initial stereotactic procedures were performed bilaterally in the thalamus. Within Cooper's large series of thalamotomies, he referred to six patients with severe motor tics on whom he performed staged bilateral ventrolateral thalamotomies. Only one patient's case was reported in detail, but this patient apparently sustained an estimated 90% improvement in motor tics and complete abolition of vocal tics without any obvious adverse side effects (43). Although another five patients were referred to, no detailed account of their postoperative courses was published (44).

In 1970, Hassler and Dieckmann reported on three patients with TS who were treated with bilateral thermocoagulation of the rostral intralaminar nuclei and medial thalamic nuclei. In these three patients, tics were noted to improve by 70%, 90%, and 100%, respectively (45). In a later publication, these investigators reported an updated experience of 15 patients on whom they had operated for TS. Adequate follow-up was present for nine of those patients, and four patients were believed to have improved between 90% and 100%, whereas five patients were improved by 50% to 80%. Few patients suffered serious adverse side effects (46).

In 1977, Divitiis et al. reported their experience with three patients with TS who underwent unilateral, right-sided radiofrequency coagulation of the dorsal medial and intralaminar nuclei (47). These investigators found complete remission in two patients, whereas a third had a minimal reduction in symptoms. This third patient subsequently underwent a contralateral procedure without significant benefit. The two patients who initially underwent right-sided procedures had remission of their symptoms for more than 1 year, but in both cases, TS symptoms returned thereafter. Both patients refused the contralateral procedure. Divitiis et al. concluded that the unilateral thalamotomy was potentially useful in treating TS. Korzen et al. in 1991 reported a single case of a patient with TS who underwent bilateral, ventrolateral thalamotomy with an excellent sustained result (48). Recently, Vandewalle reported a single case of bilateral deep brain stimulation in the medial and rostral intralaminar nuclear targets of Hassler with good results at 4 months and 1 year of follow-up (49). This approach has theoretic advantages over bilateral thalamotomy in that no permanent lesions are made.

Miscellaneous Procedures

On rare occasions, bilateral anterior cingulotomy has been combined with infrathalamic lesioning. In one reported case by Leckman et al. in 1993, there was a mild improvement in motor and vocal tics with a more significant improvement in OCD symptoms, but there were also significant side effects related to the procedure, including a variety of bulbar deficits (50).

Bilateral cerebellar dentatotomy has also been reported in a single case. Nadvornik et al. reported improvement in motor tics and complete abolition of the vocal tics in a young man, but the duration of follow-up was not mentioned (51).

Patient Selection

Surgery should be considered only in those patients with severe TS who have chronic, disabling, and treatment-refractory illness that interferes significantly with normal psychosocial functioning. All conventional pharmacologic therapies must have been tried without success before considering surgical intervention.

The severity of the patient's illness must be manifest in terms of both subjective suffering and a decline in psychosocial functioning. The duration of illness is not as important as its severity, although symptoms should generally have been unremitting for several years. Whenever surgery is contemplated, it should be undertaken before chronic or severe dysfunction causes irreversible damage to personality, employment, and family, social, or environmental supports.

The appropriate selection of patients for surgery is the most difficult aspect of the presurgical evaluation process. Patient selection is the primary responsibility of the neurologist and psychiatrist guided by the informed input of the neurosurgeon. Certain factors argue against surgical intervention and include sociopathic personalities or other axis II disorders. Impaired cognitive function and organic brain lesions demonstrated on neuroimaging may also increase the risk of complications or postoperative deficits. Advanced age and serious medical illness can also increase the risk of perioperative complications. Given that many patients with TS improve as they reach adulthood, it is probably unwise to consider surgery in children or young adults.

Preoperative Evaluation

Any patient considered for surgical intervention must be referred by his or her treating neurologist or psychiatrist who has demonstrated an ongoing commitment to the patient and who is willing to accept responsibility for future care. Medical records should be reviewed by a multidisciplinary team experienced in the use of functional and stereotactic surgery. All members of the team must agree unanimously that the patient has severe and disabling TS and has exhausted all appropriate pharmacologic interventions.

If these initial criteria are met, the patient should then undergo a more detailed outpatient evaluation. This includes a complete neurologic and psychiatric evaluation, neuropsychologic testing, EEG examination, and MRI. A family member or close personal friend should accompany the patient to provide emotional support before, during, and after hospitalization. Both the patient and this family member or friend must be fully informed of the benefits and risks of the procedure and must be able to give informed consent.

Surgical treatment of TS is not considered a substitute for careful neuropsychiatric management. Therefore, all appropriate therapies that may have given partial benefit preoperatively must be continued postoperatively.

Considerations in Surgical Treatment

Currently, the accepted therapeutic approach to most patients with TS involves a combination of pharmacologic and behavioral therapies. Most patients improve using these treatment methods, but some patients fail to respond adequately and remain severely disabled. In these patients, surgical intervention may be considered appropriate if the therapeutic result and overall level of functioning could be improved. However, there is no consensus among practitioners about the duration, intensity, or degree to which other therapies should be tried before resorting to neurosurgery.

Many neurologists and psychiatrists could accept empiric treatment in a severe, treatment-refractory patient if the available clinical data supporting a favorable outcome were substantial and convincing. However, the experience with surgical treatment of TS is limited to single case reports and small patient series that are largely anecdotal. Given this dearth of information, there is no compelling evidence that any one of the surgical procedures employed to date is superior to any other in treating TS. Therefore, decisions regarding surgery should be made with great caution, and if surgical treatment is considered, it should be associated with minimal risk.

Anecdotal experience suggests that cingulotomy alone may be particularly ineffective for alleviating tic symptoms, although this procedure may produce some relief of OCD symptoms. In addition, it appears that cingulotomy in combination with infrathalamic lesioning and bilateral thalamic lesioning may be particularly dangerous and associated with significant side effects. It remains to be seen whether bilateral thalamic deep brain stimulation can provide a safer alternative to thalamotomy with sustained clinical benefit and no neurologic side effects. Limbic leukotomy has been used for many years in patients with treatment refractory OCD and has been shown to be a relatively safe procedure without severe neurologic consequences. Limbic leukotomy appears to show some promise, especially in the most severe cases in which the compassionate use of this operation in patients with self-injurious behavior may be warranted.

Many different targets have been chosen for a wide variety of reasons. None of the published reports have used any type of prospective clinical trial design or validated quantitative assessment tools of clinical improvement in motor and global tics. In addition, the adverse effects of these procedures have not been consistently reported, and only limited information has been made available regarding the adequacy of preoperative treatment. Consequently, there is little scientific evidence to suggest that any of these procedures is particularly effective in the treatment of TS or that one procedure appears to be clinically superior to the others.

Considerable controversy thus exists regarding the exact choice of surgical procedure to be employed. There is, however, unanimous agreement that the presurgical evaluation be performed by committed multidisciplinary teams with expertise and experience in the surgical treatment of psychiatric illness. Diagnosis based on the DSM IV classification scheme is encouraged, and although it is impossible to mandate uniformly across all centers, prospective trials employing standardized clinical instruments with long-term follow-up are needed. Comparisons of preoperative and postoperative functional status remain an important parameter in characterizing outcome. All centers with experience emphasize the importance of ongoing neuropsychiatric follow-up. The operation is not a panacea and should be considered only one aspect in the overall management of these patients.

The appropriate selection of patients for surgery remains a major issue and is the responsibility of the psychiatrist, guided by the informed and expert opinions of the other members of the psychosurgical team. Ethical objections about the use of surgery for TS must be addressed by ensuring that one has informed consent from the patient and family without coercion, along with unanimous agreement among the referring and treating physicians.

Despite the advent of new and effective psychopharmacologic agents, a few patients with TS remain severely disabled, and surgical intervention may represent a final therapeutic option. Caution must be urged regarding its use, however, to ensure that indiscriminate or inappropriate application of this form of therapy does not occur. We hope that as our understanding of the neurobiologic basis of TS improves, the rationale and theoretic basis for surgical intervention will become apparent. Until then, only carefully controlled, prospective long-term follow-up studies by independent observers can improve our empiric assessment of surgery in the treatment of TS.

CONCLUSIONS

The surgical treatment of TS may be considered in certain patients with severe, disabling disease that is refractory to medical treatment. Neurosurgical treatment should be carried out only by an expert multidisciplinary team with experience in these disorders. Surgery, if employed, should be considered only one part of an entire treatment plan and must be followed by an appropriate neuropsychiatric treatment program.

REFERENCES

1. Shapiro AK, Shapiro ES, Young JG, et al. *Gilles de la Tourette syndrome,* 2nd ed. New York: Raven, 1988.

2. Bruun RD. Gilles de la Tourette syndrome: an overview of clinical experience. *J Am Acad Child Psychiatry* 1984;23:126–133.

3. Singer HS, Walkup JT. Tourettes syndrome and other tic disorders: diagnosis, pathophysiology, and treatment. *Medicine* 1991;70:15–32.

4. Alsobrook JP. The genetics of Tourette syndrome. *CNS Spectrum* 1999;4:34–53.

5. Pauls DL. The genetics of obsessive compulsive disorder and Gilles de la Tourette's syndrome. *Psychiatr Clin North Am* 1992;15:759–766.

6. Pauls DL, Pakstis AJ, Kurlan R, et al. Segregation and linkage analysis of Tourette's syndrome and related disorders. *J Am Acad Child Adolesc Psychiatry* 1990;29:195–203.

7. Walkup JT, LaBuda MC, Singer HS, et al. Family study and segregation analysis of Tourette syndrome: evidence for a mixed model of inheritance. *Am J Hum Genet* 1996;59:684.

8. American Psychiatric Association. *Diagnostic and statistical manual of mental disorders,* 4th ed. Washington, DC: American Psychiatric Association, 1994.

9. Swerdlow NR, Zinner S, Farber RH, et al. Symptoms in obsessive compulsive disorder and Tourette syndrome: a spectrum. *CNS Spectrum* 1999;4:21–33.

10. Leckman J, Zhang H, Vitale A. Course of tic severity in Tourette syndrome: the first two decades. *Pediatrics* 1998;102:14.

11. Krauss JK, Jankovic J. Severe motor tics causing cervical myelopathy in Tourette's syndrome. *Mov Disord* 1996;11:563–566.

12. Robertson MM. The Gilles de la Tourette syndrome: the current status. *Br J Psychiatry* 1989;154:147–169.

13. Pauls D, Towbin K, Leckman J, et al. Gilles de la Tourette's syndrome and obsessive-compulsive disorder. *Arch Gen Psychiatry* 1986;43:1180.

14. Pitman RK, Green RC, Jenike MA, et al. Clinical comparison of Tourette disorder and obsessive compulsive disorder. *Am J Psychiatry* 1987;144:1166–1171.

15. Green RC, Pitman RK. Tourette syndrome and obsessive-compulsive disorder. In: Jenike MA, Baer L, Minichiello WE, eds. *Obsessive-compulsive disorders: theory and management.* Littleton, MA: PSG, 1986:147–164.

16. Comings DE, Comings BG. A controlled study of Tourette syndrome. I. Attention-deficit disorder, learning disorders and school problems. *Am J Hum Genet* 1987;41:701–741.

17. Peterson B, Riddle MA, Cohen DR, et al. Reduced basal ganglia volumes Tourette's syndrome using three-dimensional reconstruction techniques from magnetic resonance images. *Neurology* 1993;43:941–949.

18. Singer HS, Reiss AL, Brown JE, et al. Volumetric changes in basal ganglia of children with Tourette's syndrome. *Neurology* 1993;43:950–956.

19. Wright C, Peterson BS, Rauch SL. Neuroimaging research and Tourette syndrome. *CNS Spectrum* 1999;4:54–61.

20. Leckman JF, Peterson B, Abderson G, et al. Pathogenesis of Tourette's syndrome. *J Child Psychol Psychiatry* 1997;38:119.

21. Ernst M, Zametkin AJ, Jons PH, et al. High presynaptic dopaminergic activity in children with Tourette's syndrome. *J Am Acad Child Adolesc Psychiatry* 1999;38:86.

22. Feinberg M, Carrol BJ. Effects of dopamine agonists and antagonists in Tourette's disease. *Arch Gen Psychiatry* 1979;36:979–985.

23. Klawans HL, Falk DK, Nausiedo PA, et al. Gilles de la Tourette syndrome after long term chlorpromazine therapy. *Neurology* 1978;28:1064–1068.

24. Klempel K. Gilles de la Tourette's symptoms induced by L-dopa. *S Afr Med J* 1974;48:1379–1380.

25. Singer HS, Butler IJ, Tune LE, et al. Dopaminergic dysfunction in Tourette syndrome. *Ann Neurol* 1982;12:361–366.

26. Singer HS. Neurochemical analysis of post-mortem cortical and

striatal tissue in patients with Tourette's syndrome. *Adv Neurol* 1992;58:135–114.

27. Brook DJ, Turjanski N, Sawle GV. PET studies on integrity of the pre- and post-synaptic dopaminergic system in Tourette's Syndrome. *Adv Neurol* 1991;58:227–231.

28. Chase TN, Foster NL, Fedio P, et al. Gilles de la Tourette syndrome: studies with the flourine-18–labelled flourodeoxyglucose positron emission tomographic method. *Ann Neurol* 1984;15[Suppl]:S175.

29. Chase TN, Godfrey V, Gillespie M. Structural and functional studies of Gilles de la Tourette's syndrome. *Rev Neurol (Paris)* 1986;142:851–855.

30. Lichter D, Majumdat L, Kurlan R. Opiate withdrawal unmasks Tourette's syndrome. *Clin Neuropharmacol* 1988;11:559–564.

31. Cohen DJ, Riddle MA, Leckman JF. Pharmacotherapy of Tourette's syndrome and associated disorders. *Psychiatr Clin North Am* 1992;15:109–129.

32. Haber SN, Wolfer D. Basal ganglia peptidergic staining in Tourette syndrome: a follow-up study. *Adv Neurol* 1992;58:145–150.

33. Devinsky O. Neuroanatomy of Gilles de la Tourette's syndrome: possible midbrain involvement. *Arch Neurol* 1983;40:508–514.

34. Como PG, Kurlan R. An open label trial of fluoxetine for obsessive-compulsive disorder in Gilles de la Tourette syndrome. *Neurology* 1991;41:872–887.

35. Sallee FR, Nesbitt L, Jackson C, et al. Relative efficacy of haloperidol and pimozide in children and adolescents with Tourette's disorder. *Am J Psychiatry* 1997;154:1057.

36. Shapiro AK, Shapiro ES. Controlled study of pimozide vs placebo in Tourette's syndrome. *J Am Acad Child Psychiatry* 1984;23:161–173.

37. Stevens H. The syndrome of Gilles de la Tourette and its treatment. *Med Ann DC* 1964;33:277–279.

38. Baker EFW. Gilles de la Tourette syndrome treated by bimedial frontal leucotomy. *Can Med Assoc J* 1962;86:746–747.

39. Baer L, Rauch SL, Jenike MA, et al. Cingulotomy in a case of concomitant OCD and Tourette syndrome. *Arch Gen Psychiatry* 1994;51:73–74.

40. Kurlan R, Kersun J, Ballantine HT, et al. Neurosurgical treatment of severe obsessive-compulsive disorder associated with Tourette's syndrome. *Mov Disord* 1990;5:152–155.

41. Robertson M, Doran M, Trimble M, et al. The treatment of Gilles de la Tourette syndrome by limbic leucotomy. *J Neurol Neurosurg Psychiatry* 1990;53:691–694.

42. Sawle GV, Lees AJ, Hymas NF, et al. The metabolic effects of limbic leucotomy in Gilles de la Tourette syndrome. *J Neurol Neurosurg Psychiatry* 1993;56:1016–1019.

43. Cooper IS. Dystonia reversal by operation on the basal ganglia. *Arch Neurol* 1962;7:132–145.

44. Cooper IS. *Involuntary movement disorders.* New York: Harper & Row, 1969:274–279.

45. Hassler R, Dieckmann G. Traitment stéréotaxique des tics et cris inarticules ou coprolaliques considerés comme phénomène d'obsession motrice au cours de la maladie de Gilles de la Tourette. *Rev Neurol (Paris)* 1970;123:89–100.

46. Hassler R, Dieckmann G. Relief of obsessive-compulsive disorders, phobias and tics by stereotactic coagulation of the rostral intralaminar and medial-thalamic nuclei. In: Laitinen LV, Livingston KE, eds. *Surgical approaches in psychiatry: proceedings of the third International Congress of Psychosurgery.* Baltimore, MD: University Park, 1973:206–212.

47. Divitiis E, D'Errico A, Cerillo A. Stereotactic surgery in Gilles de la Tourette syndrome. *Acta Neurochir Suppl (Wien)* 1977;24:73.

48. Korzen AV, Pushkov VV, Kharitonov RA. Stereotaxic thalamotomy in the combined treatment. *Zh Nevropatol Psikhiatr* 1991;3:100–101.

49. Vandewalle V, van der Linden C, Groenewegen HJ, et al. Stereotactic treatment of Gilles de la Tourette syndrome by high frequency stimulation of thalamus. *Lancet* 1999;353:724.

50. Leckman JF, de Lotbiniere AJ, Marek K, et al. Severe disturbances in speech, swallowing, and gait following stereotactic infrathalamic lesions in Gilles de la Tourette's syndrome. *Neurology* 1993;43:890–894.

51. Nadvornik P, Sramka M, Lisy L, et al. Experiences with dentatotomy. *Confin Neurol* 1972;34:320–324.

Surgery for Parkinson's Disease and Movement Disorders,
edited by J.K. Krauss, J. Jankovic, and R.G. Grossman.
Lippincott Williams & Wilkins, Philadelphia © 2001.

39

FUNCTIONAL STEREOTACTIC SURGERY OF MOVEMENT DISORDERS IN CEREBRAL PALSY

CHARLES TEO

Cerebral palsy (CP) is a nonspecific neurologic syndrome that causes abnormal control of movement early in life. It was defined in 1964 as a disorder of movement and posture resulting from a defect or lesion of the immature brain. The incidence of CP is approximately 1.5 to 2.5 per 1,000 births, with the age of onset less than 2 years. The risk is higher in low-birth-weight infants and in twin pregnancies. Although the insult may occur at anytime before, during, or after the pregnancy, most often it occurs during the perinatal or prenatal phase. Unfortunately, although asphyxia was implicated as a major cause for CP, the reduction of this complication has not reduced the incidence of this condition. CP may be classified into four types, depending on the predominant motor disability.

CLASSIFICATION OF CEREBRAL PALSY

The *spastic type* accounts for approximately 50% of patients with CP and can be further subdivided into hemiplegic, diplegic, and quadriplegic subtypes. However, this distinction is an oversimplification, and in reality we find that most children have a combination of all three subtypes and are therefore classified as mixed. These children have varying degrees of cognitive deficits, some with exceptionally high cognitive abilities. Etiologic factors include prenatal circulatory compromise, perinatal hypoxia, cerebral dysgenesis, and prematurity.

The *dyskinetic type* accounts for approximately 20% of cases of CP and is characterized by the involuntary movements of chorea, athetosis, and dystonia. The abnormal movements differentially affect the upper limbs more than the lower and are sometimes incorrectly mistaken as spasticity. The muscles of the face are also affected, with tongue

thrusting, mastication, and generalized oral motor dysfunction. The movements become more obvious with age and are sometimes observed for the first time in the third or fourth year of life. Although CP is by definition a nonprogressive condition, the abnormal movements appear to worsen slowly over the ensuing years. This type is also known as *choreoathetoid or extrapyramidal type.*

The *ataxic or cerebellar type* is uncommon in its pure form. These patients often have a mixed clinical picture and are full-term infants. They have other cerebellar signs such as dysmetria and nystagmus. The results of neuroimaging may be normal.

DIAGNOSTIC AND THERAPEUTIC APPROACHES

The diagnosis of CP is made on history and examination. Imaging is useful in excluding space-occupying lesions and other surgically correctable congenital malformations, but it plays very little role in the confirmation or classification of CP. Some magnetic resonance imaging findings are typical, such as the "status marmoratus" of dyskinetic CP. This term refers to the marbled appearance of the basal ganglia as a consequence of diffuse gliosis in the corpus striatum and thalamus. Periventricular leukomalacia is seen in the spastic-diplegic type of CP. Overall, however, magnetic resonance imaging and other forms of neuroimaging are nonspecific and contribute little to the management of CP.

Arguably the most important factor in the efficient and efficacious management of CP is the adoption of a team approach. Indeed, neurosurgical intervention, recommended without multidisciplinary input, should be strongly discouraged. The team should include a neurologist or pediatric neurologist with an interest in movement disorders, a physical therapist, preferably one who has worked with the patient for some time, an occupational therapist, a rehabilitation

C. Teo: Center for Minimally Invasive Neurosurgery, Institute of Neurological Sciences, Prince of Wales Private Hospital; Department of Neurosurgery, Sydney Children's Hospital, Sydney NSW 2031, Australia.

specialist, a nurse, a psychologist, a social worker, and, of course, the patient's parents. The surgeon should have a command of the full range of surgical options, to be able to offer the patient the most appropriate procedure.

Timing of surgical intervention is controversial. Late intervention carries the risk of patients' developing dependency, both psychologic and physical. Deformities can become fixed and irreversible, and patients may not reach their full potential. Like patients with epilepsy, patients with CP may develop a dependent personality, with no ability or desire to enter the workforce, despite the physical capacity to do so after successful surgical treatment. Conversely, early surgical intervention may remove the tone that is essential for maintaining an upright posture or even the ability to walk. Surgery is not without risk, and complications are difficult to accept in an already compromised patient whose condition may have remained stable for several more years. These issues underscore the importance of a multidisciplinary team approach to patients with CP. In general, the literature supports an earlier surgical approach to patients with CP who have been determined to be good candidates (1–3).

TREATMENT OPTIONS

The multidisciplinary approach to the child with CP offers the parents and child a comprehensive assessment of existing treatments, makes recommendations on an individual basis, tailors the treatment regimen according to response, and, after objective and preferably independent evaluation, modifies the regimen accordingly. Treatment, for purposes of this chapter, can be divided simplistically into medical and surgical therapy. Most of the discussion concentrates on functional stereotactic surgery. For completeness, medical and other surgical options are summarized briefly. The latter techniques are described more extensively in Chapter 41.

Paramedical Treatment

Paramedical therapies play a vital role in maximizing motor use and correcting abnormal patterns of movement. They can improve functionality without changing strength or tone, by simply modifying tools, improving coordination, and teaching patients to improvise. These techniques are frequently used in conjunction with orthopedic procedures.

Medical Treatment

Medical treatment consists largely of muscle relaxants. Benzodiazepines are commonly used to treat spasticity in CP. Continuous intrathecal *baclofen*, an analog of γ-aminobutyric acid, has been shown to reduce spasticity in the upper and lower extremity and to improve daily living. Oral baclofen has poor lipid solubility and has only a mild effect in cerebral spasticity. *Tizanidine*, an α-receptor

agonist, has also been shown in clinical and control trials to be as efficacious as baclofen in the management of spasticity. *Sodium dantrolene* reduces muscle contracture and increases tone and range of movement by inhibiting calcium release from the sarcoplasmic reticulum. Other agents such as alcohol, phenol, and botulinum A toxin have also been used to control spasticity locally. Although these medications play a role in reducing spasticity, they do not improve weakness or incoordination.

Surgical Treatment

Surgical treatment can be directed at the nerves, the muscles and tendons, or the bones. Selective dorsal rhizotomy (SDR) was introduced in the 1980s and became very popular in the 1990s. More recently, its widespread use has been tempered with the introduction of more sophisticated functional stereotactic operations and slow-release pumps for administration of intrathecal relaxants. Clinical studies showing significant improvement in spasticity and gait after SDR have raised some controversy. The questions that remain unanswered are the percentage of the sensory root that needs to be cut, the method by which one determines the rootlets to be cut, the importance of intensive physical therapy after surgery and its type and duration, and the contribution of physical therapy to the end result. Some investigators have questioned the efficacy of the operation and have stated that the physical therapy is the reason for the improvement noted in these patients. Before SDR, orthopedic procedures constituted the main treatment option in patients with spastic diplegia. The procedures usually involved either lengthening and release of tendons and muscles or manipulation of bony deformities. These procedures are most frequently performed in the eighth year of life.

FUNCTIONAL STEREOTACTIC SURGERY

Various types of stereotactic techniques have been used since the 1950s in the management of CP. Previous chapters highlight the relative crudity of earlier techniques and the more refined hardware available today to increase accuracy and safety of functional surgery. There are many conflicting views on patient selection and operative techniques.

Functional stereotactic surgery for spasticity is controversial. Although spasticity was once considered a definite indication for surgery of the patient with CP, most contemporary publications fail to include functional stereotactic surgery as a treatment option for spasticity (4,5). Generally, the results of functional neurosurgery for patients with spastic CP are poor. Trejos and Araya's series is an exception to this generalization, but even in this series, these patients fared less well than those with other subtypes of CP (3). Moreover, patients with paraparesis benefit less from thalamotomy than do patients with hemiparesis. This specific subgroup of patients with spastic paraparesis benefits most from intrathecal baclofen pumps or SDR.

Some patients with CP have normal or superior mentation with profound impairment of motor function, whereas the reverse may be true in others. Recent philosophy has been to ignore the degree of intellectual compromise when selecting patients for surgery. This approach contradicts previously held opinions that surgical results were directly proportional to mentation. There is no doubt that postsurgical therapy required after any procedure is enhanced with a cooperative patient, but significant improvements in quality of life can still be achieved in intellectually devastated patients who have severe contractures and abnormal movements. Nursing care can be facilitated, metabolic needs can be decreased, self-mutilation can be limited, and contractures and pressure areas can be better managed.

Rationale

It is generally accepted that patients with CP have abnormally sensitive stretch reflexes secondary to overdevelopment of the anterior horn interneurons. This occurs as a result of periventricular leukomalacia, a universal feature of CP resulting from neonatal hypoxia, retarding the normal degeneration of neuronal projections from cortical and subcortical areas to the basal ganglia and brainstem, which are copious in the prenatal stages. This failure of regression from damaged sensory cortex results in overactivity of various basal nuclei and the clinical syndrome of profound motor imbalance. Furthermore, selective and variable damage to the nuclei of the basal ganglia is also possible, depending on the stage of development at the time of the hypoxic insult. The dyskinesia of Parkinson's disease closely resembles the choreoathetoid movements of CP, and this similarity provided the primary rationale for pallidotomy in the treatment of CP.

Surgical Options

Stereotactic Dentatotomy

It was only natural to consider the cerebellum a target for the treatment of spasticity, given the marked hypotonia associated with lesions of the dentate nucleus or superior cerebellar peduncle. Initially, the aim of surgical treatment was extensive unilateral resection of the cerebellum and its deep nuclei. However, it was too imprecise, and it left some patients markedly hypotonic. Subsequently, stereotactic dentatotomy was introduced and was considered relatively effective (6).

The dentate nucleus lies in the depths of the cerebellum and, receiving impulses from the cerebellar cortex, conveys them to the thalamus. Although there is some bilateral representation, the dentate nucleus controls movement on the same side of the body, in contrast to the thalamus, which exercises control over musculature on the opposite side of the body. Therefore, lesions should be made ipsilaterally rather

than contralaterally, as with all other stereotactic procedures for movement disorders.

Before SDR and baclofen pumps were introduced, dentatotomy was the surgical treatment of choice for the spasticity of CP. Most studies favored bilateral lesions, and some included simultaneous thalamotomy or pulvinarotomy (7). Lesions are placed in the ventrolateral portion of the dentate nucleus that is targeted using a ventriculogram demonstrating the fourth ventricle. Further localization can be achieved physiologically by eliciting motor responses, chiefly of the ipsilateral axial musculature. The effect of dentatotomy may decrease over time, but the long-term improvement in spasticity varies from 25% to 30% of patients, and it may be as high as 50% if one includes those patients in whom functionality is not improved but whose nursing care is facilitated.

Currently, with the excellent results of SDR, baclofen pumps, and pallidotomy for spastic hemiplegia (see the later discussion of stereotactic pallidotomy), there is no place for this procedure in the management of spastic CP.

Stereotactic Thalamotomy

Many controversial issues surround thalamotomy for CP. Despite the introduction of this treatment option in the 1960s (8,9), indications are poorly defined. All types of hyperkinesias may benefit from thalamotomy, but specifically, tremor has been the most commonly accepted indication (10). Before the introduction of pallidotomy and deep brain stimulation, patients with hyperkinesias, both slow (athetoid) and fast (ballistic, choreic, myoclonic), were only offered thalamotomy when medical treatment failed. As our options have increased, the indications have become less clear. Certainly, thalamotomy has some beneficial effect, albeit mild and sometimes transitory, on almost all the abnormal movements of CP, but no comparative studies have addressed the advantages of thalamotomy over other surgical procedures. The most responsive symptoms in the well-documented series of Broggi et al., were, in order of frequency, tremor, large excursion hyperkinesias, and dystonias. Spasticity, as documented by other investigators, was unaffected by stereotactic thalamotomy in the long term; patients had only temporary postoperative relief.

Another issue that has yet to be resolved is that of the ideal age at which to perform surgical treatment. Arguments for early surgery are psychologic (patients' expectations rise with age), neurofunctional and neuropsychologic (the greater willingness of younger children to accept the rehabilitative process), and the greater neuronal plasticity of the very young. Conversely, if the operation can be delayed, the operation can be performed with local anesthesia, the syndrome has developed fully and is stable, one has a good idea of the patient's mental function, and the patient is more cooperative. The arguments for late surgery are tenuous. Most patients, irrespective of age, cannot undergo the procedure with local anesthesia. Furthermore, clearly the psychosocial problems of the patient with CP have not developed fully at an early age, but the motor features have invariably stabilized and are well defined at a very young age. Further deterioration of motor function in adolescence is secondary to contractures, psychologic barriers, and functional disuse. Moreover, the younger brain is more plastic, and given the high incidence of side effects (see later), patients need this plasticity to optimize the end result.

The next issue is the patient's degree of incapacity, which may be a relative contraindication for stereotactic surgery. Patients with hemiparesis fare better than patients with paraperesis, who, in turn, do better than patients with tetraparesis. However, this apparent disparity in results of thalamotomy may be a reflection of inadequacies in the ability to evaluate the patient objectively postoperatively, and therefore, it may be unfair to reject a patient on the basis of disease severity alone. Although it is difficult to grade functional gains in many of these patients, there is no doubt their hyperkinetic states are improved with thalamotomy even if this does not then translate into better function. For example, this can result in easier nursing care, fewer self-inflicted injuries, and fewer caloric needs.

In summary, the ideal patient for thalamotomy is one who has unilateral tremor, has normal or better mentation, is cooperative and young enough not to have developed psychosocial barriers, and is motivated. The least ideal patient has spastic tetraparesis or bilateral dystonia, is functionally incapacitated, is an adolescent or older, has psychosocial problems, has poor motivation, and cannot cooperate or communicate.

The literature is confusing when discussing the ideal target for thalamotomy. The following targets have been recommended: the ventralis intermedius nucleus for tremor plus athetoid movements, the ventrolateral thalamus–ventralis intermedius for tremor plus dystonia, the ventrolateral thalamus (ventrooralis anterior and posterior) alone, the ventrolateral thalamus plus the medial pulvinar for predominantly dystonia, and lateral thalamotomy plus the zona incerta. There is justification for all of the foregoing nuclei to be targeted. The nuclei of the lateral thalamus modifies inputs from the globus pallidus as well as the dentate nucleus of the cerebellum. The anterior portion of the lateral thalamus receives pallidofugal fibers and other outputs from the striatum through the ansa lenticularis and fasciculus lenticularis. Investigators have shown that destruction of these nuclei induces an alteration of the input to the motor cortex that, in turn, reduces hyperkinesia. Further reduction in large excursion hyperkinesia can be achieved by destruction of the subthalamic input into the internal segment of the globus pallidus (see later). There is substantial justification for including the pulvinar when dystonia dominates the clinical picture (11,12).

I prefer patients to have general anesthesia. Although local anesthesia has been attempted, patients find it extremely distressing, and results seem no better. Therefore, neurophysiologic testing is extremely important, although its use is limited in the unconscious patient. Microelectrode recording is extremely helpful (see Chapter 6). Stimulation of the internal capsule with the lesioning electrode is cruder, but it can offer further accuracy. Stimulation is performed using 1-millisecond square pulses and 2 to 10 Hz to elicit muscle response. The current or voltage is monitored to give an idea of the distance of the tip of the electrode to the internal capsule. Thresholds higher than 1.5 v denote a safe distance from the motor fibers. Higher-frequency stimulation to assess proximity to the sensory structures can be performed using evoked potential monitoring. I have found this technique to be unreliable and poorly reproducible.

Results of thalamotomy for CP consistently show that the more severe the degree of palsy, the more unsuccessful the procedure will be. Patients with mild hemiparesis do better than those with severe hemiparesis. I and others have found some patients may take several months to reach their full postoperative potential (13). Spasticity does not improve in the long term, and dystonia is less influenced by posterior thalamotomy than was once speculated. Both slow and rapid hyperkinesias improve with lateral thalamotomy, but unfortunately this improvement lessens with time (13,14). Therefore, 60% to 80% of patients will improve immediately postoperatively, falling to 30% to 50% after 2 to 5 years. Repeat operation has been recommended for those patients who have small lesions on their postoperative studies and who improved with the initial surgical procedure. There appears to be little added morbidity with repeat procedures. Bilateral thalamotomies can be performed on those patients with bilateral signs either simultaneously or as staged procedures. The results are comparable (1,2,15), although temporary complications appear to occur more frequently.

Complications can be categorized as motor, sensory, autonomic, and mental (14). The most common motor disturbance is temporary hemiparesis, but the most common side effect overall is depression. This is especially so when the lesion is on the left side and of the lateral part of the thalamus. It rarely occurs with posterior thalamotomy. Patients show a marked decrease in verbal and gestural initiatives, less interpersonal communication, and autonomic phenomena such as alteration of normal sleep patterns and change in appetite. The reason this occurs is unclear but is most likely multifactorial. The lateral thalamus has connections with the limbic system, the operation results in a sudden change in physical appearance and body image, and these patients may fear abandonment from caregivers. Most patients improve, although these effects can be permanent.

Stereotactic Pallidotomy

The "slow" and "fast" hyperkinetic states seen in CP resemble the dyskinesia seen in patients with Parkinson's disease who have been overmedicated. These overmedication dyskinesias have been shown in all studies to respond very well to pallidotomy. Similarly, the often crippling and painful dystonia seen in Parkinson's disease mimics the dystonia seen in severely affected tetraparetic patients with CP, and this also improves with pallidotomy. Interrupting the pallidofugal fibers going to the ventrolateral thalamus must therefore be considered a potential target in patients with CP (16). This can either be done at the level of the internal segment of the globus pallidus or the ventrolateral thalamus.

Indications for pallidotomy include hyperkinesias of all types including tremor, choreoathetosis, myoclonus, dystonia, and ballism. Patients with pure or predominantly tremor-type CP do equally well with thalamotomy, but a mixed clinical pattern should convince the surgeon to target the globus pallidus rather than the thalamus.

Pallidotomy is best performed with the patient under general anesthesia even if the child is cooperative. This is especially true if the hyperkinetic state precludes the patient from lying still on the operating table. I favor a more lateral bur hole, to avoid the lateral ventricle and the internal capsular fibers when passing the probe. Localization and targeting and microelectrode recording techniques are described in other chapters of this volume. Attempts to maximize localization of the target further using stimulation of the internal capsule and optic tract are relatively unsuccessful in my experience. The contralateral tongue, facial, and hand muscles do not twitch as consistently as they do with an awake patient. Similarly, visual-evoked responses are difficult to elicit with higher-frequency stimulation and, like motor responses, are inconsistent.

In our series of 33 pallidotomies in 24 patients with CP, 66.7% had subjective improvement, and 41.7% had subjective and objective improvement (17). Surprisingly, and contrary to thalamotomy, the group of patients with severe disease and tetraparesis did better (six of eight patients with objective improvement, or 75%) than did the mildly affected patients (three of six patients, or 50%). Many of the patients enjoyed functional gains such as the ability to feed themselves or maneuver their wheelchairs. To the short-term observer, some of the more severely affected patients did not appear to improve, but they were described as being much better by their long-term caretakers. The complication rate was 50% and included swallowing and speech difficulties, excessive somnolence, eyelid apraxia, mild hemiparesis, and acute confusional state. The permanent complication rate was 17.5%. Most side effects resolved within 2 months of surgical treatment. There was one death in this series. A patient with severe, spastic tetraparetic CP appeared to do well after simultaneous bilateral pallidotomies with improvement in dystonia and spasticity. He was tube fed before the operation with very few problems, but for several weeks after the procedure, he aspirated almost all his tube feedings and eventually died of aspiration pneumonia 6 weeks postoperatively. Despite this case, bilateral lesioning performed either simultaneously or in staged procedures did not appear to increase the complication rate.

Pallidotomy is a very effective operation for the dyskinesia and dystonia of Parkinson's disease. This has been shown conclusively. However, the same cannot be said for CP. Although previous studies reported poor results from pallidotomy for the chorea and athetosis of CP (18–20), large numbers of patients and statistical data are lacking. With the evolution of frame-based stereotaxy allowing more accurate placement of lesions and electrodes and the failure of all current medical and surgical therapies to alleviate most of the motor manifestations of CP, we are compelled to keep an open mind to new treatment options. Unilateral or bilateral pallidotomy appears to be effective in the treatment of the patient with choreoathetoid, mixed, and, to a lesser degree, spastic types of CP, regardless of the severity. As with thalamotomy, pallidotomy is not curative and may not eliminate all the movement disorder, but it can diminish the excursions of ballism, decrease the pain and discomfort of dystonia, lessen the amount of chorea and athetosis, and reduce spasticity.

Deep Brain Stimulation of the Cerebellum, Thalamus, Globus Pallidus, and Subthalamic Nucleus

Chronic stimulation of the cerebellum, usually the anterior lobe, can offer some improvement in spasticity in the patient with CP (21). There have also been reports of improvement in choreoathetoid movements, but these are not well substantiated (22). The electrodes can be placed under direct vision over the cerebellar hemispheres through a small craniectomy below the transverse sinuses or stereotactically into the subcortical regions of the anterior lobes or deeper into the brachia conjunctiva cerebelli (23). The characteristic response is one of immediate relaxation and sometimes a feeling of euphoria, even laughter. Unfortunately, relaxation is invariably transient, with a long-term success rate of only 25% to 30%. Alternating stimulation of the cerebellar hemispheres may prolong the efficacy of this procedure.

There have been very few reports on thalamic stimulation in CP. Deep brain stimulation has the advantage of reversibility should the lesion create intolerable side effects. In a brain with preexisting areas of destruction, a method that does not create any more brain damage is very attractive. The only report on the use of deep brain stimulation is in a patient with mostly tremors (24). The electrodes were placed in the thalamus, with a good result. Both tremor and chorea improved.

CONCLUSION

CP is a diagnosis given to many different clinical syndromes. Some patients have only mild tremor that barely affects their daily activities, and others are so severely affected that they are destined to a life of dependence and misery. To date, the surgical treatment of CP has been relatively ineffective. Although patients with mostly tremor have benefited from thalamotomy, most patients with choreoathetoid or dyskinetic types of CP have suffered unaided by either functional or medical therapies. Neurosurgery is on the brink of a major revolution with the development of mechanical and electronic technology and molecular genetics. We must continue to explore different therapeutic options in the hope that one day we will make a significant change in the lives of these unfortunate children. Currently, the essence of surgical treatment is the creation of destructive, stereotactically placed encephalotomies. The future will lie in the use of deep brain stimulators, genetic engineering, and brain transplantation. More important, we should strive to find means of preventing the perinatal insults leading to CP and to develop techniques for earlier detection of the compromised fetus, neonate, and infant.

REFERENCES

1. Broggi G, Angelini L, Giorgi C. Neurological and psychological side effects after stereotactic thalamotomy in patients with cerebral palsy. *Neurosurgery* 1980;7:127–134.
2. Speelman JD, van Manen J. Cerebral palsy and stereotactic neurosurgery: long term results. *J Neurol Neurosurg Psychiatry* 1989;52:23–30.
3. Trejos H, Araya R. Stereotactic surgery for cerebral palsy. *Stereotact Funct Neurosurg* 1990;54:130–135.
4. Albright AL. Spasticity and movement disorders. In: Albright AL, Pollack IF, Adelson PD, eds. *Principles and practice of pediatric neurosurgery.* New York: Thieme, 1999:1157–1173.
5. Park TS, Owen JH. Surgical management of spastic diplegia in cerebral palsy. *N Engl J Med* 1992;326:745–749.
6. Heimburger RF, Whitlock CC. Stereotaxic destruction of the human dentate nucleus. *Confin Neurol* 1965;26:346.
7. Siegfried J, Verdie JC. Long term assessment of stereotactic dentatotomy for spasticity and other disorders. *Acta Neurochir Suppl (Wien)* 1977;24:41–48.
8. Laitinen LV. Short term results of stereotaxic treatment for infantile cerebral palsy. *Confin Neurol* 1965;26:258–263.
9. Laitinen LV. Neurosurgery in cerebral palsy. *J Neurol Neurosurgery Psychiatry* 1970;33:513–518.
10. Balasubramanium V, Kanaka TB, Ramanujan PB. Stereotaxic surgery for cerebral palsy. *J Neurosurg* 1974;40:577–582.
11. Cooper IS. Motor functions of the thalamus with recent observations concerning the role of the pulvinar. *Int J Neurol* 1971;8:238–254.
12. Denny-Brown D. The nature of dystonia. *Bull NY Acad Med* 1965;41:858–869.
13. Cardoso F, Jankovic J, Grossman RG, et al. Outcome after stereotactic thalamotomy for dystonia and hemiballismus. *Neurosurgery* 1995;36:501–508.
14. Broggi G, Angelini L, Bono R, et al. Long term results of stereotactic thalamotomy for cerebral palsy. *Neurosurgery* 1983;12:195–202.
15. De Salles A. Role of stereotaxis in the treatment of cerebral palsy. *J Child Neurol* 1996;11[Suppl 1]:43–50.
16. Narabayashi H, Okuma T, Shikiba S. Procaine-oil blocking of the globus pallidus. *Arch Neurol Psychiatry* 1956;75:36–48.
17. Teo C. Pallidotomy as a treatment option for pediatric movement disorders. *Neurosurgery* 1997;41:741–748(abst).
18. Spiegel EA, Wycis HT. Effect of thalamic and pallidal lesions upon involuntary movements in choreoathetosis. *Trans Am Neurol Assoc* 1950;75:234–236.
19. Spiegel EA, Wycis HT. Pallidothalamotomy in chorea. *Arch Neurol Psychiatry* 1950;64:295–296.
20. Tasker RR. Surgical treatment of the dystonias. In: Gildenberg PL, Tasker RR, eds. *Textbook of stereotactic and functional neurosurgery.* New York: McGraw-Hill, 1998:1015–1032.
21. Cooper IS, Riklan M, Amin I, et al. Chronic cerebellar stimulation in cerebral palsy. *Neurology* 1976;26:744–753.
22. Penn RD, Gottlieb GL, Agarwal GC. Cerebellar stimulation in man: quantitative changes in spasticity. *J Neurosurg* 1978;48:779–786.
23. Galanda M, Zoltan O. Motor and psychological responses to deep cerebellar stimulation in cerebral palsy (correlation with organization of cerebellum into zones). *Acta Neurochir Suppl (Wien)* 1987;39:129–131.
24. Thompson T, Kondziolka D, Albright AL. Thalamic stimulation for choreiform movement disorders in children. *J Neurosurg* 2000;92:718–721.

Surgery for Parkinson's Disease and Movement Disorders,
edited by J.K. Krauss, J. Jankovic, and R.G. Grossman.
Lippincott Williams & Wilkins, Philadelphia © 2001.

40

INTRATHECAL BACLOFEN FOR TREATMENT OF SPASTICITY

RICHARD D. PENN

Spasticity can be caused by any damage to the central nervous system that interrupts the descending fiber tracts that control movement. It is found in many different conditions, ranging from spinal cord trauma, stroke, and cerebral palsy to multiple sclerosis and amyotrophic lateral sclerosis. With such diverse clinical settings, it is surprising that a single approach would uniformly help. In fact, *intrathecal baclofen* does reduce spasticity in all these situations.

RATIONALES

The answer to the question, what happens to the damaged motor system that creates spasticity and makes it responsive to baclofen, is not completely known, but several clues are provided by clinical and laboratory observations. First and foremost, spasticity takes time to develop. The purest example is in spinal cord injury. Typically, spasticity does not develop until several months after the injury, and when it does develop, it slowly increases. This finding is in contrast to decerebrate rigidity, which occurs almost immediately after an injury. The most plausible reason for the slow development of spasticity is that it takes time for the structural changes to occur. The loss of synapses from descending fiber tracts must be gradually replaced by new synapses coming from interneurons. Just as it takes time for fields in the sensory cortex to reorganize after loss of sensory input from a limb, so it takes time for spinal cord circuits to reorganize after loss of descending input. Fortunately, from a therapeutic standpoint, this reorganization results in new synaptic chemistry. The γ-aminobutyric acid (GABA) GABA$_b$ receptors are gradually upregulated after spinal cord injury (1). The result is the hand-in-hand development of spasticity and increased sensitivity to GABA$_b$ agonists. Baclofen, a GABA$_b$ agonist, is a water-soluble, stable medication, that resists enzymatic breakdown and is, therefore, an ideal agent to use. Reduction in spasticity with intrathecal baclofen indicates that organizational changes in the spinal cord circuits have already occurred. In this regard, normal movement is not inhibited by baclofen. Patients with hemispastic syndromes who respond to intrathecal baclofen on the affected side do not develop motor problems on the neurologically normal side. Likewise, patients being treated for pain with intrathecal baclofen did not have motor impairments, even with high dosages (2).

The key problem in treating spasticity is how to ensure that baclofen reaches the abnormal spinal synapses. Oral administration of baclofen is often effective, but as the dose is raised enough to control spasticity, central side effects appear, such as drowsiness and incoordination. In addition, very high oral doses are needed because only a small amount of baclofen crosses the blood-brain barrier. Direct delivery of baclofen to the spinal cerebrospinal fluid by drug pump has solved this problem. In this way, baclofen is concentrated at the spinal level, and central effects are reduced (3).

Intrathecal delivery of baclofen has been proven to be effective in a large number of studies, including double-blind placebo-controlled trials (see Key References). There are, in fact, no reported failures in reducing spasticity when baclofen reaches the spinal cord. This finding means that the major questions that have to be answered are how reliable are the delivery techniques, and which patients with spasticity will benefit from treatment. Only if the baclofen delivery is sustainable and suitable patients can be selected will the therapy be worthwhile.

LONG-TERM EFFECTS AND MANAGEMENT

The first three patients, who were treated with intrathecal baclofen in 1984, continue to be treated successfully. In our clinic, it is rare for patients to stop using intrathecal baclofen, and many patients have been maintained in therapy for more than 10 years. However, to provide continuous delivery requires replacement pumps and catheter repairs. Pump reliability has improved substantially since the prototype pumps became available in the early 1980s. Now, pump

R.D. Penn: Department of Neurosurgery, Mount Sinai Medical Center, New York, New York 10029.

battery life has been extended for approximately 7 years. Mechanical problems that result in pump failure occur at about 0.5% per year, so the probability of a pump's having to be replaced for mechanical failure during its expected life is about 3%. As engineering improves incrementally over time, both longevity and reliability are likely to be better.

The major difficulty in the past was with the catheter design. The first thin-wall Silastic catheter had numerous problems because of kinking, breakage, leaks, and disconnection (4). The newer, thicker-walled catheter, that requires a larger needle for placement (No. 15 Tuohy), appears much more reliable, but it is still far from perfect. It has to be properly anchored in place and its connections well secured. Long-term results have not been published, but the failure rate is much lower than with the previous thin-walled catheter. It is still subject to mechanical forces and can be dislodged from the subarachnoid space by movement in some patients, in spite of proper anchoring. Biologic problems can also occur, such as fibrous growth over the tip of the catheter within the subarachnoid space. In several patients with intrathecal catheters used for pain control, fibromas have developed causing neurologic deficits (5). The precise cause is unclear, although chronic inflammation secondary to medications or low-grade infections is suspected. This may also happen in patients with spasticity, but it has not yet been reported. Because Silastic catheters used for shunting hydrocephalous are known to deteriorate after many years in place, intrathecal catheters may age similarly. More reliable catheters and better ways to hold them in position are needed, and new biocompatible materials have to be employed.

Another consideration that could limit use of implanted pump technology is infection. If repeated refills by needle through the skin contaminated the drug reservoir, and then the cerebrospinal fluid, the result would be unacceptable. Fortunately, meningitis is rare. The reason is that between the reservoir in the pump and its outport is a bacteriostatic filter. Even with culture-positive reservoirs, patients do not develop meningitis. However, when the outside of the pump is contaminated at the time of surgery, or later by seeding, then the entire system has to be removed. No good figures are available on how often this happens, but the number of cases may be in the same range as for cardiac pacemakers, that is, 2% to 5%. In the few patients in my series who had infections of the pump pocket or catheter, we removed the system and then, after appropriate antibiotic treatment, replaced the pump and catheter. So, although infection is a definite potential problem, if it occurs, patients can continue treatment later.

PATIENT SELECTION AND INDICATIONS

The initial tests of the safety and efficacy of intrathecal baclofen in the United States were conducted exclusively on patients with severe spinal spasticity from multiple sclerosis or spinal cord injury (6–8). This was done because the best and most uniform results of oral baclofen were seen in this clinical group. That meant that United States Food and Drug Administration (FDA) approval was only for this limited indication. In contrast, the early European experience included patients with brain injury, cerebral palsy, and anoxic encephalopathy, along with cases of spinal spasticity (9). Thus, from the outset, at least in Europe, the only criterion for treatment was severe spasticity unresponsive to oral medications. The European results in nonspinal forms of spasticity have been duplicated in studies in the United States, especially in patients with cerebral palsy, and the FDA no longer limits baclofen to spinal uses (10).

Who, then, should be given intrathecal baclofen? Any patient with spasticity that can be managed effectively by control of painful stimuli, physical therapy, or oral medications is obviously not a candidate. Patients who are too small (less than 50 lb), who have high rates of infection, or who have contraindications to a surgical implant should not undergo pump implantation. Moreover, there is no sense in starting treatment if it cannot be maintained on a long-term basis for years. Cost, transportation for refills, and availability of skilled personnel are important additional considerations. The patients in whom intrathecal baclofen is not appropriate, however, may be good candidates for other surgical procedures such as posterior rhizotomy (11). This is especially the case for infants and young children with diplegia or for adults who would prefer a single intervention to being wedded to long-term drug therapy.

Once these guidelines are followed for choosing a candidate for baclofen, the key question is who in this large group will benefit enough to justify an expensive surgical intervention and long-term maintenance. Although the risks, cost, and inconvenience of drug pump therapy will diminish over time, these factors will always have to be balanced with benefits.

The best candidates are those patients with severe, incapacitating spasticity. Patients with disabling pain from spasms, patients who are bedridden because of severe spasticity and contractures in their legs, patients with marked difficulties with activities of daily living, such as self-catheterization or transfers, are particularly suited for this treatment modality. In fact, the worse the spasticity, the greater the benefit will be. In this regard, the neglected patient who has developed fixed contractures will not initially respond. Physical therapy is required, and sometimes orthopedic intervention, to gain the full benefits of decreased spasticity.

The more difficult patients to evaluate for therapy are those with residual motor function that could be impaired by reducing spasticity. Sometimes, these patients take advantage of their increased muscle tone for standing and ambulation. The fear is that too much reduction in spasticity will bring more functional problems because of loss of strength.

Often, this consideration is greatest in the patients with spastic cerebral palsy. Fortunately, because the dosage of baclofen can be titrated very accurately, such problems are rare. Sometimes, it is beneficial to increase the baclofen dosage at night and to decrease it during the day, when muscle tone needs to be increased. In a study of 24 patients, ambulation increased significantly with treatment in nine

patients with cerebral palsy and became worse in three other patients, whereas other aspects of function improved in 20 patients (12).

A test dose of intrathecal baclofen does not solve the problem of patient selection in this group. The reason is that a bolus injection of intrathecal baclofen will reduce spasticity, but not in a graded manner. The receptors are exposed briefly

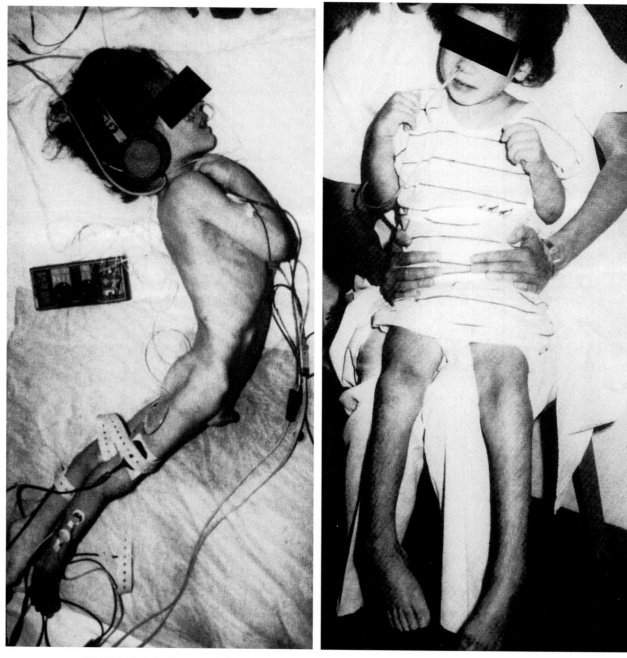

FIGURE 40.1. A: Severe opisthotonos and spasms in a 4-year-old child after a near-drowning accident. **B:** Three weeks after intrathecal baclofen treatment. The boy is able to sit, and his condition is much improved. (From Muller H, Zierski J, Dralle D, et al. Intrathecal baclofen in spasticity. In: Muller H, Zierski J, Penn RD, eds. *Local-spinal therapy of spasticity.* Berlin: Springer, 1988, with permission.)

to an extremely high amount of agonist, and the patient may become hypotonic. A more appropriate test is placement of a catheter and infusion of baclofen by an external pump for several days. This provides more time for dose adjustment. There is no absolute guideline or test for implantation in these patients. Willingness of the patient and family to work with physical therapy and to adjust baclofen doses as needed is critical. In most such cases, baclofen is considered useful by the patient, and only rarely does it need to be discontinued.

Patients who may be difficult to evaluate for baclofen are those with severe injuries to the central nervous system, whose spasticity is just one component of their motor and cognitive problems. In these cases, a bolus trial of baclofen may be more useful because one has to be sure that the complex motor disability has a true spastic element that can be helped. For example, we have tested patients with postanoxic encephalopathic conditions with mixed spasticity and dystonia and have seen little response. Conversely, patients with similar histories may have dramatic effects with baclofen (Fig. 40.1). In these cases, a trial dose of baclofen is mandatory. The earlier the intervention is done the better, before abnormal motor patterns develop or contractures occur.

In selecting patients with spasticity for baclofen treatment, it is important to achieve specific goals. The spectrum of benefit includes reduction in spasms, improvement in pain, amelioration of bladder function, reduction of movements to prevent decubitus ulcers, improved voluntary motor patterns, and better sleep. Dose adjustment may require phases of trial and error, and patients need to be fully informed preoperatively about this. In addition, variations in the patients' medical status may require dose changes, as with increased spasticity during bladder infections or decreased spasticity during an exacerbation of multiple sclerosis. Ultimately, a patient-controlled programmer may be useful for patients whose spasticity varies significantly.

Is Baclofen Useful for Other Nonspastic Movement Disorders?

The initial enthusiasm for treating generalized dystonia with intrathecal baclofen has decreased as other approaches such as pallidotomy and deep brain stimulation have emerged. In our own series of patients, we were able to help those with lower limb dystonias with intrathecal baclofen (13).

Stiff man syndrome responds well to baclofen (14). If used late in the disease, baclofen may be less effective because patients may have become bedridden with contractures. Also in these patients we have found it helpful to use diazepam orally to provide a $GABA_a$ agonist, as well as the $GABA_b$ agonist.

Another disorder with severe, and sometimes lethal, spasms is tetanus. Intrathecal baclofen given by an external pump in the acute phases of tetanus may be lifesaving (15).

CONCLUSIONS

Since its introduction in the 1980s, the long-term intrathecal infusion of baclofen has become standard treatment for many forms of severe spasticity. It is a well tolerated technique in general. It does not interfere with normal motor performance. Because it is a costly medical and surgical intervention, the benefits have to be justified by improvements in the patient's activities of daily living and comfort. As the technology improves with smaller pumps, more concentrated medication, and more trustworthy catheters, the therapy will become more widely used.

Spasticity is a condition that is often painful and interferes with normal activities. Intrathecal baclofen is a successful nondestructive treatment option, and it has been a major advance in functional neurosurgery.

REFERENCES

1. Kroin JS, Bianchi GD, Penn RD. Spinal cord transection produces a long-term increase in GABA-B binding in the rat substantia gelatinosa. *Synapse* 1993;14:263–267.
2. Latash ML, Penn RD, Corcos DM, et al. Short-term effects of intrathecal baclofen in spasticity. *Exp Neurol* 1989;103:165–172.
3. Kroin, JS, Penn RD. Cerebrospinal fluid pharmacokinetics of lumbar intrathecal baclofen. In: Lakke JPWF, Delhaas EM, Rutgers AWF, eds. *Parenteral drug therapy in spasticity and Parkinson's disease.* Canforth, United Kingdom: Parthenon, 1992:67–77.
4. Penn RD. Catheter implant systems for intrathecal drug delivery [Letter]. *J Neurosurg* 1996;84:713.
5. North RB, Cutchis PN, Epstein JA, et al. Spinal cord compression complicating subarachnoid infusion of morphine: case report and laboratory experience. *Neurosurgery* 1991;29:778–783.
6. Penn RD, Savoy SM, Corcos DM, et al. Intraspinal baclofen in the treatment of severe spinal spasticity. *N Engl J Med* 1989;320:1517–1521.
7. Loubser PG, Narayan RK, Sandin KJ, et al. Continuous infusion of intrathecal baclofen: long-term effects on spasticity in spinal cord injury. *Paraplegia* 1991;29:48–64.
8. Coffey, RJ, Cahill D, Steers W, et al. Intrathecal baclofen for intractable spasticity of spinal origin: results of a long-term multicenter study. *J Neurosurg* 1993;78:226–232.
9. Muller H, Zierski J, Penn RD, eds. *Local-spinal therapy of spasticity.* Berlin: Springer, 1988.
10. Albright AL, Barron WB, Fasick MP, et al. Continuous intrathecal baclofen infusion for spasticity of cerebral origin. *JAMA* 1993;270:2475–2477.
11. Peacock WJ, Arens LJ. Selective posterior rhizotomy for the relief of spasticity in cerebral palsy. *S Afr Med J* 1982;62:119–124.
12. Gertzen PC, Albright AL, Barry MJ. Effect on ambulation of continuous intrathecal baclofen infusion. *Pediatr Neurosurg* 1997;27:40–44.
13. Penn RD, Gianino JM, York MM. Intrathecal baclofen for motor disorders. *Mov Disord* 1995;10:675–677.
14. Penn RD, Mangieri EA. Stiff man syndrome treated with intrathecal baclofen. *Neurology* 1993;43:2412.
15. Muller H, Zierski J, Borner U, et al. Intrathecal baclofen in tetanus. In: Penn RD, ed. *Neurological applications of implanted drug pumps. Ann NY Acad Sci* 1988;531:167–173.

KEY REFERENCES

Spinal Spasticity (Multiple Sclerosis and Spinal Cord Injury)

Coffey RJ, Cahill D, Steers W, et al. Intrathecal baclofen for intractable spasticity of spinal origin: results of a long-term multicenter study. *J Neurosurg* 1993;78:226–232.

Loubser PG, Narayan RK, Sandin KJ, et al. Continuous infusion of intrathecal baclofen: long-term effects on spasticity in spinal cord injury. *Paraplegia* 1991;29:48–64.

Ochs G, Struppler A, Myerson BA, et al. Intrathecal baclofen for long-term treatment of spasticity: a multi-centre study. *J Neuro Neurosurg Psychiatry* 1989;52:933–939.

Penn RD, Savoy SM, Corcos DM, et al. Intraspinal baclofen in the treatment of severe spinal spasticity. *N Engl J Med* 1989; 320:1517–1521.

Cerebral Palsy

Albright AL, Barron WB, Fasick MP, et al. Continuous intrathecal baclofen infusion for spasticity of cerebral origin. *JAMA* 1993;270:2475–2477.

Armstrong RW, Steinbok P, Cochrane DD, et al. Intrathecally administered baclofen for treatment of children with spasticity of cerebral origin. *J Neurosurg* 1997;87:409–414.

Campbell SK, Almeida GL, Penn RD, et al. The effects of intrathecally administered baclofen on function in patients with spasticity. *Phys Ther* 1995;75:352–362.

Brain Injury

Concalves J, Garcia-March G, Sanchez-Ledesma, et al. Management of intractable spasticity of supraspinal origin by chronic cervical intrathecal infusion of baclofen. *Stereotact Funct Neurosurg* 1994;62:108–112.

Meythaler JM, McCary A, Hadley MN. Prospective assessment of continuous intrathecal infusion of baclofen for spasticity caused by acquired brain injury: a preliminary report. *J Neurosurg* 1997; 87:415–419.

Saltuari L, Kronenberg M, Marosi MJ, et al. Indication, efficiency and complications of intrathecal pump supported baclofen treatment in spinal spasticity. *Acta Neurol (Napoli)* 1992;14:187–194.

Saltuari L, Kronenberg M, Marosi MJ, et al. Long-term intrathecal baclofen treatment in supraspinal spasticity. *Acta Neurol (Napoli)* 1992;14:195–207.

Combined

Muller H, Zierski J, Penn RD, eds. *Local-spinal therapy of spasticity.* Berlin: Springer, 1988.

Surgery for Parkinson's Disease and Movement Disorders,
edited by J.K. Krauss, J. Jankovic, and R.G. Grossman.
Lippincott Williams & Wilkins, Philadelphia © 2001.

41

ABLATIVE SURGERY FOR TREATMENT OF SPASTICITY

MARC P. SINDOU
PATRICK MERTENS

Spasticity is one of the most common sequelae of neurologic diseases. In most patients, spasticity is useful in compensating for lost motor strength. Nevertheless, in many patients, it may become excessive and harmful, leading to further functional losses. When not controllable by physical therapy, medications, or botulinum toxin injections, spasticity can be improved by neurostimulation, intrathecal pharmacotherapy, or selective ablative procedures. Because hypertonia has to be reduced without suppression of useful muscular tone or impairment of the residual motor and sensory functions, neuroablative techniques must be as selective as possible. Such selective lesioning can be performed at the level of peripheral nerves, spinal roots, spinal cord, or dorsal root entry zone (DREZ).

NEUROSURGICAL PROCEDURES

Peripheral Neurotomies

Selective peripheral neurotomies were first introduced for the treatment of spastic deformities of the foot by Stoffel (1). More recently, we (3), as well as Gros and associates (2), advocated making neurotomies more selective by using microsurgical techniques and intraoperative electrical stimulation for better identification of the function of the fascicles constituting the nerve. Selectivity is required to suppress the excess of spasticity without producing excessive weakening of motor strength and severe amyotrophy. To achieve this goal, preserving at least one-fourth of the motor fibers is necessary.

Neurotomies are indicated when spasticity is localized to muscles or muscular groups supplied by a single or a few peripheral nerves that are easily accessible. To help the surgeon decide whether neurotomy is appropriate, *temporary local anesthetic block* of the nerve (with lidocaine or with

long-lasting bupivacaine) can be useful. Such a test can determine whether articular limitations result from spasticity or from musculotendinous contractures or articular ankyloses (only spasticity is decreased by the test). In addition, these tests give the patient an idea of what to expect from the operation. *Botulinum toxin injections* may also act as a "prolonged" test for several weeks or months.

Spasticity in the Lower Limbs

For spasticity in the lower limbs (4), neurotomies of the tibial nerve at the popliteal region for the so-called spastic foot (Fig. 41.1) and of the *obturator nerve* just below the subpubic canal for spastic flexion-adduction deformity of the hip (Fig. 41.2) are the most commonly used peripheral procedures.

Tibial neurotomy is performed as follows. After exposure of the tibial nerve from the popliteal region down to the soleus muscular arcade (while the patient is under general anesthesia without curarization), all the branches are individualized and are identified one by one, using the operating microscope and bipolar stimulation. Each branch (or fascicle) considered as supporting harmful spasticity on the basis of stimulation is then partially resected over a 5-mm length to prevent regeneration. Conservation of one-third to one-fifth of the fibers of each branch is sufficient to avoid loss of motor function and amyotrophy. Comparing the results of stimulation of the distal and proximal parts of the resected fibers has proved useful in controlling the effects of the operation on muscular contraction. The particular branches of the nerve to be operated on are determined preoperatively by analyzing all the components of the spastic disorder under study, according to the following schedule:

1. Equinus or ankle clonus requires section of the soleus nerve and, if necessary, the medial and lateral gastrocnemius branches.
2. Varus necessitates interruption of the posterior tibial nerve.

M.P. Sindou and P. Mertens: Department of Neurosurgery, Hôpital Neurologique P. Wertheimer, University of Lyon, 69003 Lyon, France.

421

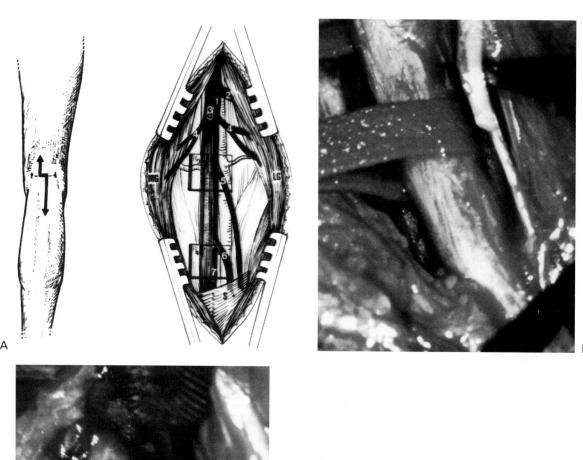

FIGURE 41.1. Selective tibial neurotomy. **A: Left:** Skin incision in the right popliteal fossa. **Right:** Dorsal view showing the tibial *(1)* and peroneal *(2)* nerves, the sural (sensory) nerve *(3)*, the medial gastrocnemius and lateral gastrocnemius branches *(4)*, the soleus nerve *(5)*, the posterior tibialis nerve *(6)*, and the distal trunk of the tibial nerve *(7)*. The distal trunk of the tibial nerve, just above the soleus arch (S), contains five to eight fascicles averaging 1 mm in diameter each; two-thirds are sensory. **B:** Operative view of the resection, more than 7 mm in length, of two-thirds of the soleus nerve (SN). **C:** Operative view of five dissected fascicles inside the distal part of the tibial nerve (TN) at the level of the soleus arch, after the epineural envelope has been opened.

3. Tonic flexion of the toes requires section of the flexor fascicles situated inside the distal trunk of the tibial nerve. Their precise identification, avoiding sensory fascicles, is of paramount importance in avoiding hypesthesia and dysesthetic disturbances as well as trophic lesions of the plantar skin.

In our series of 180 patients, tibial peripheral neurotomies resulted in suppression of the disabling spasticity with improvement of the residual voluntary movements in 82%.

In the spastic hemiplegic child, unlike in the adult, the effects of tibial peripheral neurotomies may be only transient. In our series of 13 pediatric patients followed on a long-term basis, eight had a recurrence (5).

Selective neurotomy of the branches to the *knee flexors (hamstrings)* can be performed at the level of the sciatic trunk through a short skin incision in the buttocks (Fig. 41.3). For spastic hyperextension of the first toe (the so-called permanent Babinski sign), a selective neurotomy of the branch of the *deep fibular nerve to the hallux extensor* can be useful.

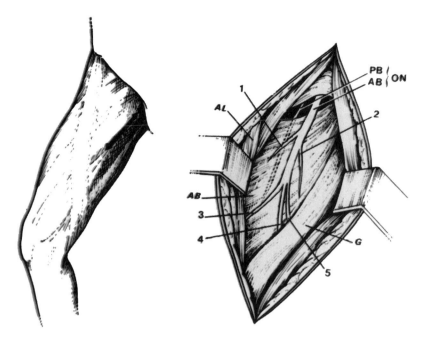

FIGURE 41.2. Obturator neurotomy. Skin incision on the relief of the adductor longus muscle. Dissection of the anterior branch (AB) of right obturator nerve (ON). The adductor longus muscle (AL) is retracted laterally and the gracilis muscle (G) medially. The nerve is anterior to the adductor brevis muscle (AB). The adductor brevis nerve *(1 and 2),* the adductor longus nerve *(3),* and the gracilis nerve *(4 and 5)* are shown. The posterior branch (PB) of the obturator nerve lies under the adductor brevis muscle (AB).

Spasticity in the Upper Limbs

Neurotomies are also indicated for spasticity in the upper limbs (4). Selective fascicular neurotomies can be performed in the musculocutaneous nerve for *spastic elbow flexion* (Fig. 41.4), as well as in the median (and ulnar) nerve for spastic hyperflexion of the wrist and fingers (Fig. 41.5).

The last procedure, which consists of sectioning the branches to forearm pronators, wrist flexors, and extrinsic finger flexors, is indicated for *spasticity in the wrist and the hand,* with the aim of opening the hand and improving

prehension. Because the fascicular organization of the median and ulnar nerves does not allow one to differentiate motor from sensory fascicles at the level of their trunks, it is necessary to dissect the motor branches after they have left the nerve trunk in the forearm. Special care must be taken with the sensory fascicles, to avoid painful sequelae.

Neurotomies of brachial plexus branches have been developed for treating the *spastic shoulder* (6). In the so-called spastic shoulder, the pectoralis major and teres major muscles are mainly implicated. Their excessive spasticity restrains the active (and passive) abduction and external rotation

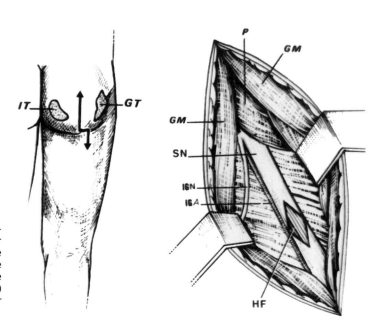

FIGURE 41.3. Hamstring neurotomy. Skin incision is between the ischial tuberosity (IT) and the greater trochanter (GT). Dissection is of the right sciatic nerve (SN), under the piriformis muscle (P), after passing through the fibers of the gluteus maximus muscle (GM). The epineurium of the nerve is opened, and the fascicles of the hamstring muscles (HF) are located in the medial part of the nerve. IGN, inferior gluteal nerve; IGA, inferior gluteal artery.

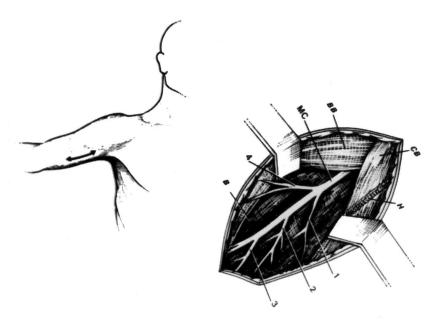

FIGURE 41.4. Musculocutaneous brachialis neurotomy. Skin incision along the medial aspect of the biceps brachii. Dissection is of the right musculocutaneous nerve (MC) in the space between the biceps brachii (BB) laterally, the coracobrachialis (CB) medially, and the brachialis (B) posteriorly. Branches to the brachialis (*1* and *2*) and to the biceps brachii (*3* and *4)* are shown. The humeral artery (H) and the median nerve are situated medially (they are not dissected).

of the shoulder. The pectoralis major nerve can be easily reached through an anterior approach to the shoulder. With the patient supine with the upper limb lying alongside the body, an incision is made at the innermost part of the deltopectoral sulcus and curves along the clavicular axis. The teres major nerve can be approached posteriorly to the shoulder. With the patient in the procubitus position and the upper limb lying alongside the body, a vertical incision is made along the inner border of the teres major. In the series of Decq and colleagues (6), surgical treatment produced a significant increase in amplitude and speed in the active mobilization of the spastic shoulder in five patients and led to better functional use.

Functional Benefit

Basically, selective neurotomies are able not only to reduce excess of spasticity and deformity, but also to improve motor function by reequilibrating the tonic balance between agonist and antagonist muscles (Fig. 41.6).

With regard to the *spastic hand,* which is a very difficult problem, a functional benefit in prehension can only be achieved if patients retain residual motor function in the extensor and supinator muscles, together with sufficient residual sensory function. If these conditions are not present, only better comfort and a better cosmetic effect can be achieved. We performed 25 median (and ulnar) neurotomies combined with tenotomies (predominantly of the epicondyle muscles) in the forearm (namely, a Page-Scaglietti operation) (7) to treat spastic flexion of the wrist and fingers, with tendinous contractures. All patients in this special group, who did not have any voluntary effective motor function preoperatively, had better comfort and a good cosmetic effect, but no significant functional benefit.

Posterior Rhizotomies

Posterior rhizotomy was performed for the first time for the modification of spasticity by Foerster in 1908 (8), after Sherrington had demonstrated in 1898 that decerebrate rigidity in an animal model was abolished by sectioning of the dorsal roots, that is, by interruption of the afferent input to the monosynaptic stretch and polysynaptic withdrawal reflexes. Its undesired effects on sensory and sphincter functions limited its application in the past. To diminish these disadvantages, several surgeons in the 1960s and 1970s attempted to develop more selective operations, especially for the treatment of children with cerebral palsy.

Posterior Selective Rhizotomy

To reduce the sensory side-effects of the original Foerster method, Gros and co-workers introduced a technical modification that consisted of sparing one rootlet of the five of each root, from L-1 to S-1 (9). On similar principles, Ouaknine (10), a pupil of Gros, developed a microsurgical technique that consisted of resecting one-third to two-thirds of each group of rootlets of all the posterior roots from L-1 to S-1.

Sectorial Posterior Rhizotomy

In an attempt to reduce the side-effects of rhizotomy on postural tone in ambulatory patients, Gros (11) and his pupils Privat et al. (12) and Frerebeau (13) proposed a topographic selection of the rootlets to be sectioned. First, preoperative assessment of spasticity useful for postural tone (abdominal muscles, quadriceps, gluteus medius) and spasticity harmful to the patient (hip flexors, adductors, hamstrings, and triceps surae) is made. Then, mapping the evoked motor activity of the exposed rootlets from L-1 to S-2 by direct

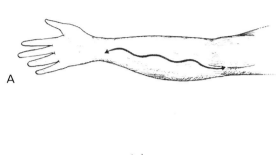

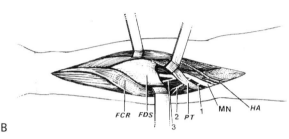

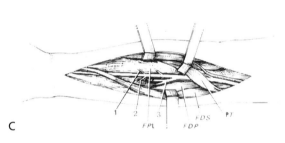

FIGURE 41.5. Median neurotomy. This procedure is slightly modified from Brunelli's technique (7). **A:** Skin incision is on the right forearm from the medial aspect of the biceps brachii at the level of the elbow to the midline above the wrist. **B:** First stage of the dissection; the pronator teres (PT) is retracted upward and laterally, and the flexor carpi radialis (FCR) is retracted medially. Branches from the median nerve (MN), before it passes under the fibrous arch of the flexor digitorum superficialis (FDS), are dissected. These branches are to the pronator teres (1) and two nerve trunks (2 and 3) to the flexor carpi radialis, palmaris longus, and flexor digitorum superficialis. **C:** Second stage of the dissection; the fibrous arch of the FDS is sectioned to allow more distal dissection of the median nerve. The FDS is retracted medially, and branches from the median nerve are identified to the flexor pollicis longus (FPL) (1), the flexor digitorum profundus (FDP) (2), and the interosseous nerve (3) and its proper branches to these muscles.

electrostimulation of each posterior group of rootlets, the rootlets to be sectioned are determined.

Partial Posterior Rhizotomy

Fraioli and Guidetti reported on a procedure of dividing the dorsal half of each rootlet of the selected posterior roots, a few millimeters before its entrance into the posterolateral sulcus (14). Good results were reported by the authors, without significant sensory deficit, the latter explained by the finding

that partial section leaves intact a large number of fibers of all types.

Functional Posterior Rhizotomy

The search for specially organized circuits responsible for spasticity led Fasano and associates to propose the so-called functional posterior rhizotomy (15). The method is based on bipolar intraoperative stimulation of the posterior rootlets and analysis of the types of muscle responses by electromyographic recordings. Responses characterized by a permanent tonic contraction, an afterdischarge pattern, or a large spatial diffusion to distant muscle groups were considered to belong to disinhibited spinal circuits responsible for spasticity. This procedure, which was especially conceived for children with cerebral palsy, has been also used by other surgical teams, each with its own technical modifications to the method (16–19).

Personal Experiences with Functional Posterior Rhizotomy

Our personal adaptation of these methods is as follows. Selection of candidates for surgery is based on a multidisciplinary approach, including the rehabilitation team, the physical therapist, the orthopedic surgeon, and the neurosurgeon, as well as, of course, the patient's family. The only patients considered suitable candidates are those in whom spasticity is responsible for a halt in motor skill acquisitions or developmental orthopedic deformities in spite of intensive physical therapy. The main goal of the surgery is clearly defined for every patient. These goals are as follows: improvement in comfort; minimization of orthopedic problems; improvement in sitting, standing, or walking; and improvement in urinary function. The muscles affected by excessive spasticity and their corresponding lumbosacral roots (i.e., those to be resected), as well as the degree of their involvement (with regard to the proportion to be resected), are determined by the multidisciplinary team. The surgical procedure is illustrated by Fig. 41.7. Our personal technique consists of performing a limited osteoplastic laminotomy using a power saw, in one single piece, from T-11 to L-1 (Fig. 41.7A). The laminae are reinserted at the end of the procedure and are fixed with wires (Fig. 41.7C). The dorsal (and ventral) L-1, L-2, and L-3 roots are identified by means of the muscular responses evoked by electrical stimulation performed intradurally just before entry into their dural sleeves. The dorsal sacral rootlets are identified at their entry into the dorsolateral sulcus of the conus medullaris. The landmark between S-1 and S-2 medullary segments is located approximately 30 mm from the exit of the tiny coccygeal root from the conus. The dorsal rootlets of S-1, L-5, and L-4 are identified by their evoked motor responses. The sensory roots for the bladder (S2-3) can be identified by monitoring vesical pressure, and those for the anal sphincter (S3-4)

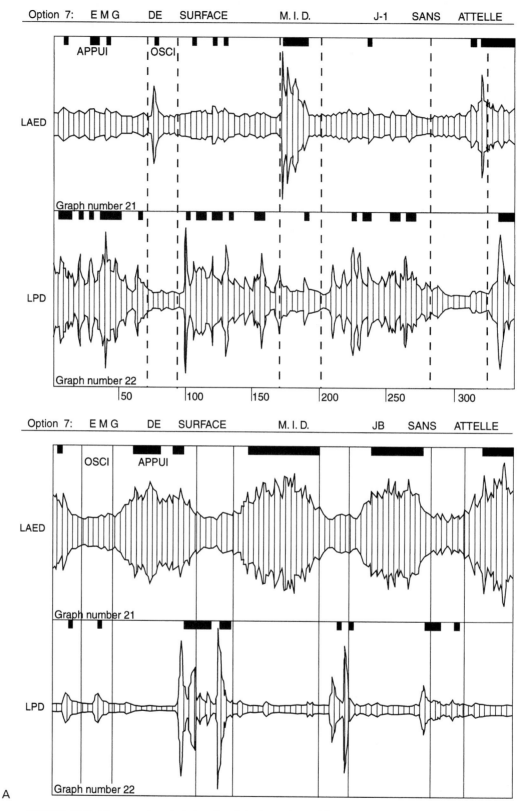

FIGURE 41.6. Movement analysis in a hemiplegic patient with a spastic foot (equinovarus) before and after selective tibial neurotomy. **A:** Surface polyelectromyography of the tibialis anterior (LAED) and the triceps surae (LPD) muscles on the spastic leg during walking. **Top:** Preoperative recordings showing desynchronized activities of the triceps surae, with abnormal cocontractions of antagonist muscles: triceps surae and tibialis anterior. **Bottom:** After selective tibial neurotomy, one sees a reappearance of muscular activities in the tibialis anterior muscle, a clear decrease in triceps surae activity, and normal alternation of contractions of these muscles (i.e., triceps surae at the end of the stance phase and tibialis anterior during the swing phase).

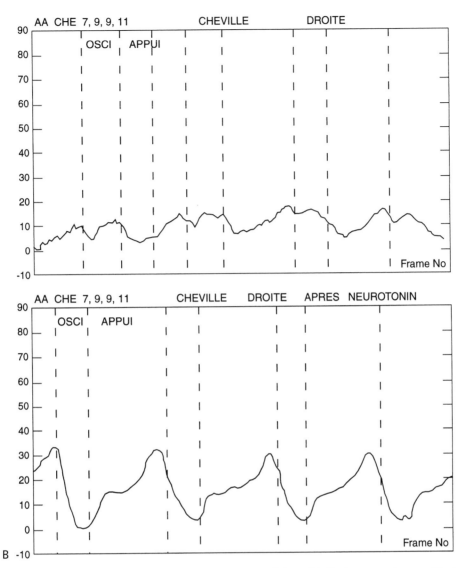

FIGURE 41.6. B: Three-dimensional movement analysis of the ankle flexion-extension amplitude during walking with the VICON system. **Top:** Preoperatively, the amplitude of the spastic ankle is limited to 18 degrees of dorsal flexion. **Bottom:** After selective tibial neurotomy, the dorsal flexion increased to 32 degrees. Thus, the tonic balance of the ankle has been reequilibrated by the selective tibial neurotomy; consequently, motor function and gait have been improved.

can be identified by rectomanometry (or simply by a finger introduced into the patient's rectum) or electromyographic recordings. Surface spinal cord somatosensory-evoked potential recordings from tibial nerve (L-5–S-1) and pudendal nerve (S1-3) stimulation may also be helpful.

For the surgical procedure to be effective, a total of 60% of dorsal rootlets must be cut, of course with a different quantity cut according to the level and function of the roots involved. Moreover, one must consider the relation of the roots to the muscles having harmful spasticity or useful postural tone in determining the amount of rootlets to be cut; in most cases, L-4 (which predominantly gives innervation to the quadriceps femoris) has to be preserved.

Until recently, we operated only on very severely affected children; those who were quadriplegic and not able to move

by themselves. Results of this series have been reported in detail elsewhere (20), and a summary is given in Table 41.1. More recently, we extended the indication to diplegic children who were able to walk. The preliminary results are satisfactory, but follow-up in this group is not yet sufficient to report the results in detail.

Outcome of Posterior Rhizotomy

The results of posterior rhizotomies obtained in children with cerebral palsy, whatever the technical modality of surgery may be, have been reported in various clinical series. We reviewed reported clinical outcomes when we reported on our own series (20). The 46 major studies were noted in our article (20). Briefly, most studies show that about 75% of

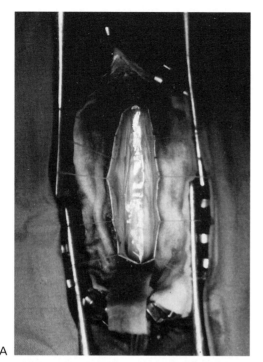

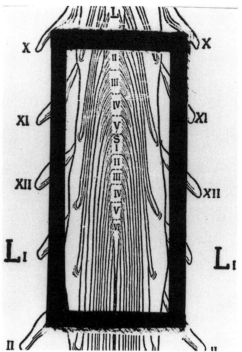

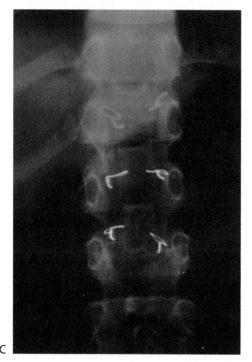

FIGURE 41.7. Lumbosacral posterior rhizotomy for children with cerebral palsy. **A:** Operative site after osteoplastic laminotomy from T-11 to T-1. **B:** Schematic topography of the thoracolumbar junction showing the origin of the lumbar and sacral posterior roots from the conus with regard to the thoracic and lumbar vertebrae. **C:** Reinsertion and fixation of the laminae with wires.

the patients had nearly normal muscle tone 1 year or more postoperatively that no longer limited the residual voluntary movements of the limbs. With intensive and continued physical therapy and rehabilitation, most children demonstrated improved stability in sitting or increased efficiency in walking. In most patients with fixed contractures, however, deformities were not improved, so complementary orthopedic surgery was advocated.

Percutaneous Thermorhizotomies and Intrathecal Chemical Rhizotomies

Percutaneous Radiofrequency Rhizotomy

Radiofrequency (RF) rhizotomies were initially performed for the treatment of pain (21). These procedures were later used in the treatment of neurogenic detrusor hyperreflexia (22) and of spasticity in the limbs (23–25). The procedure in the

TABLE 1. LUMBOSACRAL DORSAL RHIZOTOMIES IN CHILDREN WITH QUADRIPLEGIA[a]

Principal Goal	No. of Patients	Principal Goal Reached	Principal Goal Not Reached
Improvement in comfort	2	1	1
Improvement of orthopedic or joint problems	6	2	4
Improvement of sitting position	1	1	—
Improvement of standing and walking	8	6	2
Improvement of bladder function	1	0	1
Total	18	10	8

[a]Results according to principal goal reached (or not). Personal series of quadriplegic children with cerebral palsy (18 children, range of age: 5.5 to 16.5 years), who underwent lumbosacral dorsal rhizotomies and were followed-up for more than 1 year (up to 4 years in the earlier cases). A decrease in spasticity was obtained in all muscles producing harmful spasticity. Increase in range of motion was only obtained significantly on abduction and extension of the hips; deformities in the knees and feet were not so well influenced. The effects were considered satisfactory by the patients' families in 16 instances; two patients were thought to be worse. Results according to the goal defined as the main goal to be reached are summarized. Two patients had postoperative kyphosis at the level of the laminotomy.

lumbar spine is generally performed with the patient in the lateral recumbent position, with the affected side upward. The prone position would be very uncomfortable because of fixed tendons and joints resulting in abnormal postures. The entry point for insertion of the needle is about 7 cm from the midline just below the level of the intervertebral space. The needle is pushed obliquely upward to the corresponding foramen under fluoroscopic guidance to reach the target root tangentially. The RF probe is placed through the stylet, and a stimulation current is applied with an increasing voltage until a motor response is obtained in the appropriate muscular group. The probe must be repositioned if a good motor response is not obtained with a threshold of less than 0.5 v. The RF lesion is made at 90°C for 2 minutes. Then a stimulation test is applied; an increase in threshold of at least 0.2 v is desired, to ensure significant relief of spasticity. Otherwise, the procedure must be repeated. For the placement of the electrode at S-1, the needle is inserted in the midline between the spinous processes of L-5 and S-1 and is pushed laterally toward the elbow of the S-1 nerve root (without penetration of the dura). RF sacral rhizotomies can be performed at the foramen of S-1 to S-4, with cystometric monitoring for neurogenic bladder with detrusor hyperactivity. RF thermorhizotomy can be also performed in the cervical spine. The patient is in the supine position. The tip of the needle is placed in the posterior compartment of the vertebral foramen, to avoid damage to the vertebral artery. Percutaneous rhizotomies have the advantage of being less

aggressive than open procedures in very debilitated patients. It seems more appropriate for spastic disturbances limited to a few muscular groups that correspond to a small number of spinal roots (as occurs in spastic hip, which can be treated by thermorhizotomy of L2-3). The effects are most often temporary. On long-term follow-up, a high rate of recurrent spasticity is observed (5 to 9 months on average), but the preoperative level of spasticity is most often not reached, and the procedure can be repeated.

Intrathecal Chemical Rhizotomy

Intrathecal injection of alcohol was first introduced (26) for cancer-related pain, and only later was it used for hypertonia in patients with severe spastic paraplegia (27). Alcohol was subsequently replaced by phenol (a hyperbaric solution), the effects of which are easier to control (28–30). The best candidates for phenol intrathecal injections are paraplegic patients suffering from severe spasms who do not have useful residual motor, sensory, or sphincter function below the level of the lesion.

Longitudinal Myelotomy

Longitudinal myelotomy, which was introduced by Bischof (31), was elaborated by Pourpre (32) and later on by Laitinen et al. (33). In the series of 25 patients reported by Laitinen et al., 60% had complete relief of spasticity, whereas 36% showed some residual spasticity in one or both legs. Within 1 year, some muscular tone returned in most patients but seldom produced troublesome spasticity. A harmful effect on bladder function was present in 27% of the patients. Longitudinal myelotomy is indicated only in patients with spastic paraplegia with flexion spasms who have no residual useful motor control and no bladder and sexual function.

Dorsal Root Entry Zone Surgery

Surgery in the DREZ was introduced in 1972 to treat intractable pain (34). Because of its effects on muscular tone, it has also been applied to patients with localized hyperspasticity (35–38). This method, named *microDREZotomy* (MDT), attempts to interrupt the small nociceptive and the large myotactic fibers (situated laterally and centrally, respectively) selectively, while sparing the large lemniscal fibers, which are grouped medially. It also enhances the inhibitory mechanisms of fibers in Lissauer's tract and the dorsal horn (39) (Fig. 41.8).

MDT applies microsurgical incisions 2 to 3 mm deep at an angle of 35 degrees for cervical levels and at an angle of 45 degrees for lumbosacral levels (40–42). Then, bipolar coagulations are performed ventrolaterally at the entry zone of the rootlets into the dorsolateral sulcus, along all cord segments selected for the operation. The angle and depth of the surgical lesions into the DREZ and the dorsalmost layers

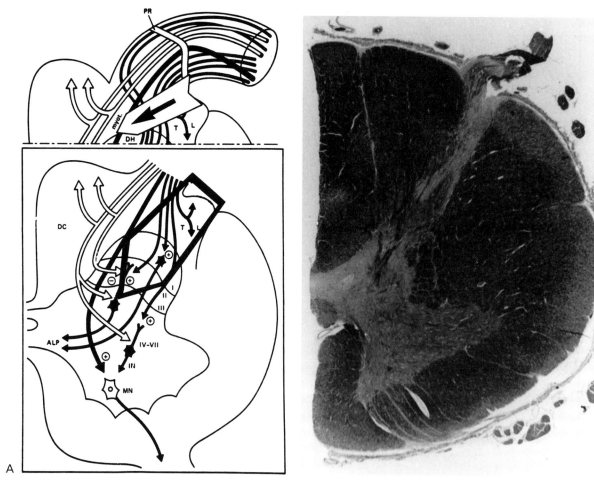

FIGURE 41.8. A: Schematic representation of DREZ area and target of microDREZotomy (MDT). **Upper part:** Each rootlet can be divided, with regard to the transition of its glial support into a peripheral and a central segment. The transition between the two segments is at the pial ring (PR), which is located approximately 1 mm outside the penetration of the rootlet into the dorsolateral sulcus. Peripherally, the fibers are mixed together. As they approach the PR, the fine fibers, which are considered nociceptive, move toward the rootlet surface. In the central segment, they group in the ventrolateral portion of the DREZ, to enter the dorsal horn (DH) through the tract of Lissauer (TL). The large myotatic fibers (myot) are situated in the middle of the DREZ, whereas the large lemniscal fibers are located dorsomedially. **Lower part:** Schematic topography of dorsal horn neuronal architecture. Note the monosynaptic excitatory arc reflex, the lemniscal influence on DH cells and interneurons (IN), the fine fiber excitatory input to DH cells and the IN, the neuronal populations in layer I and layers IV to VII contributing to the anterolateral pathways (ALP), and the projection of the IN to the motoneuron (MN). DC, dorsal column. Rexed's laminae are marked from I to VI. MicroDREZotomy *(arrowhead)* severs most of the fine and myotatic fibers and enters the medial (excitatory) portion of the LT and the apex of the DH. It should preserve most lemniscal presynaptic fibers, the lateral (inhibitory) portion of the TL, and most of the DH. **B:** Transverse hemisection of the spinal cord, at the lower cervical level, with myelin stained by Luxol fuchsin, showing the myelinated rootlet afferents that reach the dorsal column (DC). P, pyramidal tract. The *small arrow* designates the pial ring of the dorsal rootlet (diameter, 1 mm). The *large arrowhead* shows the MDT target.

of the dorsal horn have to be adapted to the shape and size of the dorsal horn, which vary according to spinal cord levels (Fig. 41.9).

For patients with paraplegia (41), the L2-5 segments are approached through a T-11–L-2 laminectomy (Fig. 41.10), whereas *for the hemiplegic upper limb* (42), a C4-7 hemilaminectomy with conservation of the spinous processes is sufficient to reach the C-5–T-1 segments (Fig. 41.11).

Confirmation and further delineation of the spinal cord levels associated with spasticity are achieved by evaluation of the muscle responses to bipolar electrical stimulation of the anterior or posterior roots. The motor threshold for stimulation of anterior roots is one-third that of the threshold for posterior roots. Then, the lateral aspect of the DREZ is exposed. Intraoperative neurophysiologic monitoring may be helpful to identify the corresponding spinal cord levels and

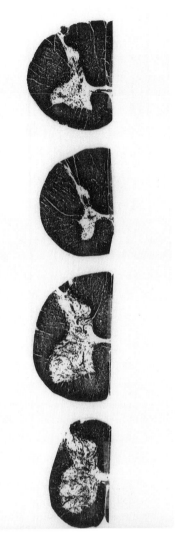

FIGURE 41.9. Variations of shape, width, and depth of the DREZ area, according to the spinal cord level (from **top** to **bottom:** C-7, T-5, L-4, S-3). At the thoracic level, Lissauer's tract is narrow, and the position of the dorsal horn is deeper. Thus, it is understandable that DREZ lesions at this level can jeopardize the corticospinal tract and the dorsal column.

to quantify the extent of MDT, to avoid impairment of long fiber tracts.

MDT is *indicated in* paraplegic patients, especially when they are bedridden as a result of disabling flexion spasms, and in hemiplegic patients with irreducible or painful spasticity in the upper limb (40–44). MDT also can be used to treat the neurogenic bladder with uninhibited detrusor contractions (43).

Our series to date has consisted of 45 cases of unilateral cervical (C-5 to T-1) MDT for harmful spasticity in the upper limb, 121 cases of bilateral lumbosacral MDT (L-2 to S-1 or S-5) for disabling spasticity in the lower limbs, and 12 cases of bilateral sacral S2-3 (S-4) MDT for hyperactive neurogenic bladder only. Effects on muscular tone could be judged only after a 3-month follow-up. A "useful" result on

spasticity that allowed withdrawal of antispasmodic medications was obtained in 78% of the patients with a spastic upper limb. A similarly useful effect was obtained in 75% of the patients with spasticity in the lower limbs.

Spasms in paraplegic patients were suppressed or were markedly reduced in 88% of cases. The results were best in patients with spasticity (and spasms) resulting from primary spinal cord lesions (useful effects on the order of 80%), and they were similar in patients with spasticity from multiple sclerosis (75%); the least improvement was observed in patients with spasticity resulting from cerebral lesions (60%). Reduction in spasticity usually leads to a significant improvement of abnormal postures and articular limitations. This was achieved in about 90% of our patients.

For the hemiplegic upper limb, the increase in articular amplitude was most remarkable for the elbow and shoulder (when not "frozen"), but it was much more limited for the wrist and fingers, especially when patients had retraction of the flexor muscles and no residual voluntary motor activity in the extensors. For the lower limb with abnormal postures in flexion, the increase in articular amplitude depended on the degree of the preoperative retractions. When the post-MDT gains were deemed insufficient because of persistent joint limitations, complementary orthopedic surgery was thought to be indicated. All five patients who had paraplegia with irreducible hyperextension were completely relieved of their spasticity. In those patients who had some residual motor activity masked by spasticity, reduction in the hypertonia resulted in improvement in muscular force on voluntary movements. Fifty percent of the patients operated on for spasticity in the upper limb had better motor activity of the shoulder and arm, but only half of those with some preoperative distal motor function obtained additional hand prehension. Only 10% of the patients with spasticity in the lower limb had significant motor improvement after surgical treatment, because most patients in this group had no functional preoperative motor function. In these very severely affected patients, the main benefits were better comfort, less pain, the ability to resume physical therapy, and less dependence in their daily life. The preoperative and postoperative assessments of these patients are shown in detail elsewhere (44).

Bladder capacity was significantly improved in 85% of the 38 patients who had a hyperactive neurogenic bladder with urine leakage around the catheter. These 32 patients who improved were those in whom the detrusor was not irreversibly fibrotic. Pain, when present, was in general favorably influenced. MDT constantly produced a marked decrease in sensation.

Because most patients were in a precarious general and neurologic state, five patients (4%) died, four who had respiratory problems and one who had bedsores. Two patients with multiple sclerosis presented with an acute but transient increase in their preexisting neurologic symptoms during the postoperative period, whereas two others had a new postoperative clinical manifestation of the disease. Another

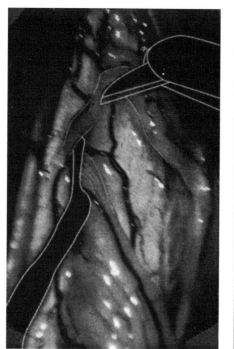 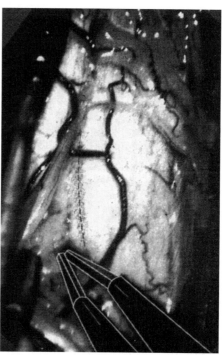

FIGURE 41.10. MicroDREZotomy technique at the cervical level. Exposure of the right dorsolateral aspect of the cervical cord at C-6. **A:** After coagulating only the tiny pial vessels, an incision, 2 mm in depth, at 35 degrees ventrally and medially, is made with a microknife in the lateral border of the dorsolateral sulcus. **B:** Then microcoagulations are performed down to the apex of the dorsal horn, with bipolar microforceps.

patient who was operated on at the cervical level had a persistent motor deficit in the ipsilateral leg postoperatively.

With rigorous selection of patients, MDT can be very effective in relieving pain and in suppressing excessive spasticity. Good long-lasting relief of spasticity was achieved in about 80% of our patients. As a result, MDT, sometimes combined with complementary orthopedic surgery, resulted in significant improvement in patient comfort and articular deformities and even enhancement of residual voluntary mobility masked preoperatively by hypertonicity.

COMPLEMENTARY ORTHOPEDIC SURGERY

Orthopedic procedures can reduce spasticity and may help to restore articular function when deformities have become irreducible. Current techniques for correcting excessive shortness of the muscle tendon assembly are *muscular disinsertion, myotomy, tenotomy, and lengthening tenotomy.* The lengthening operations most often used are (a) muscular disinsertion of the epicondylic muscles for flexed wrist and fingers (Scaglietti's procedure), (b) flexor digitorum lengthening for the hemiplegic hand, (c) tendon lengthening of the heel cord for equinus deformity of the foot, and (d) hamstring tendon lengthening combined with patellar tendon shortening. Such techniques aim at a more functional position for the

limb or limbs involved. Excessive lengthening can lead to a decrease in muscular strength. Tendon transfer has a different goal: to normalize articular orientation when it has been distorted by muscular imbalance. Transfer of spastic muscles must be avoided. If necessary, suppression of spasticity must be achieved by neurosurgical procedures before tendon transfer. A frequently performed tendon transfer is the fixation of the distal tendon of the peroneus brevis onto the tibialis anterior for equinovarus foot deformity (Bardot's procedure). Osteotomies aim to correct bone deformities resulting from growth distortion in a child (e.g., femoral derotation osteotomy to correct excessive anteversion in patients with cerebral palsy) or to treat stiffened joints (e.g., supracondylar femoral osteotomy for irreducible flexed knee). Articular surgery is indicated only when osteoarticular deformities cannot be corrected by osteotomy or tendon surgery alone. When a varus deformity of the foot is very severe and fixed, a triple hind foot arthrodesis may be indicated, with a subtalar and midtarsal procedure; with this technique, the ankle remains free. Arthrodesis must not be performed in children until they stop growing. Orthopedic surgery can be useful to correct or even to prevent irreducible deformities, to increase comfort in severely affected patients, or to improve function in those who have recovered to a satisfactory level of voluntary motor function, but only after spasticity has been reduced.

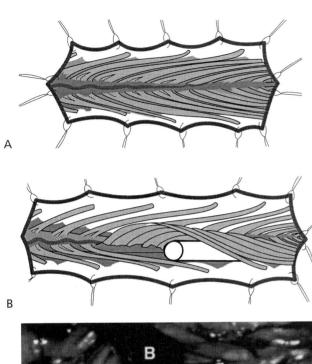

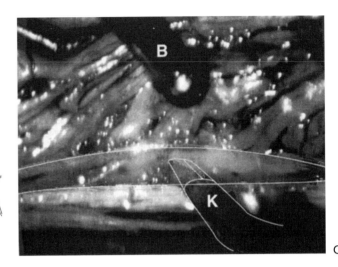

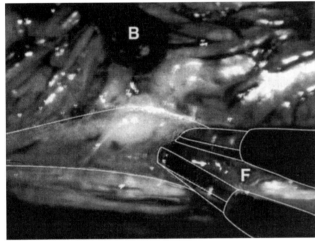

FIGURE 41.11. MicroDREZotomy technique at the lumbosacral level. **A:** Exposure of the conus medullaris through a T-11 to L-1 laminectomy. **B:** Approach to the left dorsolateral sulcus. The rootlets of the selected lumbosacral dorsal roots are displaced dorsally and medially to obtain proper access to the ventrolateral aspect of the DREZ. **C:** The rootlets of the selected dorsal roots are retracted dorsomedially and are held with a (specially designed) ball-tip microsucker (B), used as a small hook, to gain access to the ventrolateral part of the DREZ. Then, a continuous incision is performed using a microknife (K). The cut is, on average, at a 45-degree angle and to a depth of 2 mm. **D:** Microcoagulations under direct magnified vision are then applied at low intensity, inside the posterolateral sulcomyelotomy down to the apex of the dorsal horn. These microcoagulations are made by means of special sharp bipolar forceps (F), insulated except at its tip over a distance of 5 mm.

INDICATIONS FOR SURGERY

Adults

Intrathecal baclofen administration is indicated for paraplegic or tetraplegic patients with severe and diffuse spasticity, especially when the origin is spinal. Because of the reversibility of this approach, this method has to be discussed before an ablative procedure is performed. However, the range between excessive hypotonia with reduction of strength and an optimal therapeutic effect may be narrow. Intrathecal baclofen for treatment of spasticity is discussed in Chapter 40.

Neuroablative techniques are indicated for severe localized spasticity in the limbs of paraplegic, tetraplegic, or hemiplegic patients. Neurotomies are preferred when spasticity is localized to muscle groups innervated by a few peripheral nerves or by a single peripheral nerve. When spasticity affects an entire limb, MDT is preferred. Several types of neuroablative procedures can be combined in the treatment of one patient, when needed. Whatever the situation and the cause

of the disorder, *orthopedic surgery* should be considered only after spasticity has been reduced by physical and pharmacologic treatments first and, when necessary, by neurosurgical procedures.

Guidelines for surgical indications are detailed elsewhere (45,46), and they are summarized in Figs. 41.12 to 41.14. The general rule is to tailor individual treatments as much as possible to the particular patient's situation.

Children with Cerebral Palsy

In children, surgical indications depend on preoperative abilities and disabilities and eventual functional goals. For guiding indications, we have adopted the following classification into six groups, as defined by Abbott (47):

1. *In independently ambulatory patients,* the goal is to improve efficiency and cosmetic effect in walking by eliminating as many abnormally responsive neural circuits

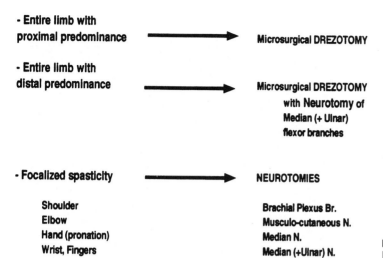

HEMIPLEGIA WITH HYPERSPASTICITY

UPPER LIMB

- Entire limb with proximal predominance ⟶ Microsurgical DREZOTOMY

- Entire limb with distal predominance ⟶ Microsurgical DREZOTOMY with Neurotomy of Median (+ Ulnar) flexor branches

- Focalized spasticity ⟶ NEUROTOMIES

Shoulder	Brachial Plexus Br.
Elbow	Musculo-cutaneous N.
Hand (pronation)	Median N.
Wrist, Fingers	Median (+Ulnar) N.

FIGURE 41.12. Guidelines for spastic hemiplegia (upper limb).

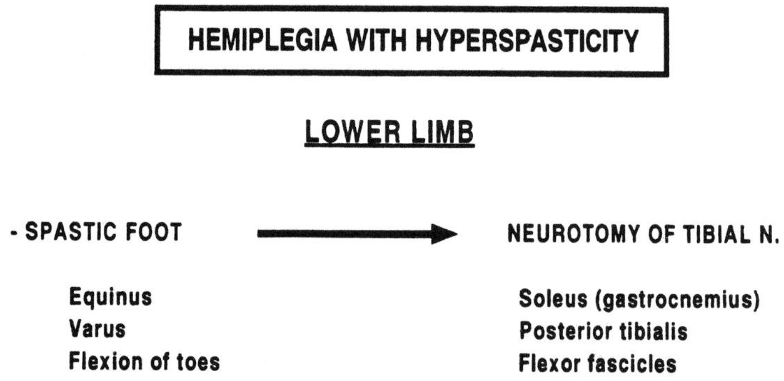

HEMIPLEGIA WITH HYPERSPASTICITY

LOWER LIMB

- SPASTIC FOOT ⟶ NEUROTOMY OF TIBIAL N.

Equinus	Soleus (gastrocnemius)
Varus	Posterior tibialis
Flexion of toes	Flexor fascicles

FIGURE 41.13. Guidelines for spastic hemiplegia (lower limb).

PARAPLEGIA WITH HYPERSPASTICITY

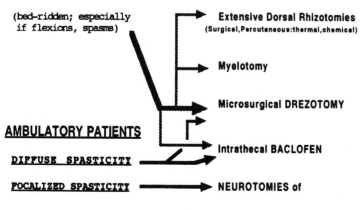

NON AMBULATORY PATIENTS

(bed-ridden; especially if flexions, spasms)

⟶ Extensive Dorsal Rhizotomies (Surgical,Percutaneous:thermal,chemical)

⟶ Myelotomy

⟶ Microsurgical DREZOTOMY

AMBULATORY PATIENTS

⟶ Intrathecal BACLOFEN

DIFFUSE SPASTICITY

FOCALIZED SPASTICITY ⟶ NEUROTOMIES of

– HIP	- Obturator N.
– KNEE	- Hamstring N.
– FOOT	- Tibial N.

FIGURE 41.14. Guidelines for spastic paraplegia.

as can be identified through functional posterior rhizotomy. Surgery is best performed as soon as possible after the child has demonstrated the ability to work with a therapist, usually between 3 and 7 years of age, and it frequently must be done in conjunction with operations on tendons because of concomitant shortened muscles.

2. For *ambulatory patients dependent on assistance devices* (canes, crutches, rollators, walkers), the goal is to lessen that dependence. A child with poor trunk control or lack of protective reaction but with good underlying strength in the antigravity muscles can safely undergo a functional posterior rhizotomy. In children dependent on hypertonicity in the quadriceps to bear weight, a limited sectorial rhizotomy is preferable. For children who are in the process of developing ambulatory skill and who need an assistance device only temporarily, it is important to delay surgical treatment until they have perfected these skills.

3. For *quadruped crawlers* (or bunny hoppers), the goal is to achieve assisted ambulation during middle childhood to early adolescence. A functional posterior rhizotomy will decrease hypertonicity in the leg musculature and will allow better limb alignment in the standing position for a child with adequate muscular strength. However, a child who exhibits quadriceps weakness can be considered for a sectorial posterior rhizotomy. Children in this group can present at a young age with progressive hip dislocation. The goal is to stop the progressive orthopedic deformity by using obturator neurotomy with adductor tenotomies or functional posterior rhizotomy.

4. For *commando (or belly) crawlers* who are disabled by severe deficiencies in postural control, the goal of posterior rhizotomy is only to improve functioning in the sitting position by increasing stability.

5. In *totally dependent children, with no locomotive abilities,* the goals are simply to improve comfort and to facilitate care. As with group 4, the preferred treatment is posterior rhizotomy, but there is also a need for exploring the efficacy of intrathecal baclofen.

6. *For asymmetric spasticity,* selective peripheral neurotomies must be considered, especially obturator and tibial neurotomies for the spastic hip and foot, respectively. For upper limb spasticity, the MDT procedure or selective neurotomies of the flexor muscles of wrist and fingers can be considered.

In summary, for children, the main goal is to stop and prevent progressive and irreversible orthopedic deformities. Lumbosacral posterior rhizotomies can be indicated for reducing the excessive general level of spasticity in diplegic patients (and even quadriplegic patients, thanks to distant effects in upper limbs). Intrathecal baclofen is an alternative, but the range between an insufficient effect and an excessive effect responsible for a global decrease in tone that impairs gait and reduces muscular strength is often very narrow in

children. Frequently, orthopedic surgery can be usefully performed in conjunction with neurologic surgery to lengthen tendons.

CONCLUSIONS

When excessive spasticity is not sufficiently controlled by physical therapy and medication, various surgical procedures are available. By suppressing excessive spasticity, correcting abnormal postures, and relieving the frequently associated pain, surgery for spasticity allows physical therapy to be resumed and sometimes results in the reappearance of, or improvement in, useful voluntary motor function. When dealing with these patients, the surgeon must know the risks of the available treatments. To minimize those risks, the surgeon needs a strong anatomic, physiologic, and biochemical background, rigorous methods to assess and quantify the disorders, and the ability to work in a *multidisciplinary team* (46).

REFERENCES

1. Stoffel A. The treatment of spastic contractures. *Am J Orthop Surg* 1913;10:611–619.
2. Gros C, Frerebeau P, Benezech J, et al. Neurotomie radiculaire sélective. In: Simon L, ed. *Actualités en rééducation fonctionnelle et réadaptation,* ser 2. Paris: Masson, 1977:230–235.
3. Sindou M, Mertens P. Selective neurotomy of the tibial nerve for treatment of the spastic foot. *Neurosurgery* 1988;23:738–744.
4. Mertens P, Sindou M. Selective peripheral neurotomies for the treatment of spasticity. In: Sindou M, Abbott R, Keravel Y, eds. *Neurosurgery for spasticity: a multidisciplinary approach.* Berlin: Springer, 1991:119–132.
5. Berard C, Sindou M, Berard J, et al. Selective neurotomy of the tibial nerve in the spastic hemiplegic child: an exploration of the recurrence. *J Pediatr Orthop* 1998;7:66–70.
6. Decq P, Filipetti P, Fevet A, et al. Peripheral selective neurotomy of the brachial plexus collateral branches for the treatment of the spastic shoulder: anatomical study and clinical results on five patients. *J Neurosurg* 1997;86:648–653.
7. Brunelli G, Brunelli F. Hyponeurotization in spastic palsies. In: Gamm I, ed. *Textbook of microsurgery.* Paris: Masson, 1988:861–865.
8. Foerster 0. On the indications and results of the excision of posterior spinal nerve roots in men. *Surg Gynecol Obstet* 1913;16:463–474.
9. Gros C, Ouaknine G, Vlahovitch B, et al. La radicotomie sélective postérieure dans le traitement neurochirurgical de l'hypertonie pyramidale. *Neurochirurgie* 1967;13:505–518.
10. Ouaknine G. Le traitement chirurgical de la spasticité. *Union Med Can* 1980;109:1–11.
11. Gros C. Spasticity: clinical classification and surgical treatment. In: Krayenbühl H, ed. *Advances and technical standards in neurosurgery,* vol 6. Berlin: Springer, 1979:55–97.
12. Privat JM, Benezech J, Frerebeau P, et al. Sectorial posterior rhizotomy: a new technique of surgical treatment of spasticity. *Acta Neurochir (Wien)* 1976;35:181–195.
13. Frerebeau P. Sectorial posterior rhizotomy for the treatment of spasticity in children with cerebral palsy. In: Sindou M, Abbott

R, Keravel Y, eds. *Neurosurgery for spasticity: a multidisciplinary approach*. Berlin: Springer, 1991:145–147.

14. Fraioli B, Guidetti B. Posterior partial rootlet section in the treatment of spasticity. *J Neurosurg* 1977;46:618–626.
15. Fasano VA, Barolat-Romana G, Ivaldi A, et al. La radicotomie postérieure fonctionnelle dans le traitement de la spasticité cérébrale. *Neurochirurgie* 1976;22:23–34.
16. Peacock WJ, Arens LJ. Selective posterior rhizotomy for the relief of spasticity in cerebral palsy. *S Afr Med J* 1982;62:119–124.
17. Cahan LD, Kundi MS, Mc Pherson D, et al. Electrophysiologic studies in selective dorsal rhizotomy for spasticity in children with cerebral palsy. *Appl Neurophysiol* 1987;50:459–682.
18. Abbott R, Forem SL, Johann M. Selective posterior rhizotomy for the treatment of spasticity. *Childs Nerv Syst* 1989;5:337–346.
19. Storrs B. Selective posterior rhizotomy for treatment of progressive spasticity in patients with myelomeningocele. *Pediatr Neurosci* 1987;13:135–137.
20. Hodgkinson I, Berard C, Jindrich ML, et al. Radicotomie postérieure fonctionnelle chez l'enfant IMC: résultats à un an post-opératoire sur 18 cas. *Ann Readapt Med Phys* 1996;39:103–111.
21. Uematsu S, Udvarhelyi GB, Benson DW, et al. Percutaneous radiofrequency rhizotomy. *Surg Neurol* 1974;2:319–325.
22. Young B, Mulcachy JJ. Percutaneous sacral rhizotomy for neurogenic detrusor hyperreflexia. *J Neurosurg* 1980;53:85–87.
23. Kenmore D. Radiofrequency neurotomy for peripheral pain and spasticity syndromes. *Contemp Neurosurg* 1983;5:1–6.
24. Herz DA, Parsons KC, Learl L. Percutaneous radiofrequency foraminal rhizotomies. *Spine* 1983;8:729–732.
25. Kasdon DL, Lathi ES. A prospective study of radiofrequency rhizotomy in the treatment of post-traumatic spasticity. *Neurosurgery* 1984;15:526–529.
26. Dogliotti A. Traitement des syndromes douloureux de la périphérie par l'alcoolisation sous-arachnoïdienne des racines postrieures à leur émergence de la moelle épinière. *Presse Med* 1931;39:1249–1252.
27. Guttman L. The treatment and rehabilitation of patients with injuries of the spinal cord. In: Cope X, ed. *History of the Second World War: surgery*. London: Her Majesty's Stationery Office, 1953:422–516.
28. Maher R. Relief of pain in incurable cancer. *Lancet* 1955;1:18–20.
29. Nathan PW. Intrathecal phenol to relieve spasticity in paraplegia. *Lancet* 1959;11:1099–1102.
30. Kelly RE. Gauthier-Smith PC. Intrathecal phenol in the treatment of reflex spasms and spasticity. *Lancet* 1959;11:1102–1105.
31. Bischof W. Die longitudinale Myelotomie. *Zentralbl Neurochir* 1951;2:79–88.
32. Pourpre MH. Traitement neurochirurgical des contractures chez les paraplégiques post-traumatiques. *Neurochirurgie* 1960;6:229–236.
33. Laitinen LV, Singounas E. Longitudinal myelotomy in the treatment of spasticity of the legs. *J Neurosurg* 1971;35:536–540.

34. Sindou M. *Etude de la jonction radiculo-medullaire postérieure: la radicellotomie postérieure sélective dans la chirurgie de la douleur*. Medical thesis, Univiersity of Lyon, 1972.
35. Sindou M, Fischer G, Goutelle A, et al. La radicellotomie postérieure sélective dans le traitement des spasticités. *Rev Neurol (Paris)* 1974;130:201–215.
36. Sindou M, Millet MF, Mortamais J, et al. Results of selective posterior rhizotomy in the treatment of painful and spastic paraplegia secondary to multiple sclerosis. *Appl Neurophysiol* 1982;45:335–340.
37. Sindou M, Pregelj R, Boisson D, et al. Surgical selective lesions of nerve fibers and myelotomies for the modification of muscle hypertonia. In: Eccles J, Dimitrijevic MR, eds. *Recent achievements in restorative neurology: upper motor neuron functions and dysfunctions*. Basel: S Kaeger, 1985:10–26.
38. Sindou M, Abdennebi B, Sharkey P. Microsurgical selective procedures in the peripheral nerves and the posterior root-spinal cord junction for spasticity. *Appl Neurophysiol* 1985;48:97–104.
39. Eccles J, Eccles R, Magni F. Central inhibitory action attributable to presynaptic depolarization produced by muscle afferent volleys. *J Physiol (Lond)* 1961;159:147–166.
40. Sindou M, Jeanmonod D, Mertens P. Surgery in the dorsal root entry zone: microsurgical DREZotomy (MDT) for the treatment of spasticity. In: Sindou M, Abbott R, Keravel Y, eds. *Neurosurgery for spasticity: a multidisciplinary approach*. Berlin: Springer, 1991:165–182.
41. Sindou M, Jeanmonod D. Microchirurgical-DREZ-otomy for the treatment of spasticity and pain in the lower limbs. *Neurosurgery* 1989;24:655–670.
42. Sindou M, Mifsud JJ, Boisson D, et al. Selective posterior rhizotomy in the dorsal root entry zone for treatment of hyperspasticity and pain in the hemiplegic upper limb. *Neurosurgery* 1986;18:587–595.
43. Beneton C, Mertens P, Leriche A, et al. The spastic bladder and its treatment. In: Sindou M, Abbott R, Keravel Y, eds. *Neurosurgery for spasticity: a multidisciplinary approach*. Berlin: Springer, 1991:193–199.
44. Sindou M. Spinal entry zone interruption for spasticity. In: Tasker RR, Gildenberg P, eds. *Textbook of Stereotactic and Functional Neurosurgery*. New York: McGraw Hill, 1998:1257–1266.
45. Sindou M, Mertens P. Indication for surgery to treat adults with harmful spasticity. In: Sindou M, Abbott R, Keravel Y, eds. *Neurosurgery for spasticity: a multidisciplinary approach*. Berlin: Springer, 1991:211–213.
46. Sindou M, Abbott R, Keravel Y, eds. *Neurosurgery for spasticity: a multidisciplinary approach*. Berlin: Springer, 1991.
47. Abbott R. Indications for surgery to treat children with spasticity due to cerebral palsy. In: Sindou M, Abbott R, Keravel Y, eds. *Neurosurgery for spasticity: a multidisciplinary approach*. Berlin: Springer, 1991:215–217.

INDEX

Page numbers *in italic* followed by "f" denote figures. Page numbers *in italic* followed by "t" denote tables.